Galip Gürel

The Science and Art of Porcelain Laminate Veneers

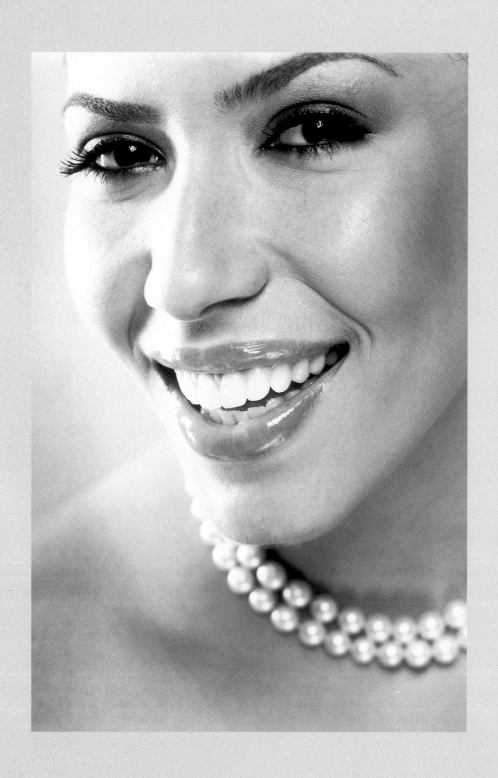

The Science and Art of

Porcelain Laminate Veneers

Galip Gürel

quintessence
books

Quintessence Publishing Co. Ltd.

London, Chicago, Berlin, Copenhagen, Tokyo, Paris,
Barcelona, Milano, São Paulo, New Delhi, Moscow, Prague,
Warsaw and Istanbul

British Library Cataloguing in Publication Data

Gürel, Galip
   The science and art of porcelain laminate veneers
   1. Dental ceramics 2. Dental veneers 3. Dentistry – Aesthetic
   aspects
   I. Title
   617.6'95

   ISBN 1850970602

© 2003 Quintessence Publishing Co. Ltd.

Illustrations: Dr. Rainer Landsee in collaboration with Zoeller & Karrer, Konstanz, Germany
Lithography: S & T scan, Berlin, Germany
Printing and Binding: Bosch-Druck GmbH, Ergolding, Germany

Printed in Germany

ISBN 1-85097-060-2

Contributors

Jean-François Roulet, Prof. Dr. med. dent.
Ivoclar Vivavent AG
Schaan, Liechtenstein

Claude R. Rufenacht, Dr. med. dent.
Periodontal Prosthesis and Esthetic Dentistry Practice
Geneva, Switzerland

Stephen J. Chu, DMD, MSD, CDT, MDT
Director, Advanced Program in Aesthetic Dentistry
Clinical Associate Professor
Department of Implant Dentistry
New York University College of Dentistry
New York, USA

Korkud Demirel
Professor of Periodontology
Department of Periodontology
School of Dentistry
University of Istanbul
Istanbul, Turkey

Frank Celenza Jr, DDS
Orthodontist, Periodontist
Clinical Associate Professor
New York University, College of Dentistry
New York, USA

Cathy Jameson, PhD
President and CEO of Jameson Management, Inc.
Davis, Oklahoma, USA

To Berna and Ali

Foreword

Not that long ago dentists were mostly relied upon for the relief of pain and the restoration of decayed teeth. Everyone dreaded a trip to the dentist. A visit was associated with pain and one frequently left the office with teeth filled with silver amalgam, the generic restoration available at the time.

Esthetics, such an integral part of our lives today, was barely at the periphery of dental concerns. There were, of course, a handful of dentists who exercised the available esthetic dental options, but these options were time consuming, expensive and, unfortunately, frequently unattractive.

Change was inevitable. Awakened to beauty by the media, the public became aware of the importance of a beautiful smile. The dental profession, conscious of this growing demand, began a search for cosmetic restorations. Change came gradually. Many techniques and materials were tried and discarded. Progress was halting, often two steps forward and one step back.

1970 saw our first major breakthrough. Tooth bonding, a technique that rapidly, painlessly and much less expensively made teeth cosmetically beautiful, was born. Bonding, however, as extraordinary as it was, had a much greater effect on the dental profession than its originators ever imagined. It was a catalyst to a revolution. Dentistry would be changed forever. Bonded bridges, porcelain laminates and, infinitely stronger and more stable, all-porcelain crowns were just its immediate derivatives. Beyond that the profession expanded its perimeters.

Improvements in maintaining teeth both endodontically and periodontically were enhanced. Missing teeth were no longer automatically replaced with removable dentures – implants often rendered dentures unnecessary. A new era had arrived – a revolution in patient care with no end in sight.

And that is why this book is so valuable and important. It has circumscribed this revolution and detailed all the important changes that have occurred in our profession.

Nonetheless, my rationale for this foreword is not my appreciation of the book, but my respect for its author and his accomplishments. Dr. Galip Gürel, involved in a profession whose values were noble but antiquated, has in a relatively short time span changed Turkish dentistry.

Esthetic dentistry, although flourishing elsewhere, was unknown in Turkey. Dr. Gürel left his homeland to learn these revolutionary techniques, but beyond learning them, he mastered them. He is currently lecturing and teaching dentists all over the world and his modern office is improving smiles daily. His efforts, beyond bolstering his reputation, have not only elevated the prestige of Turkish dentistry but have paved the way for recognition and appreciation of Turkey all over the world.

It was a monumental task Dr. Galip Gürel undertook, and after reading his book I find he has completed it exceptionally well, and I am certain that everyone who reads it will both appreciate and benefit from it.

Irwin Smigel, DDS

Acknowledgements

I have found that it is impossible truly to appreciate just how difficult it is to write a book. In fact, I now believe that only the writer, their family and those people of their inner circle can fully understand this daunting task. When I decided to undertake writing this book, I did not know how demanding and time-consuming a task it would be. The more that I researched, the deeper I was drawn into the material, and as I was drawn into it this incredible well of knowledge opened before me. It was actually difficult finally to stop myself and to filter through it all, while adding my own experiences and clinical work along with the photos and drawings to complete this book. The final task of arranging all this in the most presentable way possible in order to make it more readable for my colleagues was my most challenging undertaking. The key to this achievement was undoubtably the successful teamwork throughout this project.

To start with, I must thank my wife Berna and my son Ali for supporting me in everything that I have ever done until now. However, I want especially to thank them for their exceptional patience during my absences over the last 18 months and for the love and understanding that they have shown to me throughout the preparation of this book.

In loving memory, I would like to express my grad.tude to my grandmother Tomi, who has passed away, but remains the most influential person in my life. She brought me up and laid the foundation for all that I have accomplished in my life. My only regret is that she is not here to share this moment with me.

I am eternally grateful to my mother Güngör and my father Gültekin Gürel, my idols in the dental profession, whom I may not have been able to choose as my parents but who proved to be the greatest gift God could have given me, and who were not only the driving force in my choice of this profession but the foundations of my hard working, honesty and happiness.

I must of course extend my thanks to my dearest brother Gürcan and his family, every one of my patients, my friends and my associates for their tolerance and understanding during my obession with this book.

Being a private practitioner and lecturing all over the world, the task of writing a book that requires a lot of scientific research and clinical work to support. It could not have been accomplished without the help of my associates, who were of great assistance and support in every way. I would therefore like to extend my gratitude to those associates who have been involved in each case and who have worked closely together with me for years. I would especially like to thank Dr. Kübel Iltan, Dr. Birgül Yeruşalmi and

Acknowledgements

Dr. Talin Çitak for their limitless assistance, dedication and patience. I am also grateful to Dr. Ipek Cenkçiler, Dr. Elif Ay and Dr. Elif Özcan for their sincere efforts and support.

Dentistry, and especially esthetic dentistry, requires a solid team effort and it is for this reason that I have tried to share with you the smallest possible details about every aspect of esthetic dentistry. I have been very lucky to have many valuable colleagues, each a star in their specialty, who have made time in their extremely demanding professional lives to share with us the details of their techniques in their contributions to this book. I cannot thank each of them enough for their work in summarizing, as they have for us, their areas of specialty, which are very complex and broad topics. I have had the honor of the contributions of Prof. Dr. Roulet on adhesion, Dr. Claude Rufenacht on occlusion, Dr. Stephen Chu on color, Dr. Korkud Demirel on periodontology, Dr. Frank Celenza on orthodontics and Cathy Jameson on patient education. I cannot thank my colleagues enough for their work in making each of their specialties so pleasing and clear for us to read.

My everlasting thanks go to my dear Nancy Barlas and Laura K. Franklin, who with their knowledge and effort and unfailing drive worked with me to edit my texts into a more easily readable and understandable state.

It is impossible to separate prosthodontics from the lab technician and especially so in a book on PLVs, as each case I have shared with you ultimately is the product of a ceramic specialist. I would like to thank the ceramists with whom I work in great harmony every day in my daily practice and who have discussed each of the cases with me. These valuable colleagues and their teams deserve my sincere thanks: Gerard Ubassy, Jason Kim, Michael Magne, Adrian Jurim and Hakan Akbayar.

I am particularly grateful to my assistant Sinan Yíldírím for all his wonderfully supportive technical assistance and to my secretaries Nalan Ince and Sevtap, and to my clinical assistants, Yasemin, Filiz, Zülfiye, Nurhan and Ayse, who form the backbone of my clinic and who shouldered so much of this production process.

I would like to express my appreciation to Tamer Yilmaz for the wonderful photograph that was used for our cover and to Joelle Imamoglu for her valuable assistance and artistic flare in her design of the cover.

A very special thanks to all my supportive patients and especially those who showed exemplary patience during the photographing of their dental work and allowed me to share these photographs with you for this scientific record.

I am deeply appreciative of Dr. Rainer Landsee for his illustrations that have added so much to this book. I am also grateful to Peter Sielaff and his team for their editing and for their attention to each and every page of this volume.

I am eternally grateful to Horst-Wolfgang Haase, who was the person who originally gave me the idea of writing this book and encouraged me to undertake such a challenging project, and finally to Quintessence for arranging this collaboration.

Dr. Galip Gürel

Preface

The appreciation and pleasure that we all derive from observing anything beautiful is part of basic human nature. A beautiful image conjures positive thoughts and feelings towards someone and also provides that person with a good self-image and gives them self-confidence.

The same applies to a person's spiritual and physical esthetics. I think that the coherence of physical and esthetical appearance, as well as being at peace with oneself, is what is known as "well being". Within the foundation of all these ideas, rather than the exaggeration of artificiality, we aim to achieve a plain, more natural appearance that brings out the innate good thoughts and feelings of humans. As the natural span of life has been prolonged in our time, so have changed the concepts of "middle aged", which is now percieved as young, and "old age", which no longer seems old to us. Parallel to this phenomenon are people now in search of a younger, more attractive, dynamic and youthful appearance.

Creative people who are gifted in terms of artistic talents, with a traditional culture enriched by internationally flavored gusto and who sense and enjoy the beautiful details of living, tend to offer other people the opportunity to appreciate pleasures that are hard to explain. This is clearly seen in music, fine arts, fashion and other social activities. The aim is to present these beautiful touches and feelings to people as if they had actually been present in their lives for years.

Just as walking and running are part of man's nature, so is laughter. The most prominent expression of joy even for the blind or deaf is through their laughter. So it only follows that a beautiful smile should accompany this laughter. When we consider "esthetic dentistry" within this framework, a well-planned and beautifully achieved smile is without doubt one of the major elements in the concept of this total image of "well being".

A sparkling smile, in coherence with the lips and face, reflects a person's character and life: a smile, individual to only that person, forever present with them and so natural that it appears always to have been a part of them.

This book was written to help the esthetic dentist in treating unesthetic alignment, color, shape or form of the teeth—in other words, enhancing the smile while enforcing function and occlusion. The book examines porcelain laminate veneers, the most successful non-invasive, prosthodontic application of dentistry in this decade, with all its pros and cons. When designed and delivered properly, PLVs are not only the most sparkling, natural, man-made form of esthetic dentistry but they do not appear in any way to be anything but innate, as if they were always a part of that person and their personality.

We have used hundreds of scientific references to present to you a book on "evidence-based dentistry". After working for 15 years with my mentors and with other successful dentists from the world of esthetic dentistry, and with the support of their research and help, I have developed some new techniques which I hope will make a contribution to the PLV world – specifically, Chapter 7, which has been designed as an atlas, and the sections involving teeth preparation for APR (Aesthetic Pre-recontouring) and APT (Aesthetic Pre-evaluative Temporaries), which I feel will become a part of all general practitioners' daily applications. I believe minimum tooth preparation is one of the most sensitive steps in PLV applications. I am sure that you will read with great interest about the techniques for nearly 100% accuracy in this process.

Chapters 3, 4 and 5, on the important topics of adhesion, color and occlusion, are written by doctors who are unequaled in their field. In addition, the supporting specialties in the periodontic, orthodontic, and patient education chapters were written by specialists in those fields.

The expectations the esthetic dentist has of the lab technician mean that we must fully understand the process of the production of PLVs in the laboratory. Some of the world's foremost ceramists have prepared photographs and illustrations of pressable ceramics, feldspathic refractory die, and platinum foil—all techniques which are clearly explained in Chapters 7, 9, and 10.

After reading this book you will have a very comprehensive and in-depth knowledge of the PLV process. Esthetic dentistry is an "art form", which provides us with a youthful, pleasing, alluring and beautiful smile that can only be achieved through a combination of the esthetic dentist's perception, talent and artistic flare along with their full understanding of the patient's desires. Otherwise, all smiles would be the same prototype, with no personalization and character to them.

If you do everything right, no jobs are more rewarding than those of the esthetic dentistry team of dentist, specialist, technician and patient. I wish you all the best for successful clinical work and professional satisfaction.

Dr. Galip Gürel

Contents

Contents

Contents

Emotions...

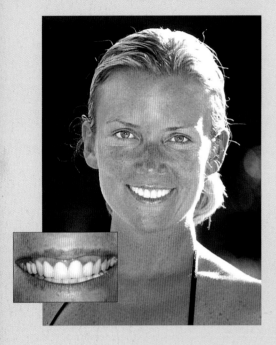

Dear Dr. Gürel,

I had an amazing experience today. I had driven to a business appointment in my city. Once I have arrived and was parked, I dropped the mirror in my car, so that I could check my hair and lipstick to make sure that I was presentable for my meeting.

"What is so amazing about that?", you may be asking. Well, when I looked in the mirror, I thought that the person looking at me was pretty. I am thirty-two years old. Other people have espoused my attractiveness. But, until today, I didn't see it. Until today, I had never seen my own reflection and been pleased. But, today, I saw a different person. Today, the person looking back at me in the mirror – me – was pretty.

The only thing that has changed is my smile. You changed my smile. I came to you for a conference about a smile makeover, and you listened to me as I told you how much I disliked my smile and my teeth. You didn't tease me, make fun of me or tell me I was foolish for thinking poorly of my teeth. You simply and caringly listened. And you performed magic!! Or at least that's what it seems like to me!

I love my smile and the porcelain laminate veneers that cover the old teeth and have given my smile a much, needed correction and lift. I feel younger, more confident, more attractive and more self-confident. How can I ever thank you? You have touched me – and my life – in a very special way. I will be forever grateful.

Sincerely,
A.Arasil

1   Esthetic Dentistry

Galip Gürel

Definition

"All human desires are in some way related to beauty."[1]

The term "esthetics" is borrowed from the Greek word "aesthesia", which means sensation or sensibility. It can be defined as "belonging to the appreciation of the beautiful". Esthete – the noun form of the same word – may be used to describe a person who enjoys or perceives a pleasant sensation. Similarly, the meaning of the term in adjective form indicates ability to respond to beauty in art or nature.[2] The relation of this term to dentistry has been differentiated from the word "cosmetic", which is derived from the Greek word "kosmos", or adornment. It is further stated that esthetic dentistry enhances the natural beauty of the mouth and face and that the term is used specifically to imply an improved relationship rather than a superficial one.[3]

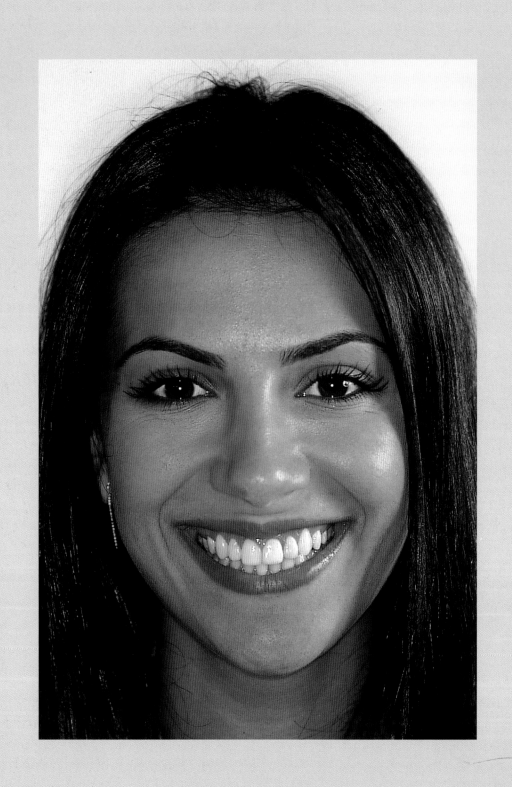

In dentistry, these phrases can be confusing. By virtue of naming anything "cosmetic", the immediate perception left in the patient's mind is the enhancement of beauty alone. However, the author believes that esthetic or cosmetic dentistry – regardless of the name – serve the same purpose. Through technological advances, it is now possible conservatively to enhance and strengthen the health and function of a patient's appearance and smile. The true understanding of all aspects of comprehensive esthetic/cosmetic dentistry and the integration of the philosophical triad of "health, function and beauty" will assist the dentist in providing optimal dental care.[4] The philosophy of esthetic dentistry can be defined as the process of providing the most convincing natural dentition possible, while maintaining it to the highest of standards.[5] Owing to the vast improvements in dental technology, materials and techniques, most of the procedures that were thought to be primarily cosmetic have been found to be quite durable as well.

In this changing world, the appearance or packaging of everything is important. A pleasing appearance is important not only socially and romantically, but also economically, for it has been found that attractive people tend to get the better jobs.[6] It is no longer a matter of conceit, but rather a necessity to pay close attention to one's appearance not only for the individual's self-confidence but also for the image he or she portrays to others. Studies on self-worth have shown that poor body image is the primary factor in self-rejection. It logically follows that the face – which is the most noticeable part of our whole appearance – has become essential to the patient's overall esthetic appearance (Fig 1-1).[7] The size and the mobility of the mouth make it the most dominant feature of the face, but it is the patient's personality, along with the strength and harmony of the other facial features, that will determine how dominant the mouth will be in the total composition.[8]

The dominance of a dental composition may be amplified by rendering it more visible. Increasing the crown size or/and using lighter teeth, placing them more anteriorly or increasing the exposed gingival length, may produce this effect. It is for that reason that the teeth and smile play a major role in whether we perceive the face of an individual as attractive or not. It is now possible for the esthetic dentist to "beautify" the patient's smile while creating a more "youthful" appearance.

Dentofacial Attractiveness

The importance of dentofacial attractiveness to the psychosocial well-being[9] of an individual has been well established.[10] As an attractive smile has always been the focal point of attention in any esthetic procedure, the esthetic dentist seeks not only to improve the esthetic appearance of the patient, but also to improve the patient's self-esteem.[11] The positive effects of a restoration on the patient's smile, appearance, self-esteem and general mental health should not be underestimated. The influence of a beautiful smile on our overall facial esthetics, well-being and self-image is quite obvious. A display of pleasing intact dentition is the key element in the creation of an attractive smile.[12]

The recognition of these factors and the increase in the number of patients seeking to improve their appearance (Fig 1-2) have compelled the dental profession to address more challenges in esthetic dentistry and to respond to the needs of their patients. The influence of the smile on facial esthetics is well recognized by society. It can be said that "better smiles are being equated with better living". In 1936, *Pilkington* defined dental esthetics as "the science of copying or harmonizing our work with that of nature, making our art inconspicuous".[13]

A beautiful smile seems to reflect a certain style of living, and the enhancement of facial beauty is one of the primary goals of patients seeking elective dental care. The lower one-third of the face has a major impact on the perception of facial esthetics, and the role of a beautiful smile is, therefore, undeniable (Fig 1-3). Once the ideal relationship between the restoration and the facial soft tissues is achieved, improvements in natural beauty can be expected to follow. With the ever-increasing importance that the media, patients, and society in general place on appearance, an

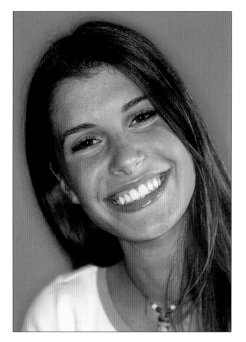

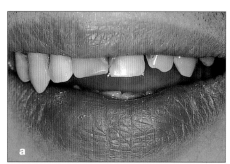

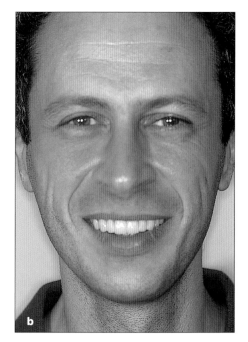

Fig 1-1 The proportional display of naturally arranged teeth always has a positive impact on a beautiful smile.

Fig 1-2a, b (a, b) Patients may present unesthetic as well as unhealthy teeth. With the new advances in materials and techniques it is now possible to treat what was once considered an impossible-looking case, thereby improving the health, esthetics and self-esteem of the patient. An unattractive smile, esthetically enhanced eight years ago. Today's materials allow us to deliver even more natural-looking teeth and smiles.

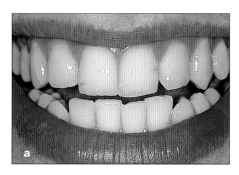

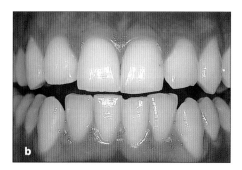

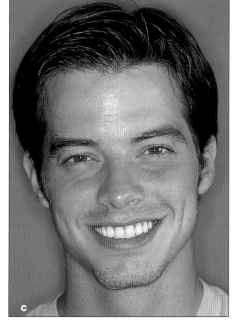

Fig 1-3a-c Facial esthetics are always related to the anterior dentition of an attractive smile (a), but even an attractive smile can be further improved with the relatively new techniques, like bleaching (Opalescence 20%, Ultradent), (b). Note the difference between the upper and lower teeth (c), and the brighter smile impact on the face.

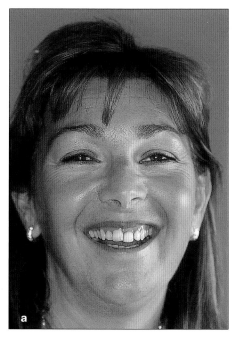
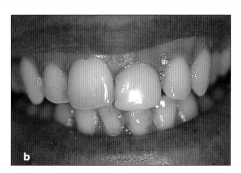
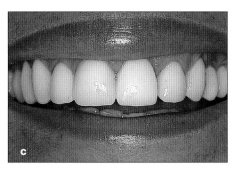
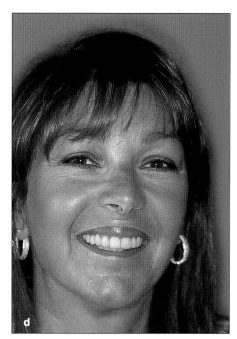

Fig 1-4a-d (a, b) Healthy teeth may be disproportionately aligned and so may not display their optimal esthetic appearance. (c) A new smile design. The irregularities of the soft and hard tissues have been corrected. The dark buccal corridors are eliminated with slightly overcontoured porcelain laminate veneers placed on the premolars. Balance, symmetry and an improved arch form have been successfully achieved.

even greater emphasis is now put on of elective esthetic dentistry. By improving deficient facial proportion and integumental form, surgeons, orthodontists and restorative dentists have the unique opportunity to address these esthetic needs while creating a pleasing smile.[14]

Need for Esthetic Dentistry

As the popularity of esthetic dentistry increases, growing numbers of patients are seeking treatment for the improvement of unesthetic anterior dentition (Fig 1-4).[15] Earlier focus on the mere restoration of carious teeth has shifted to treatment for enhancement of the esthetic appearance of already healthy teeth.[16] The professional approach to dentistry has changed rapidly. The acceleration in dental, ceramic and bonding material development has made conservative tooth preparation and restorative procedures possible that were never imaginable before (Fig 1-5). These new techniques enable the clinician to achieve cosmetic improvements and esthetically pleasing results.[17-20] Dentists are excited about

the positive impact a beautiful smile has on the social, psychological and emotional lives of our patients.

New Face or Concept of Dentistry

The entire concept of dentistry has changed dramatically over the last 30 years, and an entirely new era of restorative dentistry has begun. Practice has moved out of the classic era of dentistry, when the extraction of teeth was a common procedure, and has moved into the age of conservative restoration with minimal invasive procedures. These procedures are becoming simpler and even more conservative with every passing day. Less-aggressive tooth preparation will arrive at more predictable results. The more conservative the tooth preparation done, the fewer traumas to the teeth, and the less postoperative discomfort experienced by the patient. As esthetic procedures are generally elective procedures, clinicians should strive to make the experience as pleasant as possible for their patients. The traditional role of the dentist in the past was to correct or repair the teeth and if that

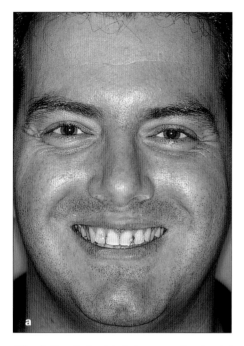
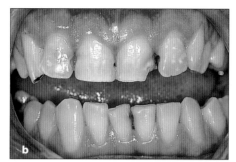
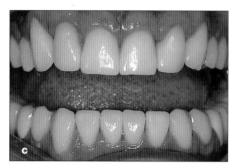
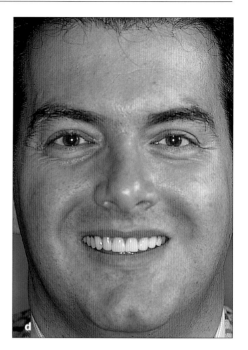

Fig 1-5a-d (a, b) Advances in dental technology now allow the clinician to improve patient appearance with minimally invasive techniques (c, d). Note that all upper and lower dentitions have been treated with porcelain laminate veneers. Even severely decayed teeth (b) can be restored successfully with porcelain laminate veneers: improving health, function and esthetics.

proved to be impossible, to remove them, leaving an older generation of people with partial or even total tooth loss.[21]

Today, the goal to retain all natural teeth intact is achievable. It is now feasible for patients to preserve their teeth through proper maintenance, good oral hygiene, the use of fluoride as a preventive measure against caries and improved restorative materials and techniques. The active preventive measures of the clinicians along with the patients' increased information and knowledge of dental care have increased the lifespan of natural teeth. Today, the dental profession strives not only to preserve healthy teeth with proper function, but also to create and enhance teeth that are esthetically pleasing as well.

Another positive factor in the patient's desire for more esthetic teeth is that by visiting the dentist to seek better appearance in their teeth, they make a trip to the dentist that they would not have made otherwise and therefore benefit by having their teeth thoroughly examined. This is one of the greatest services we, as healthcare professionals, can provide. Instead of merely imparting information to our patients concerning their oral

health, we can now provide enhancement of the quality of their smile. It improves the profession's reputation in the public eye and increases the number of patients who would otherwise not visit the dental office regularly. All of us have encountered patients who have not been to the dentist for several years but suddenly appear in the office because they are interested in "tooth whitening". Once in the office, they can be persuaded to accept other necessary periodontal or restorative treatment.[22] During the actual diagnostic examination that takes place prior to treatment, various problems that would otherwise have remained undetected and untreated can be diagnosed and treated before they become major problems (Fig 1-6).[21]

It was not very long ago that a visit to the dentist was provoked by an emergency situation, such as a painful tooth or a swollen face. Trips to the dentist were only out of necessity. Frequently, the procedures following these emergency visits were gross restorative solutions. By contrast, recent developments in dentistry have changed these visits to "want-based" treatment.[22,23] Visits to the dentist now tend to be esthetically motivat-

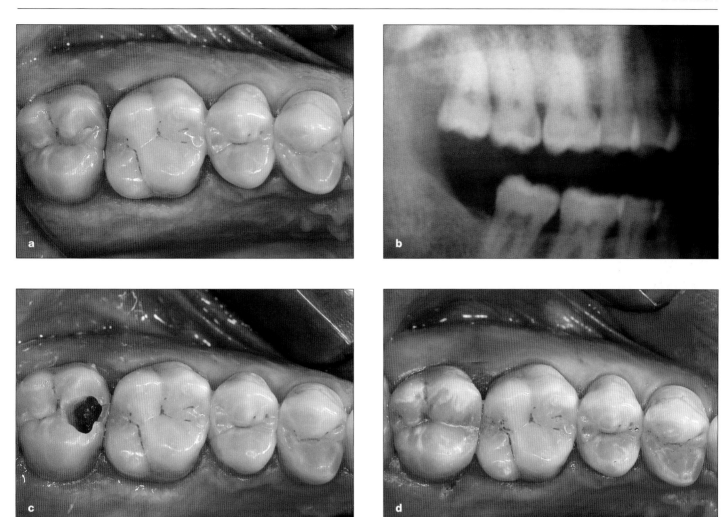

Fig 1-6a-d If the patient does not visit a dentist regularly, defects may remain undetected. Here they are discovered when the patient sought esthetic dental treatment. (a) The patient remains unaware of any interproximal defects, unless pain ensues. As no discoloration is seen on the enamel of tooth #17(2) (b), x-rays are required for detection. (c) Note the extent of the defect and (d) the restored esthetics and function.

ed. Esthetic dentistry has opened an entirely new world for most clinicians, and changed the lives of hundreds of thousands of patients in a positive way.[22] Likewise, the image of dentistry has evolved from one of pain relief and functional restorations, to the sophisticated esthetic perception the profession enjoys today.[24]

During the last decade, a large portion of the treatment protocol of dentists has entailed more and more esthetic dentistry. It is estimated that as many as 50% of individuals seeking dental care are actually seeking esthetic self-improvement.[25] In an esthetic-conscious society, where "beautiful" tends to create the image of someone "good" and "successful", individuals are prepared to invest in the improvement of their teeth and,

therefore, their appearance. Not all of these patients require major treatment and some may in fact suffice with routine procedures, such as bleaching, composites and laminate veneers to achieve the desired effect (Fig 1-7). All phases of anatomic and clinical dental practice, including orthodontics, oral surgery, periodontics and prosthodontics, may be involved in the process of esthetic dentistry. It is because these treatments can be performed with minimally prepared teeth that it is possible to enhance the existing healthy oral environment through elective procedures in contemporary esthetic practice.

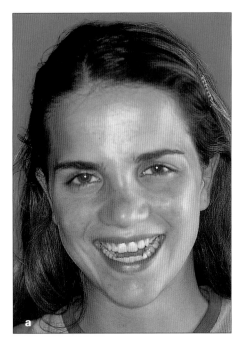
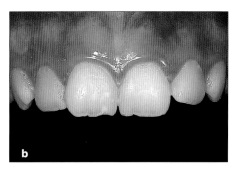
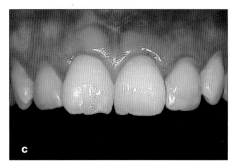
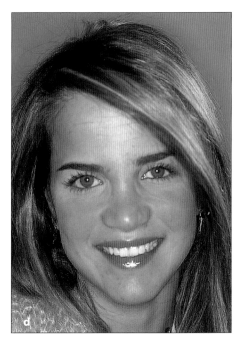

Fig 1-7a-d (a, b) To improve the esthetics, aggressive treatment methods are not always required. A patient complaining about her dark-colored, short teeth, presents requesting esthetic improvement without any invasive techniques. (c) Simple gingival surgery is performed to alter the gingival levels, thereby increasing the length of the short teeth. The teeth are bleached and the protruding maxillary left lateral incisor recontoured and restored with a composite material. Note the change in the length and color of the whole maxillary arch, as well as the change of the form and appearance of left maxillary lateral. (d) Especially for young patients, when the overall facial appearance needs to be improved, such minimal invasive techniques should be utilized. And even with these minimal changes, the whole facial beauty can be tremendously increased.

Subjective Criteria

There is nothing quite as personal as each patient's own perception of esthetics. Numerous factors, such as the region in which the patient lives, the media and fashions to which they are exposed, may all serve to influence their perception of esthetics. However, there are accepted norms by which the dentist is guided when creating an esthetically pleasing smile (see the section on Smile Design). These norms take into consideration the general appearance of the patient, including even such minute details as the specific particulars of a single tooth. However, no matter what the norms are, the preferences of the patient and their own image of their smile must be given careful consideration.[26]

When the overall dental appearance is considered, several factors of significance, such as the color, shape, position, quality of the existing restorations, and the general arrangement of the dentition should be noted, especially focusing on the particulars of the anterior teeth. Each factor may be considered individually, but all components must be both compatible and in harmony in order to produce the final esthetic result. Esthetics, as it is perceived today, not only encompasses beauty and harmony but naturalness as well. Consequently, there is no fixed standard and we must recognize that esthetic perception is influenced by the mood of the times and regional differences as well.[27] The difficulty with esthetic judgement is that the objective criteria are not always absolute. Esthetic judgement depends on the subjective feelings and interpretations of the observer, with racial, ethnic and cultural factors playing a significant role (Fig 1-8). Surprisingly enough, despite what most dentists believe, only 30%-40% of adults with nonharmonious teeth are actually unhappy with their smiles.[26] Hence, if the patient is comfortable with their existing smile, there may be no reason to change it, even if it is not the "loveliest in the world". Female patients are more likely to seek oral rehabilitation to

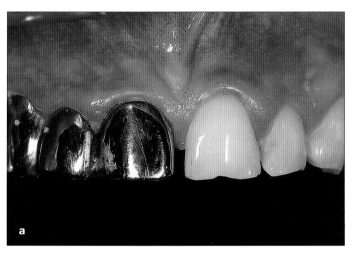 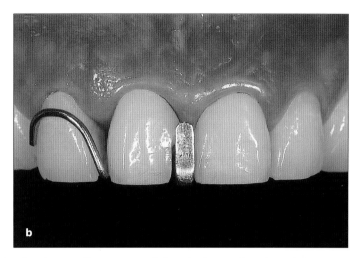

Fig 1-8a, b Esthetic judgement rests on subjective criteria depending on racial, ethnic and cultural factors. (a) Gold is still preferred in some parts of the world. (b) A variety of restorative materials can also be used. The missing part of tooth #11(8) is restored with a removable metal restoration.

improve their esthetics than male patients;[28] research shows that nearly 60% of esthetic patients are female.[29-32]

Esthetics and Function

In esthetic approaches, the patient's self-image, personality and personal relationships must be taken into consideration. A successful result is only possible when all of these factors have been included in the evaluation and treatment plan. The expansion of esthetic and cosmetic dentistry has been so extensive that it now encompasses everything related to dental appearance. There is no doubt that the great strides in adhesive materials have broadened the scope of dentistry from what was once a health and function-based practice, to a substantially more esthetic conscious style of dentistry.[33] While striving for finer esthetic appearance, careful attention to the requirements of function is essential.[34]

Therefore, it is the esthetic dentist's responsibility to provide treatment that is esthetically pleasing, functional, as well as biocompatible.[35] Esthetic dentistry is the art of dentistry in its purest form. The purpose is not to sacrifice function, but to use it as the foundation for esthetic treatments.[36] The dentist must strive to achieve final restorations that have a natural appearance and that integrate harmoniously with the proper soft tissue architecture that has been meticulously

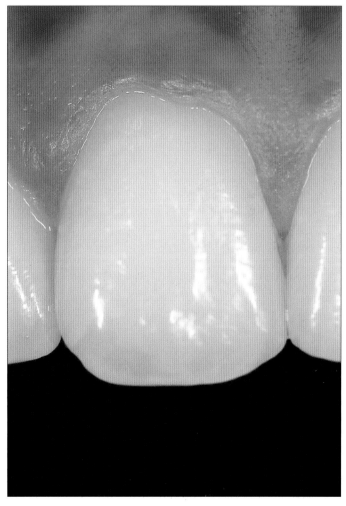

Fig 1-9 Current materials and application knowledge, combined with the artistic abilities of the dentist and laboratory technician, provide restorations that are natural in appearance and integrate harmoniously with the proper soft tissue architecture. It is difficult to differentiate this porcelain laminate veneer restoration from a natural tooth.

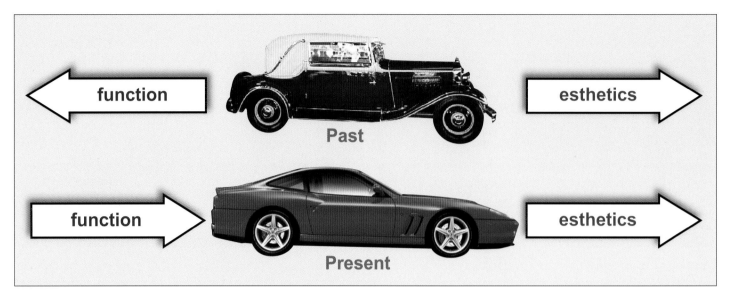

Fig 1-10 In the past, the achievement of either esthetics or function required the sacrifice of the other. Whenever function was the predominant requirement, esthetics had to be compromised. Today's materials and treatment approaches permit the clinician to achieve both goals simultaneously.

controlled throughout the restorative procedure (Fig 1-9).

When these requirements are adhered to and the desired relation between esthetics and function is achieved, the patient will feel more beautiful. Adherence to the natural morphologic state of the tooth is a prerequisite for successful esthetic results. Investigations of the functional mechanisms of the stomatognathic system have discovered that respect for tooth morphology and delicate application of a variety of parameters are required in the restorative approach to achieve good occlusion and optimal esthetic results.[37] The materials and techniques must be carefully selected to ensure that the restorations will sufficiently withstand the forces of occlusion and mastication while providing long-term function.[38]

In the past, function and esthetics often acted as two competing components in the restorative process. The overall impression was that whenever function was to be established, esthetics would have to be sacrificed; similarly, when esthetics was of prime importance, function would be compromised. These standards are no longer valid and it is now possible to improve them simultaneously. The esthetic dentist has achieved the finest form of dentistry when these two components are successfully performed in harmony

(Fig 1-10), creating restorations that are indistinguishable from the natural dentition.[39]

Personal Expectations

When we observe a person's face we judge the appearance of their smile based on the subjective evaluation of the characteristics we see.[40] The viewer's response to what is seen is actually a psychological response to the interpretation of physiological processes. This is the basic science of visual perception.[41] Whether what they see is perceived as pleasant or unpleasant will be influenced to some extent by cultural factors. As dentists, we are responsible for transforming this visual concept into the appropriate desired esthetic response. Our awareness and perception of the facial features must be continually modified, expanded, and developed.[42]

The anterior oral region and dental esthetics are of universal concern and of primary importance to all dentists. Topographic facial anatomy, which is the study of facial features and characteristics, is the method by which we recognize and distinguish one individual from another. Every individual has unique facial characteristics, including those of their smiles. According to the definition of esthetics, a smile is something very

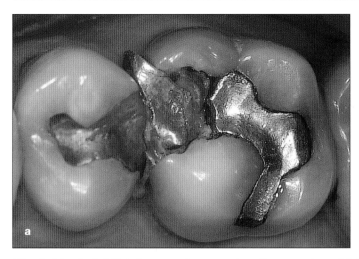 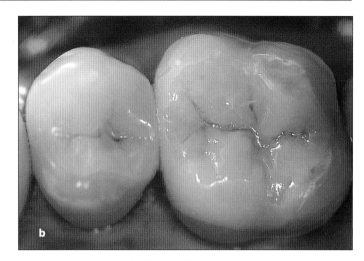

Fig 1-11a, b (a) Existing amalgam restorations replaced (b) with porcelain onlays. In the existing restorations, the emphasis was on function, sacrificing the esthetics. Note the crack lines on the amalgam. It is impossible to distinguish the porcelain onlay restorations from natural teeth, which enhances both function and esthetics.

personal, relating directly to that person's facial structure, gender, style, and character. Therefore, when considering esthetic dentistry, patients should never limit themselves to the smile they see in a photograph. Similarly, the esthetic dentist should not be restricted by specific requirements, such as those in the Golden Proportion, but rather consider them as useful guidelines to create a smile that best suits that particular patient's personal appearance (see Chapter 2). The accepted standard of "beauty" in individuals, in any society today, is subject to an incredible amount of influence from magazines, television and ethnic, racial, and environmental surroundings.[9,10] It is necessary to keep a healthy balance between the maintenance of the perfect appearance and a philosophy of life that includes physical and psychological factors.

Effects of Media and Fashion

We are all influenced by those around us. Just as we perceive and recognize a new fashion in clothing, we are also influenced by representations of beauty.[43–45] Television, magazines, motion pictures and other media contribute their daily influence. Therefore, as the perception of beauty is constantly subject to change, the concept of the "ideal" smile does not seem actually to exist.[46,47] However, the esthetic dentist cannot

become a reproducer of "trendy" smiles that are subject to the whims of the media and in constant change. Some patients arrive with requests that are impossible to fulfill and it is up to the dentist to present a reasonable treatment approach to arrive at an acceptable and achievable final result. Saying that, the concept of esthetics from the professional aspect of proportion, harmony and beauty should always be taken into consideration; however, the public eye and its perception of beauty and facial esthetics must not be excluded in the attempt to find a reasonable approach in creating a smile that is a natural extension of the patient's inherited facial state. These clinical circumstances may be encountered when a patient arrives with a stack of photographs of the latest models and film actresses or actors and requests a "smile" that will never suit his/her face or personality.

Natural-looking Restorations

The objective in the fabrication of any dental prosthesis is to provide a restoration that fits harmoniously into the facial composition, while hoping to emulate the previously existing teeth, gingiva, mucosa, soft tissue and bone as closely as possible, providing that these components previously existed in esthetic harmony. In an optimal restoration, the observer should not be

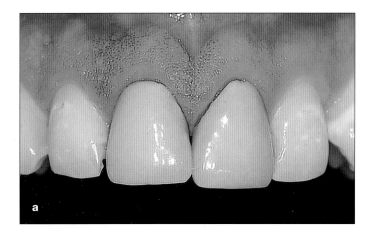
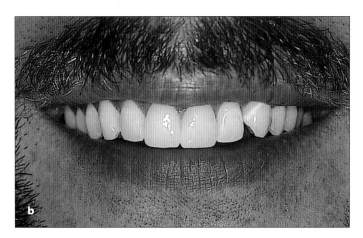
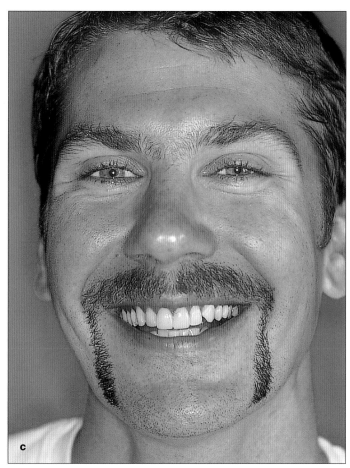

Fig 1-12a-c   (a) Iatrogenic factors may affect the smile. Two porcelain-fused-to-metal restorations exhibit an unesthetic appearance. (b) They have been replaced by all-ceramic crowns and the remaining teeth bleached. (c) Even though the asymmetrical gingival levels are not altered, an overall esthetic integration of the crowns into the facial appearance is achieved through the use of correct placement, texture, color and form. In order further to improve the esthetics, the inciso-mesial embrasure of tooth #23(11) could have been closed with a restorative material. However, since the patient has asked to retain his natural-looking smile, it is kept as it is.

able to recognize the presence of a replacement (Fig 1-11). The patient and the observer should perceive the restorative result as entirely natural.[48] The continuing esthetic evolution has fostered a growing need for materials and application techniques that can augment the armamentarium for esthetic design. Some patients may complain that their new restorations are not "esthetically pleasing" owing to the fact that their friends or relatives failed to notice their new teeth from "miles away". The reason for this is that we have succeeded in achieving esthetic harmony by adhering to the natural morphologic state. Some patients may go as far as to ask the clinician to spoil this naturally pleasing smile. Therefore, it is essential to keep in mind that "esthetic values" vary not only from nation to nation but from individual to individual as well.[49,50]

The author's philosophy on natural-appearing esthetics is that even if treatment necessitates drastic changes in the dental composition, it should not be obvious to the observer that alterations were made but rather the observer should simply recognize a very positive improvement in the smile and overall facial appearance (Fig 1-12).

Ceramics

The utilization of porcelain as a restorative material began a new era in esthetic dentistry. By today's standards, the early porcelains were rather primitive and of low value. Upon recognition of the potential use of porcelain in esthetic dentistry, various modifications and enhancements were made to render the material applicable for dental restorations. The history of porcelain follows a specific direction in approach.[51] The first major improvement in esthetic materials, especially in the translucency of all porcelain crowns, was introduced by *Vines* et al. in 1958.[52] He developed porcelain powders suitable for vacuum firing or low-pressure air firing. *Weinstein* et al. first discovered the bonding of porcelain-to-gold alloys by means of vacuum firing in the early 1960s.[53] In addition to these developments, the introduction of gap-graded finer powders, that could be vacuum fired, started a new era in dental esthetics. Owing to the ability to layer and carve porcelain, clinicians and laboratory technicians became more aware of the esthetic significance of light transmission as well as the changes in refractive indices and reflection from opaque porcelains.[54]

In 1965, *McLean* and *Hughes* described sintered alumina that was originally used for the fabrication of crowns, small fixed partial dentures, and individual and custom-built pontics for use in restorative dentistry in the form of prefabricated profiles.[55] Owing to excessive shrinkage, it was impossible to manufacture custom-made high alumina copings for porcelain crowns. The first commercial porcelain was marketed in 1966, and more than 30 years after its introduction porcelain still remains on the market today.[51] In 1968, *MacCulloch*, who first described the methods used for making artificial teeth, veneers and crowns in glass ceramic, utilized this approach.[56] The desired shade modifications, however, were only possible with surface colorants that had a tendency to erode after a certain period of time. Despite its esthetic appearance, porcelain was prone to fracture and required direct resin bonding with an acid-etch technique.

In the 1970s, colorless metal ceramic crowns were fabricated with newly improved techniques, and commercial shoulder porcelains were developed. They had higher firing temperatures and increased resistance to pyroplastic flows that caused minimal distortions when the veneer porcelains were fired.[51] At that time, the goal of eliminating the gold coping and replacing it with

high-strength ceramic was not yet achieved. In 1976, *McLean* and *Sced* developed the first commercially possible foil-reinforced crown system.[57] The dental porcelain could be strengthened by the dispersion of ceramic crystals of high strength and elastic modulus within the glassy matrix. McLean and Hughes used this method to develop the first aluminous porcelains for the fabrication of crowns.[55] These reinforced porcelains had strengths of up to 180 MPa – approximately double that of the more conventional feldspathic materials. Electroforming and the use of tin oxide coatings for the attachment of a conventional metal-bonding porcelain was reported by *Rogers* in 1979, and a number of foil systems were marketed in the 1980s.[58]

Slip casting, or the science of preparing stable suspensions and fabricating structures, was accomplished by building a solid layer on the surface of a porous mold where the capillary forces absorb the liquid. *Sadoun* refined *Count von Schwerin's* slip casting technique[59] in a paper given at the International Conference on Dental Ceramics held at Leeds Castle, England in 1989. These changes produced high-strength coping, and was marketed under the name of In-Ceram. It was not a pure ceramic and represented a step forward in achieving strengths of up to 630 MPa.[60] In-Ceram made it possible for the laboratory technicians to make advancements in the esthetics of anterior crowns, without losing strength. Undoubtedly, this work deserves a notable place in the history of dental ceramics.

In 1993, *Anderson* and *Oden* described a technique for manufacturing individual all-ceramic crowns made up of densely sintered high-purity alumina.[61] However, the color of sintered alumina may vary according to the firing conditions, presenting a serious disadvantage. Similarly, when compared to regular or aluminous dental porcelains, the sintered alumina is a more difficult material to control.

At the Dental Institute of the University of Zurich, Wohlwend developed and marketed a material for the bonding of porcelain that used the principle of leucite crystal dispersion.[62] This material, Empress, consists of leucite crystals that are only a few microns in size and are produced by controlled crystallization in a special glass that contains nucleating agents.

Ceramic materials have now become the mainstay of esthetic dentistry. Rapid advances in the quality of ceramics and ceramic technology have made it possible for the manufacturers to emulate nature more effectively than ever before. Despite the rapid advances in ceramic technology, the ultimate failure or success of a ceramic restoration is related directly to the expertise of the dentist and his team of technicians. Ceramic material that is used for all ceramic restorations is bonded to the teeth without the support of a metal substructure. Typically, it is reinforced porcelain, designed to withstand the forces of occlusion.[63]

Porcelain Laminate Veneers

Translucent ceramics were first used for clinical purposes as early as 1862, and ceramic veneers were used more frequently in the 1920s and 1930s.[64,65] In 1938, *Pincus* actually attempted to use a denture adhesive to bond the veneers to the teeth,[66] but at that time they were too fragile, as the adhesives available were neither strong nor durable.[67] In 1955, *Buonocore* published an article describing the "acid-etch technique",[68] where a micro-chemical "interlock" was achieved through "acid-etching" the enamel and forming a resistant bond between the composites and inorganic enamel. Subsequently, transparent luting resins replaced the plaque zinc oxyphosphate cement for ceramic inlays. Without any disturbance from an opaque material, light transmission improved, and esthetically pleasing results were achieved.[69]

All-Ceramic versus Porcelain-Fused-to-Metal Restorations

From the initial introduction of porcelain, the use of it in porcelain-fused-to-metal (PFM) applications has achieved the most popularity. Through the years, this system has proved to be beneficial

not only for use in the posterior region but also in the anterior, where esthetics are an especially important issue. Even today, there are a considerable number of dentists who are still using PFMs in the anterior regions to achieve better esthetics. However, this technique, or the metal used, impairs the transmission of light.[70] If the gingival tissues are thin, the marginal soft tissues near the metal collars that have been placed subgingivally may appear to be dark (Fig 1-13). Since the ceramic layer is quite thin and opaque, this is a common occurrence, interfering with the transmission of light through the labial gingival tissues, owing to the shadows created by the porcelain-fused-to-metal restorations with labial butt joint designs. When there is no metal coping, natural teeth, all-porcelain jackets, and cast glass ceramic crowns allow light transmission. All-ceramic restorations require the removal of large amounts of sound dental tissue in order to provide adequate space for the placement of the jacket crown of optimal thickness over the prepared tooth.[70,71]

Until the 1980s, esthetic dentistry was concerned primarily with the close replication of the tooth structure. In the last two decades, several modifications of porcelain-fused-to-metal crown restorations were developed and incorporated within the all-porcelain systems.[53,72] The improved physical properties of these systems, combined with advancements in adhesive technology, such as enamel bonding,[68] dentin bonding,[73] porcelain etching, and silanization[74,75] facilitated the reproduction of new prosthodontic treatment modalities.[76] Clinicians, ceramic technicians, manufacturers, and researchers have striven to produce a substitute artificial enamel, intimately bonded to the dental tissue, for teeth that lack shape, color, or structure, while attempting to retain the maximum amount of healthy intact tooth structure and not exceeding a reasonable financial expenditure.[77]

PLVs

With the recent increase in patients' demands for esthetic restorations in the anterior as well as

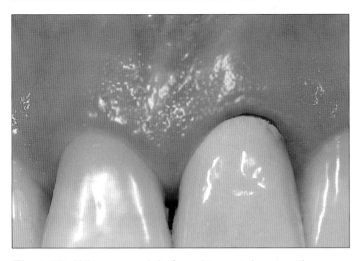

Fig 1-13 When porcelain-fused-to-metal restorations are used on dentition with thin gingival tissue, the dark color of the metal may create a reflection, thereby creating an unesthetic appearance.

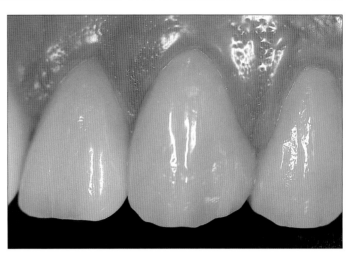

Fig 1-14 Research has shown that when porcelain laminate veneers are properly prepared, produced, and finished, an increase of the crevicular fluid decreases the plaque index and plaque bacteria vitality. Note the gingival health around the biologically integrated porcelain laminate veneers.

the posterior regions, it has become necessary to develop new materials that combine the strength and the resistance that are essential in the posterior region, along with the esthetic qualities desired in the anterior region.[78] Porcelain laminate veneers (PLVs) have become the esthetic alternative to ceramic crowns and the traditional porcelain-fused-to-metal.[79] Smiles can be transformed painlessly, conservatively and quickly with dramatic, long-lasting results with the successful use of the porcelain laminate veneer. Porcelain veneers are now the restorative choice for esthetics in numerous clinical circumstances that would have resulted in the use of full crowns in the past. Tissue response is excellent, and the finished surface is very similar to the natural tooth. Veneers exhibit natural fluorescence and absorb, reflect, and transmit light exactly as does the natural tooth structure. Patients are highly enthusiastic about these restorations that represent a conservative treatment that enhances patient self-image.[3]

The subsequent introduction of special acid-etching techniques improved the long-term retention of veneers.[80-82] *Horn*[83] and *Simonsen* and *Calamia,*[84] for example, increased interest in porcelain veneers. They were influential in demonstrating that the bond strength of hydro-

fluoric acid-etched and silanated veneer to the luting resin composite is generally greater than the bond strength of the same luting resin to the etched enamel surface.[75]

Minimal Tissue Response

Perhaps one of the most important advantages of porcelain laminate veneer is that the periodontal reaction is minimal. The smoothly finished margins help to maintain good periodontal health and oral hygiene (Fig 1-14).[85,86] Various studies have been performed. One of them established that the porcelain-fused-to-metal tissue response is similar to that of the veneers; yet, another found that there was considerably less inflammation with porcelain veneers than with porcelain-fused-to-metal (PFM) restorations.[28,31] In another particular study, *Kourkouata* et al. found that after the porcelain veneer restoration was completed, there was an increase in cervicular fluid; similarly, there was a significant decrease in plaque index and plaque bacteria vitality.[87] When selecting a treatment, longevity is a major concern. A more invasive procedure will result in a higher risk to the tooth and ultimately a more expensive treatment.

Ceramic and metal-ceramic crowns require a considerable removal of the natural tooth structure, thereby increasing the risk. The subsequent increase in interest in less invasive procedures is therefore inevitable.

State of the Art

The dental profession has always been in search of restorations that have a "natural" appearance but are, at the same time, long lasting. In the past, the lack of appropriate dental materials rendered this impossible.[35] However, advances in porcelain veneers and bonding materials now offer a variety of selections in treatment, with long-lasting restorations and improved quality in esthetic results.[3,88-101]

Porcelain veneers are to be considered the "state of the art" in esthetic dentistry, providing abundant advantages over any previous form of veneer system. They are excellent in terms of their appearance and durability, and the actual procedure does not disturb the soft tissue or the adjoining periodontium. Since their introduction almost 20 years ago, porcelain veneers have become the flagship of most esthetics-based practices.

Strength

Owing to their ceramic thinness (0.3-0.5mm), the porcelain veneers can be easily fractured before they are even bonded, similar to kitchen or bathroom tiles. However, once bonded on a solid foundation, they integrate with the tooth structure and become extremely durable, in vitro and in vivo. If all conditions have been adhered to and the appropriate bonding composite has been selected, the dentist will achieve successful results. The patient's satisfaction is bound to be high as this medium ensures long-term maintenance, good gingival health and excellent oral hygiene. Prior to the recent popularity of porcelain laminate veneer application; full crowns were the earlier esthetic restorations for the anterior region. Preparation for full crowns involved removal of

large amounts of enamel, and these invasive procedures often adversely affected the periodontal tissues and pulp.[102-104] When it was proven that function and esthetics could be achieved with porcelain laminate veneers and without the removal of large amounts of intact tooth structure, porcelain veneers became the restorative material of choice in addressing the most challenging aspects of esthetic dentistry by integrating the individual restorations into the adjacent natural dentition.

Enamel Replacement

Recent major breakthroughs in bonding materials and their predictable retention of porcelain to the tooth surface have added an entirely new dimension to the field of esthetic dentistry.[105,106] The introduction of multi-step total etch adhesive systems was made possible by the progress made in the bonding to the enamel and dentine capabilities.[102-104] Porcelain laminate veneer restorations, bonded with the latest generation of adhesive systems, are capable of achieving biological compatibility and function, while attaining a comparable esthetic result. We all agree that the natural human enamel would be the best restorative material to use, if that were possible[79] – but porcelain laminate veneers, being the closest material to natural human enamel, are the least destructive to the adjoining tissues. These characteristics have established the porcelain veneers as the preferred restorative material preserving the enamel, which is ultimately the most valuable part of the tooth. Numerous authors have suggested that the a minimal thickness for tooth preparation for ceramic veneers should be no more than 0.5 mm.[64,65,107] In practice, however, the actual approximate thickness of a porcelain laminate veneer is 0.4 to 0.7 mm, which closely resembles that of the natural tooth enamel. As the quality of porcelain veneers has improved, their popularity has increased, owing to the technique's ability to preserve larger portions of the natural enamel by offering a conservative alternative to full coverage crowns.

Biological Acceptance

Evaluation of published data has shown that porcelain laminate veneers are biologically acceptable to the body owing to their increased chemical stability, lesser cytotoxicity and reduced risk of causing irritation or sensitivity.[108,109] Other advantages of porcelain veneer that have been supported by studies include the reduced plaque build-up and its easy removal.[110-113] Even the bacterial plaque vitality on these surfaces was found to be considerably reduced.[114] *Quirynen* et al. found that only minimal plaque is retained by the porcelain veneers, less than on any other type of material, including natural enamel. The reduced plaque retention is a direct result of the smoothly glazed surface of the porcelain that discourages plaque adherence.[115] The positive effects of porcelain veneers on the marginal gingival tissues are supported by extensive studies and cannot be negated.[30,31,65,81,116]

Application and Case Selection

Although all techniques may have their limitations, porcelain laminate veneers have remained the most esthetic of all the ceramic materials. Awareness of the porcelain characteristics and a careful selection of the cases will enhance the overall success of the restorative treatment.[117] Ceramic veneers may be applied in any number of instances, ranging from the restoration of small proximal lesions and moderate incisal chipping to the cosmetic repairs of developmental defects on the facial surface of the tooth or even to the otherwise intact anterior teeth that have been damaged by severe staining. They have also been successfully used to close diastemata, correct misalignment, and to cover discolored or misshapen teeth. For esthetically unacceptable teeth, porcelain laminate veneers offer a restorative technique using ceramic material that has an enamel mass and translucency to ensure a natural esthetic result with a conservative preparation.

In the more severe clinical circumstances that involve fractured incisors and nonvital teeth, the improvements made in the development of adhesion offer the porcelain veneers as a viable alternative treatment.[118] Along with the revolution in materials, the actual tooth preparation procedures have changed considerably as well. Extensive guidelines are now available to prepare the tooth for partial coverage. Application can be determined by the amount of remaining tooth structure, removal of diseased dental structures, and the space available for a restoration that provides not only form but function as well (see Chapter 7).[119]

Longevity

The union of etched enamel and porcelain, combined with the bonding composite resin-luting agent with a silane coupling agent, enables the dentist to perform restorations that are solid as well as long lasting. The long-term data is encouraging and reports a high success rate for this form of treatment. Materials used in the 1980s are now considered primitive, whereas the restorations made with laminate veneers even 15 years ago have shown a high rate of success, increasing interest and widespread acceptance[68,120,121] (Fig 1-15). Porcelain laminate veneers are continually gaining respect as the best and most durable restorative treatment, while patients and dentists alike are delighted with the esthetic results and the minimal tooth preparation required.[31,66,122-125] As esthetic dentists are becoming increasingly confident of its application to a variety of clinical cases, the survival rate of laminate veneers reported in literature ranges anywhere from 18 months to 15 years.[85] *Friedman* reports in another study that of the 3,500 porcelain veneers that were placed over a 15-year period, 93% of the cases were successful.[126]

Translucency

Since ceramic restorations allow the transmission of light in a manner similar to that of the natural tooth structure, most of these systems offer the potential for superior esthetics. The inherent translucency of the material itself is the superior

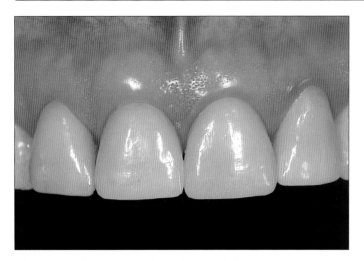

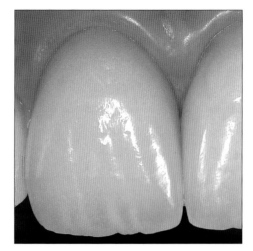

Fig 1-15 The longevity of porcelain laminate veneer restorations has been demonstrated by their service in function and esthetics for years, even though the quality of the earlier material is not comparable to that available today. Note the current status of porcelain laminate veneers that were placed 12 years ago.

Fig 1-16 Using a translucent layer during the laboratory stage can enhance the depth and vitality of the veneers. With adequate communication of information from the clinician, a skillful laboratory technician can judge the amount of translucency porcelain that should be applied over the veneer surface, especially the incisal edges (Technician *Gerard Ubassy*).

characteristic of porcelain laminate veneers. It adds depth of translucency and light transmission to the restored tooth, regardless of the depth of its application (Fig 1-16).[127] These translucent materials allow light to be transmitted into the tooth without causing undesirable tissue darkening adjacent to the restorations. If the shade of the porcelain is close enough for a clear resin composite to be used for cementation, impressive results can be achieved.[128]

Porcelain Laminate Veneers versus Composite Restorations

It is possible to use composite restorations instead of porcelain laminate veneers to cover up tooth discolorations or unesthetic forms. However, the longevity of composites is questionable as they are susceptible to discoloration, marginal fractures and wear. Consequently, any esthetic result requiring long-term durability will be compromised;[129,130] while porcelain veneers are superior in esthetic quality and longevity. The biocompatibility and nonporous surface of the porcelain that prevents plaque adherence has increased its popularity and usage.[131] Fur-

thermore, the applicability of the supragingival preparation technique, used in most veneer restorations, ensures excellent periodontal health. As a result, the porcelain laminate veneers have an important role as a solution to both functional and esthetic challenges.

Functional Corrections

In addition to esthetic restorations, porcelain veneers are a favorable choice for treatment of occlusal deficiencies and for the reestablishment of correct guidance during excursive movements.[132] As *Friedman* reports, porcelain veneers provide functional strength as well as esthetic results.[133] Porcelain laminate veneers can be used as an alternative treatment to guarantee the least reduction of the tooth structure while achieving the most perfect fit. Clinical and laboratory fabrications should be performed in concert to provide a result that is both functional and esthetic.

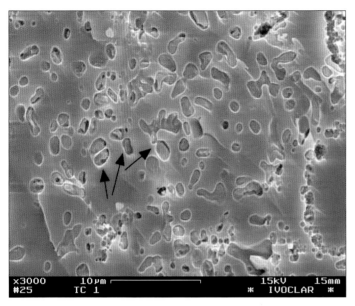

Fig 1-17 First generation of Empress reinforced with leucite crystals.The leucite crystals are responsible for strength. They reflect and scatter the light through the glass matrix, which helps keep the vitality and translucency.

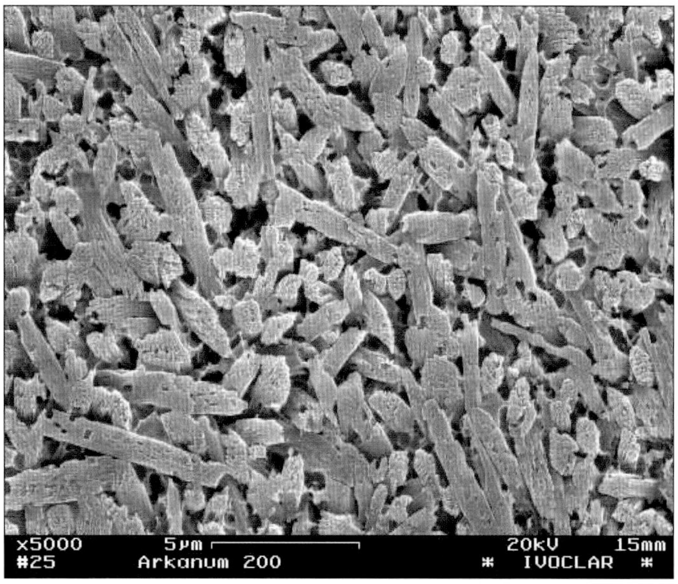

Fig 1-18 Surface of lithium dissilicate after being treated with HFA. A high amount of crystal can be seen, which will stop crack propagation. These crystals not only make the porcelain stronger but it keeps the translucency.

Porcelain Materials for Veneers

Several porcelain materials can be used for the fabrication of veneers and they can be classified into five groups: castable glass ceramic; heat-pressed ceramic; computer-aided manufacturing (CAD/CAM) processed factory produced ingots; feldspathic porcelain baked in the traditional water-slurry method; and feldspathic porcelain over foil-matrix with refractory die technique. Each system has its own advantages and disadvantages.[127] The feldspathic porcelain is the most commonly used porcelain today (either fabricated over the refectory die or the platinum foil) as well as the pressable ceramics. Their esthetic qualities and results may vary. Most veneers can be made from both pressable ceramics and the low-fusing feldspathic porcelain with the platinum foil technique.[134,135]

Pressable Ceramics

Pressable ceramics were successfully launched onto the market approximately 10 years ago. Since their introduction, many similar products have been introduced and have since flooded the market. This was a consequence of the acceptance and reliability of the system of pressable ceramics made of pre-sintered ingots, offering a variety of advantages (Fig 1-17).

The ingots are made of a silicate glass matrix and sometimes contain a crystal phase range, depending on the type of product. The mechanical and physical results of this material show their best results in vivo. In later stages, new developments like Empress 2 even increased the mechanical and optical benefits (Fig 1-18). This product line represents a new type of material, which does not resemble the Empress leucite glass-ceramics.

The following simplified definition of glass-ceramics should help distinguish them from other related materials such as glasses and sintered ceramics/porcelains: "a glass-ceramic is a glassy crystalline material that consists of at least one glass phase and one crystalline phase. The base material for the product is glass, in which crystals are formed by controlled nucleation and crystallization. The finished glass-ceramic product is characterized by at least one type of special crystal that is embedded in at least one glass matrix."

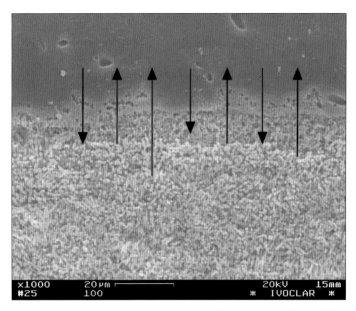

Fig 1-19 Layering technique for Empress 2. The SEM picture shows the perfect interface of which the layering porcelain fluor apatite is diffused into the core material lithium dissilicate.

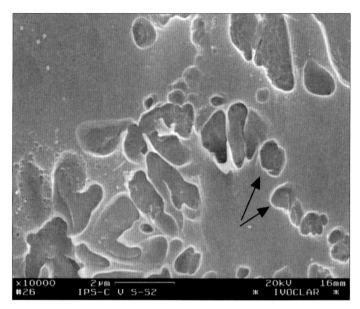

Fig 1-20 The matrix of a feldspathic porcelain with a high amount of glass. Some single crystals are visible. Crack propagation can be easier owing to the high amount of glass matrix. These materials are highly translucent.

Methods

To produce restorations with the Pressable System, special equipment is required. It is very important to adhere to one system-brand and that your choice includes all the requested tools. The pressing machine, special investment and ingots, as well as additional items such as die material for shade control, are all key points. The more complete the system is, the safer and more exact the results will be.

The technician will simply model the object in wax and invest it. The muffles are preheated and, depending on the restorations, either one or two or multiple ingots will be placed into the muffle. The pressing procedure today is fully automatic and controlled with hi-tech electronics. The technician gets the best fitting object after divesting the muffle, which, depending on the chosen technique, may only need to be painted or layered (Fig 1-19).

Advantages
1. Safe
2. Highly esthetic
3. Less work time
4. Firm fit

5. Long-term success
6. Large indications

Disadvantages
1. Relatively high equipment costs

Feldspathic Porcelain

The use of 0.3 mm thickness is possible with feldspathic porcelain, allowing the esthetic dentist to remove only a minimal amount of the natural enamel in preparation. However, this quality can prove disadvantageous as its very thinness renders the veneer brittle, and porcelain particles may cause micro porosities that create low flexural strength[127] (Fig 1-20).

Refraction Die Method (RDM)

Just as with the foil technique, RDM is not a technique that has been reinvented or offers a modern lab high-end technology, but rather gives the technician a solution that avoids the use of extra hardware. It is worth considering as its correct usage offers attractive esthetic results.

These products are mostly made from sinter porcelain. The materials themselves do not generally carry crystals in high quantity if the origin is natural amorph raw material. The porcelain ceramics used for this material do not commonly show outstanding physical properties.

The method consists of duplicating the die by using addition silicones or other accurate, precise impression materials. To pour out the impression, refractory, phosphate-bonded material will commonly be used. Although setting time and the sintering process in preheating furnaces are time consuming, they are crucial steps.

Finally, to apply the ceramic on the die we have to immerse the model in water and seal the surface. The next steps are to build up the dentin, modifiers and incisals according to each case. The firings, including correction, staining and glazing are always done without removing the object from the die. Only at the end can the refractory die be removed by using glass beads in the sandblaster. The final fit must be rechecked on the master model.

Advantages
1. Low hardware costs
2. Highly esthetic results
3. Creativity

Disadvantages
1. Technique sensitive
2. Time-consuming
3. Shrinkage/fit
4. Limited indications

Foil-Matrix Technique

The foil-matrix technique has been used for decades and was one of the first in this field. Several published articles and technical instruction books explain the technique in detail.

Platinum foil is used as a support for core porcelain. The core material requires reinforcement, with products such as aluminous core porcelains. The following layers are dentin enamel porcelain, which is compatible to the reinforced core.

The foil-matrix technique does not require a large quantity of expensive tools. The technician must accurately apply a thin (0.025 mm) foil which must be adapted perfectly and squeezed tightly at the joints. The core porcelain has to be applied and baked. The thickness of core porcelain after firing determines its stability and strength. There will always be shrinkage that will require compensation as well as some difficulties in the marginal fit that are unavoidable.

Advantages
1. Low hardware costs
2. Quick
3. Acceptable esthetic

Disadvantages
1. Limited indications
2. Quiet opaque core
3. Handling must be trained

The greatest flexural strength is found in the castable glass ceramic and heat-pressed leucite-reinforced ceramic, when the thickness is no less than 0.5 mm.[136]

Computer aided design/milling (CAD/CAM)

In comparison to all the other systems, the CAD/CAM or copy-milling techniques create a mean interfacial gap between the actual tooth structure and the restoration that is considerably wider than that of the other systems.[137,138]

This technology for metal-free restorations has become increasingly popular and reliable. In the last few years, several systems have shown that CAD/CAM-produced restorations are accurate enough to be used in the modern clinic. Different material compositions have been used.

Aluminum reinforced matrix, zirconium and leucite ceramics were the most frequently used materials in the past. Some CAD/CAM systems have been used in the dental clinic (Cerec).

Next-generation CAD/CAM units are being introduced, and will be able to prepare any kind of geometry; the indications for which they can be used are virtually limitless.

Owing to the large size of this unit, access to the equipment is generally scanning or through

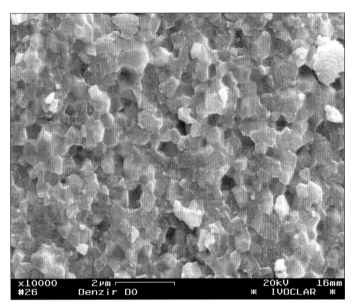

Fig 1-21 Picture of a highly reinforced zirconium dioxide with over 1,000 Megapascal flexural strength. Due to the special means of production, this material can also keep its translucency. Note the compact structure of the material. Under normal circumstances chances of crack propagation is minimal.

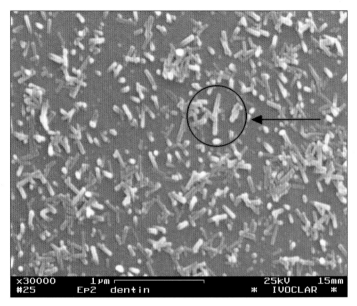

Fig 1-22 For CAD-CAM produced framework such as in the figure, layering material does need to be developed. The picture shows a material with fluor-apatite crystals which is one of the possible choices. The geometry of these crystals is similar to natural enamel in scattering and breaking the light.

the impression or die. A specialist will feed the clinical information into the software with all the related details concerning the preparation parameters. Centers will be set up so that all the necessary information about each case can be collected, produced and distributed.

The results are perfectly fitting restorations, of exactly 5 micron. Outstanding results can be expected. These new materials, which are colored and translucent, will join compatible layering ceramic to conclude the restoration. This technique is very promising as it excludes the human fault rate with the production of a core or frame.

On the other hand, it gives technicians the chance to concentrate their creativity totally on the build-up (Figs 1-21 and 1-22).

Advantages
1. High esthetic
2. Quick
3. Very large indications
4. Safe

Disadvantages
1. Units are expensive

Porcelain Selection

In clinical practice, the personal experience and esthetic performance of the clinician play major roles in the selection of porcelain and in the final outcome. However, no matter which porcelain material is used, when they are applied properly, most of the materials exhibit high strength. The techniques adopted and the ceramic materials employed by the technician also affect the final esthetic outcome. Some technicians may produce only a small number of ceramics each day – care which is reflected in the restorations. By contrast, others prefer more straightforward fabrication and the potential for high-volume production, and this will influence their choice of techniques and materials. In the hands of a talented ceramist, satisfactory results can be achieved. The choice will depend on the commitment of the dentist, their adherence to excellence, and the financial circumstances of the patient.

Technical Sensitivity

The unique characteristics of this particular restorative treatment and its application require special consideration. The highly technical sensitivity of the porcelain laminate veneers may present a so-called "downside" (see Chapters 7, 9 and 10). The success of the porcelain veneers is related directly to the expertise of the technical application, just like other new techniques that are used in dentistry today. Meticulous attention to the correct sequence of application will ensure successful results. When properly utilized, these techniques present several distinct advantages. The reliability and longevity of porcelain laminate veneers mean they will become more popular and have a vital role in esthetic dentistry. This increasing popularity will place demands for further development of the technical preparation, application, and especially of the color matching and masking methods.[139-145]

The Esthetic Dentist

Esthetics, more than any other area in dentistry, is based on individual perception.[146,147] The rationale of the clinician is generally the most important factor in success. Sound scientific knowledge alone is not enough to ensure the success of any prosthodontic procedure and indeed the wisdom of a dentist is required. Sensible selections of suitable physiologic or morphologic variations that are appropriate for each individual are primarily the responsibility of the clinician. Sensibility is not innate; it must be acquired through diligent training and continuous observation.[148] A dentist must therefore acquire and develop the artistic talents necessary to perform the most delicate procedures. The esthetic dentist must have not only a good technical understanding of artistic principles, such as the shaping of teeth and the creation of illusions, but also the knowledge and expertise in their application to clinical esthetic dentistry. The goal should be to establish a biologically compatible dentition that is esthetically acceptable to the patient.[149,150]

Creativity and technical skills are required to become an accomplished esthetic dentist and to attain successful therapeutic results. An accomplished clinician must be able to design a smile or modify a flawed display in such an artistic way that the patient perceives it as pleasing and attractive.[36] A creative manipulation of tooth dimensions and color can change the smile dramatically (Fig 1-23). Artificial materials can be used to create an illusion, and the contrivance of reality may be used to create a restorative change that is perceived by each patient as beautiful. The advent of bonding has furnished the resources to attach composite resins and porcelain in their numerous shades to the tooth surface, enabling the concealment of imperfect teeth by creating an esthetic illusion.[151,152]

The Esthetic Dentist as a Designer

As a successful architect takes various aspects into consideration while designing a building, similarly the esthetic dentist must focus not only on form and function but also the personality, gender, occupation and even the life-style of the patient. The smile is a reflection of that individual. It is important, therefore, to communicate with the patient about all aspects of the treatment. The clinician must fully comprehend what any particular procedure will mean for that particular patient. The anticipated final result must be absolutely clear to the clinician and if deemed necessary, the esthetic dentist should not hesitate to refer a patient to a colleague for a second opinion or treatment. This will establish positive patient/dentist relations, and it is an ethically correct approach. As the quality and standards of esthetic dentistry improve, so will the image and reputation of the esthetic dentist.[36] The dentist must be aware of the limitations of each technique and the materials used. They must personally have superior knowledge of tooth preparation and of the specific material used as well as the ability to be able to execute the finishing touches for the best possible result.[153] Excellence has been defined as "the possession of good qualities or skill in an eminent or unusual degree". In striving for perfection, the esthetic dentist should be willing to expect excellence as a final result.[154]

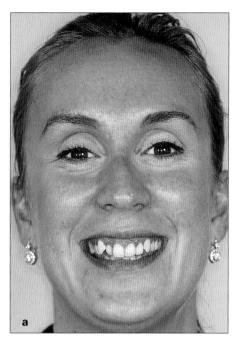
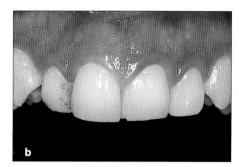
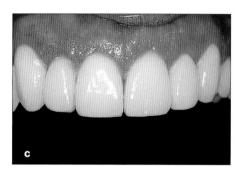
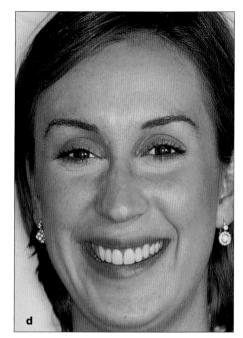

Fig 1-23a-d View of an unattractive smile with healthy teeth (a). The final result should be visualized at the first appointment: (b) If gingival alteration is required, a periodontist may be consulted in advance; (c) when the gingival asymmetries are leveled adequately, the vertical dimensions of the tooth are adjusted accordingly; (d) porcelain laminate veneers are used to correct the third dimension and the bucco-lingual discrepancies. A natural smile is achieved that blends into the facial composition, even though the PLVs applied 9 years ago were monochromatic.

The techniques adopted and material to be used are ultimately the decisions of the clinician. An awareness of the quality of material and its suitability for the particular patient must be determined prior to the initiation of treatment. Sound judgement, a desire to improve one's technical skills, and keeping abreast of the new products that are available should be combined with the most important quality a dentist can possess, the vision or perception of natural esthetics. If the design is successful, there should be no "whiter than white" color emanating from the dentition, or excessive length that can be seen from miles away. When the restoration combines proper function and harmony with its environment, an esthetic pleasure should be felt when observing the smile.

Advanced Training

Until the dentist is familiar with new products or "advanced materials", discretion should be exercised in their use. The new and changing concepts involved in esthetic dentistry, along with the rapid advancements made in the field of restorative materials, require "being up to date" while continuing one's training and education. Failure correctly to apply new techniques that the field now offers may be a cause for dissatisfaction or disappointment.[155] The basics of dentistry are taught in the universities; however, a good dentist who wants to advance in their field must keep up with the continuing advancements in the profession as well as with their training. As long as the field of dentistry produces new materials, ideas and techniques the dentist must further his/her knowledge of the on-going technology.

Creating Natural-looking Smiles

When considering an approach for a new smile design, the dentist undertakes the creation of a new but natural esthetic effect. With each restoration, the patient must be considered as a whole, instead of focusing merely on one or two teeth. Each tooth exists as part of the mouth and face, assisting in creating a smile that reflects the patient's personality.[156] To create a restoration, harmony in the size, shape and arrangement of the teeth are required in order to enhance each patient's facial features. When the teeth, the surrounding soft tissue and the patient's facial characteristics are taken into consideration, a three-dimensional canvas is examined. The dentist must be aware of the ratio between the anterior teeth and the surrounding tissue and analyze them to arrive at the desired result.[36]

A combination of only a few teeth may create an impact larger than the sum of the parts and an esthetic case may vary from a simple esthetic contouring of a corner of a single tooth to the complete recreation of a new smile involving the entire dentition.[156] The mouth and its physiological make-up for each individual patient must be studied carefully by the esthetic dentist, analyzing and anticipating any problems that may arise in carrying out the treatment.

No matter what treatment is undertaken, all patients believe that esthetics is the issue of primary importance even though they may not express this belief. A pleasing smile is important to the patient's morale and self-esteem while the loss of it will negatively affect self-image.[12] The anatomic structure may sometimes affect the function and therefore the esthetics. In such cases, owing to functional disorders, restorations may not be as durable as expected. An inability to achieve an optimal esthetic result may be apparent even from the start and the patient must be informed of the possibility of a compromised esthetic outcome prior to the commencement of treatment in order to prevent postoperative dissatisfaction and arguments (see Chapter 14).

Examining the Smile

When a patient arrives for esthetic treatment, they are usually enthusiastic and motivated about beginning the process. Unfortunately, they frequently arrive with a diagnosis of their own, and the esthetic dentist must be careful not to be influenced by it. It is essential that the dentist knows the relation between diagnosis and treatment planning, as well as the patient-driven difference, when diagnosing an esthetic case. It is not recommended to begin planning the treatment procedure without full knowledge of the reasons that caused the esthetic problems. Once the correct diagnosis is made, the dentist has a sound base on which to discuss the details with the patient and to propose an appropriate treatment plan.

While making these plans, the dentist should listen to what the patient says about their postoperative expectations; respect their ideas and arrive at the best treatment plan suitable for that particular patient. In treatment evaluation, facial muscles and characteristics are an important consideration. Photography can be a great help better to examine the smile in its various forms of laughter, smiling and speech. Unesthetic conditions, such as asymmetric gingival crests, blunted papilla or inflamed and uneven gingival lines may distract from the overall esthetic image; therefore, the importance of esthetic conditions and their relation to appearance cannot be overlooked. The dentist must believe in the final outcome of the treatment plan. The patient's new smile will be carrying the dentist's signature and will be the best source of new referrals. The patient's satisfaction with the final result in terms of both appearance and function is of vital importance. Dissatisfaction with either of these will not only be harmful to the patient's ego but also to the dentist's professional reputation.

The professional responsibilities of an esthetic dentist entail more than the correction of functional or pathologic irregularities. They require that the dentist be skillful, and also fully aware of each patient's particular problems. A complete understanding of the patient's needs, personality and psychological state will result in a more ready acceptance of the proposed treatment plan.[157]

An important element in the success of any such treatment is attention to detail. Inevitably, it is the fine details that will produce a superb result, while the same techniques applied without attention to detail may produce only average results.[36] It is the dentist who invests time in esthetic dentistry, who has the necessary artistic feeling, the eye and hand coordination, and the eye for detail that will separate him or herself from their peers.

Understanding the Patient

Some patients are "result oriented" and cannot be bothered with time-consuming imaging, discussions or long explanations. The responsive dentist must get to the point quickly, summarize the situation and make use of the appointment time. On the other hand, there are the patients who are more emotional, rather disorganized, and not interested in the details but who are quite ready to make a quick decision. It is necessary for the dentist to explain everything to the patient in an enthusiastic way and illustrate the narrative with photographs.[158] As the perception of beauty may differ from individual to individual, so it may differ from culture to culture and from one racial group to another. Basic principles of visual perception need to be developed to determine the response.

Perception

When we are consciously looking at something, the brain is trained to focus immediately on a particular object. In fact, the mind's eye tends to focus on one important object and ignore the surrounding features. When the mouth opens, and the teeth come into view, the brain automatically focuses on the teeth. However, as most people tend to speak to each other usually at a conversational distance, their attention is not focused on every detail of each individual tooth, but rather on the total symmetry, line, proportion, form and size. An esthetic dental observer must learn to focus on a particularly obvious feature of the oral region[12] (see Chapter 2).

Careful observation and the ability correctly to perceive the tooth is a matter of training where only a small degree of error is acceptable. However, errors in the perception of morphology are possible no matter how great the care exercised. Errors such as these may result from the failure of the eye to perceive an object correctly.[159] The esthetic dentist must correctly perceive what is seen in order to form the right morphology and to correct any error that may otherwise lead to serious problems.[159]

Morphological Thinking

The actual phenomenon of visual perception has not been seriously studied as a part of dental methodology. However, dental techniques and the anticipation of problems regarding possible misperceptions should be part of these studies. For that reason, it may help to take a closer look at how visual misperceptions may affect morphologic restorations. Our objective is to create artificial teeth that are as natural in appearance as possible; therefore, focusing our morphologic thinking based on natural teeth.[159] The esthetic dentist needs a keen eye that can readily distinguish natural teeth and their distinct differences one from another. Once this "eye" has been developed, the chances of successfully creating a natural-looking dentition will be greater.[159] Esthetic dentists should have a vision that leads them to strive for leadership in dentistry acquired through personal excellence, education, and integrity positively to affect the health, function, and beauty of mankind.[160]

Teamwork

Elective esthetic dentistry may be defined as the "art form" within the field of dentistry. In order to offer the highest level of patient care, the restorative team must be able to provide treatment that is not only biocompatible and functional but also predictably esthetic. As the field of esthetic dentistry continues to expand, it is essential to retain the quality of natural-looking restorations, harmoniously integrated with proper soft tissue architecture, that have been carefully and meticulously controlled throughout the duration of the restorative procedure.[35] The aim of the esthetic team should be to provide the best products and services available today, with team coordination in the diagnostic phase of the esthetic rehabilitation. The role of the esthetic dentist is to understand the needs of the patient and to formulate a plan that includes not only esthetic considerations, but also occlusal, periodontal and functional requirements, while successfully relating this information to and coordinating with the specialists.

The Specialists

Successful esthetic treatment demands a competent professional team of devoted and skilled specialists. Today, we have built stronger bonds with our fellow specialists in an effort to create treatment options that address health considerations and the esthetic desires of patients. Health issues should never be compromised for the sake of beauty. This is especially important when addressing the demands of capricious patients who present unreasonable or impossible requests that only a skilled team of professionals will be qualified to handle (Fig 1-24). It is of the utmost importance to establish and maintain communication and cooperation between the patient and the technical team, so that the available options can be discussed and the appropriate treatment selected.[36]

The esthetic dentist may be considered as the captain of the team, responsible not only for meticulous artistry and skill but also for the coordination of the team. Each member of the dental team must be aware of their responsibility to one another and to their individual work. Awareness of the team's individual limitations is as important as the awareness of its qualifications. The dentist, acting as the orchestra conductor, along with the team of specialists and technicians, must provide an esthetically pleasing concert. The specialized team members may have varied perceptions of the treatment for a particular esthetic case. The role of the team captain is to select a plan and communicate the concepts to the specialists.

The esthetic dentist may want simply to alter the asymmetric gingival levels (see Chapter 6). For most of the periodontologists, the treatment is limited to tissue health only, unless it has been agreed that the gingival levels be altered. This is also an example of changing the perception of a specialist.

The same thing may happen when orthodontics enters into treatment planning. For most orthodontists, their esthetic goal is achieved when the incisal edges of the incisors are equilibrated. However, as a part of the "esthetic treatment plan", the captain may want the intrusion of one of these incisally-equilibrated anteriors in order to alter an asymmetric gingival level without a periodontal approach (see Chapter 11). This treatment will naturally distort the already well-aligned incisal edge positions of the natural teeth. However, once the gingival levels are aligned, the altered incisal levels resulting from this treatment can be balanced with the help of the porcelain laminate veneers. Mutual respect and encouragement for constructive criticism are required under these circumstances.

The Dental Technician

It should be emphasized that the laboratory technician has a major role in the success of this delicate restorative procedure, especially in the case of porcelain laminate veneers. The success of this team is directly related to the technician's powers of observation, artistry, and the technical discipline of the other members of the team of dentists and specialists (Fig 1-25). The technician is one of the most influential members of the team and deserves most of the credit in properly finished porcelain laminate veneers.

The Patient

The patient, who is the most important member of the team, is frequently overlooked. A successful team needs to integrate the patient into the team as a responsive, contributing member to maintain the motivation and synergy. Consequently, any esthetic restorative treatment also exerts a collaborative effort between the esthetic dentist, the team and the patient. The patient must receive comprehensive information from the dentist regarding the scope, the details and the limitations of the various treatment options, in order to base their decision on a solid understanding of the situation. The patient will appreciate a true collaborative effort and fulfillment of the dental and laboratory team's responsibilities.[161]

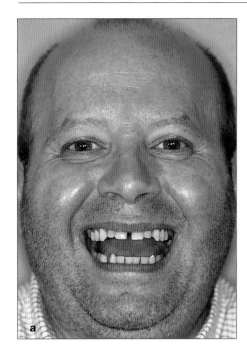
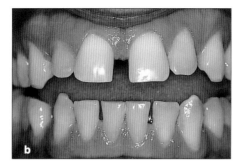
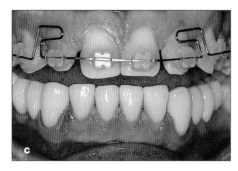
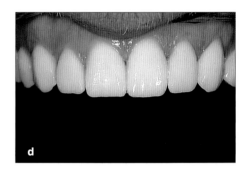
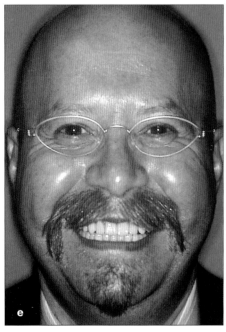
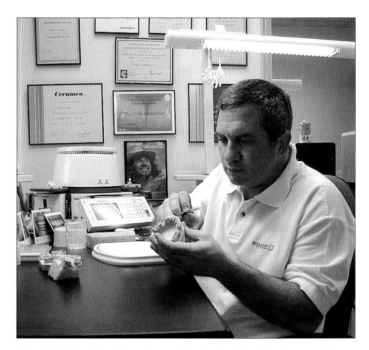

Fig 1-24a-e (a, b) Successful teamwork is essential in achieving success in esthetic dentistry; (c) the diastemata are closed by orthodontic means, and some spaces are deliberately opened in other areas in order to create a space for a pontic; porcelain laminate veneers are used to treat the mandibular arch first (d), then continued to the maxillary arch (e). Note the total impact of a beautiful smile, that improves the alignment of the teeth as well as the self-image of the patient.

Fig 1-25 In the laboratory, the technician's observations, communicated information, and artistic talent and skill combine to achieve the optimal definitive restoration. View of the author's in-house laboratory and his chief technician Mr. Hakan Akbayar at work.

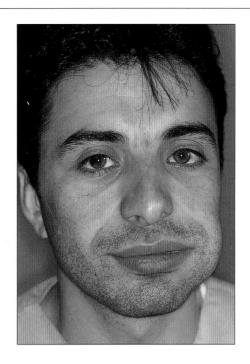

Fig 1-26 Patients who do not visit a dentist regularly may do so only when pain is already present. In such cases, the treatment suggested by the dentist for pain relief is usually accepted.

The Staff

It is not only the specialists, but the hygienist, receptionist and the assistants who play important roles. They should share the same vision and passion as the other team members, because in terms of communication the patient tends to spend more time during the treatment with the hygienist and the dental assistants than with the dentist. The staff will ask questions and share some of their expectations, since the patient is unable to speak while the dentist is working in the oral environment. When the dentist leaves the surgery, they have time to speak to the assistants and hygienist about the procedure and may need answers to some questions that have arisen. Therefore, the entire team must be well informed on everything the procedure entails and be able to answer any questions. The synergy that is created through these efforts will have a positive effect on the patient and the rest of the team (see Chapter 14).

Communication

The needs and motives of esthetic dentistry are different from conventional dentistry. Under normal circumstances, a patient visits the dentist either for a routine check-up or the treatment of a specific dental problem. If there is a tooth defect, a fractured tooth, discomfort or swelling that requires attention, a patient seeks treatment that is probably standard procedure, and there is no "need" for the dentist to confer with the patient (Fig 1-26). This clinical situation may be called "need" dentistry.[22] Most of these treatments will be "dentist driven" and the patients are often in pain or discomfort and feeling relief is their primary concern. Whatever treatment plan the dentist offers will be accepted, as there is a desperate need for something to be done to reduce the pain.[22]

However, if the patients are seeking some form of esthetic improvement, they will arrive with ideas of their own concerning how they want to see themselves upon completion of the treatment. We now face a number of totally different patient expectations, and the treatment has changed from "need" dentistry to "want" dentistry.[22]

It is essential to develop a rapport with the patient, especially in esthetic dentistry. This rapport enables the dentist to discern what the functional and esthetical needs are in order to agree on an appropriate procedure. In addition to being successful in the treatment, the dentist must also be able to articulate and impart their procedural plans to the patient in such a way that they fully understand what they are about to experience. This is an additional aspect of the responsibilities to their patients, and it requires that they maintain a high level of consciousness. This aspect is important in all types of dentistry, but particularly so in esthetic dentistry.

Patient Communication

Personal communication between the dentist and patient is of the utmost importance. This rapport should be established at the first appointment and continue throughout the treatment to ensure success.[39] The field of esthetic dentistry is growing rapidly and prospective patients are becoming increasingly aware of the various innovative procedures available to them. The first meeting between the dentist and patient is vitally important to the success of the prosthetic treatment. The positive attitude of the dentist, along with the comprehensive diagnostic and communication techniques used, builds the patient's confidence in the dentist and the team and helps to establish the communication that is necessary for attaining optimal results. Patients who have developed a good rapport with their dentist also become excellent sources for referrals.[79]

The First Visit

The first visit will set the tone for the relationship between the patient and dentist. It is vitally important, therefore, to make it a positive experience for the patient. If a good relationship is initially established, it will aid in developing trust and make any other stages of the treatment process easier.[36] In private practice, most patients arrive with questions about the cost of the treatment and the time involved. Some may be hesitant to inquire, especially about the cost. In offices where patients visit on a referral basis, the reluctance does not present a problem, as the patients arrive with a general idea of the approximate expendi-

tures anticipated. In the author's experience, it is best not to use external marketing tools but rather to focus on internal marketing, which means a display of quality work supported by patient education. It will take longer to become well known compared to surgeries that have external marketing. However, as years pass and satisfied patients result in increasing referrals, a more respectable image develops.

It is important for the dentist to be a good listener and to be meticulous in recording all the pertinent information. The first appointment will also include a preliminary clinical examination. To ensure the complete confidence of a patient, the dentist must fully comprehend the motives of the patient, accurately grasp the particular dissatisfaction with the dentition, and properly interpret the changes desired. If the dentist is completely honest with the patient and conceals nothing that the procedures may entail, the patient will feel confidence in the dentist and the team, and the rapport between them will strengthen.

Success or Failure

This cooperation and communication between the patient and the dentist will determine the success or failure of the treatment. The esthetic dentist needs to be completely "in tune" with the attitude of the patient, the verbal requests, and the less-obvious nonverbal cues. The dentist who is able to generate a confident, competent and observant attitude makes the patient feel relaxed, and inspires confidence in him or herself and in the proposed treatment. The dentist's perception of a desirable smile and the style of design should be discussed with the patient and be considered along with the patient's personal thoughts on their appearance. The patient may wish to reinstate the appearance that has been established over a long period of time or may request an alteration that is totally unrealistic for their face. Perhaps one of the most difficult tasks is to select the right treatment in order to achieve success in esthetic dentistry. The ability to say "no" will save the dentist sleepless nights and it should also be remembered that one setback can easily erase many brilliant and successful procedures.[79] If the esthetic dentist and patient find it difficult to agree on the objectives, it is in the best interests of everyone not to begin the treatment.

Patient Expectations

The other extreme of the clinical circumstances might be that the dentist may interpret esthetic attitudes based on their own opinions and references, rather than on the expectations of the patient.[162] This can result in a "standardized" sense of beauty, which the dentist may attempt to achieve through unnecessary restorations, causing unneeded stress. The Pocket Oxford Dictionary defines esthetics as "philosophy of beauty", and in reality the perception of beauty varies from individual to individual. There are specific criteria that dentists use to determine one tooth or one smile as more pleasing than another. However, dentists must be aware that the esthetic understanding of the patient may not be the same. The result, which may be esthetically pleasing to the dentist, may not be esthetically pleasing to the patient (Fig 1-27).[163]

The human being is a complicated creature and therefore an art as subjective as dental esthetics can be a very complicated matter. Patients arrive with their own distinct personality, family background, and own social environment. They have their own fears and desires that will affect the way they perceive their treatment. Sometimes dissatisfaction with treatment may stem from insecurities and problems. Sufficient knowledge of the individual's circumstances helps in treatment planning for potentially difficult situations. The social surroundings, as well as the family of the patient, must also be taken into consideration as they have an influence on the patient and the perception of the outcome.[79]

When the patient arrives for the first consultation they may be confused and undecided about what they actually want. It is vital that the dentist guides them and helps them to refine and formulate their particular desires, not only for the sake of their own personal satisfaction but also to avoid remaking the prosthesis owing to any possible misunderstanding. The dentist's objective should be to minimize the problems that may arise

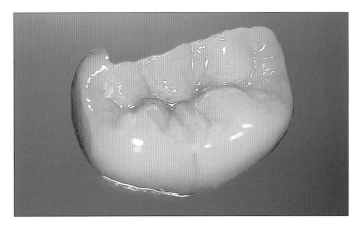

Fig 1-27 Dedicated clinicians and technicians achieve restorations that closely mimic nature. The figure presents a posterior porcelain onlay with the layering and staining effects to emulate nature. Many patients, however, may not like such effects.

from the patient's unrealistic expectations. Some patients seek extreme results to ensure that attention is drawn to their restorations. It is the dentist's responsibility to determine exactly what kind of appearance the patient wants and he or she must then correctly understand and interpret the terminology the patient uses. The self-image and treatment expectations of the patient should be thoroughly understood by the dentist in order to achieve the desired effect.[36]

Unrealistic Expectations

It is not uncommon for patients to arrive with expectations that are literally impossible to deliver, and it is up to the dentist to enlighten and educate the patient, while maintaining a healthy rapport at all times. There are a several considerations to remember. It is important to determine whether the patient intends to change the position and shape of hard and soft tissues through aggressive preparations or if they only require a change in tooth color. The dentist should ask the patient to complete a detailed questionnaire concerning esthetic considerations (see Chapter 14). This questionnaire acts as a supplement to standard medical questions, pinpointing esthetic possibilities and improving dentist–patient communication. It must be supported by careful clinical examination and detailed information from their dental history.[164]

To be an effective communicator, the dentist must be willing to listen to all possible fears and doubts of the patient concerning the proposed treatments. Each method considered for the treatment should be explained in detail and demonstrated, if necessary. The dentist should be optimistic but should not allow the optimism to interfere with the facts of the actual treatment. Always encourage the patient to bring photographs and share visual images better to illustrate and to generate understanding. Some patients may have a fixed image in mind and these subjective expectations may reduce or eliminate the possibility of an objective and attainable treatment.[152]

There comes a point in the communication when the dentist has to make a decision. It is unwise to accept a request just because the patient wants it, and especially because the final result will carry the dentist's signature on that particular smile. The other choice is to offer objective criteria and combine the patient's and the dentist's expectations, that being perhaps the most challenging aspect of esthetic dentistry. The third solution is to be able to say NO to the demanding patient who has unrealistic expectations.

New Diagnostic Tools

Innovative diagnostic tools are available today that expedite the process and aid in communication. Internet and video conferencing reach across distances, while intraoral cameras and transmission of photographs offer information readily available for viewing, which also saves time while clarifying and illustrating the patient's condition. Although it does not replace actual communication with the patient, these diagnostic tools serve as an adjunct to the traditional restorative process.[165] In order to get an accurate image of the anticipated final restoration, a composite mock-up should be prepared. The closer the shades, resins and thicknesses are to the expected final restoration, the better the patient's perception of the final outcome will be. In cases that involve extensive reduction, closure of diastemata, or realignment with veneers, the use of a model or mock-up is essential (Fig 1-28).

A successful alteration, presented in a composite model, allows the patient to see an approximation of the final result. It is also an important exercise for the inexperienced dentist. In time, the dentist will be able to visualize the achievable final result. The experienced dentist uses composite models primarily for the benefit of the patient.[165] The author has found that the use of composite models strengthens the relationship between dentist and patient by allowing the patient to see and feel the final outcome on a three-dimensional scale, as well as testing it for pronunciation. It usefully expedites the preoperative procedure. Nevertheless, neither good communication skills nor the use of models is a guarantee that the patient will accept the proposed esthetic treatment.

Case Acceptance

The visual stimulus can help motivate the patient to arrive at a decision. However, if the patient does not have enough self-confidence, it is useful to have them bring along a friend, relative or someone who can voice an opinion and be involved in the decision-making process, while providing support and reassurance. If the patient cannot make a decision at that moment, the mock-up composites can be secured in a more retentive manner, allowing the patient to leave the office with them in place. It should be explained to the patient that these composites should be used only for an esthetic and not a functional trial. The patient should be advised that they might fall out at any time, and that he/she should not eat or apply force to them. The techniques for removing these devices should also be shown to the patient, so that if one mock-up becomes detached, the others can be removed to prevent the strange look of having a single unaesthetic tooth.

It is better to have these trials and explanations preoperatively rather than have your patient voice negative feelings after the procedure has been completed. The dentist acts almost like a psychologist, allowing the patient to express observations and opinions before and after the treatment, thereby avoiding unnecessary confrontations. An important factor to remember is

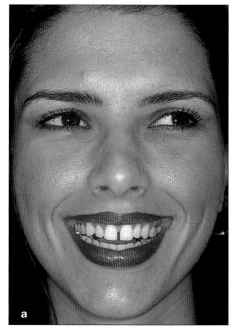
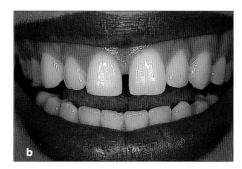
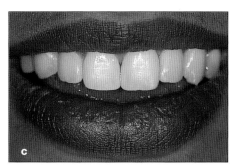
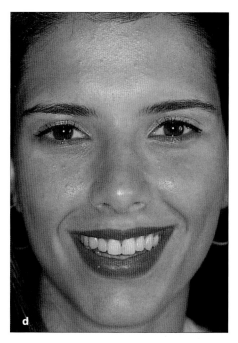

Fig 1-28a-d (a, b) While closing a diastema, both dentist and patient should review the final outcome before the final PLVs are made. (c) Composite mock-ups are simpliest and fastest. In this way the end result can be seen from the first appointment. The patient gains a full perception, including the triangular shape of the papilla between the teeth involved. (d) The final PLVs mimic the contours of the composite mock-up. Through natural integration, teeth look extremely natural.

that the patient's outlook and opinions are subjective from the outset, and it may be difficult for the dentist to influence the patient. Through preliminary discussion and attentive listening to criticism, time can be saved and subsequent unnecessary problems avoided. Unless all aspects of the treatment about to be undertaken are fully understood by the dentist and patient, the treatment should not be initiated.[36]

The area of color is a sensitive one. Despite the dentist's expertise, it is improbable that the patient will submit to the dentist's advice. The use of shade guides for the patient is, therefore, advisable. If the dentist is to place porcelain laminate veneers that have to be the same color as the patient's remaining intact teeth, the matter is a straightforward case. The entire responsibility rests with the dentist and the dental technician to produce veneers that match the color of the remaining teeth precisely. However, if the procedure is a completely new smile design, one that includes all maxillary and mandibular anterior teeth, the patient's ideas should be taken into consideration during the decision-making stage of

the new color. The patient should then sign the shade selection, since the topic of color is a tricky one indeed, as dentists often discover through years of experience.[79]

The Esthetic Consultation

It is important to set out on the right foot. The initial examination must be thorough, with emphasis on periodontal health, caries, possible orthodontic corrections, occlusion, esthetic requirements, and the economic details of these procedures. A good rapport must be developed with the patient, and a plan made that explains all the various techniques to be used. Techniques, such as bleaching, cosmetic recontouring, porcelain veneering, direct resin bonding, or any other necessary procedures should be explained to the patient. Finally, the verbal presentation should be written as a treatment plan, with all pertinent details included and a copy should be prepared for the patient.

Clinical examples are often required to illustrate the application of visual perception to the intraoral environment in order fully to comprehend why dentition, when in harmony with the facial features, creates a beautiful smile. An excellent way of communicating with the patient is through visual presentation on a three-dimensional basis. A simple presentation of some "before" and "after" cases can be enlightening. "Before" and "after" three-dimensional acrylic models or wax-ups of the patient's dentition, including color, serve to illustrate the visual effect.[166] It is the dentist's responsibility to assist the patient in formulating their often confused and unrealistic desires into realistic and achievable expectations and goals, so avoiding having to remake the prosthesis due to dissatisfaction.[79]

In search of a "media smile", some patients place great importance on the symmetry and alignment of the dentition and gingiva. Other contributing factors, such as cultural preferences, age and gender must be considered as well. The lip length should be considered, as the gingival asymmetries may be neglected in the case of a low lip line. However, even though a low lip line hides the gingival margins or asymmetries, some patients may still insist on altering the gingival levels. Or, as in the case of tetracycline discoloration, the placement of a supragingival margin can upset the patient even though the only way of seeing the margin is by lip retraction. Effective communication is essential prior to undertaking the restoration.[79]

Preoperative Evaluation

The preoperative evaluation must begin with a complete examination that includes all details concerning color, characterization and value, from the gingival to the incisal aspects. Written notes should be taken of any undesirable characteristics that may need special attention at the time of the final veneer preparation. The actual selection of the veneers will depend upon the agreement between the patient and the dentist. When designing the prosthesis, several factors must be taken into consideration. The extension of the lip movement during function and the coronal portions of the teeth that are visible at that time, along with consideration of the patient's age,

are all important factors. As various observers may perceive the same image differently, the dental team must be aware of the potential problems that can arise when the perceptions of the patient, the dentist, or dental technician differ. It is possible that the patient may even request a certain appearance that is unsuitable, unachievable, or esthetically not optimal.[167]

Esthetic perceptions may differ owing to a lack of communication, as can be observed when some patients remain passive and allow the dentist to design a smile for them without themselves making a contribution. The actual notion of how the patient perceives their own smile may be complex, and even if an esthetic need for treatment exists, the patient may actually be content with their existing smile. Therefore, for each specific case, the dentist must understand the underlying reasons why that particular individual is seeking treatment and what result is ultimately anticipated. Alteration in any existing dental condition must be initiated only after all the needs of that particular patient have been explored and he/she has accepted all points in question.

The Risks and Benefits

The risks and benefits of any treatment should be thoroughly discussed by the patient and dentist. Even though there may be a clinical indication for a porcelain veneer treatment, it does not necessarily have to be carried out. However, once the decision is made, a full and detailed written approval from the patient should be obtained. When only verbal descriptions are used as the basis for treatment decisions, there is a considerable area for subjective interpretation. To avoid subsequent misunderstandings, exercise the proper use of visual images, models and photographs as aids in designing the restorations.

"Before" Pictures

Preoperative images serve as illustrations for the patient and dentist to clarify the differences between the initial problem and the applied solution. Extensive preoperative photographs of the patient's dentition are useful, as patients tend to forget their original appearance and often need to be reminded. One-to-one and full-face Polaroid photographs, printouts, or digital photography should be taken prior to the treatment. The photographs are essential in order properly to communicate with the technician, and once the case is completed, some of them should be retained in the office with the patient's records and others given to the patient who may wish to show them as evidence of the improvement. Photographs of a successful treatment, to be shown either by the patient or dentist, may serve as proof of their skill in future referrals.[165]

Patient Education

Regardless of their education or social status, most patients have little knowledge of the advancements in dental technology or the treatment techniques available. In addition to their lack of clinical information, patients are exposed to advertisements in magazines or other mass media concepts of what is "beautiful". It is therefore the dentist's responsibility to educate patients about the various techniques available today in esthetic dentistry, the current materials, and the minimally invasive treatments (see Chapter 14). Some patients may arrive with already formulated ideas and expectations about the treatment, ranging from a simple single tooth replacement to a radical change in the position, shape or color of the entire dentition. Others may arrive for a consultation or routine check-up and only find out then that they may have esthetic disorders of which they had not been previously aware. Precious time will be saved by preliminary discussion and good communication skills.

Symmetry exists if the right and left sides are mirror images of each other, despite any variations in their shapes. In restorations, dentists usually prefer to allow more irregularities than do the patients, since they provide an illusion of a more natural appearance. Dentists tend to like longer maxillary incisors, whereas patients do not. It is best to discuss these subtle points with the patient and to develop their awareness. Almost all patients are looking for a "whiter" smile, or at least a lighter color than their existing teeth. This is especially true when they are seeking complete esthetic rehabilitation through a full mouth restoration.

If a patient has been dreaming of a perfect smile, with all-white teeth and perfect arrangement, there may be a shock in finding that the actual result of the restoration is a more natural, subtle version, with slight irregularities and a moderate whiteness of the teeth. Unless the patient has been prepared for this by their discussions with the dental team, they may be disappointed and dissatisfied. There is no doubt that this subtle variety in the arrangement of the dentition will enhance the natural look of their appearance, but it is important for the patient to understand this prior to the treatment; otherwise they may be unhappy and reject the results.[168]

Patients generally tend to select very light colors because they cannot imagine what that color will look like when actually applied to their teeth.[36] To aid in the selection of color, various dental manufacturers produce shade guides. Unfortunately, these shade guides are the size of a single tooth, and it is difficult for the dentist to explain to the patient that this shade will appear quite differently and much lighter when applied to all their teeth. The size, proportion and position of the tooth or teeth in the arch are some of the details that influence the perception of color, and an explanation of this phenomenon to the patient prior to the commencement of treatment is necessary. To enforce verbal communication, colored waxes are used for composite wax-ups to refine the patient's esthetic perceptions. Computer imaging is also becoming increasingly important in illustrating the anticipated result.

Computer Imaging

The magic of computers and the introduction of color monitors, digital and intraoral cameras, electronic graphic tablets, and the mouse, have enabled the dental industry to advance in leaps and bounds. With the help of computers the dentist can illustrate on screen what he/she plans to do, and the patient can see immediately what the restorations will look like. The image can be printed out, saved in the computer, or saved in video form for future reference. Some systems enable the clinician to create two images side-by-side: one the original for the initial reference and the other for simulation of various restorative procedures. Almost anything can be simulated – from bleaching, to crowning, to repairing fractured teeth, tooth lengthening, orthodontic work, or veneering. Imaging can be used for the simplest procedures, such as a gingivoplasty to correct a gummy smile, or for major orthognathic surgery, such as maxillary/mandibular realignment.[169]

Developing communication skills is important, and imaging is one way to improve them. Imaging has the potential to increase the acceptance of treatment plans that may otherwise have left question marks in the patient's mind and delayed treatment decisions. Some patients like to be able to see imaging, while others are interested only in the basic clinical facts, and here the personality of each patient becomes the deciding factor. Imaging is just one of those tools that are beneficial in illustrating and visualizing the potential results prior to treatment.

Interactive imaging is quite different because it is performed with the patient at the dentist's side. "Before" and "after" images can be somewhat limited, whereas interactive imaging enables real communication on all levels. The prints can be sent directly to the laboratory to hasten the process.[169] There are now dental laboratories that specialize in computer imaging. Dentists can email their patient's "before" pictures with a prescription of the alteration required, and the laboratory can perform the imaging. The image of an actual porcelain veneer built-up may be prepared and sent within one hour.

Imaging is not a simple system to implement and requires special considerations. The equipment is costly and requires additional personnel and adequate space. It takes time to perform the actual imaging and it is essential to provide a comfortable atmosphere in which to do it. Training the staff may be time-consuming while the capability to produce detailed imaging that may be impossible to reproduce clinically, may lead to unrealistic expectations and result in patient dissatisfaction.

Composite Models or Mock-ups

If tooth color and shape are to be enhanced by porcelain veneers, composite models are extremely useful. A major problem with diagnostic tools is that they provide only a two-dimensional plane. This limitation makes it difficult for the patient to imagine the profile, position of the lips and the effects that the restoration will have on the occlusal plane and phonetics. In order to produce undetectable porcelain veneers, careful observation of the dentition from all angles is vital and an eye for detail is essential. As Yamamoto has stated, we must train our eyes to observe the natural teeth and educate our hands to express exactly what our eyes perceive.[170] Composite models can be helpful for those patients who seek restorations to mimic natural dentition and the supporting soft tissues. Prior to the treatment for misaligned and malformed anterior teeth, non-bonding composite additions can be effective for illustration of the final esthetic outcome. Optimized transference techniques are effective and valuable procedures that can be used to produce the perfect replica of the definitive restoration. This procedure provides for comfortable communication between the dentist and patient, and allows the artistic creation of the smile to take place through a trial-and-error designing process, until the dentist and patient are mutually satisfied.

When preparing the models, it is to the advantage of the dentist to use the same shades and veneer thickness planned for the final restorations. If the model is properly finished and polished, with close attention paid to the details of shape and texture, it can serve as a useful preview of the final result. This is especially important in determining the effect on the patient's smile, realigning the teeth with veneers, and in reducing or closing diastemata. In the case of the more demanding patients, the dentist must be honest in explaining to the patient that the clinician, the technical team, the dental materials, and the application techniques all have their limitations.

References

1. Rufenacht CR. Morphopsychology. In: Rufenacht, CR. Fundamentals of Esthetics. Chicago: Quintessence, 1990: 11-31, 59-64.

2. Frush JP, Fisher RD. Introduction to dentogenic restorations. J Prosthet Dent 1955;5:586-595.

3. Nasedkin JN. Current perspectives on esthetic restorative dentistry. Part 1. Porcelain laminates. J Can Dent Assoc 1988;54:248-256.

4. Okuda WH. Resolve to recommit to excellence. AACD J 1997;Winter:2.

5. Stein H. Aesthetic color reproduction. Indep Dent 1999; July/August:65-66.

6. Goleman D, Goleman TB. Beauty's hidden equation. Am Health 1987;March.

7. Patzer GL. The Physical Attractiveness Phenomena. New York: Plenum Publishing, 1985.

8. Lombardi RE. The principles of visual perception and their clinical application to denture esthetics. J Prosthet Dent 1973;29:358-382.

9. Guerini VA. History of Dentistry from the Ancient Times until the Time of the Eighteenth Century. New York: Milford House, 1969.

10. Jarabak JR. Management of an Orthodontic Practice. St Louis, MO: Mosby, 1956.

11. Mack MR. Perspective of facial esthetics in dental treatment planning. J Prosthet Dent 1996;75:169-176.

12. Renner RP. An Introduction to Dental Anatomy and Esthetics. Chicago: Quintessence, 1985:241-272.

13. Pilkington EL. Esthetics and optical illusions in dentistry. J Dent Assoc 1936;23:641-651.

14. Mack MR. Perspective of facial esthetics in dental treatment planning. J Prosthet Dent 1996;75:169-176.

15. Peumans M, Van Meerbeek B, Lambrechts P, Vanherle G. Porcelain veneers: A review of the literature. J Prosthet Dent 2000;28:163-177.

16. Reinhart JW, Capiulonto ML. Composite resin esthetic dentistry survey in New England. J Am Dent Assoc 1990; 120:541-544.

17. Brown LJ, Swango PA. Trends in caries: Experience in US employed adults from 1971-74 to 1985: Cross-sectional comparisons. Adv Dent Res 1993;7:52-60.

18. Johnson BD, Mulligan K, Kiyak HA, Marder M. Aging or disease? Periodontal changes and treatment considerations in the older dental patient. Geriodont 1989;8:109-118.

19. White BA, Caplon DJ, Weintraub JA. A quarter century of changes in oral health in the US. J Dent Educ 1995;59: 19-57.

20. Marcus SE, Drury TR, Brown LJ, Zion GR. Tooth retention and tooth loss in the permanent dentition of adults: United States, 1988-1991. J Dent Res 1996;75 (special issue): 684-695.

21. Morley J. The role of cosmetic dentistry in restoring a youthful appearance. J Am Dent Assoc 1999;130:1166-1172.

22. Hornbrook DS. From the editor. AACD J 1997;Fall:2.

23. Rinaldi P. Simplifying anterior esthetics in the general practice. Contemp Esthet Rest Pract 2001;April 2001:1-6.

24. Smigel I. The non-surgical facelift. Contemp Esthet Rest Pract 2000;October:12-14.

25. Goldstein RE, Fritz M. Esthetics in dental curriculum. J Dent Ed 1981;45:355.

26. Goldstein RE, Lancaster JS. Survey of patient attitudes toward current esthetic procedures. J Prosth Dent 1984; 52:775-780.

25. Goldstein RE. Esthetics in Dentistry. 2nd ed. Hamilton, ON: BC Decker Inc, 1998:3-15.

27. Roulet J-F. Operative dentistry versus prosthodontics. In: Fischer J, Esthetics and Prosthetics. Chicago: Quintessence, 1999:101-120.

28. Karlsson S, Landahl I, Stegersjö G, Milleding P. A clinical evaluation of ceramic laminate veneers. Int J Prosthodont 1992;5:447-451.

29. Shaini FJ, Shortall ACC, Marquis PM. Clinical performance of porcelain laminates veneers. A retrospective evaluation over a period of 6.5 years. J Oral Rehabil 1997;24:553-559.

30. Kourkuata S, Walsh TF, Davis LG. The effect of porcelain laminate veneers on gingival health and bacterial plaque characteristics. J Clin Periodont 1994;21:638-640.

31. Pippin DJ, Mixon JM, Soldon-Els AP. Clinical evaluation of restored maxillary incisors: Veneers vs. PFM crowns J Am Dent Assoc 1995;126:1523-1529.

32. Peumans M, Van Meerbeek B, Lambrechts P, Vuylsteke-Wauters M, Vanherle G. Five-year clinical performance of porcelain veneers. Quintessence Int 1998;29:211-221.

33. Chiche GJ. The evolution of prosthodontic treatment. Pract Periodont Aesthet Dent 2000;12:94.

34. Rufenacht CR. Principles of Esthetic Integration. Chicago: Quintessence, 2000:169-240.

35. Trinkner TF, Roberts M. Anterior restoration utilizing novel all-ceramic materials. Pract Periodont Aesthet Dent 2000;12:35-37.

36. Goldstein RE. Esthetics in Dentistry. 2nd ed. Hamilton, ON: BC Decker Inc, 1998:3-15.

37. Lee R. Esthetics and its relationship to function. In: Rufenacht CR. Fundamentals of Esthetics. Chicago: Quintessence, 1990:137-210.

38. Fischer J. Esthetics and Prosthetics. Chicago: Quintessence, 1999:1-30.

39. Pietrobon N, Paul S. All ceramic restorations: A challenge for anterior esthetics. J Esthet Dent 1997;9:179-186.

40. Zide MF. Evaluation of facial esthetics. JDC Dent Soc 1981;55:27.

41. Lombardi RE. The principles of visual perception and their clinical application to denture esthetics. J Prosthet Dent 1973;29:358-382.

42. Renner RP. An Introduction to Dental Anatomy and Esthetics. Chicago: Quintessence, 1985:187-233.

43. Graber LW, Lucker GW. Dental esthetic self-evaluation and satisfaction. Am J Orthod 1980;77:163.

44. Hershon LE, Giddon DB. Determinants of facial profile self-perception. Am J Orthod 1980;78:279.

45. Spradley FL, Jacobs JD, Crowe DP. Assessment of the anterio-posterior soft-tissue counter of the lower facial third in the ideal young adult. Am J Orthod 1981;79:316.

46. Brigante RF. Patient assistant esthetics. J Prosthet Dent 1981;46:14.

47. Brisman AS. Esthetics: A comparison of dentists' and patients' concepts. J Am Dent Assoc 1980;100:345.

48. Fischer J, Esthetics and Prosthetics. Chicago: Quintessence, 1999:1-31.

49. Rosenthal L, Rinaldi P. The aesthetic revolution: Minimum invasive dentistry. Dent Today 1998;17:1-4.

50. Nathanson D. Current developments in aesthetic dentistry. Curr Opin Dent 1991;1:206-211.

51. McLean JW. Evolution of dental ceramics in the twentieth century. J Prosthet Dent 2001;85:61-66.

52. Vines RF, Semmelman JO, Lee PW, Fonvielle FD. Mechanisms involved in securing dense, vitrified ceramics from pre-shaped partly crystalline bodies. J Am Ceram Soc 1958;41:304-308.

53. Weinstein M, Katz S, Weinstein AB. Fused porcelain-to-metal teeth. US patent 3052,982 (1962).

54. McLean JW. The science and art of dental ceramics. The nature of dental ceramics and their clinical use. Quintessence Int 1979;1:47.

55. McLean JW, Hughes TH. The reinforcement of dental porcelain with ceramic oxides. Br Dent J 1965;119:251-267.

56. MacCulloch WT. Advances in dental ceramics. Br Dent J 1968;124:361-365.

57. McLean JW, Sced IR, The bonded alumina crown. 1. The bonding of platinum to aluminous dental porcelain using tin oxide coatings. Aust Dent J 1976;21:119-127.

58. Rogers OW. The dental application of electro-formed pure gold. 1. Porcelain jacket crown technique. Aust Dent J 1979;24:163-170.

59. Schwerin GB. German patents 274039 and 276244 (1910).

60. McLean JW. New dental ceramics and esthetics. J Esthet Dent 1995;7:141-149.

61. Anderson M, Oden A. A new all-ceramic crown. A dense-sintered, high-purity alumina coping with porcelain. Acta Odont Scand 1993;51:59-64.

62. Wohlwend A. Vefahrenund ofen zur Herstellung von Zahnersatzteilen. European patent 0231773 (1987).

63. Miller M. Reality 2000. Houston: Reality Publishing, 2000;4:1-88.

64. Calamia JR. The etched porcelain veneer technique. NY State Dent J 1988;54:48-50.

65. Calamia JR. Clinical evaluation of etched porcelain laminate veneers. Am J Dent 1989;2:9-15.

66. Pincus CR. Building mouth personality. J South California Dent Assoc 1938;14:125-129.

67. Qualtrough AJE, Wilson NHF, Smith GA. The porcelain inlay: A historical view. Oper Dent 1990;15:61-70.

68. Buonocore MG. A simple method of increasing the adhesion of acrylic filling materials to enamel surfaces. J Dent Res 1955;34:849-853.

69. Kern M, Thomson VP. Tensile bond strength of new adhesive systems to Inceram ceramic. J Dent Res 1993; 72:369. Abstract 2124.

70. McLean JW. The science and art of dental ceramics. Bridge design and laboratory procedures in dental ceramics. Chicago: Quintessence, 1980;2.

71. Geller W, Kwiatkowski SJ. The Willi's glas crown: a new solution in the dark and shadowed zones of esthetic porcelain restorations. QDT 1987;11:233.

72. Lehner C, Mannchen R, Scharer P. Variable reduced metal support for collarless metal-ceramic crowns: A new model for strength evolution. Int J Prosthodont 1995;8:337-345.

73. Krejci I, Lutz F, Mörmann W. Zahnfarbene adhäsive Restaurationen im Seitenzahnbereich. Zürich: Eigenverlag PPK, 1998.

74. Rochette AL. A ceramic restoration bonded by etched enamel and resin for fractured incisors. J Prosthet Dent 1975;33:287-293.

75. Calamia JR, Simonsen RJ. Effect of coupling agents on bond strength of etched porcelain. J Dent Res. 1984; 63:179.

76. Studer S, Zellweger U, Scharer P. The aesthetic guidelines of the mucogingival complex for fixed prosthodontics. Pract Periodont Aesthet Dent 1996;8:333-341.

77. Magne P, Perroud R, Hotges JS, Belser UC. Clinical performance of novel-design porcelain veneers for the recovery of coronal volume and length. Int J Periodont Rest Dent 2000;20:440-457.

78. Rosenthal L. Clinical advantages of pressed ceramic restoration technology. Pract Periodont Aesthet Dent 1996;supplement.

79. Touati B, Miara P, Nathanson D. Esthetic Dentistry and Ceramic Restorations. New York: Martin Dunitz, 1999:161-214.

80. Strassler HE, Weiner S. Abstract reporting 96.4% success with 196 veneers up to 13 years, average 10 years. J Dent Res 1998;77:233.

81. Kihn PW, Barnes DM. The clinical longevity of porcelain veneers at 48 months. J Am Dent Assoc 1998;129:747-752. Ceramco color logic veneers work well.

82. Yaman P, Qazi SR, Dennison JB, Razzooq ME. Effect of adding opaque porcelain on the final color of porcelain laminates. J Prosthet Dent 1997;77:136-140.

83. Horn HR. Porcelain laminate veneers bonded to etched enamel. Dent Clin North Am. 1983;27:271-284.

84. Simonsen RJ, Calamia JR. Tensile bond strength of etched porcelain. J Dent Res. 1983;62:297. Abstract 1154.

85. Strassler HE, Nathanson D. Clinical evaluation of etched porcelain veneers over a period of 18 to 42 months. J Esthet Dent 1989;1:21-28.

86. Rucker ML, Richter W, Macentee M, Richardson A. Porcelain and resin veneers clinically evaluated: 2-years result. J Am Dent Assoc 1990;121:594-596.

87. Korukent S, Walsh TF, Davis LG. The effect of porcelain laminate veneers on gingival health and bacterial plaque characteristics. J Clin Periodont 1994;21:638-640.

88. Horn HR. Porcelain laminate veneers bonded to etched enamel. Dent Clin North Am. 1983;27:671-684.

89. Clyde JS, Gilmore A. Porcelain laminate veneers. A preliminary review. Br Dent J 1988;164:9-14.

90. Levin RP. The future of porcelain laminate veneers. J Esthet Dent 1989;1:45.

91. Goldstein RE. Diagnostic dilemma: To bond, laminate, or crown? Int J Periodont Rest Dent 1987;7:9.

92. Sorensen JA, Torres TJ. Improved color matching of metal-ceramic restorations. Part 3. Innovations in porcelain application. J Prosthet Dent 1988;59:1-7.

93. Sheets CG, Taniguehi T. Advantages and limitations in the use of porcelain veneer restorations. J Prosthet Dent 1990;64:406.

94. Chpindel P, Cristou M. Tooth preparation and fabrication of porcelain veneers using a double-layer technique. Pract Periodont Aesthet Dent 1994;6:19-30.

95. Christensen GJ. Have porcelain veneers arrived? J Am Dent Assoc 1991;122:81.

96. Christensen GJ. Porcelain veneer update 1993. CRA Newsletter 1993;17.

97. Christensen GJ, Christensen RP. Clinical observations of porcelain veneers: A three-year report. J Esthet Dent 1991;3:174-179.

98. Nixon RL. Mandibular ceramic veneers: An examination of diverse cases integrating form, function and aesthetics. Pract Periodont Aesthet Dent 1995;1:17-28.

99. Strassler HE, Nathanson D. Clinical evaluation of etched porcelain veneers over a period of 18 to 42 months. J Esthet Dent 1989;1:21-28.

100. Zappala C, Bichacho N, Prosper L. Options in aesthetic restorations: Discolorations and malformations. Problems and solutions. Pract Periodont Aesthet Dent 1994;6:43-52.

101. Fischer J, Kuntze C, Lampert F. Modified partial-coverage ceramics for anterior teeth: A new restorative method. Quintessence Int 1997;28:293-299.

102. Nakabayashi N, Kojima K, Masuhara E. The promotion of adhesion by filtration of monomers into tooth substrates. J Bio Mat Res 1982;16:265-273.

103. Van Meerbeek B, Vanherle G, Lambrechts P, Braem M. Dentin- and enamel-bonding agents. Curr Opin Dent 1992;2:117-127.

104. Pashley DH, Ciucchi B, Sano H, Horner JA. Permeability of dentin to adhesive agents. Quintessence Int 1993;24:618-631.

105. Horn HR. Porcelain laminate veneers bonded to etched enamel. Dent Clin North Am. 1983;27:671-684.

106. McLaughlin G. Porcelain fused tooth. A new esthetic and reconstructive modality. Compend Contin Educ Dent 1984;5:430-435.

107. Weinberg IA. Tooth preparation for porcelain laminates. NY State Dent J 1989;55:25-28.

108. Anusavice KJ. Degradability of dental ceramics. Adv Dent Res 1992;6:82-89.

109. Schafer R, Kappert HF. Die chemische Löslichkeit von Dentalkeramiken. Dtsch Zahnärtzl Z 1993;48:625-628.

110. Newcomb GM. The relationship between the location of sub gingival crown margins and gingival inflammation. J Periodont 1974;45:151-154.

111. Janenko C, Smales RJ. Anterior crowns and gingival health. Aust Dent J 1979;24:225-230.

112. Chan C, Weber H. Plaque retention on restored teeth with full-ceramic crowns: Comparative study. J Prosthet Dent 1986;56:666-671.

113. Olsson J, van der Heijde Y, Holmberg K. Plaque formation in vivo and bacterial attachment in vitro on permanently hydrophobic and hydrophilic surface. Caries Res 1992;26:428-433.

114. Hahn R, Weiger R, Netuschil L, Bruch M. Microbial accumulation and vitality on different restorative materials. Dent Mater 1993;9:312-316.

115. Quirynen M, Bollen CML. The influence of surface roughness and surface-free energy on supra- and subgingival plaque formation in man. A review of literature. J Clin Periodont 1995;22:1-14.

116. Walls AWG. The use of adhesively retained all porcelain veneers during the management of fractured and worn anterior teeth. Part 2. Clinical results after five-year follow-up. Br Dent J 1995;178:337-339.

117. Cornell DF. Ceramic Veneers: Understanding their benefits and limitations. QDT 1998;21:121-132.

118. Besler UC, Magne P, Magne M. Ceramic laminate veneers, continuous evolution of indications: J Esthet Dent 1997;9:197-207.

119. Sulikowski AV, Yoshida A. Clinical and laboratory protocol for porcelain laminate restorations on anterior teeth. QDT 2001;24:8-22.

120. Calamia JR. Etched porcelain facial veneers: A new treatment modality based on scientific and clinical evidence. NY J Dent 1983;53:255-259.

121. Horn HR. Porcelain laminate veneers bonded to etched enamel. Dent Clin North Am. 1983;27:671-684.

122. Dunne SM, Millar J. A Longitudinal study of the clinical performance of porcelain veneers. Br Dent J 1993;175:317-321.

123. Nortbo H, Rygh-Thoresen N, Henaugh T. Clinical performance of porcelain laminate veneers without incisal overlapping. Three years' results. J Dent 1994;22:342-345.

124. Reid JS, Murray MC, Power SM. Porcelain veneers: A four-year follow-up. Rest Dent 1988: 60,62-4,66.

125. Jordan RE, Suzuki M, Senda A. Clinical evaluation of porcelain laminate veneers. A four-year recall report. J Esth Dent 1989;1:126-137.

126. Friedman MJ. A fifteen-year review of porcelain veneer failure. A clinician's observations. Compend Contin Educ Dent 1998;19:625-636.

127. Giordano RA, Pelletier L, Campbell S, Prober R. Flexural strength of an infused ceramic, glass ceramic and feldspathic ceramic. J Prosthet Dent 1995;73:411-418.

128. Pameijer JHN. Onlays: Is gold still the standard? In: Degrange M, Roulet J-F. Minimally invasive restorations with bonding. Chicago: Quintessence, 1997:139-152.

129. Peumans M, Van Meerbeek B, Lambrechts P, Vanherle G. The five-year clinical performance of direct composite additions to correct tooth form and position. Part 1. Esthetic qualities. Clin Oral Invest 1997;1:12-18.

130. Peumans M, Van Meerbeek B, Lambrechts P, Vanherle G. The five-year clinical performance of direct composite additions to correct tooth form and position. Part 2. Marginal qualities. Clin Oral Invest 1997;1:19-26.

131. Eichner K. Einfluss von Brückenzwischengliedern auf die Gingiva. Dtsch Zahnärztl Z 1975;30:639.

132. Mahonen KT, Virtanen KK, An alternative treatment for excessive tooth wear. A clinical report. J Prosthet Dent 1991;65:338-340.

133. Friedman M. Multiple potential of etched porcelain laminate veneers. J Am Dent Assoc 1987;115 (special issue):831-878.

134. McLaughlin G, Morrison JE. Porcelain fused to tooth: The state of the art. Rest Dent 1988;4:90-94.

135. Wildgoose DG, Winstanly RB, Van Noort R. The laboratory construction and teaching of ceramic veneers: A survey. J Dent 1997;25:119-123.

136. Dalloca LL, Demolli, U. A new esthetic material for laminate veneers: IPS-Empress. QDT 1994;17:167-171.

137. Isenberg BP, Essig ME, Leinfelder KF. Three years clinical evaluation of CAD-CAM restorations. J Esthet Dent 1992; 4:173-176.

138. Heymann HO, Bayne SC, Sturdevant JR, Wilder AD, Roberson TM. The clinical performance of CAD-CAM-generated ceramic inlays. J Am Dent Assoc 1996;127: 1171-1181.

139. Davis, BK, Aqulinio, SA, Lund, PS, Diaz-Arnold, AM, Denehy, G. Subjective evaluation of the effect of porcelain opacity on the resultant color of porcelain veneers. Int J Prosthodont 1990;3:567-572.

140. Davis BK, Scott JO, Johnston WM. Effect of porcelain shades on final shade of porcelain veneers. J Dent Res. 1991;70:475. Abstract 1671.

141. Davis, BK, Aqulinio, SA, Lund, PS, Diaz-Arnold, AM, Denehy, G. Subjective evaluation of the effect of porcelain opacity on the resultant color of porcelain veneers. Int J Prosthodont 1990;3:567-572.

142. Mörmann WH, Link C, Lutz F. Color changes in veneer ceramics caused by bonding composite resin. Acta Med Dent Helv 1996;1:97-102.

143. Davis BK, Papcum LJ, Johnston WM. Effect of cement shade on final shade of porcelain veneers. J Dent Res 1991;70:297. Abstract 250.

144. Davis BK, Johnston WM, Saba RF. Kubelka-Munk theory applied to porcelain veneer systems using a colorimeter. Int J Prosthodont 1994;7:227-233.

145. Meijering AC, Roeters FJ, Mulder J, Creugers NH. Patients' satisfaction with different types of veneer restorations. J Dent 1997;25:493-497.

146. Smigel I. Chancing facial contour with expert application of porcelain laminates. Dent Today 1988;7:5.

147. Rosenthal L, DiPilla RP. A simple technique for impression making, bite registration and fabricating provisionals. Post Grad Dent 2000;7:2-7.

148. Rufenacht CR. Principles of Esthetic Integration. Chicago: Quintessence, 2000:63-169.

149. Gwinnett AJ. Effect of Cavity disaffection on bond strength to dentin. J Esthet Dent. 1992;4 (special issue): 11-13.

150. Rosenthal L. The state of the art in porcelain laminate veneers. Part 1. Simple cases. Esthetic Dent Update. 1991;2:5.

151. Tao S, Lowental U. Some personality determinants of denture preference. J Prosthet Dent 1980;44:10-12.

152. Geller W. A timeworn concept: reality or utopia? Pract Periodont Aesthet Dent 1998;10:542-544.

153. Morley J. Critical elements for the preparation and finishing of direct and indirect anterior restorations. Contemp Esthet Dent 1997;3:1-6.

154. Glick K. In search of excellence. AACD J 1997;Fall:3.

155. Morley J. Critical elements for the preparation and finishing of direct and indirect anterior restorations. Contemp Esthet Dent 1997;3:1-6.

156. Golub-Evans J. Unity and variety: Essential ingredient of a smile design. Curr Opin Cosmet Dent 1994;2:1-5.

157. Levin RP. Patient personality assessment improves case presentation. Dent Ecom 1988;78:49-50,52,54-55.

158. Levin RP. Patient personality assessment improves case presentation. Dent Ecom 1988;78:49-50,52,54-55.

159. Yamamoto M, Miyoshi M, Kataoka S. Special Discussion. Fundamentals of esthetics: contouring techniques for metal ceramic restorations. QDT 1990/1991;14:10-81.

160. Crispin BJ. Segmented Reconstruction. AACD J 1997; Winter:42.

161. Drago CJ. Clinical and laboratory parameters in fixed prosthodontic treatment. J Prosthet Dent 1996;76:233-238.

162. Goldstein RE. Study of need for esthetic in dentistry. J Prosthet Dent 1969;21:589-598.

163. Feeley RT Cosmetics and the esthetic patient and laboratory communication. Oral Health 1995;85:9-12,14.

164. Levinson N. Psychological facets of esthetic dentistry: A developmental perspective. J Prosthet Dent 1990;64: 486-491.

165. Baratieri LN. Esthetics: Direct Adhesive Restoration on Fractured Anterior Teeth. São Paulo: Quintessence, 1998:270-312.

166. Moskowitz M, Nayyar A. Determinants of dental esthetics: A rationale for smile analysis and treatment. Compend Contin Educ Dent 1995;16:1164,1166,1186.

167. Cornell DF. Ceramic veneers: Understanding their benefits and limitations. QDT 1998;21:121-132.

168. Shillingburg Jr HT, Hobo S, Whitsett LD, Jacobi R, Brackett SE. Fundamentals of Fixed Prosthodontics. 3rd ed. Chicago: Quintessence, 1997;419-432.

169. Miller M. Reality 2000. Houston: Reality Publishing, 2000;Imaging Systems 14:315-324.

170. Yamamoto N. Metal-Ceramics: Principles and Methods of Makoto Yamamoto. Chicago: Quintessence, 1985.

2 Smile Design

Galip Gürel

Introduction

Esthetic dentistry is a delicate combination of scientific principles and artistic abilities. Mathematical parameters used by the dentist and the laboratory technician combine to produce an attractive esthetic appearance. However, these geometric laws must not be used mechanically; instead, they must act as guidelines for each clinical restoration.[1,2] Esthetic judgement is not an entirely objective criterion; the dentist must also consider the subjective concerns of the character and the life-style of the individual patient when designing a natural smile. Taking these criteria into account, the dentist and the dental team must then incorporate their own personal artistic abilities and their subjective feelings to create a smile. The creativity of the procedure makes each case unique and the dentist's job pleasingly varied and rewarding.

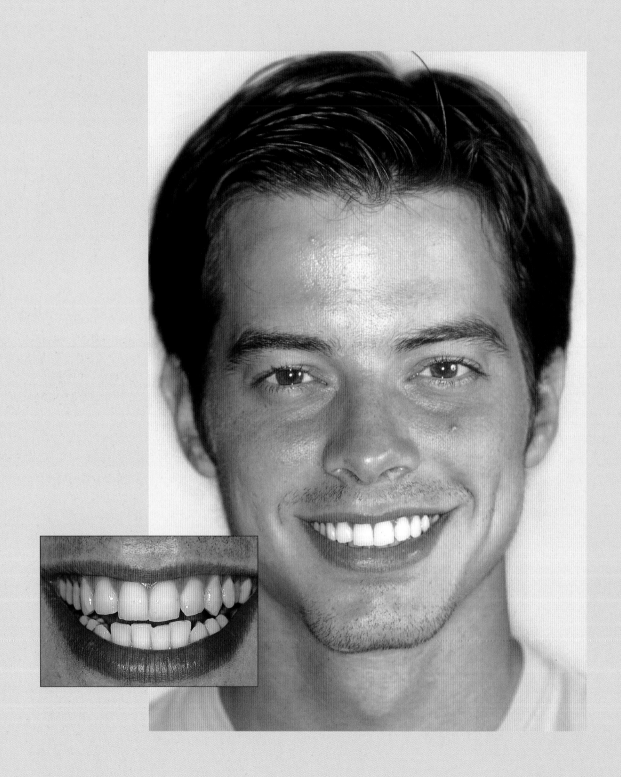

No two humans are alike in appearance and character and therefore each restoration should be designed according to a particular individual's needs and characteristics. This personalization is especially important in the restoration of the anterior teeth. With the increasing patient interest in esthetic dentistry, a need for a more thorough understanding of the esthetic principles has become apparent. The objective of this chapter is to review the "keys and pathways" to achieving a pleasant smile.

The primary elements of a beautiful smile are the teeth and therefore a sound knowledge of individual tooth forms and anatomy is the foundation of any treatment. The teeth are aligned and related to each other and to the surrounding soft tissues that act as their frames. To have a better feeling of what a beautifully designed smile is, the inner and outer edges of the individual outlines must be examined. Artists draw within a measured frame that is further defined with inner outlines and imaginary reference points, relating the parts to each other and, in turn, to the original frame. Esthetic dentistry is not very different from an artist's eye.[3-5] To achieve the best esthetic results in dentistry, we also should use "frames", "from the inside out": the line angles and axial inclinations that frame a single tooth, the gingival edge that frames the teeth, the lips that frame the teeth and gingiva, and, finally, the face that frames all these components and acts as the master or the original frame in which all the components interact in a natural or optimally restored dentition to present a pleasing and esthetic smile.

Other issues of concern are the objects, such as the teeth and gingiva, that can be termed as "static", and the lips and facial soft tissues that can be termed as dynamic or "mobile". To achieve a pleasant smile, some imaginary vertical or horizontal reference points must be used to relate these parts to each other in addition to certain phonetic references. These reference points may be the mid-line, the facial mid-line, the lip line, the commissural line, or the interpupillary line. All these structures exist in certain proportions and relations to one another and should never be isolated, but instead perceived as a whole in their total composition, and unique for each individual.

The pleasant smile is perceived as harmonious only when the various lines, proportions, and structures are in visual balance with each other. The already existing status of the smile can be improved by changing these proportions, creating illusions, and minimizing the negative visual tension produced by improperly aligned teeth, gingiva, and the lips. To have a more thorough understanding of every element and the related factors, attention to detail must be exercised in all visual aspects of the dentition, analyzing each one separately and carefully.[6,7]

Mid-line

The facial mid-line is located in the center of the face, perpendicular to the interpupillary line.[8-11] It has been defined as a vertical line, drawn through the forehead, nose columella, dental midline, and chin.[5] It has also been referred to as the imaginary line that runs vertically from the nasion, subnasal point, interincisal point and the pogonion.[13] Heartwell defines the dental mid-line as an imaginary vertical line that does not necessarily coincide with the facial mid-line. The lingual papilla or the labial fraenum may be used as a placement landmark.[14] Ideally, the papilla between the maxillary central incisors coincides with the mid-line of the face.[15]

Observing the dynamics of a smile is the best way to visualize the dental mid-line. The space between the two maxillary central incisors appears most pleasing when observing the anterior dentition in a smile. Preferably, it should be centered between the left and right sides of the face. However, that does not necessarily mean that the dental mid-line will always coincide with the other features of the face.[16] In research conducted by *Bodden, Miller* and *Jamison,* it was statistically demonstrated that the maxillary mid-line coincided with the mid-line in 70% of cases, using the lip's philtrum as a reference guide. Their research revealed that slight deviations in the central mid-line did not necessarily compromise esthetics.[17] Moreover, it was found that the maxillary and mandibular mid-lines did not coincide

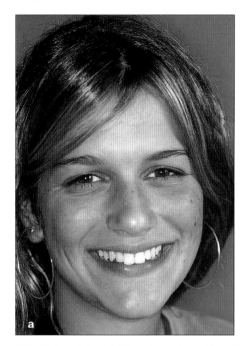
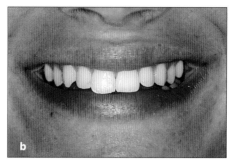
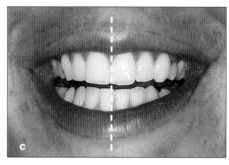
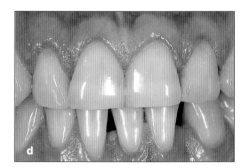

Fig 2-1a-d (a, b) The dental mid-line is placed on the imaginary line, which is actually the facial mid-line in 70% of cases. (c) The mid-line can be slightly deviated to the right or left, when the lips" philtrum is used as a reference. This is true for 30% of the population. Slight deviations do not create visual tension nor do they affect the esthetics negatively. (d) A high percentage of the patients (as much as 75%) have mandibular mid-lines that do not coincide with the maxillary.

in 75% of the cases, demonstrating that the lower mid-line is not suitable as a reference for the maxillary mid-line placement (Fig 2-1). However, as the mouth does not stay in a static position and the mandibular teeth are not that visible, this mismatch does not create an esthetically unpleasant appearance. Actually, this aspect is more important for the dentist because in the cases where the maxillary mid-line is lost (owing to tooth extraction, etc.), the dentist should avoid reliance on the mandibular mid-line in order to assess the maxillary mid-line.

Johnston et al. write: "In white and non-white groups of adults, the dental mid-lines of each group were found to match in less than 30% of the cases. However, as the mandibular teeth are not usually exposed while smiling, the mismatch of mid-lines does not affect the natural esthetic dentition. In esthetics, the mandibular mid-line is not of great importance. The visualization of the middle point often becomes difficult, owing to the narrowness and uniform size of the mandibular incisors."[18]

The parameters of symmetry and balance of the facial and dental mid-lines are the vectors for our esthetic appraisal. Not all patients have symmetric faces; they may even have chins or noses that are not centered, making it impossible to use them as landmarks for the facial mid-line. The left and right sides of the face, with all their variations, are not precise guides for a geometrical division.[19] The natural appearance of the face as a whole does not influence our visual perception of the dental mid-line, even if the philtrum is off-center. However, if there is an overlap of the maxillary central incisors, or spacing owing to diastemas, they may affect the facial median line in relation to the mid-line. The dental mid-line should be right in line with the precise mid-line of the smile, which is in the center and coinciding with the symmetry of the dental composition.

Owing to the focus of attention that is naturally given to the face, any deviations in the maxillary dental mid-line in relation to the facial mid-line, as in the case of slanting, have the potential of creating a negative overall effect on the smile. The appearance of order and organization is made possible with a vertical dental mid-line.[20] The mid-line between the facial mid-line and maxillary central incisors should coincide whenever pos-

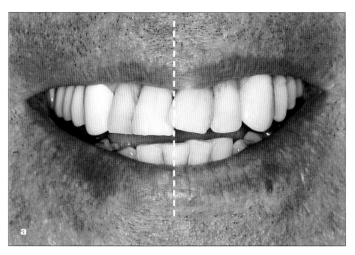 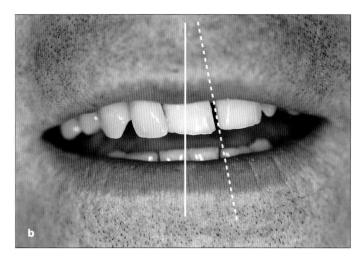

Fig 2-2a, b (a) A slanted mid-line, or a dental mid-line that is placed obliquely in relation to the facial mid-line, will always distort the symmetry, even when placed in exactly the correct position. (b) It looks even more unpleasant when it is slanted and shifted to the side at the same time.

sible.[21,22] In cases where the dental and facial mid-lines do not match, or are far apart, the dental mid-line should be kept perpendicular to the pupillary or horizontal lines, to prevent the illusion of asymmetry owing to an excessive right or left shift of the dental mid-line. Once it is straight, the composition will appear symmetrical or at least pleasing. Even if the mid-line is placed in the precisely correct position, and if it should happen to be oblique in relation to the facial mid-line, it will disturb the symmetry (Fig 2-2).[20] In any restored dentition, slanting is an unacceptable major flaw.[18] Therefore, the mid-line, which is the center of attraction, should be as perpendicular as possible to avoid any distortion.

Incisal Length

The incisal edge of the maxillary central incisor is the most important determinant in the creation of a smile. Once it is set, it serves to determine the proper tooth proportion and gingival level; therefore, setting the place of the incisal edge is especially important. Elongation of the incisal edge is often indicated to correct incisal wear, inadequate tooth display, or a displeasing tooth or crown proportion. To correct excessive tooth display, or

a displeasing tooth or crown proportion, shortening the incisal edge may sometimes be required to compensate for unesthetic elongation created by periodontal recession. The position of the incisal edge acts as the parameter upon which the rest of the treatment is built. Several reference teeth serve as the reference point for the correct incisal edge position for the remaining teeth.

The self-image of the patient and a desire for a dynamic and youthful appearance will determine just how prominent or noticeable a smile is desired.[23] The age and gender of the patient, along with the length and curvature of the upper lip, will determine the length of the incisal edge.[24] Average anatomic crown length values for the maxillary central incisor range from 10.4 to 11.2 mm.[25] For young patients who do not have fully erupted teeth, a semi-permanent restoration, such as a composite application, is preferable .

Once the eruption is complete, a definitive restoration can be performed to establish the tooth length. A central incisor that is not visible when the lips are at rest, but can be seen when smiling, tends to render an older appearance to the dentition. Similarly, a young smile can be achieved when the upper front teeth are lengthened. Therefore, one of the most important factors in dental esthetics is the visibility of the teeth when the mandible and lips are at rest. It is not only the form and position of the teeth, but the

Incisal edges showing through the lips at rest position

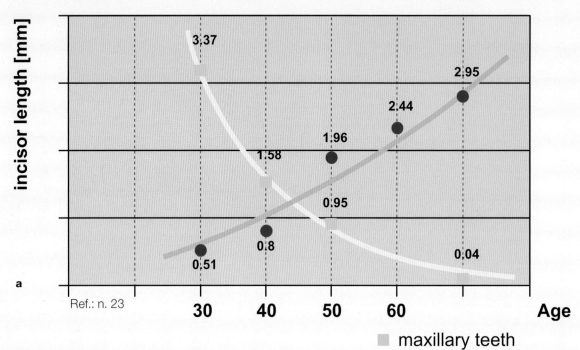

Ref.: n. 23

■ maxillary teeth

● mandibular teeth display

1. lip line 30 years (3.45 mm)
2. lip line 40 years (1.60 mm)
3. lip line 50 years (0.95 mm)
4. lip line 60 years (0.50 mm)
5. lip line 70 years (0.20 mm)

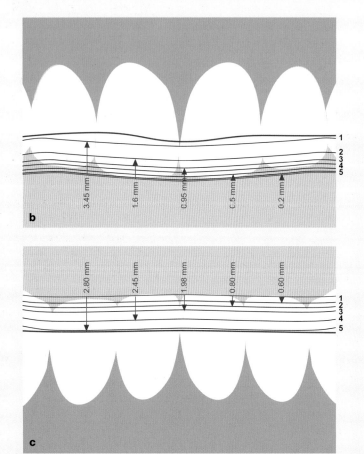

1. lip line 30 years (0.60 mm)
2. lip line 40 years (0.80 mm)
3. lip line 50 years (1.98 mm)
4. lip line 60 years (2.45 mm)
5. lip line 70 years (2.80 mm)

Fig 2-3a-c (a) The diagram showing the inverse proportion of tooth display between the maxillary and mandibular incisors, related to age.[45,116] (b) As people age, less incisal length is displayed. The reduced display is owing to the sagging of the upper lip, and the reduction is further increased by the incisal tooth wear. (c) In the mandibular arch, even though some incisal wear does exist, the lower tooth display increases as the muscle tone of the lower lip decreases and sags down owing to gravity.[89]

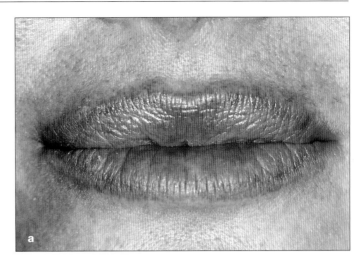

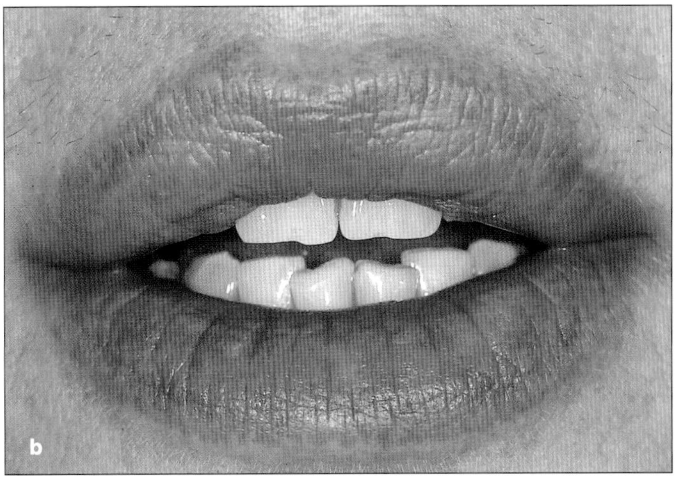

Fig 2-4a, b (a) While seated in an upright position, the patient is asked to repeat the "M" sound several times. In so doing, the lips relax, and the dentist can readily observe the incisal edge position of the lips at rest. When the "M" sound is pronounced, the lips come together. (b) After the "M" sound, the lips part in the rest position.

muscle tone and skeletal build-up that are important as well.[29]

It may happen occasionally that the incisal edge has been compromised, or that it is necessary partially to rebuild erupted central incisors. The difficulty is in determining the size of the tooth, as there is no defined landmark from which to proceed. Without this tooth of reference, the dentist must use the upper and lower lips, and the exposed portion of the teeth as the reference points.

When the mouth is slightly open, approximately 3.5 mm of the incisal portion of the maxillary teeth is visible in a 20-year-old person, while the mandibular teeth are barely visible. As age increases, the muscles become lax and slowly diminish the display of the maxillary incisors, while the visibility of mandibular incisors increases. The dentofacial plane that is exhibited in youth is permanently changed, and although it may vary from individual to individual, the degrading process

is unfortunately irreversible. This laxness first appears at approximately the age of 30 to 40 years and continues to increase with each passing year.

A study has shown that there may be many variables in the lip length and, therefore, in the visible length of the incisal teeth, depending on gender, racial factors and age. In the young female, the exposure of the maxillary central incisors can be as much as 3.40 mm, with a minimum of 0.5 mm for mandibular incisor exposure. Between the ages of 30 and 40 years, mandibular incisor exposure increases while the maxillary tooth length exposure decreases (Fig 2-3).[45]

Tooth exposure is determined by muscle position, yet the restorative dentist often disregards it. Phonetic values, and the experience of the clinician, were often the determining factors for the prosthodontist when deciding the relationship between the lips and the incisal edges. It was assumed that these factors could determine the

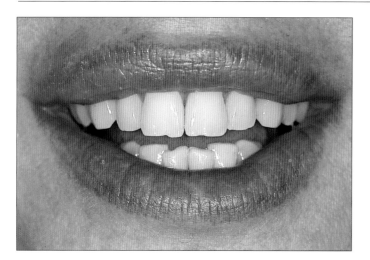

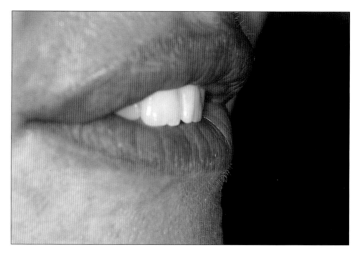

Fig 2-5 The position of the incisal edges during the "E" sound is another important parameter. Under normal circumstances, a pleasing incisal edge position is centered between the upper and lower lips when the patient is asked to say "Eeeeee".

Fig 2-6 "F" and "V" sounds are used to locate the length of the incisors and the buccal lingual position of the incisal edges. While reducing these sounds, the incisal edge should be gently contracting the vermillion border of the lower lip. The length of the incisal edges can be observed from the facial aspect and from the profile the buccal lingual placement of the incisors can be evaluated.

correct position of the maxillary anterior incisors in the vertical plane.

The lips and teeth have a different position and relation for each sound that is made. The evaluation of the relationship between both dental arches and the lips will be the instrumental approach in determining this point of reference. The clinician is not basing the decision solely on esthetic factors, but also on the relation of the incisal edge to the anterior guidance and phonetics. This is especially true in determining the length of the maxillary incisors, which play an important role in the anterior guidance and phonetics. While seated in an upright position, the patient is asked to produce the "M" sound several times. When the lips relax, the dentist can observe the incisal edge position of the lips at rest. After pronunciation ceases, the lips return to the relaxed rest position for evaluation. Repetition of this sound will enable the patient to relax between producing each sound, allowing the dentist to evaluate the amount of incisal tooth displayed in the rest position (Fig 2-4).[25]

The amount of incisal tooth display may vary from individual to individual. The length of the display depends on the length of the upper lip and the age of the patient.[45] The "E" sound is another important parameter when evaluating the length of the teeth and the incisal line. The maxillary teeth should be displayed halfway between the upper and lower lip lines while forming this sound (Fig 2-5). The patient is asked to say "Eeeeee" for a few seconds so that the dentist can observe the position of the maxillary incisors.

The length and the lingual tilt of the incisal third of the maxillary central incisors are used to determine the fricative "F" and "V" sounds. To produce these sounds, the maxillary incisors must press against a slightly retracted lower lip partially to block the remaining air stream. The wet-dry line of the vermilion border of the lower lip is the location of the incisal edge for the maxillary incisors in most individuals. The correct labiolingual position and the length of the anterior teeth should enable the patient to produce the "F" sound by placing the incisal edges against the inner edge of the vermilion border of the lower lip (Fig 2-6).[30–33] During this evaluation, the buccolingual placement of the upper maxillary incisors is also evaluated. The "F" and "V" sounds should also be used to determine the superior/inferior length of the incisal edge.[33]

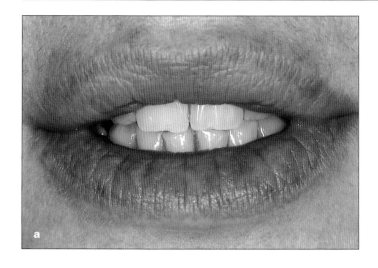

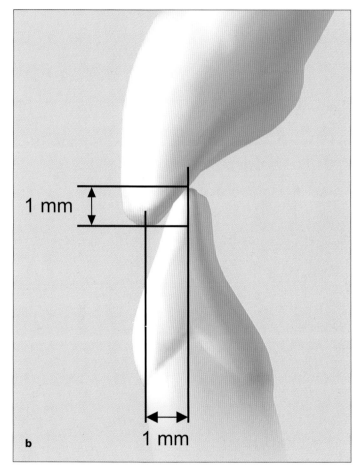

In cases where porcelain is used in the form of onlay veneers for premolars and molars and for the purpose of correcting the vertical height of dimension, the pronunciation of the "S" sound is of crucial importance. The vertical dimension of speech is determined by the "S" sound formation, when all teeth should be in light contact.[34] During the pronunciation of the "S" sound, the incisal edges of the mandibular incisors establish occlusal contact with the maxillary incisors owing to their position, which is 1 mm behind and 1 mm below the edges of the maxillary teeth (Fig 2-7).[32]

While the maxillary teeth can be placed according to these parameters, minor differences in the height of the central and lateral incisors add vitality and dynamics to the total frame. The lateral incisors should be approximately 1 mm above the gently curved horizontal line that is shared by the incisal edges of the maxillary central incisors and the cusp tips of the canines. The positioning of the incisal edge is open to subjectivity, and the input of the patient is vital for the final decision.

Composite resin models or mock-ups of the desired length, computer imaging, diagnostic waxing, provisional restorations, and trial porcelain laminate veneer tooth set-ups should be used as aids and guides for communication with the patient (Fig 2-8). Assessment of the desired crown length and a preview of the proper incisal edge are some of the factors aiding in the final decision. To achieve attractive maxillary central incisor proportions, the gingival position must be adequate; and if it is not, it can be surgically or orthodontically altered (see Chapters 11 and 12).[24]

Fig 2-7a, b (a) The "S" sound is used to determine the vertical height of dimension. (This is used for fabrication of complete dentures while checking the vertical height.) For the veneers, this parameter is used to check the relation of the maxillary and mandibular teeth. (b) The mandibular incisals should be in gentle touch with the palatal surfaces of the mandibular incisors, being 1 mm behind and 1 mm below.

Zenith Points

The so-called zenith points are the most apical points of the clinical crowns; which are the height of contour. Their positions are dictated by the root-form anatomy, cementoenamel junction (CEJ), and the osseous crest, where the gingiva is scalloped the most. The zenith points are generally located just distal to a line drawn vertically through the middle of each anterior tooth. The lateral

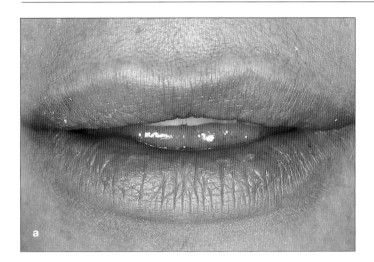 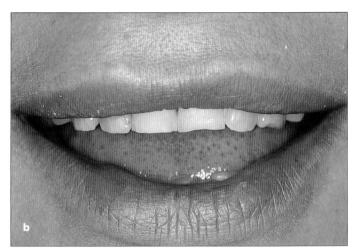

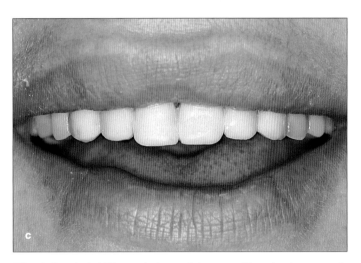 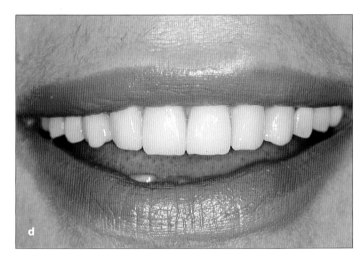

Fig 2-8a-d (a) The relation of the maxillary incisors to the upper lip. The teeth are short and can barely be seen when the lips are in rest position. (b) A rough composite model ("mock-up") is built, following the references explained above. It is a good communicative and educational tool. (c) The provisionals prior to polishing. After the preparation, the patient is dismissed. The provisional restorations are a helpful in-patient evaluation of the eventual restoration for functional and esthetic purposes. If the patient is pleased with the evaluation, the definitive porcelain laminate veneers can be fabricated. (d) The definitive restoration (porcelain laminate veneers), a beautiful and youthful smile. The incisal edge position is centered exactly where it should be, allowing the functional moves and apprising. Asking the patient to repeat the "M", "E", "F", and "S" sounds can identify this exact position.

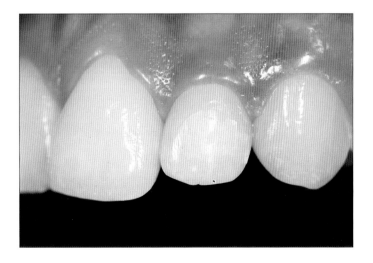

Fig 2-9 The zenith points are the most apical points of the clinical crowns. They are usually placed distally, when viewed from the facial aspect. Only the lateral incisors do not abide by this rule; in the laterals, they are placed centrally.

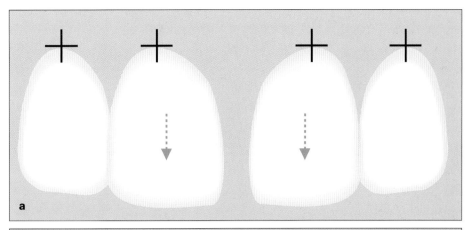

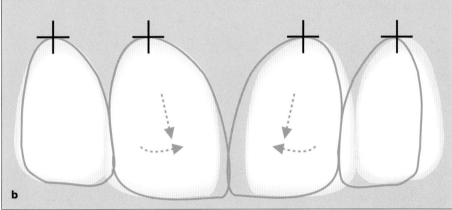

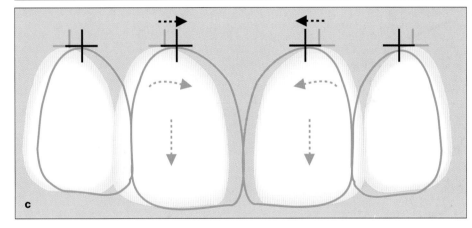

Fig 2-10a-c When closing diastemas, the zenith points should be repositioned to avoid a mesially tilted appearance. (a) Preoperative view of the zenith points in their originally correct position—slightly distal to the central incisors and in the middle of the laterals. (b) When the diastema is closed, the distal portions of the central and lateral incisors are cut down and porcelain is added to the mesial aspects of the incisors for a proportional restoration (see Chapter 9). (c) Together with the veneers, the zenith points should be moved mesially to where they should be when the diastema is closed. This can be achieved with minor gingival alteration at the time of, or prior to, the tooth preparation. The illustration shows the mesially shifted zenith points with the new veneers.

incisors are one exception to that rule, as their zenith points are placed more centrally or on the mid-line of the tooth margin (Fig 2-9).[35–37] The positions of the zenith points gain importance when closing diastemas or changing the distal or mesial tilted position of the teeth. In the case of diastema closure, if the zenith points are not moved mesially from their originally existing positions, the finished porcelain laminate veneers may give the perception of being mesially tilted. In addition, the extreme distal positions of the gingival zeniths will result in an exaggerated triangular

form.[38] To prevent these occurences and to create an illusion of bodily shifted central incisors towards the mid-line, the zenith points should also be moved mesially (Figs 2-10 and 2-11).

These are examples of moving the zenith points horizontally. In the case where the tooth needs to be shown longer or more tapered at the gingival 1/3rd, the zenith points can be moved apically (Fig 2-12). Such an apical movement obtains a triangular shape. An equilateral triangle will always appear longer in height than in width and this also proves that a tapered tooth

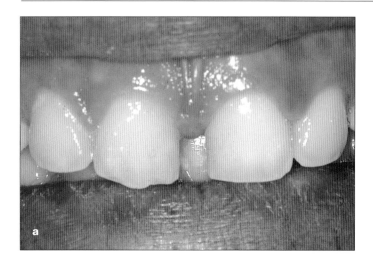
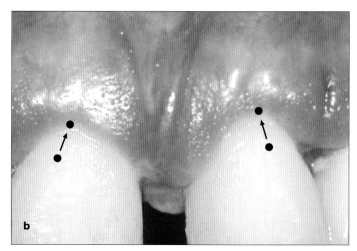
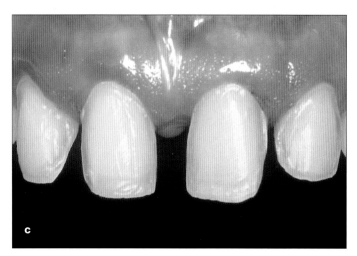
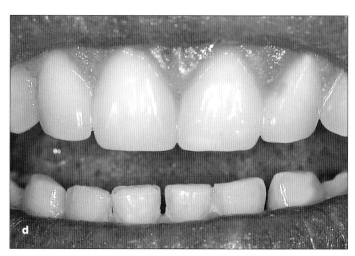

Fig 2-11a-d (a) Preoperative view of a diastema case, where the zenith points are located at their original positions. (b) The "gummy smile" is corrected by placing the gingival tissues apically. The positions of the zenith points are altered horizontally forwards, in the mesial direction. (c) The distal portions of the central and lateral incisors and the canines, by adding porcelain to the material used. Combined with a mesial shift of the zenith points, a pleasing natural effect is created. (d) Postoperative view of the horizontal shift of the zenith points. Even though large gaps have been closed with porcelain veneers, the final outcome is natural.

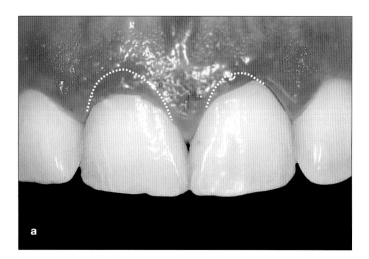
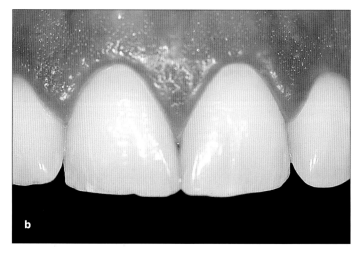

Fig 2-12a, b (a) Short teeth can be made to appear longer by carrying the zenith points further apically. (b) This rounded shape of the gingival portion is changed into a more triangular shape. The rounded gingival silhouette of the incisals is broken and an illusion of longer teeth is created.

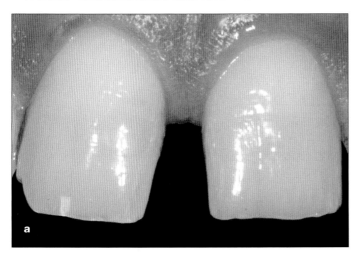 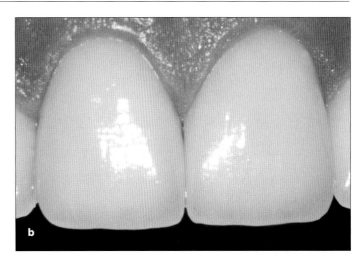

Fig 2-13a, b (a) When a diastema is present, the papilla has a blunt shape. (b) If properly treated, it can regain its natural crisp triangular form. View of a blunt, horizontally aligned appearance of the papilla is altered with custom-designed porcelain laminate veneers.

design will make the tooth seem longer than it is. This procedure should therefore be used with shorter teeth, where elongation towards the apical direction is required. Consequently, zenith points can enhance the perception of the tooth axis as well as the length and the gingival shapes, which can be achieved by horizontal or vertical alterations.

Gingival Health and Interdental Embrasures

The gingiva is normally pale in color and extends to the cementoenamel junction, forming a static frame for the teeth.[38] Healthy interdental papillae should be thin and terminate on the tooth in a knife-edged contour. The interdental papillae should form a pyramid-shaped confluence of the gingiva margin of the adjacent teeth (Fig 2-13).[24] The level of healthy gingiva is dictated by the position of the alveolar bone beneath it.[39-42] Healthy gingiva lies 3 mm away from the intact bone on the facial aspect and the tip of the stable papilla maintains a distance of 5 mm from the intercrestal bone (see Chapter 6).

The notions of "beautiful" or "ugly" are subjective ones. However, in the case of the health of the tissue, they are objective. The gingiva must always be healthy and sound (Fig 2-14). The initiation of prosthodontic treatment should be postponed until the health of the gingival tissue has been sufficiently reinstated. The postponement will allow the clinician to assess the inflammation and devise treatment and it will also allow the clinician to examine the position of the gingiva when the hypertrophic soft tissue shrinks. Once in a healthy state, the tissue must be scalloped to follow the contours of the underlying bone. The papilla should be formed to fill the interdental embrasures in a crisp triangular shape, and the design of porcelain laminate veneers should complete the closure. The esthetic harmony can be reinstated only with a healthy dentogingival complex (see Chapter 12).[44]

In some patients, healthy gingiva may show irregularities or asymmetries whereas in other cases gingival asymmetry can be the result of hypertrophic inflammation that will disappear after a routine periodontal treatment or prophylaxis. As the gingiva acts as a frame for the teeth, such irregularities will affect the final esthetic result, especially in patients with high and medium lip lines.

Trauma at an early age may impede normal tooth eruption. It may cause altered passive

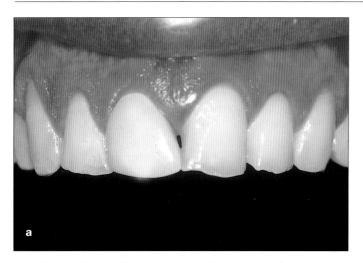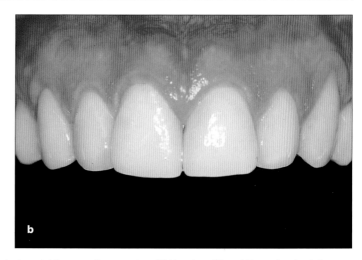

Fig 2-14a, b (a) The initiation of the prosthodontic treatment should be postponed until the health of the gingival tissue has been reinstated. The postponement will allow the clinician to assess the inflammation and devise treatment; it will also allow the clinician to see the position of the gingiva when the hypertrophic soft tissue shrinks. (b) Once the tissue has returned to its healthy state, the gingival scallops, the position of the papilla, the zenith points, and gingival asymmetrics are evaluated and porcelain laminate veneers are applied (11 years post-operative view).

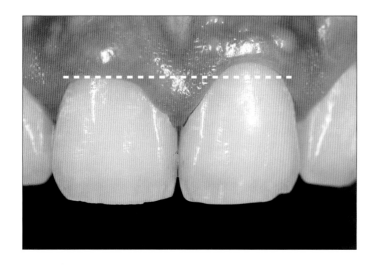

Fig 2-15 The tooth may migrate incisally. If the cause is wear the tooth may erupt towards the area of wear, bringing the gingival tissue down incisally. This makes the tooth appear shorter and creates a gingival asymmetry.

eruption and result in abnormal habits and wear owing to bruxism. It is important for the dentist to obtain a thorough dental history that will help him/her to discover the factors that may have caused the gingival asymmetries (Fig 2-15). For these particular cases, the gingival levels should be altered with special care (see Chapter 12). There may also be some introgenic factors that cause the scalloped formation of the gingiva to disappear.[44] In order for the mind to register a horizontal line, a simple movement of the eye is required, whereas the registration of an undulating line demands an up and down ocular movement, which may not leave time for the apprecia-

tion of its characteristics, required to generate an esthetic appeal.[44] Such an unscalloped horizontal gingival architecture should be altered, in order to achieve an undulating appearance, by moving the zenith points apically.

Gingival Levels and Harmony

The gingival line runs parallel to the bipupillary line, which should be parallel to the canine line with a tangent through the incisal edges of both

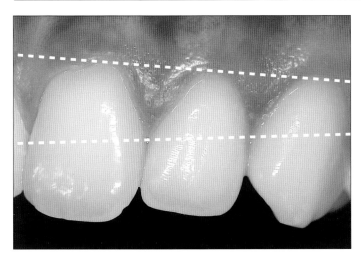

Fig 2-16 The tips of the papilla gradually follow a pattern in the apical direction, when proceeding from the anterior towards the posterior dentition, thus the volume of the gingival embrasures is getting smaller.

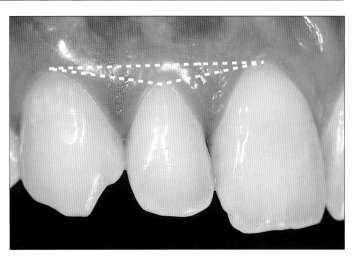

Fig 2-17 Nicely scalloped gingival contours. The pleasing relationship of the gingival levels (previously determined by the zenith points) should create a shallow reverse triangle (*Magne P*). The apex of the triangle (zenith point of the lateral incisor) is 0.5 to 1 mm, positioned incisally.

canines. The appropriate position and curvature of the incisal edges in conjunction with the lower lip line, and the determined correct length of the maxillary teeth, will determine the correct vertical position of the gingival line.[9,45]

The most incisally positioned portion of the gingiva is the tip of the papilla between the maxillary central incisors, which gradually assumes a more cervical position to the canine, premolar, and molar (Fig 2-16).[46] The width and height of the gingival arcade, which is to be the triangle between the zenith points and the tip of the papilla, depend upon the corresponding gingival morphotype, forming a high or low scalloped gingiva.[47]

When the zenith points of the maxillary incisors and the canines of a natural smile are followed, it is readily observed that they are not aligned on an imaginary straight line. Usually, the zenith points of the lateral incisors are 0.5 to 1 mm below those of the central incisors and canines, while the zenith points of the canines and central incisors remain on the same horizontally drawn imaginary line. This relationship of the zenith points actually forms a type of an imaginary triangle (Fig 2-17).

The angles or the depth of this triangle do not follow any rules. Any kind of triangle in which the zenith of the lateral incisors stays below will usually reflect a pleasant relationship. If the teeth

are aligned on a straight line, it is an indication of high lateral zenith point placement and in some cases this display is a reversed or inverted triangle, where the gingival level of the lateral incisor is placed even more apically than the central incisor and the canines, creating an unesthetic configuration. This will affect the gingival harmony, but also result in short lateral incisors, with relatively correct proportions. If the laterals are lengthened without altering the gingival level, long laterals with the correct incisal edge position but unpleasant proportions will appear (Fig 2-18). There may be irregularities when the gingival level of the canine or central incisor is placed above or below these indications.

As observed posteriorly, gingival gradation can occur. Gingival gradation is a gradual decrease in height of the gingival outline from the canine back to the second molar.[48] This event is displayed in an architectural gradation in perspective. Owing to the palatal inclination of the premolars, the gingival tissue may be perceived as longer than it actually is.

Another condition that creates unpleasant esthetics is the appearance of a "gummy smile". It is important to determine its etiology as it may be caused by any variety of problems. It may be associated with the overgrowth of the maxilla (Fig 2-19) or it may also be owing to a high lip line

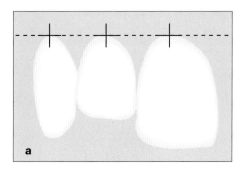

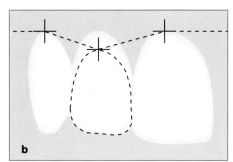

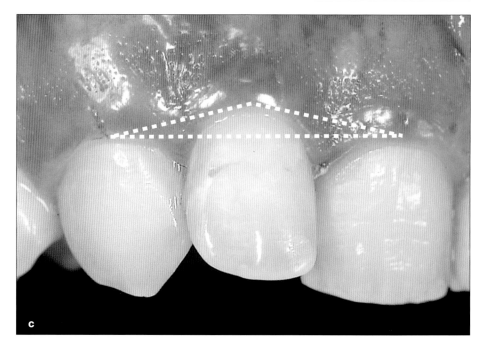

Fig 2-18a-c (a) When the zenith points are level, the gingival harmony is distorted. If the lateral incisors have not erupted properly, the length of the lateral incisors is shorter. (b) An attempt to correct the length of the lateral incisor without changing the position of its zenith point incisally will result in a longer tooth and a loss of proportion. (c) When the apex of the lateral incisor is placed more apically, the gingival relationship is totally distorted. This may happen owing to a facially positioned lateral incisor that forces the gingival level apically.

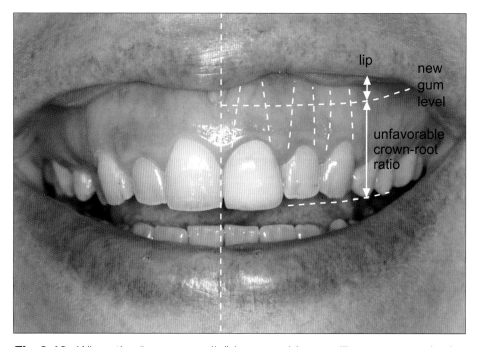

Fig 2-19 When the "gummy smile" is caused by maxillary overgrowth, the choice of the treatment is maxillofacial surgery. The gingival display exceeds 10 mm; any effort to treat this case merely by periodontal means will result in nonproportional root-crown ratios.

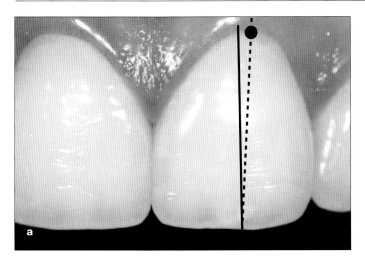 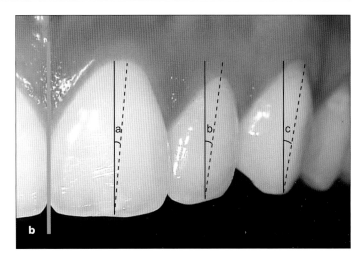

Fig 2-20a, b (a) The tooth axis of the central incisors may be positioned slightly distally towards the apex when compared to the vertical midline. (b) In comparison to central incisors, the laterals exhibit a more distal inclination towards the apex. The lateral incisors are asymmetric in a pleasing smile and can display different axial inclinations. The angle, formed between the imaginary axis of the central lateral aspect, may be different on both sides. Note that angles a < b < c.

or altered passive eruption, which can be the primary cause for the appearance of short clinical crowns and excessive gingival display. Altered passive eruption is the condition that exists during tooth eruption, in which the gingival margin fails to recede to the cervicoenamel junction. This condition occurs in approximately 12% of the population.[49-53] A "gummy smile" or excessive gingival display can be corrected by orthognathic surgery, orthodontics, or periodontal osseous surgery.[61,63,64]

To alter unesthetic gingival disharmony, the dental specialty of esthetic periodontics has developed esthetic approaches since the early 1980s which include the removal of excessive gingiva, bone and new root coverage procedures (see chapter 12).[40,54-57] Techniques such as ridge augmentation have been included,[42,58-60] as well as site development for esthetic dental implants, and various types of gingival alterations.[25,61] The development of osseous grafting for repair of isolated esthetic deformities continues. These procedures are of critical importance to the success of creating a beautiful smile. Restorative dentists must understand the treatment options and refer patients to their periodontal team for consultation.[62]

Consequently, mucogingival surgery has been redefined as "periodontal plastic surgery" to correct or eliminate anatomic, developmental, or traumatic deformities of gingiva or alveolar mucosa.[61] As previously mentioned, the only true alteration of the gingival levels is dictated by the actual incisal positions of the maxillary anterior teeth.[65]

Tooth Axis

In an esthetic smile, the direction of the anterior teeth and the long axis follow a progression as the teeth are viewed from the mid-line towards the posterior area, creating a harmonious smile framed by the lower lip when the maxillary anterior teeth tip medially.[9] The axis of the central incisors is usually slightly tilted distally towards the apex of the tooth when compared to the mid-line, perpendicular to the interpupillary line (Fig 2-20). The most pleasing position of the central incisors labiolingually exists when the labial surface of the incisors is positioned vertically or with a slight labial axial inclination. Variations of this position will occur in individuals with different skeletal types and facial profiles.

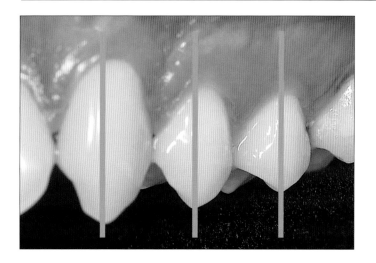

Fig 2-21 Canines and premolars follow a vertical tooth axis when viewed from the lateral aspect. However, when they are observed from the facial aspect, owing to their lingual inclinations towards the incisal edges, they impart the appearance of a distally tilted tooth towards the apex. The position of the canine dictates the front–back progression of the smile.

When the lateral incisors are considered, it is observed that the lateral incisors are inclined somewhat more distally towards the apical than the central aspect. Similarly, in most of the pleasing natural smiles, the mesiodistal axial inclination as well as the anteroposterior position of the lateral incisors is placed asymmetrically.

The canine tends to be even more distally inclined when viewed from the facial aspect. However, when viewed from the side, it has a long axis in a vertically or slightly distalled position in the dental arch (Fig 2-21). The best way to analyze tooth axis position of the canine is to relate it to certain facial formations. In the majority of cases, it follows a parallel line drawn from the corner of the mouth to the corner of the eye when smiling and, in turn, runs parallel to the vertical side of the vestibular frame.[44]

Interdental Contact Areas (ICA) and Points (ICP)

The broad zone in which two adjacent teeth appear to touch is called the interdental contact area (ICA). Observation suggests that the 50-40-30 rule, indicating the relationship between the anterior teeth, applies to 50% of the length of the maxillary central incisors and is defined as the ideal connector zone.[66] This means that 40% of the length of the central incisor is the ideal con-

nector zone between a maxillary lateral and central incisors. When viewed from the lateral aspect, the prime connector zone between a maxillary canine and a lateral incisor is about 30% of the length of the central incisor (Fig 2-22a).[66]

In cases where the teeth are too long, it may be best to increase the vertical contact area and thereby keep the embrasures (both gingival and incisal) as narrow as possible.[67] This will enhance the perception of a relatively wider and, therefore, a relatively shorter incisor. The contact area can also be lengthened apically to close the interdental embrasure, if enough papilla cannot be obtained (Fig 2-23).[67]

The most incisal aspect of the contact area is called the contact point. After this point, the two adjacent teeth diverge, and the medial-distal contacts turn to incisal edges. When we consider the appropriate shape of the incisal teeth and their esthetically correct alignment, it is obvious that the interdental contact points move apically as they proceed towards the posterior area (Fig 2-22b). The contact point of the two central incisors is located in the most incisal area, owing to the almost right-angled relation of their incisal and mesial line angles. Because of the relatively rounded corners of the distoincisal aspect of the central incisor and the mesioincisal aspect of the lateral incisor, this contact point is placed more apically between the two. This contact point may display different heights, owing to their natural asymmetric position and form of the lateral incisors.

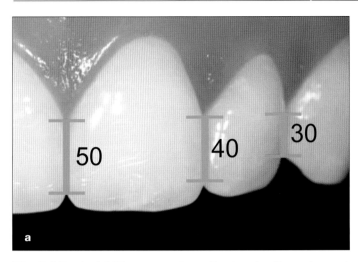
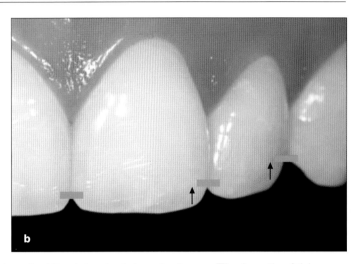

Fig 2-22a, b (a) The zone where the two teeth are in contact is called the interdental contact area. The length of this area is not the same between the incisors. The longest contact area is between the central incisors; the shortest contact is between the lateral incisor and the canine, still following a pleasing pattern. (b) The points where the interdental contact areas end, and the incisal and distal surfaces of the teeth begin to converge at the incisal edges, are called the interdental contact points. They move apically as the teeth proceed from the central incisors to the posterior area.

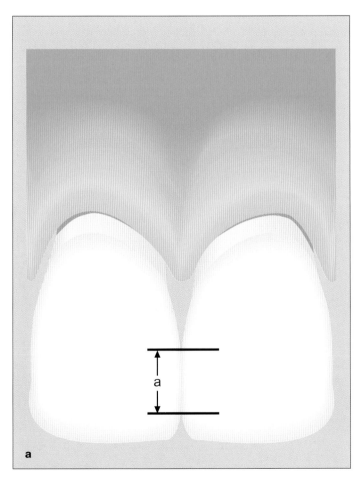
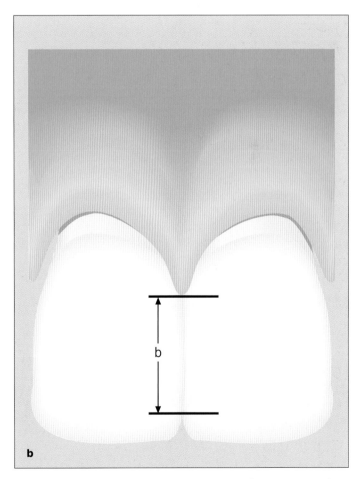

Fig 2-23a, b (a) At times, owing to the lack of adequate bone support, the new papilla cannot be generated to close the unesthetic space that appears between the teeth. (b) In such cases, the interdental contact can be moved apically to close the gap.

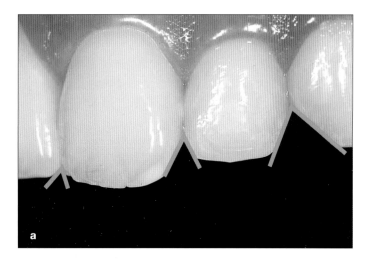

Fig 2-24a-c (a) The interdental embrasure is the smallest and sharpest in the central incisors. Continuing the observation posteriorly, the embrasures become larger and wider. Owing to the asymmetric positions of the lateral incisors, the embrasures may differ between the central and lateral incisors and the canines. (b) The size of the embrasures increases between the premolars. An angle of 90 degrees can be seen in young, unworn dentitions. (c) The incisal edge position of the lateral is placed 0.5 to 1 mm apically compared to central and canine in young dentitions.

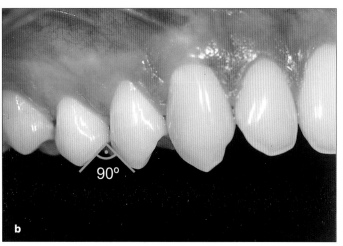

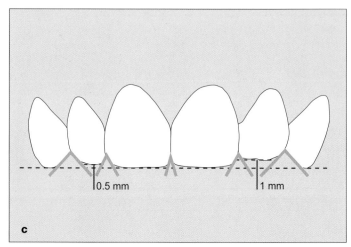

The contact points of the more-rounded corner of the distoincisal portion of the lateral incisor and the almost triangular shape of the mesioincisal corner of the canine should be placed even more apically. The same routine can be applied towards the premolars.

Incisal Embrasures

When the dental arches separate, as in speaking or in a smile, a dark area can be seen in the anterior region between the incisal edges of the maxillary and mandibular teeth. This negative space creates a contrast with the teeth that enhances the appearance of the incisal embrasures.[68] An attractive smile is defined by the pattern of silhouetting that is created by the contrast of the darker background of the oral interior, along with the edges and separations between the maxillary and anterior teeth. As the dentition progresses away from the mid-line, the size and volume of the incisal embrasures increase.

The incisal embrasures between the central incisors are the smallest in area and the sharpest in angle (Fig 2-24). Owing to the symmetric nature of the central incisors, this forms a triangle with the narrowest angle on the top. The incisal embrasures between the central and lateral incisors are larger than the incisal embrasures between the centrals, with a relatively wide angle. A pleasing smile can be achieved with relatively symmetric central and asymmetric lateral incisors. This also applies to the nature and shape of the incisal embrasures between the central and lateral incisors. These triangles should not always be symmetrical on each side, but should vary in shape (Fig 2-24c).

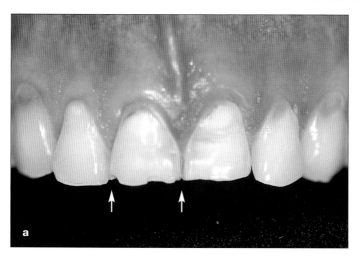
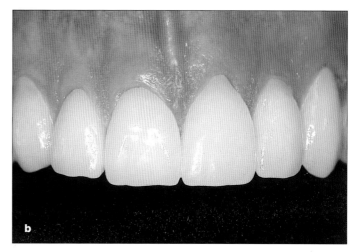

Fig 2-26a, b (a) In the aged or worn dentition, caused by the incisor loss of length, the incisal embrasures become smaller or may even disappear. (b) To create a youthful smile, these teeth have to be lengthened and the embrasures re-created.

The largest of the incisal embrasures exists between the lateral incisor and the canine. The triangle here exhibits different characteristics related to the gender of the patient. The lateral incisors of females tend to have a more rounded incisodistal corner than those of males, creating a wider canine embrasure space in women than in men. The teeth become larger in the posterior region, and the angle that forms the contact point reaches almost 90 degrees between the canine and the premolars. These contact points and incisal embrasures are important factors in determining a youthful smile. When teeth abrade from the incisal aspect by wear and age, the contact points slowly disappear, beginning from the central incisors and then the lateral, finally resulting in an aged smile (Fig 2-25).

The embrasures may also affect the perception of the length, width, and the incisal edge. A change in the shape of the incisal edge can alter the illusion of reduced or increased width. If the mesioincisal and distoincisal corners are more rounded than they should be, the tooth will be perceived as longer than its original length (Fig 2-26).[67] With the alignment of dental elements, provided with well-marked incisal spaces, an apparent reduction of the anterior segment is promoted, whereas the absence of interdental spaces in the incisal alignment (i.e. worn dentitions) simulates a straight line and results in the apparent enlargement of the anterior segment.[44]

Individual and Collective Tooth Dimensions

Relative tooth dimensions, as opposed to the original tooth form, have an input on the smile. When restoring the dentition, the primary objective is to achieve the most natural state possible, while respecting the patient's esthetic preconceptions. The maxillary central incisors are especially important in determining the size and shape of the anterior dentition and its overall visual effect. Disproportionately shaped teeth, i.e. teeth that are too long, too short, too wide or too narrow in relation to the proportion as a whole, may create facial disharmony.

Dominance

Dominance is the primary requisite for providing unity, and unity is the primary requisite for providing composition.[69] Dominating elements are supported by similarly dominant subsequent elements, bringing vigor to the composition. Consequently, in faces adorned by a beautiful smile, the dominance of the mouth exceeds the dominance of the eyes. In a harmonious anterior dentition, the maxillary central incisors dominate in shape, size and position (Fig 2-27).

A consistent arch form and correct proportion to the facial morphology are essential in the pleasing dentition. The proportion must be in harmony with the strong or weak features of

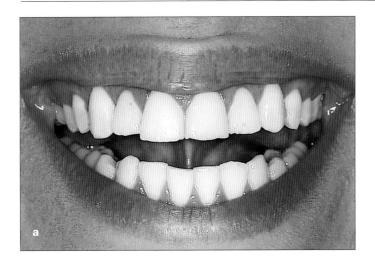

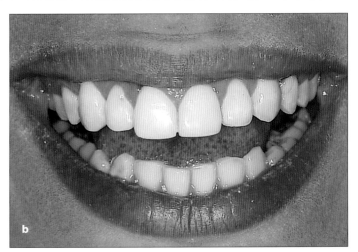

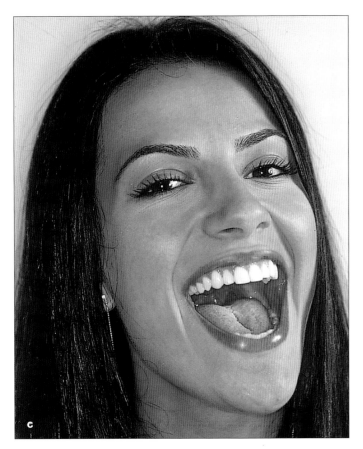

Fig 2-26a-c (a) In cases where there is loss of the vertical length, the embrasures become smaller (when teeth lose their individual proportions, they appear to be smaller and wider). (b) If the teeth cannot be lengthened incisally, owing to functional disturbances or the patient's wishes, the incisal embrasures and the contact points can be carried apically, making the incisal 1/3rd of the tooth narrower and creating the illusion of longer teeth. Also, note the esthetic tooth recontouring on the incisal edges. (c) The whole impact of a beautiful smile on the face.

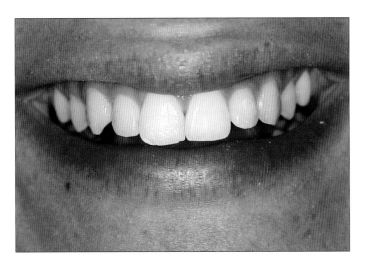

Fig 2-27 Relative tooth dimensions. In a pleasing smile, maxillary central incisors dominate the anterior dentition in shape, size and position.

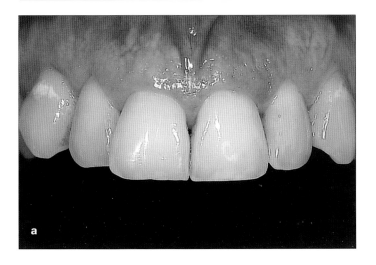

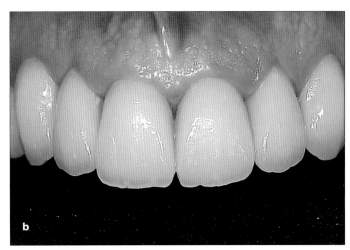

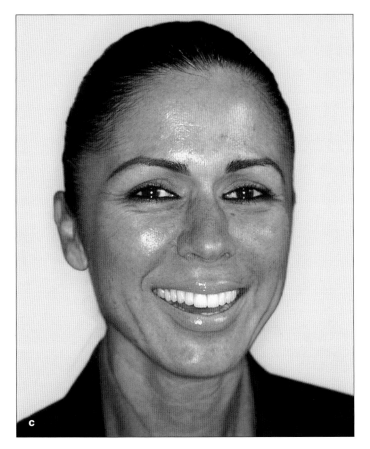

Fig 2-28a-c The canine is placed too bucally, disturbing the flow of an otherwise possibly pleasing smile. (a) In some patients, even though the canine is placed on its correct arch form, it is rotated and displays the distal half, which is not pleasing. (b) Full arch treated with PLVs. The canines usually dictate the total width of the smile, even though only their mesial halves can be seen. The character and width of the buccal corridor are similarly influenced by the appearance of the canines. (c) The positive impact of a balanced smile on the facial appearance.

the individual's facial characteristics.[20,70-74] To achieve an esthetically pleasing smile, the dentist should first decide on the appearance of the central incisors, followed by the laterals and the canines. Whether in a natural or a treated dentition, the appearance of the maxillary central incisors is of critical importance to the pleasing smile. In a pleasing anterior dental composition, the canines are also vitally important teeth as they form the junction between the posterior and anterior arch segments and support the surrounding

facial muscles by means of their position and investing tissues. The size and character of the buccal corridor created when a person smiles are controlled by the size and position of the canines (Fig 2-28).

The proportion of the anterior teeth, displayed in the total width of the smile, is affected by the position of these teeth. Only the mesial half of the canine can be seen from the frontal view of the most pleasing anterior dentitions. The distal half of the tooth is usually in line with the buccal sur-

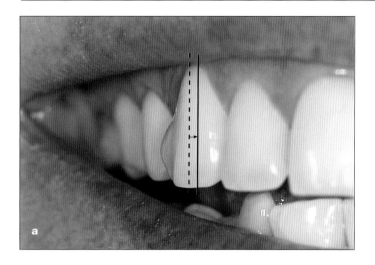

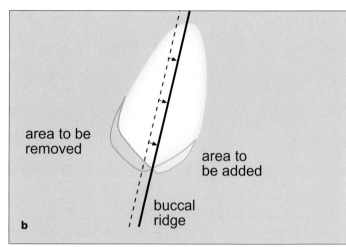

Fig 2-29a, b (a) If the canines look stronger, the buccal ridge has to be moved mesially. This will lessen the excess of the mesial half of the canine. (b) While performing the above function, the incisal edge has to be modified (*Zappala C*). The longer mesial incisal edge has to be shortened horizontally, while the distoincisal edge should be moved towards the apical area.

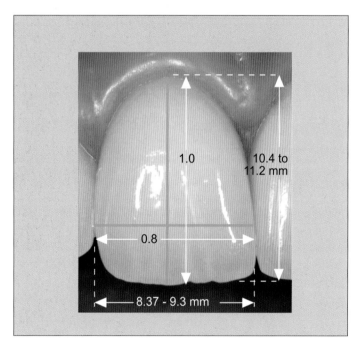

Fig 2-30 The central incisor has a proportion by itself, such as 1 to 0.7, 0.8, giving it a somewhat more rectangular silhouette. In most cases, the width of the central incisors ranges from 8.37 mm to 9.3 mm, whereas the length differs from 10.4 mm to 11.2 mm.

faces of the maxillary posterior dentition, as the canine turns in the arch. The cervical aspect is prominent as opposed to the cusp tip. Sometimes viewed from the facial aspect, even though the tooth axis of the canine follows its natural path, the canine may still look larger (see below, Single Tooth Proportion). The way to overcome this problem is to carve the buccal ridge towards the mesial aspect to eliminate the excess width of the cuspid (Fig 2-29).[67]

Single Tooth Proportion

The central incisor, as a tooth alone, should have a widthheight proportion within itself. The most pleasing width-to-length ratio for maxillary central incisors is approximately 75% to 80% in a pleasant smile. However, it has been reported that it can vary between 66% and 80%.[75] Put another way, a relation of 10:8 in lengthwidth is reasonable for the maxillary central incisors. An 85% width-to-height ratio will give a square appearance, whereas a 65% width-to-height ratio will make the teeth appear longer. There are some individuals who have a pleasant smile despite disproportionate teeth. Therefore, the elements discussed above should not be accepted as an absolute rule.[76] In a number of studies, the mesiodistal diameter of the maxillary central incisor was anywhere from 8.37 to 9.3 mm, [26,28,77,78] and the crown length was in the range of 10.4 to 11.2 mm (Fig 2-30).[26–28]

$$\frac{S}{L} = \frac{L}{S+L} = \frac{2}{1+\sqrt{5}} = 0.618$$

Fig 2-31 The mathematical formula of the golden proportion.

Golden Proportion

The most influential factors in a harmonious anterior dentition are the size, shape and position of the maxillary central incisors. Proportion is the key to a pleasing dentition, and it should be consistent with the patient's facial features, whether they be strong or weak. In order to appear pleasing, the maxillary central incisors must be in proportion to facial morphology and consistent to the arch. The dentist must allow natural variations in form and position, and ensure that the central incisor is in harmony with the facial outline and profile forms.[20,70–73] *Lombardi* suggests that we view the patient as a whole when seeking to achieve harmony. To achieve facial harmony, the overall anterior dental composition must be approached as a whole picture, with the facial features as their frame.[79] It is only through the application of specific laws, whether knowingly or unknowingly, that visually appealing proportional relationships can be achieved.[44] Beauty is connected to numerical values, as in the relationship of harmony between two parts. Pythagoras described it as it is presented in Fig 2-31.

In dentistry the term "golden proportion" is a mathematical theorem concerning the proportions of the dentition. It is considered as the only mathematical tool for determining dominance and proportion in the arrangement of the maxillary teeth from the frontal view.[80,81] *Lombardi* was the first actually to apply this equation to dentistry[82] and *Levin* developed the principles of visual perception and their application to dental esthetics.[81] It was found that certain proportions

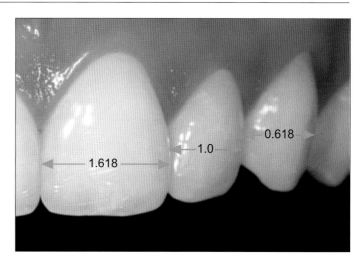

Fig 2-32 If the golden proportion has to be followed strictly, the ratios between the widths of the incisors should be 1.618 for the central, to 1 for the lateral, and 0.618 for the canine. The author suggests using those numbers and proportions only as valuable parameters, since in real life, symmetric and proportional smiles hardly ever exist.

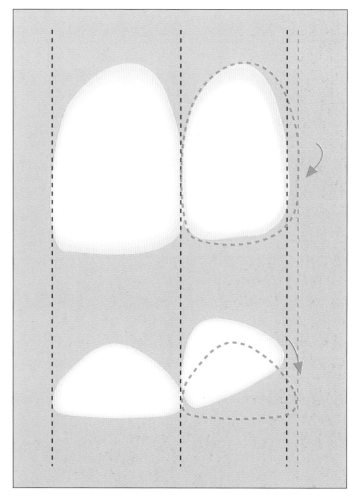

Fig 2-33 The position of the lateral incisor can affect its facial display: if the distal aspect of the lateral incisor is lingually positioned, the tooth will look narrower than its actual size (see *Goldstein*, Esthetics in Dentistry).

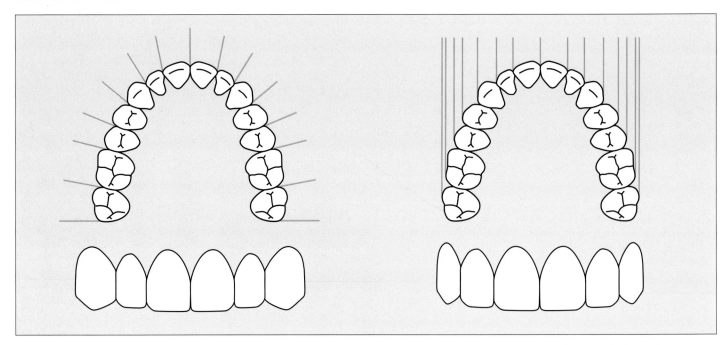

Fig 2-34a, b (a) If the teeth were to display their actual size, the distance from canine to canine would have been considerably wider and their related proportions would have been different. (b) The perception of tooth size is different when viewed from the facial aspect, owing to the placement of the teeth in the dental arch (*Ward*, Proportional smile design).

were more appealing than others, and beauty was equated with these proportions.[66] To some extent, these proportions can be defined, taught and used as the basis for the dentist's artistic plans.[83] According to this rule, if the width of each anterior tooth is approximately 60% of the size of its adjacent anterior tooth then it is considered esthetically pleasing.[84] It follows logically that if the width of the lateral incisor is 1, the central should be 1.618 times wider and the canine 0.618 times narrower (Fig 2-32).

A proportional relationship between the teeth alone is not enough to attain successful results, there must also be a proportion between the size of the teeth and the face.[85] Generally, there is an obvious contrast in the size of the lateral and central incisors when viewing the natural anterior dentition. The contrast is created by their respective positions and the differences in their mesiodistal widths, when observed from the facial aspect (Fig 2-33).[95] The distal surface of the lateral incisors is less visible, owing to their rotation in the arch, whereas the most dominant anterior teeth in the dental arch, the maxillary central incisors, can be seen in their full size.[82] It is not the actual size of the teeth, but the perceived size that these pro-

portions were based upon, when viewed from the anterior aspect (Fig 2-34).[76]

The effects of optical illusions and perspectives may lead us to perceive an object as deformed or in geometric shape when it is observed from a particular position. As distance from the perceived object increases, the objects observed seem to diminish in size, and their appearance differs from reality. Therefore, it can be said that a shape is never perceived as it really exists.

If the original definition of the golden proportion is applied to dentistry, the anterior teeth would display a relationship that is perfect and uniformly the same for everyone. Even though it sounds reasonable, it is very difficult to apply this rule because in reality patients have different arch forms as well as different lip and facial proportions. *Lombardi* stated that the "strict application of Golden Proportion is too limiting for dentistry, owing to the differences in the shape of the dental arch",[82] and he suggested using a continuous proportion, not necessarily limited to the 62% proportion. In this concept of "repeated ratio", the ratio of the widths established between central and lateral incisors must be used as the viewer proceeds distally.

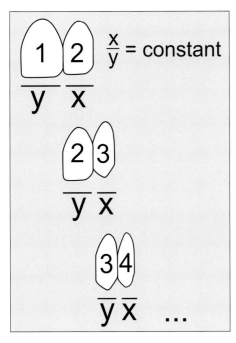

Fig 2-35 The epigraphic definition of tooth proportion, when the successive widths of two different teeth are viewed posteriorly (*Ward*, proportional smile design).

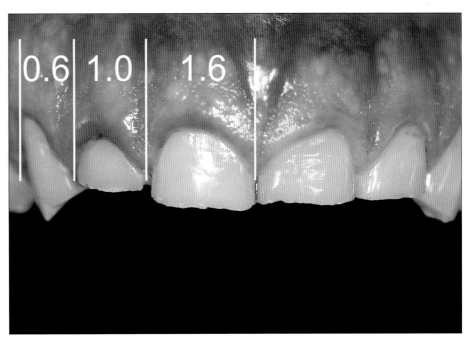

Fig 2-36 The proportions that dictate only the width of the teeth do not mean much unless they are somehow related to the height of the teeth. The teeth may still exhibit the exact golden proportions horizontally, but, owing to their short height, they may appear unesthetic.

Recently, the "recurring esthetic dental proportion" concept was introduced.[86] It states that the proportion of the successive widths of the teeth, as viewed from the frontal aspect, should remain constant as one moves distally (Fig 2-35) and rather than being locked into using the 62% proportion, the dentist may use a proportion of their own choice, as long as it remains consistent, while moving distally. The use of a recurrent esthetic proportion gives greater flexibility and is supported and enhanced by recent research conducted on the evaluation of beautiful smiles.[87] It has been found that the majority of the proportions of beautiful smiles do not coincide with the exact golden proportion formula. In this particular research, the proportions showed distinct differences between males and females, and the canines displayed a larger width in females than in males. This finding makes it clear that the strict observations of laws and rules may not only limit creativity, but may also lead to failure, considering the individual and cultural environment of the observer. Perhaps it is best to say that the golden proportion rarely exists in any natural dentition and overly strict adherence to it in order to achieve the ideal smile may be detrimental and limit cre-

ativity.[88] In the actual formulation and application of these laws and rules a marriage of science and emotion is required.[44]

Another downside of the golden proportion, as mentioned, is that it indicates only the width. However, it is generally agreed that the width alone does not mean much. Its perception is related directly to the height–width ratio and the objects next to them (Fig 2-36).[86] Therefore, the height-width ratio of the tooth within itself defines the perception of width and the natural progression of these proportions.[44] The natural smile is expected to be in harmony with the face, exhibiting different facial characteristics and dimensions. The concept of an ideal anterior dentition, or a formula to achieve harmony with a particular facial type, does not exist, and the patient's own perceptions, along with cultural and social influences, must be free to combine with the dentist's artistic abilities to achieve the finest results.[16] These formulas must be used only as guidelines and tools that the dentists integrate with their own artistic abilities and imagination.[83]

The notion of an esthetically correct standard arrangement of teeth was found to be completely inaccurate, and patients began to request

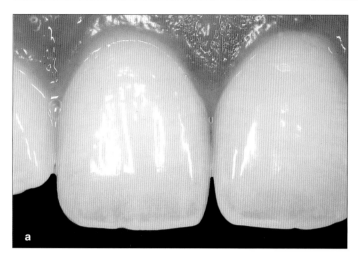 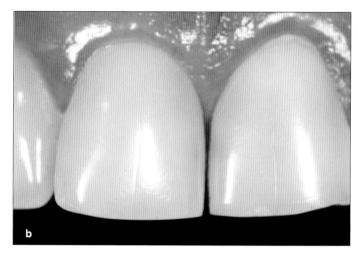

Fig 2-37a, b (a) Dentition of a 16-year-old teenager. (b) Aged tooth. Surface texture is affected by age. Young teeth exhibit a roughened surface texture, whereas the aged teeth have a relatively smooth surface. Children have a characteristic surface texture.

customization rather than standardization for their prosthetic restoration. Essentially, the patients themselves were responsible for the idea that beauty is best represented through the diversity that exists in the natural dentition. Accordingly, porcelain laminate veneers were fabricated with an increased focus on the charisma of the results rather than on their form and geometric alignment. These are the characteristics that impart the youthful appearance to the smile. It can usually be seen in the proportions existing in young dentitions and smiles when compared to aged dentitions. Therefore, care should be given to evaluating the patient's age, facial appearance, style and personal expectations. An important goal of the esthetic dental treatment is to restore the dentition to the most natural state possible, within the patient's esthetic preconceptions.

Tooth Character

Surface Texture and Contour

The challenge to emulate nature and establish oral harmony is a thoroughly complex issue, particularly in anterior restorations. Knowledge of the interplay of shape, function and surface texture is the basis for esthetically appealing restorations.

Surface texture affects the size, shape and position of the teeth. In esthetic restorations, the surface texture of the anterior teeth and their enamel, which becomes abraded in time, are the important factors to consider. The natural teeth of young children have a characteristic roughened texture, whereas adult teeth tend to have a smooth surface texture (Fig 2-37). This smooth texture is owing to the erosion of the enamel over a period of time.[89] Young teeth always look brighter than aged teeth. As the enamel of adult teeth becomes thinner, the hue of the dentine becomes more distinct, and the value decreases owing to the smoothened surface texture.[90] In a restored tooth, surface exturing must be similar to the adjacent natural tooth to allow the interplay of light that produces pleasant color matching.

Visual Perception

A contrast in color, shape and size allows the deflection and reflection of light from the dental surfaces and this visual perception of these reflections is somehow related to following rules:

1. The greater the contrast the greater the visibility.
2. Visibility increases with an increase in light reflection.
3. Visibility diminishes as light deflection increases.[44]

An esthetic effect can be created in dental treatment by using artificial materials to create an illusion. This illusion can be enhanced by artifice and reality in order to satisfy the patient's own perception of their image.[90]

Illusions

Certain conditions may alter the perception of teeth by creating illusions in the oral environment:

1. Depth can be created with shadows.
2. Prominence can be increased with light.
3. Length can be emphasized with vertical lines.
4. Width can be emphasized with horizontal lines.

Tooth contouring and color manipulation are optical principles applied in dentistry. Tooth contouring can be achieved through the manipulation of the natural grooves, angles, incisal or gingival inclines, and incisal edges, whereas the manipulation of color is performed on selected tooth surfaces, natural locations, gingival inclines and interdental areas.[91] In any restoration, the surface of the tooth's morphology is influenced by this relationship, especially in the issue of brilliance.[92] Young teeth with unworn enamel always exhibit a high surface texture with increased brightness. If the surface of the tooth or restoration is macro- and micromorphologically roughened, it will diffuse the reflected light.

The light reflected by the dental surfaces alters the perception of the size and color and the perception of the depth of a tooth on the dental arch. Teeth will seem closer, wider and lighter if the amount of light reflected is increased. Brighter teeth (therefore with high texture) appear larger and closer to the eye, and so in order to create the illusion of bringing a tooth forward, the surface texture can be increased, thereby increasing the value of the tooth. If the tooth must appear darker and more distant, the surface texture should be kept as smooth as possible. Variation in the reflection of light is required to make the teeth appear brilliant, and it can be achieved with convexities or cavities breaking up the surface. The brilliance exhibited in young teeth is enhanced by the surface texture, and if the value of the tooth needs to be increased, this high texture is a necessity. The natural anatomic surface must be carefully observed, and the dentist must try to achieve the same reflection of light that is reflected by the non-restored adjacent teeth surfaces.[93]

The technician should be knowledgeable of the compatibility of the porcelain selected for the planned surface texture.[94]

Misperceptions

In the case of the misperception of a crown contour, owing to a change in their outline form, it is observed that the lesser the contour, the smaller the tooth appears, and the esthetic dentist must be careful to guard against the possibility of any such misperceptions.[85]

Sometimes a tooth may look wider, even if its height and width are the same. This phenomenon is owing to the surface configuration of that tooth. Occasionally, the developmental grooves of the incisors follow a wider trajectory. In such cases, even though the tooth has the correct proportion, it is perceived as thick in width and relatively short. Altering the already existing mesial and distal line angles can also change the length perception of the tooth. The tooth can be perceived as longer if the mesial and distal line angles are moved towards the center of the facial surface (Fig 2-38).[95] Owing to wide gingival 1/3rds, the teeth may display a rough and square appearance. If the display of the smooth lines is broken, the gingival 1/3rd of the tooth appears narrower. The next step in creating a narrow appearance at the gingival 1/3rd is to prepare the tooth accordingly. These sites should be prepared somewhat deeper in order to create space for the technician, who will want to create the same effect with the porcelain laminate veneers (see below, Tooth Preparation and Fig 2-39).

An outline form misperception can be corrected, as in the case of central incisors where one is narrower than the other. To impart a wider appearance on the narrower incisor, a sharper curve is made in the distal line angle than that of the opposite tooth. If the crown's width appears to be too great, the tooth's distal outline should be shaped

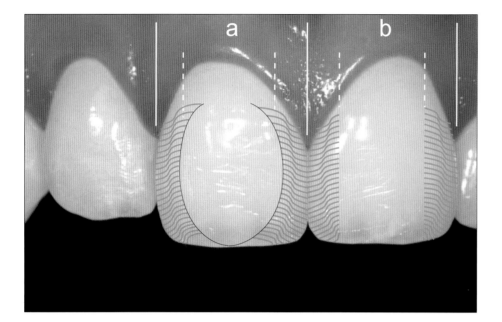

Fig 2-38 When the tooth appears wider (a), the vertical developmental grooves are moved closer, i.e. the already existing mesial and distal line angles are moved towards the center of the tooth to create the illusion of a longer tooth (b). If this procedure is insufficient, the mesioincisal and distoincisal corners of the tooth are rounded to enhance the lengthening effect.[67]

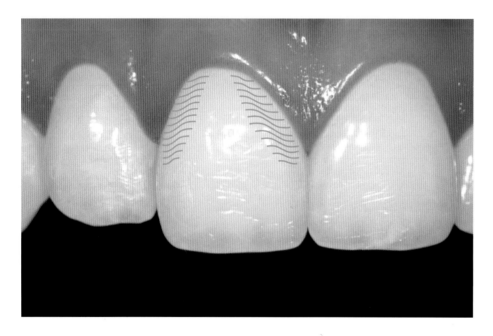

Fig 2-39 If the tooth appears wide, it can be modified from its gingival third, by breaking the mesiodistal line angles in that area. This will create a more triangular shape, thereby giving the illusion of a narrower tooth form.[67]

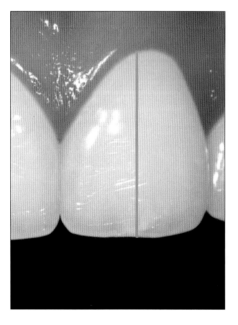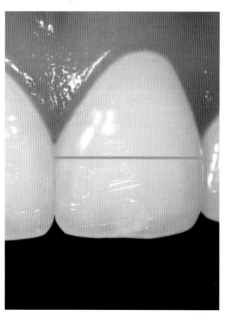

Fig 2-40 Vertical lines impart a narrow appearance to the objects, whereas the horizontal lines enhance the perception of the width. Two teeth of the same size may be perceived differently, owing to delicately placed horizontal or vertical grooves or internal stains in ceramic restorations.

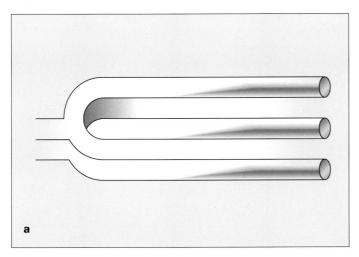
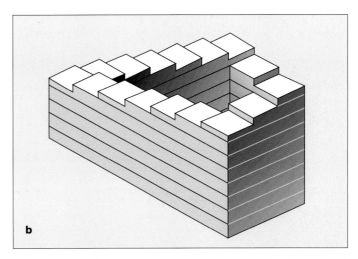

Fig 2-41a, b Power of illusion. Using the line angles, changing the internal angles and using shadows and different kinds of light reflections, creates illusions that can fool our eyes. (a) Even though there are only two extensions of the main bar, it can be perceived as having two or three prongs, depending on which side of the picture you start looking at. (b) If you keep on climbing the stairs you will do so forever!

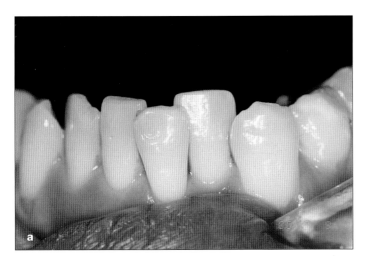
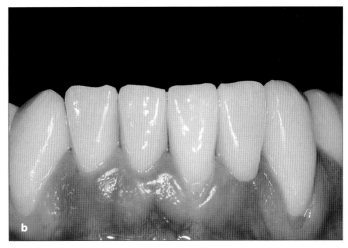

Fig 2-42, b A complicated case with crowded mandibular anteriors. Even though it seems very difficult to enhance the esthetics with porcelain laminate veneers, it is not. With careful treatment planning, delicate preparation and skillful application of porcelain laminate veneers and by using some illusive effects, the case can be treated as if there had been no crowding before.

to have a gentler curve, thereby making it appear smaller.[85]

The proportion or the orientation of the teeth can be changed readily by the influence of either vertical or horizontal lines. These can be achieved by using either different colors in different planes or by enhancing the vertical or horizontal grooves related to the surface texture. Dominance of the vertical lines will impart a longer and narrower appearance to the tooth, and the existence of horizontal lines will let the viewer perceive the tooth as wider (even if both teeth are identical) and shorter when viewed from the facial aspect

(Fig 2-40). If the adjacent teeth are characterized, and the teeth in question lack characterization, they may appear artificial, causing a high reflection of light. If the shade reflection areas that control the light used to create illusions are employed properly, the restorations will appear to be natural.[95]

Changing the line angles, surface texture and lightening can create illusions that play tricks on ones eye (Fig 2-41). In this way it is being possible to correct crowded teeth, even though it seems impossible to correct with porcelain laminate veneers to begin with (Fig 2-42).

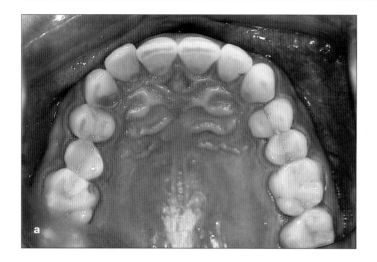

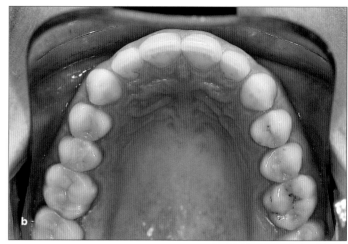

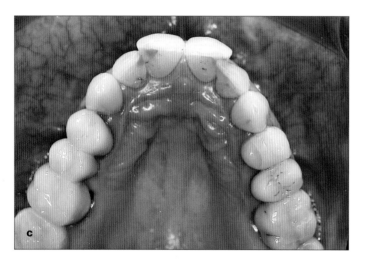

Fig 2-43a-c (a) Square dental arch. The maxillary incisors assume a position almost in line with the canines. (b) Ovoid dental arch. The central incisors appear along or across the curvature, whereas lateral incisors and canines are aligned with the curvature. (c) Tapered dental arch. A variety in tooth positions range from the V-shaped central incisors to the other anterior teeth that exhibit marked rotations or overlaps.

Shape and Position of the Teeth

To achieve esthetic harmony and support for the facial muscles and lips, the incisors must be correctly shaped and positioned. The perception of the tooth shape is related to the shape of the dental arch. There are three broad geometric categories of the overall alignment of the dental arch: ovoid, square, and tapered, which can be seen in numerous variations (Fig 2-43).[91] When observing the square alignment, the anterior teeth have quite literally a square appearance, with the incisal edges of these teeth basically identical and without much variation between them. It is as if the two canines have erupted parallel, and the tooth axis is straight without any labiolingual or mesiodistal inclination. The anterior triangular teeth are tapered within a triangular arch, and are protrusively inclined, while the central incisors are often labially displaced. An oval dental arch is usu-

ally made up of oval teeth, with the central incisors slightly labially displaced, and the posterior teeth on a generally contracted tooth axis with a lingually inclined incisal edge. The central incisors tend to have a distal surface that is rotated lingually.[16] Their edges are longer than those of the lateral incisors, and they also differ. The dentist is able to recognize this pattern through years of clinical observation of the natural structure of teeth.[91]

When a single incisor or a pair of incisors is being restored, adherence to the tooth's natural form is important. If homologous teeth cannot be used as a reference, then teeth from other groups may lend information as to the general shape of the tooth that was lost. The morphologic shape of the face, including the characteristics of gender and age, are useful in developing tooth form.[96]

Tooth Arrangement

The dental arch and position of the anterior teeth will determine the appearance of the lips and cheeks. If the dental arch is made too small, wrinkling of the skin may appear in the skin above the cheek and upper lip, as the arch is now unable to support the muscles. Similarly, axial inclinations of the teeth must also be carefully considered.[85]

Color of Teeth

The perception of the color of the teeth is influenced by the tooth's shape and its morphologic placement over the arch. Although there may not be great variation in the color of a single tooth, when the entire dental arch is carefully observed, it can be readily seen that there is a considerable variation in the color.[97] There tends to be a pattern in shade and color from the mid-line of the maxillary teeth. The brightest teeth in the smile are the maxillary central incisors, and although the lateral incisors are similar in hue, they are lower in color value. Of all the anterior teeth, the canines have the highest chroma saturation and the lowest value. The first and second premolars, although lighter and brighter than the canines, are quite similar to the lateral incisors in value (Fig 2-44).[98] In creating a natural appearance, it is vitally important to reproduce shade progression in any anterior dentition, even when the patient requests the lightest colors.

Characterization Via Colors

To create a natural reproduction with ceramic restorations, varying patterns of translucency must be followed. Throughout the life span, teeth are in a constant state of change. In youth, the teeth are more textured, lighter, brighter, and have a lower saturation. They also have a gingival margin at approximately the cementoenamel junction, along with light characterization that often has white hypoplastic lines or spots (Fig 2-45).[85]

Depending on the age of an individual, the amount, location and quality of translucency vary. At times, the enamel of young teeth may appear transparent, owing to their exhibition of an abundance of incisal translucency. However, after years of function, the highly translucent enamel is lost as the incisal edges wear. The facial enamel becomes thinner through daily functions, such as tooth brushing and eating, thereby allowing the dentine to dominate the shade of the tooth. Consequently, the teeth of older individuals tend to be lower in value and higher in chroma than those seen in younger adults (Fig 2-46).

The decision of the depth and extent of the enamel of the translucent porcelains used in restoration will be dictated by the pattern of translucency.[96,99-101] The sum of chromas that are contained and distributed over the entire tooth surface determines the mean value from which the "basic hue" or color of the tooth is identified. The color of natural teeth is related directly to the correlation of enamel, dentin and light that appear during the light wave refraction and reflection process. The high chromic saturation of the inner dentin body and low translucency are the source of the "basic hue". The varying chromas of the "basic hue" are based on intensity and can be located in different areas of the tooth, such as the middle, cervical and incisal thirds. The translucent regions of the tooth, which are a part of the "chromatic map", actually originate from the enamel that is free of interposed dentin. The cervical third contains the highest chroma, as the highest degree of saturation is found there, owing to its thinner enamel and more visible color. At the middle third, the chromas are a slightly lower. In unworn teeth at the incisal third, opalescence that is created by the translucency of the incisal and intraproximal enamel gradually replaces the "basic hue" chroma.[92]

The inner dentin body and the external enamel layer of the tooth upon illumination create the fluorescence and opalescence phenomenon. The factors determining tooth color are the varying saturation levels, which are related directly to the thickness of the inner dentin body and the translucent areas of the enamel.[92] The 3-dimensional color of the tooth that is perceived by

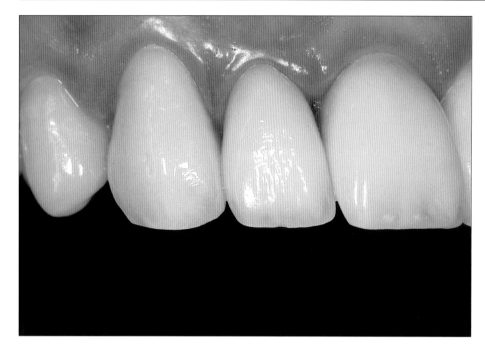

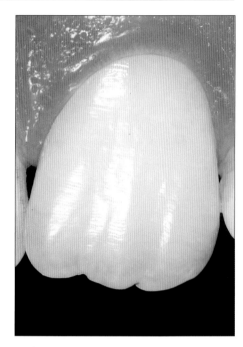

Fig 2-44 The smile is enhanced with 10 maxillary veneers (ceramist *G. Ubassy*). Through close communication with the patient, the progressive pattern of color change is explained. Since the patient also wants to have the natural tooth gradation, the veneers are produced in a natural way.

Fig 2-45 Young teeth are more textured, lighter, and brighter, with low color saturation. They exhibit transparent incisal edges. The enamel surface is semi-translucent, with a slightly irregular surface. Owing to the thicker enamel and translucency, the teeth look grayish white in certain areas.

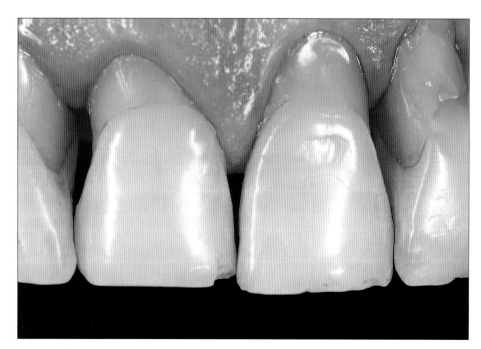

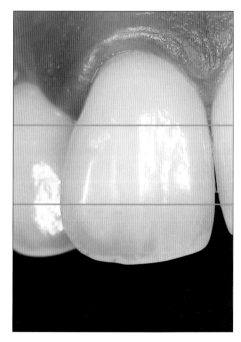

Fig 2-46 As the teeth age, the enamel becomes thinner, allowing the dentin to dominate the shade of the tooth. The value decreases, and the chroma increases.

Fig 2-47 The intensity of the basic hue can be different in various areas of the same tooth. The cervical third contains the highest chroma and the lowest value, whereas the slightly lower chromas are at the middle third. The transition to transparency at the incisal 1/3rd minimizes the chroma, thereby letting the opulence effects to take place at the incisal edge.

the eye, consists of delicate fluorescence and sophisticated opalescence. Fluorescence is the ability to absorb light energy and empty it in a different wavelength that creates value in the tooth. Therefore, if the value needs to be increased, more fluorescence should be added. In performing any restoration, the ultimate goal of the dentist is to make the artificial prosthesis appear natural (Fig 2-47).

To achieve a natural look, these substitutes should be created with the age, gender and personality of the patient in mind. When the restoration of an older patient is in question, the dentist must consider the fact that older teeth are naturally smoother, darker, and have a higher saturation or chroma. In the case of the lower incisors, the older teeth often exhibit flat, broad incisal edges that show a dentin core.

Life-style

As already mentioned, not only the surrounding tissues of the dentition, but the personality, character and life-style of a patient must be evaluated as a whole, as all these factors can directly affect the color of the teeth. For individuals who use red lipstick, the treatment (in terms of color) must be designed accordingly. As described by *Steven Chu* (Chapter 5), colors have complementary peers. The complementary color for red is green. Therefore, if the porcelain laminate veneers are produced without taking the patient's lipstick preference into consideration, when that patient uses red lipstick, the teeth will be appear greener than they actually are. To compensate for this effect, the porcelain laminate veneers must be in harmony with the red color of the lips, and red pigments should be added to porcelain.

Europe Versus North America

Another cultural point to be considered is that, until recently, Europeans favored teeth that are genetically normal, whereas Americans have always placed more value on whiter teeth. However, with the advent of bleaching, even Europeans are changing their values with a preference for whiter teeth.[102] As more and more individuals use bleaching, the proportion of whiter teeth has increased, thereby changing the entire perception of dental health. The fact that white teeth appear to be cleaner and fresher is enough to persuade any individual of their desirability. Therefore, although imitation of nature is a priority for the dentist, sensitivity to the changes in dental treatments and the possibilities that they offer, along with the change of perception that they bring with them, must always be a consideration in treatment selection. Patient perception will always tend to favor whiter colors and higher values.[92] The knowledge, experience and the personal artistic skills of the dentist will result in a full understanding of the color phenomenon. Quality laboratory work is necessary to create natural porcelain laminate veneer restorations with natural tooth arrangement and proper proportions.

Sex, Personality and the Age Factor

Lombardi has described anterior estheticism as the personality, age and gender of the person as it is reflected in the shape and form of that individual's teeth.[82] Clinical investigations by *Frush* and *Fisher*[20,70–74] concerning the sex, personality and age (SPA) factor arrived at the norms for these investigations (Fig 2-48).[79]

The masculine or feminine characteristics have an important effect on the esthetics of a pleasing smile. In Western culture, femininity can be expressed in terms of delicacy and softness, whereas masculinity can be expressed in terms of vigor and angularity. *Frush* and *Fisher* describe femininity in the female form as the roundness, smoothness and softness that is typical in a woman.[74] Masculinity, on the other hand, according to *Frush* and *Fisher*, is the "cuboidal, hard, muscular, vigorous appearance, which is typical of men". The aging signs seen in the facial features that often reflect masculine or feminine

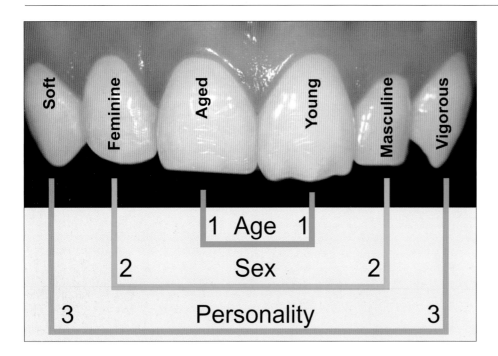

Fig 2-48 The classic chart from Lombardi, illustrating the SPA factor. Every characteristic of a single tooth may carry evidence concerning the patient's age, sex, and personality. However, when designing a new smile, factors such as cultural background, the expectations of the patient and their lifestyle, as well as the dentist's artistic ideals and values, are to be taken into consideration.

traits, can also be seen in the contours and positions of the natural dentition. If the incisal edges of the maxillary incisors, and especially the lateral, appear more rounded, than the effect is a delicate, feminine pleasing smile. These rounded softer lines add to the delicate nature of the facial features of a female.[103]

The incisal edges and transitional line angles of feminine teeth are rounded, while the edges tend to be translucent. In addition, the white hypoplastic striations can be used to give the effect or illusion of delicacy.[104] In the case of males, square incisal edges that appear to be blunt can enhance the masculine appearance.[103] This does not mean that all the features of a male's dentition will appear according to the categories listed for masculine teeth, and, similarly, neither will the female's. It is common to find that people tend to exhibit various features of both sexes in the same dental arch.[104] There are many factors related to the interpretation of these features. Our cultural background, personal artistic ideals and esthetic values are all to be taken into consideration.[105]

The rotation of the lateral incisor's mesial surface, outward and beyond the distal surface of the central incisor can create a more delicate or softer position of the lateral when observed. Similarly, the lateral incisor may appear quite the opposite,

or appear in a hard position, when it is located behind the distal surface of the central incisor.[103] In individuals of all ages, changes of character, position or color of the teeth are reflected in their dentition (see Incisal Length). When we think of the canine teeth, aggressive cartoon characters come to mind. Canines are thought of as the teeth of a ferocious animal or an antisocial person's indication of hostility and anger.[106]

The design of canines may take the passive–aggressive factor into consideration, when the tone of the appearance is selected. A tooth that is longer than the ones next to it and has a pointed incisal edge will appear more aggressive. A frontal view may display a height of contour or a flat profile. A small incisal embrasure between the lateral and cupid teeth can exaggerate an aggressive look. A passive cuspid may show no aggression at all. In such cases, the tooth is usually the same length as the adjacent tooth or even shorter. The passive cuspid may have a blunt rounded tip and a convex profile, often exhibiting large incisal embrasures between the laterals and canines that create a passive appearance.[107]

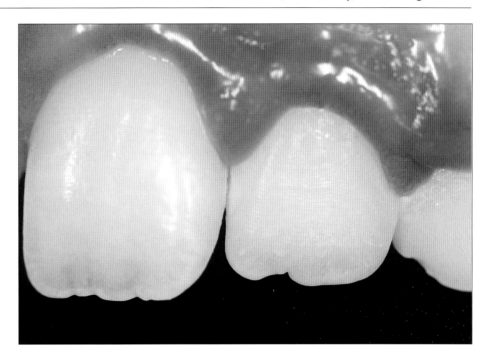

Fig 2-49 Shortly after the eruption of the permanent dentition, the cervical line lies well beneath the gingival tissue, and the clinical crown looks square or rounded.

Young Teeth

In the younger patient, the anatomic crowns are not fully exposed shortly after the eruption of the permanent dentition, and the cervical line is well below the gingival tissue. Consequently, young unworn crown teeth tend to have a triangular or square morphology that looks almost like a square or round crown (Fig 2-49). Enamel has a refractive index of 1.62 and appears bluish white or gray when exposed to light, and presents vitality. The labial surfaces of the unworn incisal edges may appear darker owing to the thickness and translucency in this region. The underlying color of the dentin of the natural tooth affects the overall color and may cause the dentition to appear yellow or gray white. The enamel surface of a youthful dentition is semitranslucent, hard and shiny with a slightly irregular surface. Younger teeth often have white hypoplastic lines and have a lower saturation light characterization, owing to lower chroma, with a more textured, lighter, brighter and higher value. They have smaller gingival embrasures and a gingival margin at the dentoenamel junction. They also have significant incisal embrasures. The intraoral color is influenced by the color reflected onto the dental arch from the soft tissues around the tooth.[108]

Aged Teeth

Aged teeth appear triangular, even if they are square or rounded by nature. As the gingival tissues recede, the root becomes narrower than the crown and comes into sight. Aged teeth may be shorter incisally but longer gingivally, which means that less tooth will be visible when smiling. Little incisal embrasures appear on the worn incisal edges, whereas the gingival embrasures widen owing to the recession of the gingiva. Flat broad incisal edges and a dentin core are characteristic of the lower incisors. These fine details are of the utmost importance for a thorough understanding of the teeth by skilled dentists, so that their artistic skills can be used to create the necessary illusions in order to achieve a successful result.

Functional, parafunctional and occlusal wear of the enamel surface will result in changes related to age. These changes can be observed in the maxillary central incisors, canines and mandibular anterior teeth. Generalized attrition results in posterior wear of the dentition as well. Broadening of the contact areas occurs from the interproximal enamel wear between the anterior and posterior teeth, and there can be up to a 1 cm decrease in the overall anteroposterior dental arch length, as the wear becomes advanced

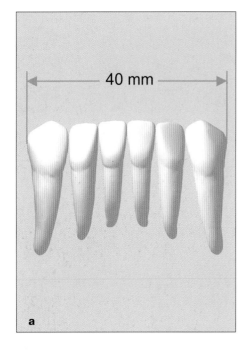
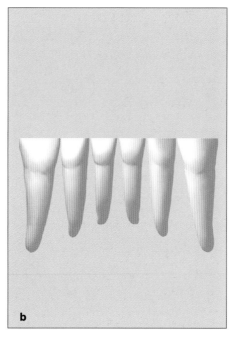
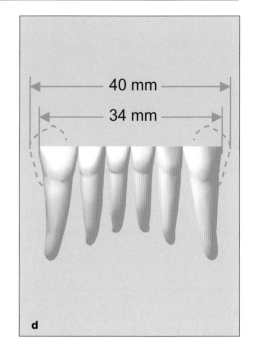

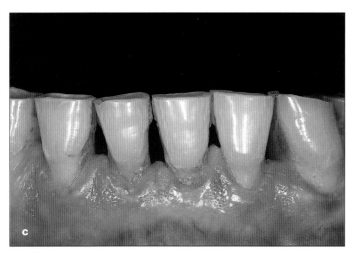
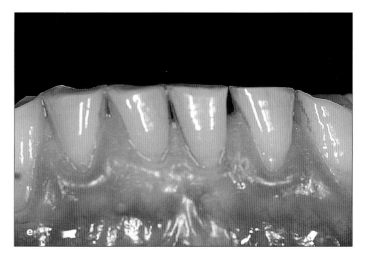

Fig 2-50a-e (a, b) Owing to wear, the length of the mandibular teeth reduces (c, d, e). As this continues to a level more apical than the "interdental contact point" (ICP), the teeth drift towards the lingual in order to preserve these contacts by narrowing the dental arch.

with age (Fig 2-50).[109] This excessive wear can eventually lead to narrowing of the teeth. For class I classification, the incisal edges of the maxillary central incisors tend to wear more cervically, affecting the lingual, rather than the labial enamel. Eventually, the maxillary central and lateral incisors will exhibit the same incisogingival length.[85] As the incisal wear continues, the lateral and central incisors and canines wear evenly, creating a flat incisal silhouette (Fig 2-51). This silhouette is quite characteristic of an aged occlusal plane without the incisal embrasures. Unlike the youthful smile that becomes flat and broad owing

to the steep curve of the occlusal plane, the aged smile is affected by the dental attrition and changes in the tissue elasticity and facial muscle contractility.

Little or no incisal wear is characteristic of a class II incisor relationship. In patients with class II occlusion, and parafunctional habits such as bruxism or tooth grinding, the labial surfaces of the incisors tend to wear cervically. The patient's position is determined according to the individual's occlusal type, and the canine's wear-patterns tend to be similar or not flat.[103]

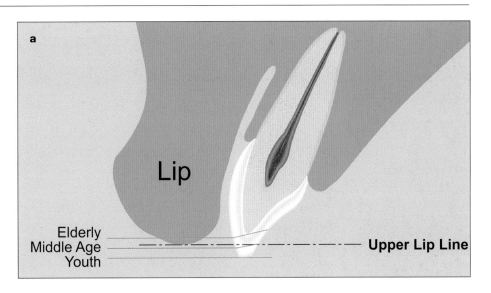

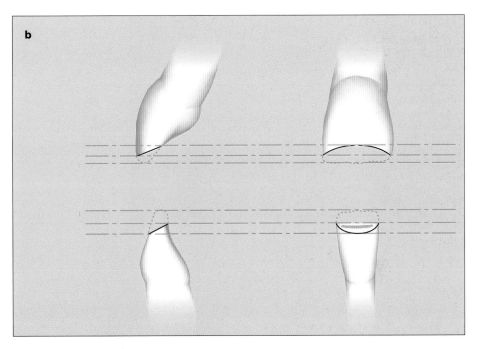

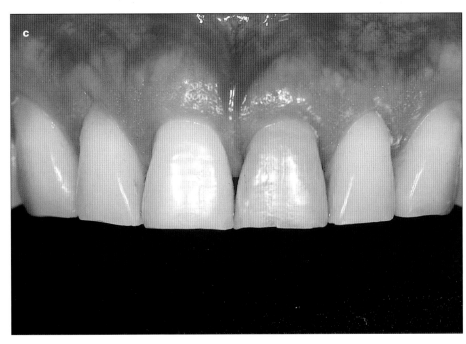

Fig 2-52a-c (a) Owing to wear, changes in tooth display occur during aging. (b, c) The loss of overall vertical dimension of occlusion will accelerate the maxillary and mandibular tooth wear.[131]

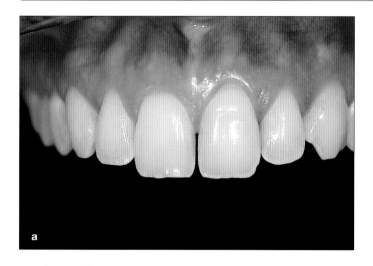
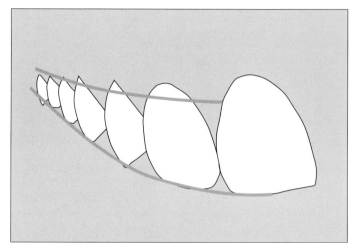

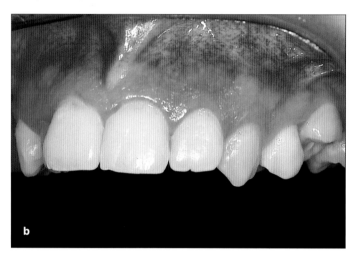
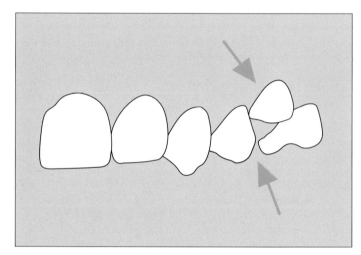

Fig 2-53a, b (a) A typical gradation effect. The larger the object, the nearer it appears to be. The natural smile has a pleasing front–back progression in terms of vertical relations. The perception of this progression requires the alignment of facial outlines and those of the incisal edges. (b) Unproportional gingival or incisal levels and the tooth inclinations and distinct color differences may distort this harmony.

The translucent enamel is lost over years of wear and function. The enamel layer becomes thinner from simple daily functions, such as tooth brushing and eating, and as a result, the dentine begins to dominate the shade. Although the reason for these changes is not fully understood, daily oral habits allow the pigments and ions to be absorbed into the teeth; in time, combining with the decreased enamel thickness, they dominate the shade of the dentition that becomes progressively darker. Changes in the underlying dentine, owing to aging or pathologically related color changes, also contribute to this phenomenon. Similarly, unlike young teeth, aged teeth exhibit higher chroma and less value.[96,99,100] The translucent porcelain, and the depth and extent of the

enamel built into the restoration, will depend on the effects that needed to be incorporated related to how young the smile should be designed.[101]

These changes affect not only the appearance of the teeth, but also their function. Higher surface stains and increased crown flexibility are caused by the progressive thinning of the enamel. It is possible to re-establish a youthful smile, and the appearance and function of the crown, through the restoration of the lost tooth volume. In preservation of the remaining elements of the tooth, enamel should be the priority in any treatment approach, and the degree of success of the final outcome is related directly to such preservation. Although many of the techniques used in porcelain veneer preparation actually expose the dentin, enamel preservation is possible through specific techniques (see Chapter 7). As the process of aging takes place, teeth tend to drift to the middle of the face; and over a period of time crowding of the dentition becomes progressively worse.[111]

Gradation

There is a natural bilateral progression in the size and shape of the teeth from the central incisor to the most visible posterior tooth, as can be observed when the maxillary dental arch is viewed from the anterior aspect. When viewing two separate but similar objects from a distance, the one closest will appear to be the larger of the two. Despite having the same occlusogingival length, when the teeth are closer to the viewer as in the case of the central incisors, they appear larger; however, when they are further away, as in the case of the premolars, they appear smaller. In the posterior progression of the teeth, the lateral incisors and the canines tend to be proportionately reduced in size. This effect, which aids in creating an illusion and results in a pleasing dentition, is referred to as "the principle of gradation of size".[108] Any other similar structures should be introduced and aligned accordingly, creating a gradual reduction in size when viewed from the closest to the farthest. The contour and alignment of the buccal surface, incisal third, and the alignment of the incisal mesiobuccal inclines are very important. At a secondary level, the lower rate and the gingival third are the prerequisites for the front–back progression (Fig 2-52).[91]

The gradation effect may be distorted if there are colored or distorted restorations, improperly placed teeth, or differences in tooth and gingival length. The key tooth in the arch form determines this natural transition that creates the front–back perception. The most important elements in achieving this transition are the canine and the premolar positions in the buccal corridor and the gradation effect that they create. The gingival area is very important in such restorations. Frequently,

it is not given the necessary consideration, and can even destroy the illusion of the front-to-back gradation. When performed improperly and when the illusion of gradation is impaired, the viewer's attention is drawn directly there in an effort to see what is actually esthetically wrong in the dentition. When viewing a smile, it is not only the teeth that should be considered, but also the illusion of depth and distance, along with the gradual elevation of the maxillary posterior occlusal plane as the teeth are followed posteriorly.[108]

The amount of light or illumination that strikes the teeth is an important aid in the illusion effect. In altering tooth illumination, the gradation effect is made possible by the negative space created by the buccal corridor or lateral negative space that exists between the buccal outline of the posterior teeth and the corner of the mouth. An illusion of depth is created in such a manner. The prosthodontist is able to manipulate these elements to enhance the characteristics of that particular patient's personality. The dark anterior "negative" space creates a clear contrast between the incisors and the lower lip in the anterior region and this color contrast, in turn, adds a dynamic external appearance[68,91,106] influenced by the width of the vestibule and the variances in the width of the arch form of the teeth.[95]

A bilaterally equal buccal corridor appears in the posterior teeth area. When smiling, this region between the buccal surfaces of the teeth on one side, and the internal surface of the cheek and the angle of the mouth on the other side, appears to darken posteriorly. The buccal corridors are occluded by the buccolingual position of the maxillary canines, emphasizing this effect. Patients are not aware that this negative space needs to be emphasized, and yet this is the key to achieving harmony in the smile. The harmonious proportionate relationship between the facial features and the smile itself is made possible by this space.[91]

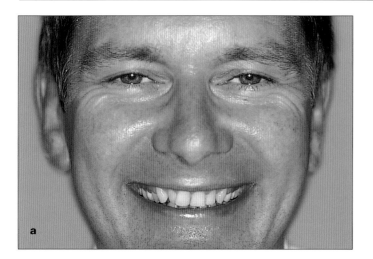

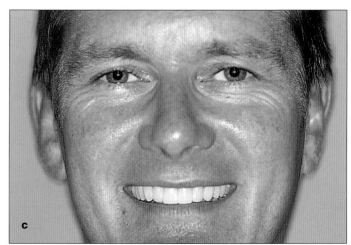

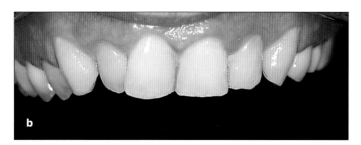

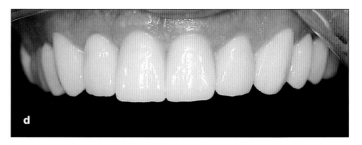

Fig 2-53a-d (a) The symmetry and balance were lost in this case, creating a negative visual tension. The disharmony of the teeth beyond the central incisors, horizontally and vertically, influences this negative tension. (b) To relieve the tension and disharmony, the gingival levels that were placed incisally must be altered apically. Following periosurgery, the vertical alignments of the premolars are corrected to improve the gradation effect. Note the extremely short premolars resto red with porcelain laminate veneers, as opposed to the natural pleasing vertical length. To provide balance and fill the buccal corridor, the lingually tilted short premolars have been slightly contoured with porcelain laminate veneers. When applied on the central incisors, symmetry is achieved. The central incisors provide the symmetry; the posterior segment provides the balance. (c, d) Balance is instated with the vertically and horizontally altered posterior teeth perception. The overall effect of the smile is totally integrated within the whole face.

Symmetry and Balance

When speaking about the esthetic beauty of a composition, symmetry and balance should always be considered. Symmetry may be explained as the harmonious arrangement of several elements with respect to each other[106] and which can be observed on both sides of a central axis. If the object displays a mirror image on both sides of the center, it can be said to have "static" symmetry. "Dynamic" symmetry refers to the condition in which two very similar but not identical halves are opposed.[106] Such minor deviations and irregularities will impart a more vital, dynamic and natural effect to the smile. Diversity adds charisma, and is an important part of beauty. A specific geometric alignment cannot create

the same effect. Recognition of these characteristics has caused the restorations of individual teeth to evolve from being similar to one another to being more individualized in their appearance.[112] The nature of the human body presents a dynamic rather than a static form of symmetry, and it should be taken into consideration and applied during the fabrication of anterior restorations as well.[79,113]

Balance must be diffentiated from symmetry. Balance can be observed as the eyes move distally from the center, which is in contrast to symmetry that is centrally located. In balance, objects that are farther from the center grow in importance and weight. The elements of balance should not be alike; however, when observed, they should display a comfortable, relaxing visual tension.

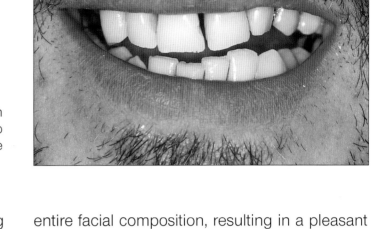

Fig 2-54 When the imaginary lines, drawn from the zenith points or the cusp tips of the canines, are not parallel to the pupillary line or horizon, an unpleasant smiling line occurs.

Balance can also be defined as the stabilizing result from the exact adjustment of opposing forces.[114] If balance cannot be achieved, the equilibrium of the composition cannot be maintained. The equilibrium and balance can be reinstated either by moving the causative element towards the line of forces until the magnitude of the visual tension is released, or by introducing an opposite element along the line of forces (Fig 2-53).[114] Since the central incisors tend to be the main focus, their asymmetry may have a negative effect on the smile, as in the case of overlapping central incisors that occupy more facial position, or in the cases where one of them is rotated facially, distorting the perception of symmetry. There are various types of asymmetric problems. Sometimes a canine may be more facially inclined or the mesial incisal angle of the central incisors may be rotated towards the opposite sides. Any of the anterior teeth may be inclined, abraded or rotated so that asymmetry occurs.[114]

Although the patients may not realize it, their perception of an attractive smile subconsciously expects a certain amount of facial symmetry. It is not enough for the smile alone to be symmetric, but the smile must also be in harmony with the facial components.[24] This pleasant relation between the teeth and lips is possible when the alignment of the commissural line (that connects the corners of the mouth) and the imaginary line (that connects the incisal tips of the maxillary canine teeth) is parallel. When these two lines are parallel to the infraorbital line and perpendicular to the facial mid-line, they reflect positively on the entire facial composition, resulting in a pleasant smile, otherwise the whole composition will be distorted (Fig 2-54). Ideally, the dental mid-line is in the center of the smile and is determined by the nature of the symmetry of the dental composition.

Smile Line

The Smile

Facial expressions are a part of our nonverbal communication, along with the less descriptive hand and body gestures. The most vivid of all our facial features is the smile,[108] as it is an extension and expression of the person as a whole. The beauty of a person's face is enhanced by a pleasant smile and reflects the virtues and qualities of that person's character.[91] The smile is one of the most expressive forms of nonverbal communication and it can convey countless emotions, from the small grin of embarrassment to the wider smile of happiness and enchantment to the full-teeth dazzling smile of exhilaration. It may last for a fleeting moment or remain intense, but it reveals the emotions of happiness and joy.[68] As each stage of human life lengthens owing to better nutrition and medical care, a middle-aged person is no longer considered old and, therefore, the period of time deemed "youth" has been extended, physically and psychologically.[91]

As more and more emphasis is placed on youth, it has become a challenge for the esthetic dentist to restore the aged smile. A youthful smile makes an individual feel young and improves their self-esteem. From a cultural standpoint, a prominent smile with bright teeth is synonymous with youth and dynamism.[115] In a young smile, the maxillary anterior teeth are more visible than their mandibular counterparts.[45,116] A more dynamic and youthful smile is created when the incisal embrasures become larger as the contacts are more gingivally located (see Interproximal Contacts) towards the posterior.[89] When observing a patient preoperatively, the esthetic dentist should always evaluate each case individually, since the determination of an older patient to have a young smile may lead us to create unnatural smiles.

Young smiles are whiter and brighter owing to the thickness of the enamel that keeps the darker hue of the dentin partially blocked. The heavy surface texture of the teeth scatters light, creating the perception of high value in color. Certain principles that have been explained are related to essential and structural beauty and therefore must be used in the restoration of the older individual in order to restore esthetics.[91] As beauty has always been related to youth, the media have constantly emphasized this relationship and they have created a demand for a restoration of youth.

From the patient's point of view, an anterior restoration with a perfect marginal fit and great biocompatibility of material with the surrounding healthy gingiva, may have no value unless the smile he or she expects to see is there. Even if the restoration is performed perfectly from the technical point of view, if the facial integration of the restoration is unsatisfactory (i.e. if the patient is not satisfied with the new smile), all the efforts of the dentist and the dental technician from the beginning of the case will be disregarded by the patient.[91] With the steady increase in the popularity of esthetic dentistry, smile design discipline has become an increasingly important aspect of the esthetic plan. In addition to the artistic touch, clinicians must also combine adherence to the principles used in smile design to improve the esthetics of any anterior procedure. The smile is outlined by a pleasant curvature of the upper and lower lips. The position of the angle of the mouth determines the degree of exposure of the gingiva, the width of the buccal corridor and the degree of exposure of the posterior and anterior teeth.[91]

The smile is perceived as beautiful when the fundamental dental and facial elements adhere to esthetic principles, and a harmonious integration into the patient's morpho-psychological profile creates an emotional psychological reaction.[91] The dentist who wants to create a smile design must closely observe the intact smile, the dominant position of the maxillary central incisors, and the art of the esthetic integration of the maxillary incisors in proper proportion to the face. The patient will exhibit a pleasing smile only when the quality and health of the gingiva and dental elements, together with the relation between teeth and lips, are harmoniously adapted to the face.

When smiling, the teeth are fully visible when the upper lip meets the apex of the gingiva showing the central incisors and leaving the gingiva less noticeable.[117] The teeth should be displayed to the first molar and the maxillary anterior incisal curve parallel to the lower lip. Personality traits like warmth, calmness and kindness are integral parts of what makes up an attractive smile.[91] The impact of a smile is not determined solely by the teeth but also by occlusal and engineering issues.[118] Sometimes the perception of a naturally pleasing smile with beautifully altered gingival levels and restored dentition may be distorted by the negative tension of the lips. Asymmetry, as in the case of individuals with paralysis of the lips, can be the cause of an undesired result despite all the necessary steps that have been taken to achieve the desired smile. The way in which people perceive a smile can vary from culture to culture: in North America, for example, where dental crowding is found to be very unattractive,[119] while the Europeans, on the other hand, tend to find certain irregularities quite acceptable.[121,122]

The Lips

The teeth, visible in laughter and in speech, are framed by the lips.[106] A harmonious morphologic and esthetic relationship is sought for the

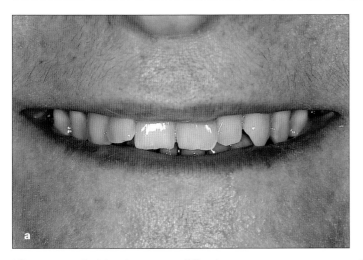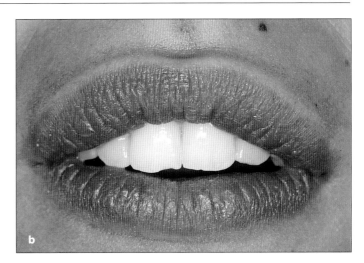

Fig 2-55a, b Lip sizes may differ from person to person, affecting the appearance of the smile.

dental elements that are framed by the lips. The lips are centered in the lower third of the face and consist of nerves, vessels, labial glands and alveolar tissue. The enclosing oribicularis oris muscle joins the lips superiorly to the base of the nose, laterally by the nasolabial sulci and inferiorly by the mentolabial sulcus. When compared to the upper lip, the lower lip has a tendency to be wider, fuller, longer and more elastic.[16] A vertical depression, called the "philtrum", is located on the upper lip. It proceeds superiorly on the facial skin from the tubercle of the upper lip and runs to the base of the nose. The philtrum is one of the most important landmarks when the placement of the dental mid-line is of concern (see Figs 2-1 and 2-5) The variations in lip posture may depend on racial and/or gender differences, especially in size, contour, shape, position, and in the range of exposure of the natural dentition (Fig 2-55). These variations may also occur owing to the shape, length and activity of the lips and their support, which is based on the position of the alveolar process and teeth.

When viewing a patient with class I skeletal relation and a natural detention from a lateral aspect, the external contour of the upper lip is projected beyond the lower lip. In other more severe cases such as class III malocclusion, where the lower lip may protrude beyond the upper, or the class II malocclusion, when the mandible is in a physiologic rest position with the upper lip protruding well beyond the lower,

greater variations of the lips can be observed (Fig 2-56). In action or at rest, the volume of the lips, along with their length and shape, have an important role in determining tooth shape and spatial arrangement. The degree of lip protrusion or retrusion and their effect on the facial profile is important.[123–127] The dentition and the alveolar bone furnish the total anatomic support of the lips, while the maxillary anterior teeth support the lower half of the upper lip. It is actually the tooth position, as opposed to the position of the incisal edge, that establishes the position of the upper lip,[126] and this has been supported in studies that have found that in 70% of cases the support comes not from the incisal 1/3rd but the gingival 2/3rds of the maxillary incisors.[127] The maxillary teeth are the primary support for the upper lip, but it can vary according to the type or shape of the lip. The position of the lips has a greater effect on the thinner, protruding lips than those that are vertical, thick or retruding.[128]

The support of the lower lip is derived from a balance of the alveolar process and the mandibular teeth. Lip design, when approached from the morphologic aspect, is a combination of sentimental, cerebral and instinctive action, and it is related directly to its dentoalveolar support with which it is connected. The tonicity and strength of the muscular support are important, and the facial musculature will be affected by any changes made to the dentoaveolar support. Aging has a considerable effect on the muscle tone, and a

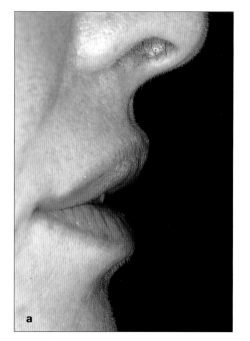
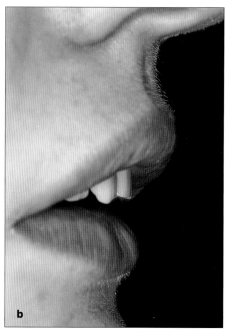
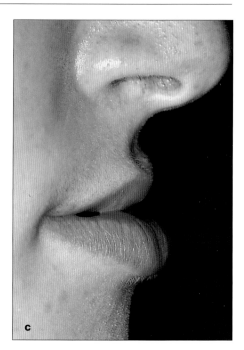

Fig 2-56a-c The lip profiles can be affected by the occlusion relationships. (a) Class I (b) Class II (c) Class III.

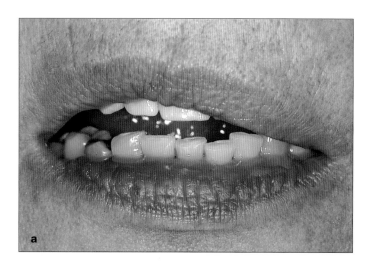
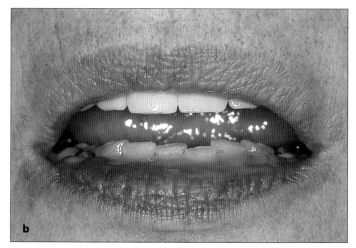

Fig 2-57a, b If the muscle tone is lost, the lips may sag owing to gravity. (a) A patient with an incisal line asymmetry; the lips are sagging towards the right. This may happen owing to the position of the head, if the smile line is to be verified with the patient on the dental chair with her head tilted to the right. (b) The same patient, with the same incisal line, in an erect position. The normal relation between the upper lip and the incisal line can now be properly observed. Note that no asymmetry actually exists.

general reduction of the tonicity and gravity causes the upper lip to elongate in the older patient. Consequently, when the lips are parted, the mandibular incisors become more prominent, and the maxillary incisors become less visible.[45] Different positions of head posture can easily change the vertical or horizontal display of lips owing to the weaker muscle tone.

Clinically, one of the most common mistakes made is the attempt to evaluate the incisal edge position when the patient is lying on the chair. This is true especially when working with older patients who have lost lip muscle tone. Owing to the working position of the dentist when the patient is lying on the chair, the only way for the dentist to see the patient directly from the facial aspect is to ask him/her to turn their head towards the side. However, owing to muscle sag and gravity, the upper lip will move towards the side of the face that has been turned. It will usually be to the right if the dentist is sitting at a 10 o'clock position. The right lateral and central incisors #7 and #8 (#12 and #11) will show more incisal edge than the left central and lateral incisors #9 and #10 (#21 and #22), because the left side of the upper lip will tend to cover the latter. The result will be an artificially inclined incisal edge position, which may mislead the perception of an inexperienced dentist. To overcome this problem, the patient should be seated in an upright position with their feet on the floor, facing the dentist and with their head perpendicular to the horizon (Fig 2-57).

Photographs from the patient's younger days will help the dentist to understand the previous tooth form and arrangement; however, they will have little use when planning the anterior smile and especially the position of the lips. The dentist must be sensitive to the patient's age and make the patient feel positive about the realistic changes that will take place.

Lip Lines (Upper and Lower)

The upper and lower lips influence a pleasing smile. A functional equilibrium exists between the forces and the compensatory action of the cheek musculature and the lips and therefore determines the natural tooth position. Dynamic oral movements are related to tooth support, and a relaxed tooth posture is present and independent of the tooth and alveolar process.[127]

The volume, shape and length of the lips are important parts in assessing the teeth when the lips are at rest or active.[103] The upper lip line has a significant correlation with the maxillary anterior teeth display as well as the gingiva. The lip line, its length and its curvature may vary, depending on the age of the patient and the anatomy of the face. This line also affects the level of tooth exposure when at rest. In close relation to this line is the incisal edge of the maxillary and mandibular teeth. At the same level to the bipupillary and occlusal plane is a parallel line to the angles of the mouth that confirms that the lip lines are horizontally lined up in a pleasing manner.[106] Before any restorative procedure is initiated, the lip position should be evaluated.

By their display of gingiva, the lip lines can be classified in three groups – high, medium (Fig 2-58a, b) and low (Fig 2-59a). A low lip line covers the gingiva and a considerable portion of the anterior teeth. In such cases, it is difficult to see the incisors when the lips are at rest. In fact, when the patient speaks, these teeth can barely be seen. The anterior teeth may be displayed when the patient is in full smile. For the teeth to be seen, it may be necessary to lengthen the crowns if the crown–root ratio and occlusion permit. The dentist may have to perform a major alteration in the proportions to establish a balance between the length of the lip line when at rest and when smiling (Fig 2-59).[103] In such cases, the dentist may have problems while trying to lengthen the maxillary incisors, and the result may be overlengthened teeth. It may be difficult at times to see the anterior teeth when the lips are at rest position even if the central and lateral incisors are lengthened. In the cases with gingival asymmetry, the advantage of the low lip line is that the gingival levels do not have to be altered, as they will not be seen even in a strained smile. Therefore, if the gingival levels are not symmetric, or the papilla is missing, these levels do not have to be esthetically altered and extreme care should be given to ensure the maximum health of the gingival at all times, even though it will be hidden. The low lip line should not become a cover for poor dentistry, by hiding the gingival one-third of the restorations and the gingiva.

The classification of medium lip line applies to the lips where 1-3 mm of the incisal edges of the incisors are seen at rest. When in a full smile, the level of the upper lip extends apically to a level where the tips of the papilla and a small portion of the gingiva are displayed. A medium lip line is considered to be the most preferable.

The high lip line can be seen on a small percentage of the patients, where more than 4-5 mm of the gingiva is exposed during a moderate smile.[25] Treatment of the high upper lip line is limited. A high lip line may often appear aggressive owing to the large display of gingiva. It will adversely affect individuals who have maxillary protrusion or strong infraorbital facial musculature.[91]

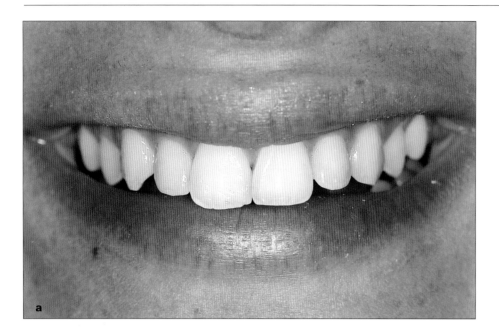

Fig 2-58a, b Varied lip lines display different tooth lengths and gingiva; for creating a pleasing smile (a) the medium lip line is the best. (b) High or low lip line may create esthetic problems.

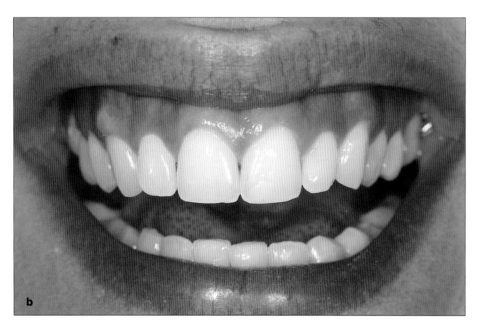

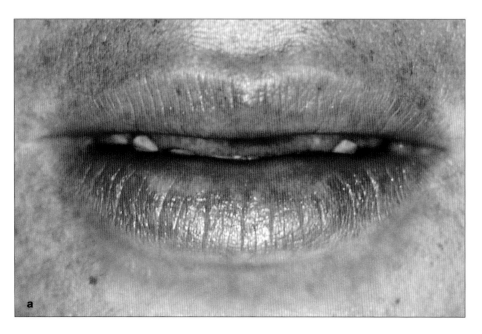

Fig 2-59a-i (a) Low lip line with relatively short teeth. It is not possible to see the teeth when lips are at rest or half smiling (b, c). The short length of the maxillary anteriors. The silicon index from the wax-up indicates how the teeth should be elongated. (d) The teeth are covered with the esthetic pre-evaluative temporaries (APT) (see Chapter 7) before the AMT (actual material preparation). The patient can now visualize the new length and color of her teeth. And the preparation is done over the APT. (e) Finished porcelain laminate veneers and their relation to the upper lip. Note that, even in half smile, the incisals of the anterior incisors can easily be seen. (f, g) The lip support of the porcelain laminate veneers. The upper lip stays retruded before the restoration. (h, i) the very positive impact of the new smile on the face.

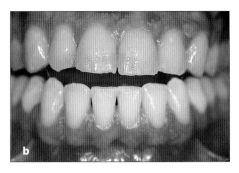
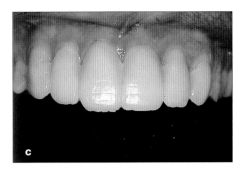
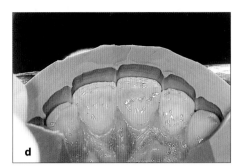

Fig 2-59b-d

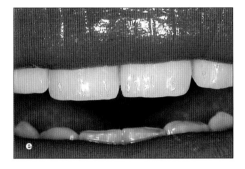
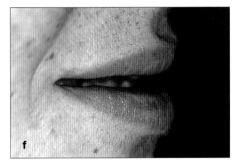
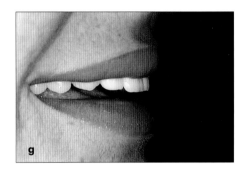

Fig 2-59e-g

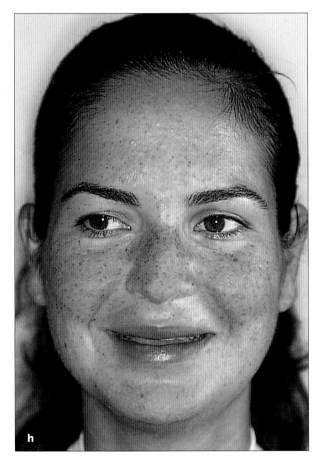
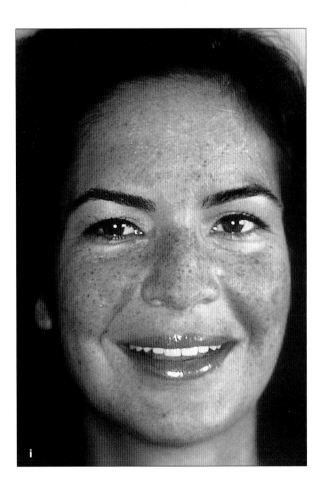

Fig 2-59h, i

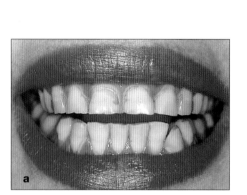
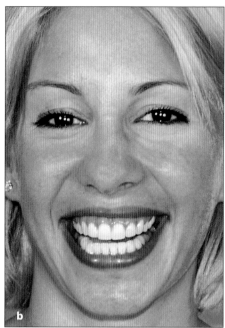
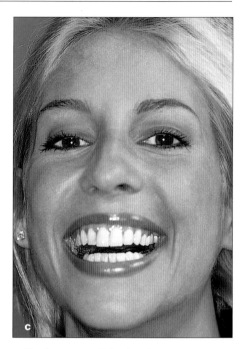

Fig 2-60a-c (a) Dark and short teeth are treated with 10 maxillary and 10 mandibular porcelain laminate veneers. (b) Owing to small and dark-colored teeth, the patient had lost the habit of smiling entirely, and the actual smile line is misjudged. Instead, the existing false smile line is taken into consideration. Since the patient liked the new appearance of the newly veneered dentition, the habit of smiling reinstated itself naturally, displaying more gingiva. (c) After 2 years, a simple gingivectomy was performed to alter the gingival levels to suit the new true smile line. The veneers are replaced accordingly. The new smile line does not exhibit any undesirable gingival tissue.

In medium and high lip lines, if the gingival display is unpleasant, such as in the case of the "gummy smile", or if gingival asymmetries are present, they should be carefully altered by the means of ortho, perio, or orthognatic surgery. The alteration should be performed only when the conditions allow and according to the esthetic demands of the patient. Even if the porcelain laminate veneers are designed esthetically, the gingival asymmetries will distort the final smile (see Chapter 10).[129] Sometimes the patient forgets how to smile owing to the unesthetic nature of their existing teeth. So even if they are asked to give a full smile, they think they are smiling extensively but they are not. Care should be paid to this aspect while restoring such cases, since after the porcelain laminate veneers are inserted, the patient will enjoy their bright and energetic appearance and start smiling more and more. And in some cases the dentist can end up wit a semi-gummy smile, which did not exist before (Fig 2-60). Therefore, this false smiling line that exists in the beginning must be carefully evaluated.[94]

Smile Line

The smile line is the lower margin of the upper lip that limits the visibility of the teeth.[130] This line also follows the edges of the maxillary anterior teeth that follow the curvature of the inner border of the lower lip. A pleasing smile is achieved when the angles of the mouth are parallel to the bipupillary line and the occlusal plane, with the tips of the canines barely touching the lower lip.[91] The lower lip curves upward and posteriorly to the corner of the mouth where it meets the upper lip. The viewer's attention is drawn to the dentition that is framed in the upward curve of the lips. As the viewer's eye is attracted to the elevation of the lower lip, it is focusing on the occlusal and incisal planes. The visible maxillary teeth have a connecting or incisal line convex, caudal and incisal that runs parallel to the upper margin of the lower lip.[91] This line can vary from individual to individual, and it is more pronounced and convex in females (Fig 2-61).

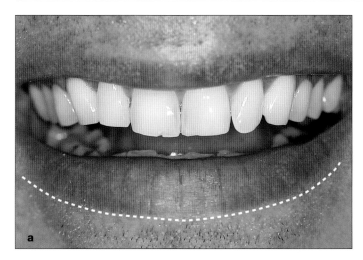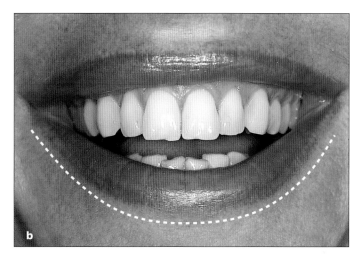

Fig 2-61a, b In a pleasing smile, the incisal edges of the incisors follow convex curvature, which is parallel to the lower lip. (a) The lower lip in men is fairly straight (b) when compared to the female lip. That creates a smile line that is flattering in males.

Conclusion

Esthetic procedures have the ability to alter the entire appearance of the patient by providing them with a beautiful smile. The patient gains not only a positively improved appearance, but also a potential moral "boost" that acts positively on their mental health and self-esteem. Any restoration to be performed must take into account the personality of the patient, and interpret and integrate it into the procedure. The importance of psychological factors that may enhance or affect the esthetic appearance should never be underestimated.

Although the dentist should always have a solid knowledge of the parameters that set a beautiful smile, they must also interpret and apply their own artistic skills in order to obtain a pleasing smile that is facially integrated.

References

1. Jenny J, Proshek JM. Visibility and prestige of occupations and the importance of dental appearance. J Can Dent Assoc 1986;12:987-989.

2. Dale BG, Aschheim KW. Esthetic Dentistry: A Clinical Approach to Techniques and Materials. Philadelphia, PA: Lea and Febiger, 1993:81-98.

3. Ramadan FA, Harrison JD. Literature review of the effectiveness of tissue displacement materials. Egypt Dent J 1970;16:271.

4. Nemetz EA, Seibly W. The use of chemical agents in gingival retraction. Gen Dent 1990;38:104-108.

5. Donovan TE, Gandara BK, Nemetz H. Review and survey of medicaments used with gingival retraction cords. J Prosthet Dent 1985;53: 525-531.

6. Gwinnett AJ. Moist vs dry dentin: Its effect on shear bond strength. Am J Dent 1992;5:127-129.

7. Moskowitz M, Nayyar A. Determinants of dental esthetics: A rationale for smile analysis and treatment. Compend Contin Educ Dent 1995;16:1164-1186.

8. Powell N, Humphreys B. Proportions of the Aesthetic Face. New York: Thieme-Stratton, 1984:2,4-9,50.

9. Lombardi RE. The principles of visual perception and their clinical application to denture esthetics. J Prosthet Dent 1973;29:358-382.

10. Cipra DL, Wall JG: Esthetics in fixed and removable prosthodontics. The composition of a smile. J Tenn Dent Assoc 1991;71:24-29.

11. Moskowitz M, Nayyar A. Determinants of dental esthetics: A rationale for smile analysis and treatment. Compend Contin Educ Dent 1995;16:1164-1186.

12. AAOMS. Dentofacial deformities: Evaluation guide 1986; 2:9.

13. Lejoyeux J. Prothèse Complète. 3rd ed. Paris: Maloine, 1979.

14. Heartwell CM. Syllabus of Complete Dentures. Philadelphia, PA: Lea and Febiger, 1968.

15. Faes R. Natürliche and künstliche obere Frontzahne. Schweiz Monatsschr Zahnheilkunde 1941;51:785-801.

16. Renner RP. An Introduction to Dental Anatomy and Esthetics. Chicago: Quintessence, 1985:241-273.

17. Miller EC, Bodden WR, Jamison HC. A study of the relationship of the dental midline to the facial median line. J Prosthet Dent 1979;41:657-660.

18. Johnston CD, Burden DJ, Stevenson MR. The influence of dental midline discrepancies on dental attractiveness ratings. Eur J Orthod 1999;21:517-522.

19. Rufenacht, CR. Fundamentals of Esthetics. Chicago: Quintessence, 1990:67-134.

20. Fruch JP, Fischer RD. The dynesthetic interpretataion of the dentogenic concept. J Prosthet Dent 1958;8:560-681.

21. Morley J, Eubank J. Macroesthetic elements of smile design. J Am Dent Assoc 2001;132:39-45.

22. Latta GH. The midline and its relation to anatomic landmarks in the edentulous patient. J Prosthet Dent 1988;59:681-683.

23. Miller LL. Porcelain crowns and porcelain laminates. Problems and solutions. Quintessence International Symposium (1991). New Orleans.

24. Chiche GJ, Pinault A. Esthetics of anterior fixed prosthodontics. Chicago: Quintessence, 1994;13-32,53-74.

25. Allen EP. Use of mucogingival surgical procedures to enhance esthetics. Dent Clin North Am 1988;32:307.

26. Shillingburg Jr HT, Kaplan MJ, Grace CS. Tooth dimensions. A comparative study. J.South Calif Dent Assoc 1972; 40:830.

27. Bjorndal AM, Henderson WG, Skidmore AE, Kellner FH. Anatomic measurements of human teeth extracted from males between the ages of 17 and 21 years. Oral Surg Oral Med Oral Pathol 1974;38:791.

28. Woelfel JB. Dental Anatomy: Its Relevance to Dentistry. 4th ed. Philadelphia, PA: Lea and Febiger, 1990.

29. Qaltrough AJE, Burke FJT. A look at dental esthetics. Quintessence Int 1994; 25:7-14.

30. Pound E. Personalized Denture Procedures. Dentists Manual. Anaheim, CA: Denar, 1973.

31. Dawson PE. Determining the determinants of occlusion. Int J Periodont Rest Dent 1983;3:9.

32. Heinlein WD. Anterior teeth: Esthetics and function. J Prosthet Dent 1980;44:389-393.

33. Robinson SC. Physiological placement of artificial anterior teeth. Can Dent J 1969;35:260-266.

34. Pound E. Let "S" be your guide. J Prosthet Dent 1977; 38:482.

35. Stein RS, Kuwata M. A dentist and a dental technologist analyze current ceramo-metal procedures. Dent Clin North Am 1977;21:729-49.

36. Kay HB. Esthetic considerations in the definitive periodontal prosthetic management of the maxillary anterior segment. Int J Periodont Rest Dent 1982;3:45-59.

37. Stein S. Periodontal dictates for esthetic ceramometal crowns. J Am Dent Assoc 1987;Dec (special issue):63E-73E.

38. Moskowitz M, Nayyar A. Determinants of dental esthetics: A rationale for smile analysis and treatment. Compend Contin Educ Dent 1995;16:1164-1186.

39. Miller Jr PD. Root coverage using a free soft tissue autogenous graft following citric acid application. 1. Technique. Int J Periodont Rest Dent 1982;2:65-70.

40. Langer B, Langer L. Subepithelial connective tissue graft technique for root coverage. J Periodont 1985;56:715-720.

41. Coslet G, Rosenberg E, Tisot R. The free autogenous gingival graft. Dent Clin North Am 1980;24:651-682.

42. Abrams L. Augmentation of deformed residual edentulous ridge for fixed prosthesis. Compend Contin Educ Dent 1980;1:205-214.

43. Tarnow DP, Magner AW, Fletcher P. The effect of the distance from the contact point to the crest of bone on the presence or absence of the interproximal dental papilla. J Periodontol 1992;63:995-996.

44. Rufenacht CR. Principles of Esthetic Integration. Chicago: Quintessence, 2000:63-168.

45. Vig RG, Brundo GC. The kinetics of anterior tooth display. J Prosthet Dent 1978;39:502-504.

46. Wheeler RC. Complete crown form and the periodontium. J Prosthet Dent 1961;11:722-734.

47. Weisgold A. Contours of the full crown restoration. Alpha Omega 1977;70:77-89.

48. Narcisi EM, Culp L. Diagnosis and treatment planning for ceramic restorations. 2001;45:127-142.

49. Berscheid E, Walster E, Bohrnstedt. G. Body image. The American body. A survey report. Psychol Today 1973; Nov:119-131.

50. Calamia JR. Clinical evaluation of etched porcelain laminate veneers. Am J Dent 1989;2:9-15.

51. Strassler HE, Nathanson D. Clinical evaluation of etched porcelain veneers over a period of 18 to 42 months. J Esthet Dent 1989;1:21-28.

52. Brodbeck U. Scharer P. Ceramic inlays as lateral tooth restorations. Schweiz Monatsschr Zahnmed 1992;102:330-340.

53. Yamashita A. A Dental Adhesive and its Clinical Application. Tokyo: Quintessence, 1983.

54. Bjorn H, Free transplantation of gingiva propla. Sven Tandlak Tidskr 1963;22:684.

55. Holbrook T. Ochseinbein C. Complete coverage of the denuded root surface: A one-stage gingival graft. Int J Periodont Rest Dent 1983;3:8-27.

56. Miller Jr PD. Concept of periodontal plastic surgery. Pract Periodont Aesthet Dent 1993;5:15-20.

57. Langer B, Calamia LJ. The subepithelial connective tissue graft. A new approach to the enhancement of anterior cosmetics. Int J Periodont Rest Dent 1982;2:22-33.

58. Rosenthal L. The smile lift: A new concept in aesthetic care. Part 1. Dent Today 1994;13:66, 68-71.

59. Seibert JS. Reconstruction of deformed, partially edentulous ridges, using full thickness onlay grafts. Part 2. Prosthetic/periodontal interrelationships. Compend Contin Educ Dent 1983;4:549-562.

60. Seibert JS. Reconstruction of deformed, partially edentulous ridges, using full thickness onlay grafts. Part 1. Technique and wound healing. Compend Contin Educ Dent 1983;4:437-453.

61. Miller PD. Regenerative and reconstructive periodontal plastic surgery. Mucogingival surgery. Dent Clin North Am 1988;32:287-306.

62. Rosenthal L, Jacobs JE. The periodontal-prosthetic-esthetic connection. Con Esthet and Res Prac Jul/Aug 1999:1-4.

63. Rosenthal L. State of the art advanced porcelain laminate veneers. Part 2. Esthet Dent Update 1991;2:97-101.

64. Rosenthal L, Rinaldi P: The aesthetic revolution: Minimum invasive dentistry. Dent Today 1998;17:42-44,46-47.

65. Gerber A. Complete dentures. 8. Creative and artistic tasks in complete prosthodontics. Quint Int 1975;2:45-50.

66. Morley J. A multidisciplinary approach to complex aesthetics restoration with diagnostic planning. Prac Perio Aesth Dent 2000;12:575-577.

67. Goldstein RE. Esthetics in Dentistry. 2nd ed. Hamilton, ON: BC Decker Inc, 1998:133-186.

68. Matthews TG: The anatomy of a smile. J Prosthet Dent 1978;39:39-34.

69. Rufenacht CR. Fundamentals of Esthetics. Chicago: Quintessence, 1990:13-48.

70. Frush JP, Fisher RD. Introduction to dentogenic restorations. J Prosthet Dent 1955;5:586-595.

71. Frush JP, Fisher RD. How dentogenic restorations interpret the sex factor. J Prosthet Dent 1956;6:160.

72. Frush JP, Fisher RD. How dentogenic restorations interpret the sex factor. J Prosthet Dent 1956;6:441-449.

73. Frush JP, Fisher RD. The age factor in dentogenics. J Prosthet Dent 1957;7:5-13.

74. Frush JP, Fisher RD. Dentogenics: Its practical application. J Prosthet Dent 1959;9:914.

75. Gillen RJ, Schwartz RS, Hilton TJ, Evans DB. An analysis of selected normative tooth proportions. Int J Prosthodont 1994;7:415.

76. Baratieri LN. Esthetics: Direct Adhesive Restoration on Fractured Anterior Teeth. São Paulo: Quintessence, 1998:35-56.

77. Moores CFA, Thomsen SO, Jensen E, Yen PKJ. Mesiodistal crown diameters of the deciduous and permanent teeth in individuals. J Dent Res 1957;36:39.

78. Mavroskoufis F, Ritchie GM. Variation in size and form between left and right maxillary central incisor teeth. J Prosthet Dent 1980;43:254.

79. Lombardi RE. A method for the classification of errors in dental esthetics. J Prosthet Dent 1974;32:501.

80. Heymann HO. The artistry of conservative esthetic dentistry. J Am Dent Assoc 1987; (special issue):14E-23E.

81. Levin EL. Dental esthetics and golden proportion. J Prosthet Dent 1978; 40:244-252.

82. Lombardi RE. The principles of visual perception and their clinical application to denture esthetics. J Prosthet Dent 1973;29:358-382.

83. Richer P. Artistic Anatomy. New York: Watson-Guptill, 1971.

84. Borissavlievitch M. The Golden Number. London: Alec Tiranti, 1964.

85. Yamamoto M, Miyoshi M, Kataoka S. Special Discussion. Fundamentals of esthetics: contouring techniques for metal ceramic restorations. QDT 1990/1991;14:10-81.

86. Ward DH. Proportional smile design using the recurring esthetic dental proportion. Dent Clin North Am 2001;45:143-154.

87. Sterrett JD, Oliver T, Robinson F, Fortson W, Knaak B, Russell CM. Width/length ratios of normal clinical crowns of the maxillary anterior dentition in man. J Clin Periodont 1999;26:153-157.

88. Preston JD: The golden proportion revisited. J Esthet Dent 1993;5:247-251.

89. Shillingburg Jr HT, Hobo S, Whitsett LD, Jacobi R, Brackett SE. Fundamentals of Fixed Prosthodontics. 3rd ed. Chicago: Quintessence, 1997; 419-432.

90. Tao S, Lowenthal U. Some personality determinants of denture preference. J Prosthet Dent 1980;44:10-12.

91. Rufenacht CR. Fundamentals of Esthetics. Chicago: Quintessence, 1990:9-31, 59-67, 67-134, 329-368.

92. Vanini L. Light and color in anterior composite restorations. Pract Periodont Aesthet Dent 1996;8:673-682.

93. Goldstein RE. Esthetics in Dentistry. 2nd ed. Hamilton, ON: BC Decker Inc, 1998:123-133.

94. Dale BG, Aschheim KW. Esthetic Dentistry: A Clinical Approach to Techniques and Materials. Philadelphia, PA: Lea and Febiger, 1993:69-78,128-149.

95. Goldstein RE. Esthetics in Dentistry. 2nd ed. Hamilton, ON: BC Decker Inc, 1998:133-186.

96. Heymann HO. The artistry of conservative esthetic dentistry. J Am Dent Assoc 1987; (special issue):14-E-23E.

97. Golub-Evans J. Unity and variety: Essential ingredient of a smile design. Curr Opin Cosmet Dent 1994;2:1-5.

98. Goodkind RJ, Schwabacher WB. Use of a fiber-optic colorimeter for in vivo measurements of 2830 anterior teeth. J Prosthet Dent 1973;29:358-382.

99. Brisman A, Hirsch SM, Paige H, Hamburg M, Gelb M. Tooth shade preferences in older patients. Gerodontics 1985; 1:130-133.

100. Winter RR: Achieving esthetic ceramic restorations. J Calif Dent Assoc 1990; 18: 21-24.

101. Kessler JC: Dentist and laboratory: Communication for success. J Am Dent Assoc 1987;115:97E-102E.

102. Feigenbaum NL. More than one reality. Pract Periodont Aesthet Dent 1999;11:136.

103. Touati B, Miara P, Nathanson D. Esthetic Dentistry and Ceramic Restorations. New York: Martin Dunitz, 1999:139-161.

104. Bruce A Singer. Fundamentals of esthetics. In: Dale BG, Aschheim KW. Esthetic Dentistry: A Clinical Approach to Techniques and Materials. Philadelphia, PA: Lea and Febiger, 1993:5-13.

105. Renner RP. An Introduction to Dental Anatomy and Esthetics. Chicago: Quintessence, 1985:187-233.

106. Strub JR, Türp JC. Esthetics in dental prosthetics. In: Fischer J, Esthetics and Prosthetics. Chicago: Quintessence, 1999:11.

107. Morley J. Smile design. Specific considerations. CDAJ 1997;25:636.

108. Renner RP. An Introduction to Dental Anatomy and Esthetics. Chicago: Quintessence, 1985.125-166,187-233, 241-272.

109. Lammie GA, Posselt U. Progressive changes in the dentition of adults. J Periodontol 1965;36:443-454.

110. Richardson ME. A preliminary report on lower arch crowding in the mature adult. Eur J Orthod 1995;17:251-257.

111. Touati B. Defining form and position. Pract Periodont Aesthet Dent 1998;10:800-803.

112. Tripodakis A-P. Dental Esthetics: "Oral personality" and visual perception. Quintessence Int 1987;18:405-418.

113. Geller W. Dental Ceramics and Esthetics. Chicago, 15 February 1991.

114. Goldstein RE. Change your Smile. 1st ed. Chicago: Quintessence, 1984.

115. Wichmann R. Über Die Sichbarkeit der Front- und Seitenzähne. ZWR 1990;99:623-626.

116. Cosmetic periodontics. Reality Now 2001;3:43.

117. Morley J, Eubank J. Macroesthetic elements of smile design. J Am Dent Assoc 2001;132:39-45.

118. Graber LW, Lucker GW. Dental esthetic self-evolution and satisfaction. Am J Orthod 1980;77-163.

119. Albino JE, Cunat JJ, Fox RN, Lewis EA, Slakter MJ, Tedesco LA. Variables discriminating individuals who seek orthodontic treatment. J Dent Res. 1981;60:1661-1667; Shaw WC, Lewis HG, Robertson NR. Perception of malocclusion. Br Dent J 1975;138:211-216.

120. Prahl-Andersen B, Boersma H, van der Linden FP, Moore AW. Perceptions of dentofacial morphology by laypersons, general dentists, and orthodontists. J Am Dent Assoc. 1979;98:209-212.

121. Burstone CJ. The integumental profile. Am J Orthod 1958; 44:1.

122. Subtelny JD. A longitudinal study of soft tissue facial structures and their profile characteristics, defined in relation to underlying structures. Am J Orthod 1959;45:481.

123. Tweed CH. The diagnostic facial triangle in the control of treatment objectives. Am J Orthod 1991;55:651.

124. Peck H, Peck S. A concept of facial esthetics. Angle Orthod 1970;40:284.

125. Maritato FR, Douglas JR. A positive guide to anterior tooth placement. J Prosthet Dent 1964;14:848.

126. Pound E. Applying harmony in selecting and arranging teeth. Dent Clin North Am 1962;6:241.

127. Crispin BJ, Watson JF. Margin placement of esthetic veneer crowns. Part 2. Posterior teeth visibility. J Prosthet Dent 1981;45:389-391.

128. Burstone CJ. Lip posture and its significance in treatment planning. Am J Orthod 1967;53:262-284.

129. Yamamoto M. Metal-Ceramics: Principles and Methods of Makoto Yamamoto. Chicago: Quintessence, 1985:410.

130. Burstone CJ. Lip posture and its significance in treatment planning. Am J Orthod 1967;53:262-284.

131. Yamamoto M. Metal-Ceramics: Principles and Methods of Makoto Yamamoto. Chicago: Quintessence, 1985:410.

3 Adhesion

Jean-François Roulet, Uwe Blunck, Ralf Janda

Introduction

Adhesion has completely changed dentistry for two reasons:

- adhesion seals dentin completely, thus preventing microorganisms access to the pulp,[1]
- with adhesion, dentists do not need to rely on macroretention using undercuts or the large parallel surfaces of indirect restorations.

This shift from macroretention to microretention has promoted aesthetic and minimal invasive dentistry. Treatments we offer these days, such as bonded veneers, were unthinkable fifty years ago.[2,3]

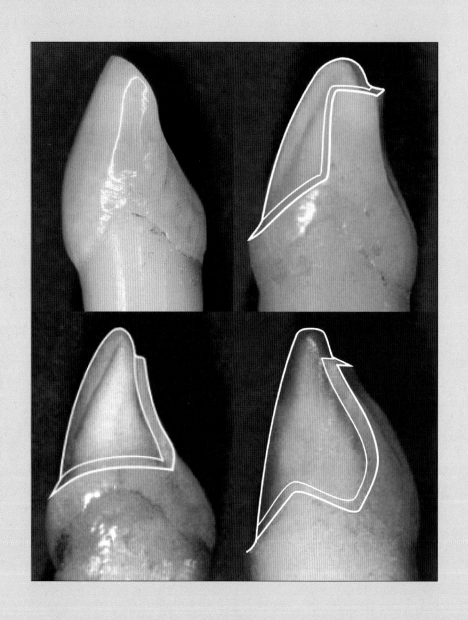

Substrates

Enamel

Enamel is the best mineralized tissue in the body. It consists of 95% w/w or 86% v/v of inorganic substances, mostly hydroxyapatite.[4,5] The water content is minimal and in contrast to bone, dentin and cementum, most of the water in enamel is bound to the crystals as a hydration layer. Only about one-quarter of the water is free within the organic component. The organic part consists of solvable and unsolvable proteins and a few carbohydrates and lipids (Figs 3-1a and b).[6] The distribution of these organic components differs from area to area and is seen as the remains from the enamel matrix as it is produced by the ameloblasts. The inorganic component is mostly apatite, especially hydroxyapatite. Some calcium carbonate is also found. Fluorides are usually present in enamel, especially in the surface layers, a little less in attrition zones. The highest fluoride concentrations are found in the most superficial 50 μm of enamel. There the concentration varies between 300 and 1,200 ppm as a function of the fluoride exposition of the individual. This is important to realize, since it is known that fluoroapatite is less soluble, and so superficial, unground enamel is more resistant to etching.

Enamel is produced by the ameloblasts, which are responsible for its structure. Corresponding to the ameloblasts and their Tomes' processes, where the enamel matrix is released from the ameloblasts, the enamel is structured in rods. These enamel rods start at the dentino-enamel junction and end approximately 30 μm under the enamel surface, where so-called "prismless enamel" is found. There the crystallites are all densely packed and oriented perpendicularly to the surface.[7,8] The rods show a curved pattern from the center to the periphery, where they are usually arranged more or less perpendicularly to the surface. Their diameter is around 5 μm, but they have an irregular shape, which is often misinterpreted. In cross sections they may appear as a keyhole type or as a horseshoe type.[9,10] This structure is seen best if the enamel is etched with phosphoric acid (Fig 3-2).

These patterns occur because of the next substructure of enamel: the hydroxyapatite crystallites. They are produced right after the secretion of the enamel matrix. The first appearance seems to occur not as a continuum, but in discrete phases, which result in a striation of the enamel (Retzius lines). Later on the enamel undergoes a maturation, in which the crystals grow from initially 15 Å (thickness) x 300 Å (width) x 800–1200 Å (length) to much larger ones (350 Å x 800–1000 Å x 1600 Å). These are densely packed in mature enamel.[11,12]

Within the prisms, the orientation of the crystallites follows well-defined patterns, which are seen as a consequence of the mechanism of

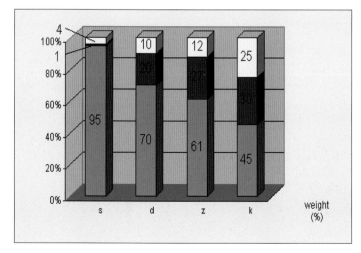

Fig 3-1a Composition of the mineralized tissues of the body by weight.

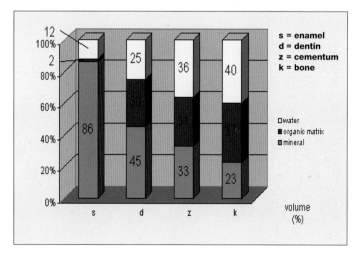

Fig 3-1b Composition of the mineralized tissues of the body by volume (*Schröder*, Orale Strukturbiologie).

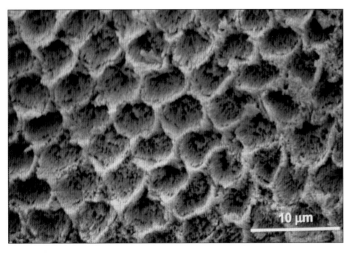

Fig 3-2 Enamel, cross section perpendicularly to the prism long axis. Etched with 37% phosphoric acid (SEM).

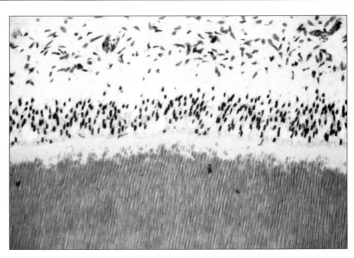

Fig 3-3 Odontoblastic layer with predentin and mineralized dentin (HE stain).

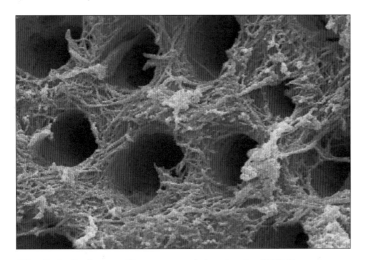

Fig 3-4 Collagen fiber network in dentin (SEM).

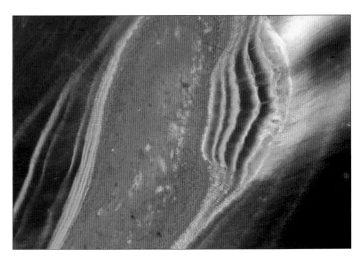

Fig 3-5 Enhanced dentin production (secondary dentin) as result of irritation. (Special stain, courtesy of *H. Stich*.)

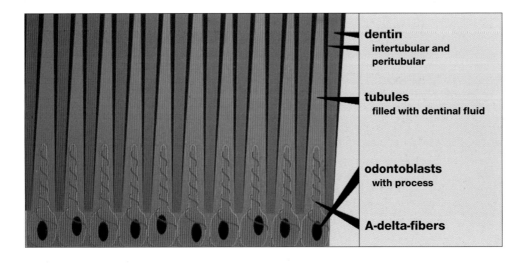

dentin
intertubular and
peritubular

tubules
filled with dentinal fluid

odontoblasts
with process

A-delta-fibers

Fig 3-6 The structure of dentin.

the enamel production. The optical axis (c-axis = length axis) of the crystallites follows distinctive patterns, with most of the crystallites being oriented within the length axis of the prism. The difference in orientation within the prism makes the different pattern in cross sections (horseshoe v. keyhole). Since the solubility of crystals is different from their steric orientation (in the c-axis they are less soluble), etching of enamel produces an extremely rough and thus enlarged surface (Fig 3-2). The crystallites are embedded in a gelatinous, unstructured matrix, which consists only of 1–2% of the total volume.[6] Since in the prismless enamel of the enamel surface all crystallites are oriented perpendicularly to the surface, this surface enamel is more resistant to etching than ground enamel, where deeper layers are exposed.

The number of prisms per surface area varies from the more centrally located enamel towards the surface.[13,14] At the tooth surface there are approximately 20,000–30,000 prisms per mm^2. At the dentin-enamel junction the density is approximately 10 % higher. These numbers correspond well with the number of odontoblasts.

Dentin

The general composition of dentin is quite different from enamel and much closer to the composition of bone (see Fig 3-1). Dentin is produced for the whole life from the odontoblasts lining the pulpal wall. This process starts during tooth formation at the dentin-enamel junction. Odontoblasts form first a collageneous matrix, called predentin, which is mineralized later on (Fig 3-3). The predentin consists of collagen b-fibrils and a basic substance rich in mucopolysaccarides. The fibrils build up a network which is mainly oriented perpendicularly to the length axis of the odontoblastic process (Fig 3-4). The calcification of the dentin occurs in the form of globuli, where the apatite crystals are laid down. The size of the crystals is small (20-25 Å width, 200-300 Å diameter, and 300–600 Å length).[10] The shape is needle- or platelet-like.[15] As in enamel, the mineralization does not occur continuously, but in a rhythmic pattern, which leaves a striation of the dentin (v.

Ebner lines). On their move away from the dentin-enamel junction, the odontoblasts leave a cellular processus behind, which remains attached to the cell. In a second phase, this odontoblastic process is used as a transport medium to build up the calcification of the wall of the odontoblastic canal leading to the highly mineralized peritubular dentin.[16] Owing to this configuration, dentin is a vital tissue, able to react against insults such as caries or other trauma (Fig 3-5). Therefore it is difficult to characterize dentin as a substrate—it is extremely inhomogeneous and variable with regard to circumstances, such as position in relation to the pulp, age and external trauma.

Overall, the structure of dentin can be described as follows (Fig 3-6). The odontoblastic process is embedded in liquid, which is in a tube (dentinal tubulus) of highly mineralized dentin called peritubular dentin. These tubes are bonded together by less-mineralized dentin called intertubular dentin. Since the arrangement of the tubuli is centripetal, the quantity per surface area varies. Most (c. 45,000 per mm^2) are found close to the pulp, while in the periphery, at the dentin-enamel junction, the number is significantly decreased, to 20,000 per mm^2.[17,18] Owing to the liquid contained in the tubuli, and the collagen content, dentin is a wet substrate; the closer we come to the pulp the more fluid from the tubules we have to expect.

The odontoblastic process also contains nerve fibers close to the body of the odontoblastic cell which are responsible for the transmission of the sensation of pain.[19–21] Every fluid movement within the odontoblastic process is transduced into pain.[22] This is the mechanism of painful tooth necks. Any process causing fluid movement within the tubulus, e.g. desiccation, temperature change or osmotic processes, will cause pain. After trauma or constant irritation, dentin may become sclerotic due to Ca-phosphate deposition within the odontoblastic process.[23–28] However, constant acid attacks may dissolve these protective "plugs".

Owing to its structure per se, and to pulpal physiology, the pulpal-dentin complex is very well equipped to fight any chemical and bacteriological insult.

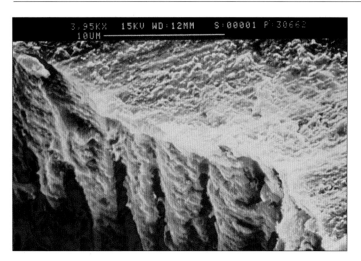

Fig 3-7 Smear layer of prepared dentin (SEM).

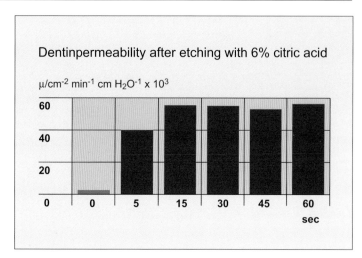

Dentinpermeability after etching with 6% citric acid

μ/cm^{-2} min^{-1} cm H_2O^{-1} x 10^3

Fig 3-8 The permeability of dentin and acid etched dentin.[36]

- Within the pulp there is a slightly higher pressure (approximately 30 cm H_2O) than in the environment. As a consequence, at open tubules there is an outward flow of the pulpal fluid within the tubuli, which means that every toxic agent must diffuse against this fluid stream.
- As mentioned above, tubules may calcify as a defending mechanism.
- Dentin is an excellent buffer; therefore it can absorb considerable quantities of acid.
- If any toxic agent may reach the pulp it will first encounter the very well vascularized sub-odontoblastic layer, where dilution can act as a countermeasure against toxic harm.
- Furthermore, the defense mechanisms are carried through blood vessels, being present in abundance in the subodontoblastic layer.

There is another issue which must be considered if dentin is to be used as a substrate for bonding: the smear layer, which is created after every instrumentation (Fig 3-7). This porous layer of about 1–7 μm is composed of hydroxyapatite and altered collagen.[29-32] The morphology and the thickness of the smear layer depend on the type of the instrument, the way it is used and on the site of the dentin.[32,33] It closes the dentinal tubules and prevents the seepage of dentinal fluid.[34] However, its most important feature is that it prevents contact between the substrate dentin and any potential adhesive. The smear layer can be easily removed by acid etching; however, this procedure also removes the smear plugs in the tubules, thus increasing the dentin permeability (Fig 3-8).[35,36]

Ceramics

First it should be mentioned that ceramics are defined as having a crystalline structure, unlike glass, which is not crystalline at all. For dental applications, pure glassy materials (i.e. fused-to-titanium "ceramics"); glassy materials with a certain amount of incorporated crystals, for instance, leucite or lithium disilicate (i.e. fused-to-metal "ceramics", e.g. Empress I, Empress II); and pure crystalline ceramics - real ceramics (i.e. aluminum oxide, zirconium oxide and glass-phase containing modifications thereof) (e.g. InCeram-Alumina, InCeram-Zircon) are used. However, all these types of glasses, glass ceramics and "real" ceramics are, in dentistry, covered by the general term "ceramic". Today different types of ceramics are available in order to manufacture ceramic restorations (Fig 3-9).

All ceramics can be subdivided as follows:
- silicon oxide (SiO_2)-based ceramics
- aluminum oxide (Al_2O_3)-based ceramics
- aluminum oxide-based ceramics reinforced with zirconium oxide (ZrO_2)
- pure aluminum oxide ceramics
- pure zirconium oxide ceramics.

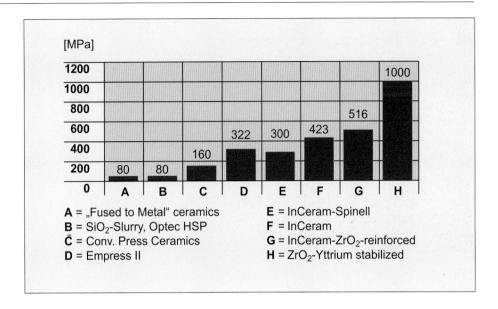

Fig 3-9 Strength of different ceramic types.

These ceramics not only differ in strength owing to their structure, but also in opacity. As a rule, silicon oxide-based ceramics are the most transparent, since they consist of a larger glass phase and only a small crystalline phase. Therefore they are able to create the best esthetics and are also able to pick up the color of their surroundings ("the chameleon effect"). To sum up, with an larger crystalline phase the strength of a ceramic material increases, but unfortunately so does its opacity. For this reason, Empress II, which provides the highest strength of all of today's silicon oxide-based ceramics, contains approximately 60% lithium disilicate crystals. However, its transparency is less compared with the conventional silicon oxide-based ceramics.

The strongest ceramics known for dental applications are aluminum oxide and zirconium oxide ceramics. They are 100% crystalline but also very opaque. Spinell, which is an aluminum oxide-based material, provides for its special crystalline structure (Spinell-structure) a significantly better transparency compared with pure aluminum oxide, but not as good as the silicon oxide-based ones. However, opacity might be a desired characteristic if severely discolored teeth must be masked with veneers. For this reason only silicon oxide-based ceramics will be considered in the following paragraphs.

A further differentiation is possible by considering the manufacturing method which depends on the respective ceramic (Table 3-1). Apart from those already mentioned, there are other techniques, such as sonoerosion, burnout and subsequent sintering, etc., which could be used to manufacture veneers.

Silicon oxide-based ceramics are characterized by a glass phase, which contains crystals (e.g. tetra silica mica, leucite, lithium disilicate). By etching away the glass phase it is possible to visualize the structure (Fig 3-10). They can be processed according to the slurry technique as well as to the press technique. However, the slurry technique is no longer used very often for this ceramic type. Optec HSP (Jeneric/Pentron Inc., USA) is, for instance, a ceramic processed on a refractory material.[37] The majority of silicon oxide ceramics is processed according to press techniques, which have several advantages, especially with regard to strength, homogeneity and fit.

Well-known ceramics of this type are:
- Empress I (Ivoclar/Vivadent AG, Liechtenstein)
- Empress II (Ivoclar/Vivadent AG, Liechtenstein)
- Finesse All Ceramic (Dentsply/Ceramco, USA)
- Carrara Press (Elephant, The Netherlands)
- Cergo (Degussa-Dental, Germany)
- Optec OPC (Jeneric/Pentron Inc., USA).

Silicon oxide ceramics are also machined, as is the case with the Cerec System (Sirona AG, Germany, Cerec-Blocks: Vita, Germany). However, other machining systems (e.g. Celay (Mikrona AG, Switzerland), DCS Precident System (DCS

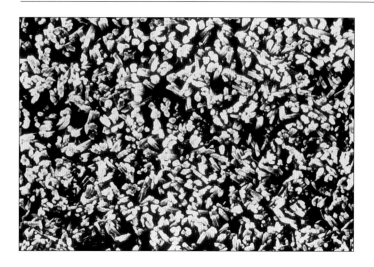

Fig 3-10 Structure of a silicon dioxide based ceramic (Dicor). The glass phase is etched away, exposing the tetra mica silica crystals (SEM).

Table 3-1 Types of ceramics and processing techniques

| Type of ceramic | Processing techniques | | | |
	Slurry	Press	Machined	Casting
SiO_2	X	X	X	X
Al_2O_3			X	
Al_2O_3 glass modified			X	
Al_2O_3 glass infiltrated	X		X	
Al_2O_3 ZrO_2-reinforced	X		X	
$MgAl_2O_4$ Spinell	X			
ZrO_2 YTZP			X	

Dental AG, Switzerland) or DigiDent (Girrbach, Germany)) can be used. Table 3-1 lists casting as a processing technique, too. Between 1985 and 1995 this technique was very popular and successful. It is known under the trademark Dicor (Dentsply International Inc., USA). Dicor was the first really acceptable all-ceramic system which provided good esthetics as well.[38,39] However, production was stopped in the last years of the twentieth century because the product has been substituted by ceramics providing higher strengths and improved processing and esthetic properties. Today the strongest dental silicon oxide ceramic known is Empress II, with a flexural strength of more than 300 MPa.[40] High-strength, non silicon oxide-based ceramics are quite opaque and, therefore, not suitable for the

manufacture of ceramic veneers. We will not discuss these materials as possible substrate for bonding within this chapter.

Adhesive Technique

Basic principles of adhesion

To achieve a good bond between two different materials, several prerequisites need to be fulfilled. To accomplish adhesion, the two substrates must come into very close contact. Only if the molecules are approached in a nanometer range intermolecular forces may be built up. For solid substrates this is almost impossible, because of

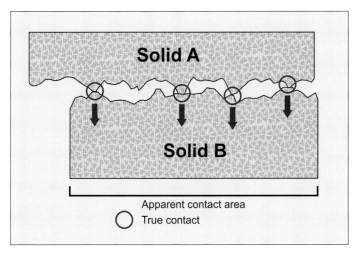

Fig 3-11 Intimate contact of two solids. Difference between true contact area and apparent contact area.

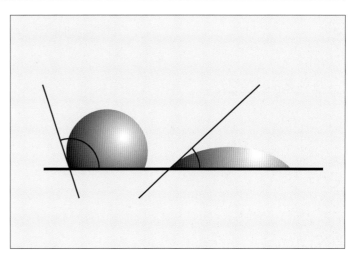

Fig 3-12 Contact angles of wetting (low contact angle, right) and non-wetting (high contact angle, left) liquids on a surface.

the surface morphology. Therefore, there is a large difference between the apparent contact area and the area of true contacts (Fig 3-11). This is the reason only small forces may be obtained with this mechanism – for example, two glass plates in close contact. This problem is solved by filling in the gaps left with an adhesive. The adhesive must be capable of getting into intimate contact with both surfaces – i.e. wetting them perfectly – which is only possible if the surface characteristics are compatible with the adhesive. For the mostly hydrophobic resins, which are used as enamel adhesives or restorative materials in dentistry, high surface energies and perfectly dry surfaces are required. This is shown with the contact angle. If the surface matches the wetting liquid, then the liquid tries to cover a surface as large as possible (low contact angle, Fig 3-12). If there is a mismatch, then the surface will try not to accept the liquid (high contact angle, see Fig 3-12).

Furthermore, the design of the adhesive configuration must be optimized to reduce interfacial stress. The larger the surface, the better. This rule is very favorable for the bonding of veneers, where very large surfaces are available for bonding.

Bonding to enamel

Almost fifty years ago, *M. G. Buonocore* published an article in which he showed that it is possible to bond acrylic resins to enamel, if the enamel is etched with phosphoric acid and rinsed and dried prior to the application of the resin.[41] This opened the road for the first steps in adhesive dentistry: the reliable bond to enamel. Untreated enamel has a very low surface energy and is therefore not suitable for bonding. Furthermore it is covered by a biofilm consisting of glycopolysaccharides from saliva. By removing this biofilm and etching the enamel with 37% phosphoric acid, two changes occur which are very favorable for bonding:[42] the surface energy of the enamel is increased considerably and, owing to selective dissolution, a microretentive surface is created that can be optimally penetrated by the hydrophobic diacrylate resins, which are the matrix of composite resins and which are used as enamel-bonding agents.

Therefore, enamel bonding is mainly a micromechanical interlocking of resin with the enamel surface. Resin may penetrate into undercuts or may shrink during polymerization on top of rodlike structures created by the etching process. This can only occur if all traces of humidity are eliminated, which is seen when the etched enamel becomes chalky in its appearance. All traces of water and other contamination (saliva, blood

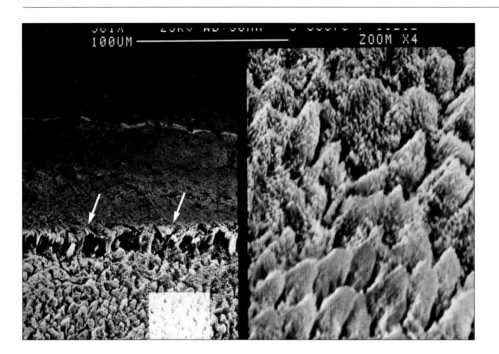

Fig 3-13 Substance loss created by etching enamel for 30 seconds (SEM).
left side, bottom: enamal is etched;
top: unetched enamel, the height of the ledge (arrow) is indicating the substance loss;
right side: higher magnification of etched enamel.

sulcus fluid) would compete with the hydrophobic resins and of course win the race. With appropriate technique, approximately 30 MPa of bond strength may be obtained, if the enamel prisms are cut more or less perpendicularly before etching and bonding.

The 37 % phosphoric acid seems to be the best compromise between substance loss and histological changes of the surface morphology. Etching for 30 seconds creates approximately 10 μm of substance loss (Fig 3-13).

The classical enamel bonding technique consists of precisely etching the enamel with a phosphoric acid gel[43] for 30 seconds, then rinsing vigorously with a water-air spray to remove all precipitates and finally, carefully and completely drying the enamel surface with a blast of air before applying the hydrophobic enamel bonding agent.

Bonding to dentin

Bonding to dentin has proven to be more complex and difficult. Reliable materials and techniques were offered to dentists only after it was realized that a permanent bond to dentin is possible if a micromechanical bond is achieved[44] (Fig 3-14). Two important approaches were changed in the treatment philosophy.

1. Dentin must be etched, which does not harm the pulp.
2. Hydrophilic resins must be used which are able to penetrate into the etched dentin surface despite its moist condition.[45]

To accomplish an appropriate micromechanical bond to dentin, which yields approximately 30 MPa, the following fundamental steps are required.

1. Etch the dentin surface in order to decalcify the surface for a few microns depth. By this means the collagen fibers are denuded and ready to be used as retention for the components of the adhesive system. In this phase it is important not to desiccate the dentin because then the collagen fibers would collapse and stick together, hindering the proper penetration of any components of the adhesive system.[46] On the other hand, if the dentin is kept too wet, then the so-called "over wet phenomenon" occurs, which means that the components of the adhesive system are diluted too much, again hindering sufficient penetration of monomers.[47] The preferable acid is phosphoric acid, which should be applied for not more than 15 seconds. If the dentin is over etched, then the etching is too deep and, again, the monomers may not penetrate fully the demineralized zone, yielding poor bond and probably facilitate nanoleakage (microleakage within the hybrid

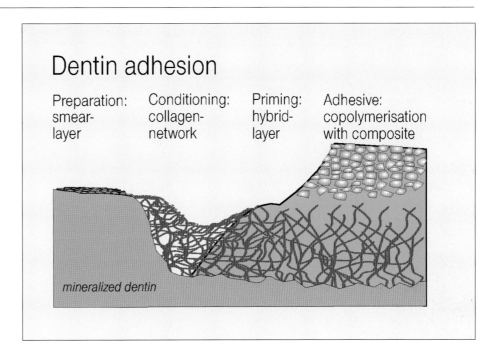

Dentin adhesion

| Preparation: smear-layer | Conditioning: collagen-network | Priming: hybrid-layer | Adhesive: copolymerisation with composite |

mineralized dentin

Fig 3-14 Principle of bonding to dentin.

layer). Sclerotic dentin should be etched for 30 seconds.

2. The etched dentin surface must be primed, i.e. penetrated with hydrophilic or amphiphilic monomers. These monomers are only able to penetrate into the wet collagen network. This penetration is possible either by the extreme hydrophilic character of the monomer (e.g. HEMA) and/or is supported by hydrophilic solvents such as acetone or alcohol. Penetration requires time, so it is very important to follow precisely the time indicated in the instructions issued by the manufacturer.[48] Usually, priming is finished by gently drying the surface with air, in order to evaporate the solvent excess.

3. The primed dentin surface is now ready to accept the adhesive, which is usually more hydrophobic and must be compatible with the composite resin of the reconstruction or the luting composite. At this stage the resin-infiltrated dentin is very fragile. It is therefore mandatory to polymerize this layer prior to applying the restoration.[46] If this is not done, the polymerization shrinkage of the overlaying composite will destroy the hybrid layer right away.

In order to facilitate the use of adhesive systems, manufacturers have tried to combine some steps. This has lead to different classes of adhesives, which are very different in their application

(Fig 3-15). There are two separate approaches regarding the conditioning process of enamel and dentin—the "total-etch technique" and the use of "self-etching bonding" systems. Within the first group we find products like Optibond FL (Kerr) and Scotchbond MP (3M Espe), which include the separate application of primer and adhesive after etching enamel and dentin simultaneously. This group of products is also called "multi-step adhesive systems". In order to simplify the application, a group of one-bottle adhesives in combination with the total-etch technique can be identified, also described as "etch and prime-bond". With these products (e.g. One Coat (Coltène), Optibond Solo Plus (Kerr), Prime & Bond NT (Dentsply), Scotchbond Single Bond (3M Espe) and Excite (Vivadent)), the manufacturers use a primer-adhesive, i.e. a mixture of hydrophilic and hydrophobic monomers. The problem with this mixture is to combine the function of a primer (to facilitate the penetration of the bonding system into the etched dentin) with the function of the adhesive (to level the cavity surface for a perfect adaptation of the composite resin).

There is also the growing group of products acting as so-called "self-etching bondings". The idea is that by being acidic enough to condition enamel and dentin, these primers can penetrate into the demineralized surface during the condi-

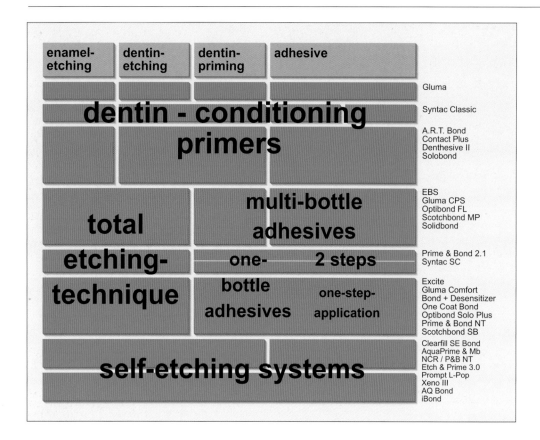

enamel-etching	dentin-etching	dentin-priming	adhesive	
				Gluma
				Syntac Classic
dentin - conditioning primers				A.R.T. Bond Contact Plus Denthesive II Solobond
total etching-technique	**multi-bottle adhesives**			EBS Gluma CPS Optibond FL Scotchbond MP Solidbond
	one- bottle adhesives	**2 steps**		Prime & Bond 2.1 Syntac SC
		one-step-application		Excite Gluma Comfort Bond + Desensitizer One Coat Bond Optibond Solo Plus Prime & Bond NT Scotchbond SB
self-etching systems				Clearfill SE Bond AquaPrime & Mb NCR / P&B NT Etch & Prime 3.0 Prompt L-Pop Xeno III AQ Bond iBond

Fig 3-15 Simplification of adhesive systems.

tioning process. Therefore, because one has never to rinse away the acid, all the problems of desiccated or over wet dentin should be solved. However, there is some concern regarding the reliability of bonding to enamel with these products. Although the acidity of these systems is not sufficient to create pronounced etching patterns (Fig 3-16), the bond strength to cut enamel is not statistically different from enamel surfaces etched with phosphoric acid. However, bonding to uncut enamel is statistically lower by using self-etching adhesives than after acid-etching.[48,49]

One group of products within the self-etching bondings can be described as "etch-prime and bond" (e.g. AquaPrime & MonoBond (Merz), Clearfil Liner Bond 2V (Kuraray) and Clearfil SE Bond (Kuraray)) with separate application of the self-etching primer and the adhesive.

Another group, etch-prime-bond, can be called self-etching adhesives and should be the ultimate simplification regarding the application of adhesive. This group again can be divided into two subgroups. Because of the required high acidity there is a problem regarding shelf life of the adhesive resins. Therefore, in one subgroup the components must be stored separately, forcing the dentist to mix the solution directly prior to application (e.g. Etch & Prime 3.0 (Degussa), Futurabond (Voco), Prompt L-Pop (3M Espe), One Up Bond F (Tokuyama) and Xeno III (Dentsply). Some manufacturers have proposed a number of intelligent mixing devices (Fig 3-17) (e.g. Prompt L-Pop) to facilitate this mixing procedure. Despite their simplicity, they have not yet completely fulfilled expectations. The other subgroup of self-etching adhesives solved the shelf life problem by further developments of monomer systems which do not need to be mixed and can be applied directly from the bottle (e.g. AQ Bond, Sun Medical) and iBond (Heraeus Kulzer).

As we have mentioned, it is important that such resin-impregnated dentin layers are stabilized by polymerization before a composite resin is placed on top, so as to prevent debonding at the interface due to the polymerization shrinkage of the composite. For precise veneers, inlays and crowns this poses a problem, since pooling of the bonding agent may prevent a precise relocation of the ceramic piece into the cavity. There are two ways out of this situation.

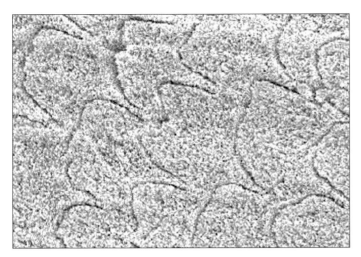

Fig 3-16 Etching pattern in enamel created by a self-etching primer (SEM).

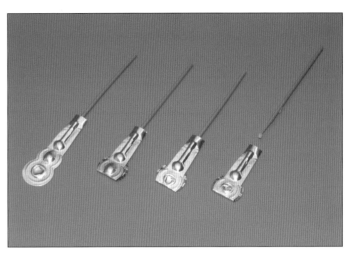

Fig 3-17 Mixing device for self-etching adhesive (Prompt-L-Pop).

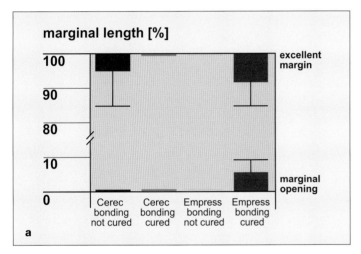

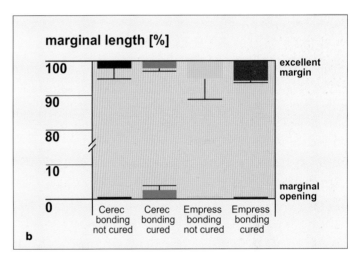

Fig 3-18a, b Margin quality of ceramic inlays bonded to teeth with Etch & Prime. (a) Box plots show the enamel composite interface. (b) Box plots show the dentin composite interface (*Clotten, Blunck, Roulet,* Influence of a simplified application technique).

1. The dentin is sealed right after the cavity preparation and then the enamel finishing line is cleaned again to make sure that it is resin free prior to the impression. At the next appointment the cavity is cleaned carefully with pumice before the veneer/inlay/crown is luted with an adhesive technique.[50]

2. The dentin must be sealed with an adhesive of very low viscosity which does not interfere with the restoration, even if it is polymerized prior to the insertion of the veneer/inlay/crown. *Clotten, Blunck* and *Roulet*[51] have demonstrated that with such a technique it is possible to obtain an excellent margin quality in vitro with ceramic inlays (Fig 3-18a and b).

Bonding to ceramics

A reliable bond of composites to ceramics is also achieved by micromechanical retention. Feldspathic (silicon oxide) ceramics and lithium silicate ceramics contain a glass phase[38,39,52] that can be etched with hydrofluoric acid[53-55] or similar compounds,[39] exposing the crystallites contained in the ceramic to create microretentions. Based on chemical knowledge, hydrofluoric acid etching is only possible with SiO_2-based ceramics or glasses according to the reaction equation:

$$6\ H_2F_2 + 2\ SiO_2 \longrightarrow 2\ H_2SiF_6 + 4\ H_2O$$

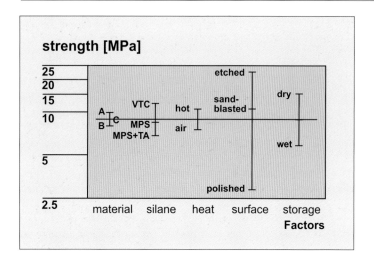

Fig 3-19 Factors influencing the ceramic-composite bond (*Roulet, Söderholm, Longmate,* Effects of treatment and storage conditions).

The etched surface can be wetted and penetrated by resins which provide a strong micromechanical bond to the ceramic. Sufficient bond strength is only reached if the resin used is able to penetrate deeply the microretentions created by the etching process. Ceramics tend to cover themselves with a monomolecular layer of water (from the humid environment), thus silanization of the surface increases "wettability" and bond strength.[55,56] Silanes need to be hydrolyzed to be reactive.[56] However, once activated (by acetic acid), they become unstable, because they tend to build up dimers, trimers, tetramers, etc., which are not reactive any more.[57] The more active a silane, the shorter is the shelf life. The best way to handle this problem is to use a two-component silane, which is activated by mixing with acetic acid prior to application. Preactivated silanes have a limited shelf life, especially after the bottles are opened and give access to water. Since this surface treatment is crucial for the clinical behavior, it is highly recommended to dentists to perform the conditioning of the ceramic's inner surface immediately prior to the insertion of the restoration. Only with this approach can one exclude any surface contamination, which would jeopardize the bonding of the ceramic restoration to the tooth. *Roulet, Söderholm* and *Longmate*[58] have clearly demonstrated that the most important factor for bond strength is the roughening of the ceramic surface (Fig 3-19).

The aforementioned chemical reaction cannot occur with high-strength alumina or zirconia ceramics since they do not contain a silicon oxide phase. Therefore, they cannot be roughened by etching with hydrofluoric acid. For this reason special treatments are indicated for these types of ceramic. Roughening is performed by sandblasting, usually with Al_2O_3. Furthermore, this roughened surface must be silica coated in order to make it "wettable" for the resin by silanization. This is done either by a tribochemical process (Rocatec, Coe Jet, 3M/Espe, Germany), where silica-coated particles are blown onto the surface with a high energy.[59-62] A further very effective method is flaming of the surface with a silane-enriched butane flame. There are two techniques: Silicoater[59,63,64] and PyroPen.[65] However, special glues (e.g. Panavia Ex) have also been successfully tested to bond zirconia ceramic.[62,66]

Product Recommendation for Bonding Veneers

Veneers are characterized by two specific features: they are usually very thin and transparent and they are bonded mostly (but not exclusively) to enamel. These two characteristics determine which bonding/luting systems should be selected. Since enamel is the prime target for bonding, reliable enamel bonding should be used. However, dentin may be involved too. Therefore, any

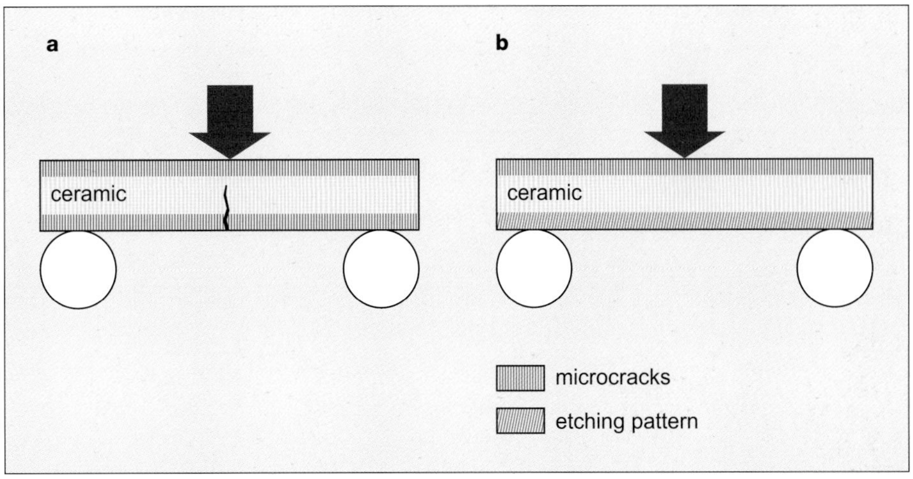

Fig 3-20a, b Crack propagation in a ceramic beam. (a) If the beam is under load, the lower side is under tensile stress, where cracks are initiated. (b) By etching the lower side of the beam the initial cracks are eliminated. Furthermore, the infiltrated composite, which is less brittle, decreases crack initiation.

total bonding system (i.e. any system where enamel and dentin are separately etched with phosphoric acid), such as etch, bond, prime systems or etch and prime-bond systems, are to be preferred. The ceramic must be etched and silanated immediately prior to insertion in order to optimize the "wettability" of the ceramic surface for diacrylate resins. The use of a two-component silane is recommended. From the luting composite, low-viscous light-cured systems should be preferred, because veneers are usually very thin and translucent. Only if very opaque veneers are to be cemented should one consider a dual-cured luting resin, especially since it is well known that these materials tend to show a yellow-brownish discoloration over time, owing to their higher amine content.

As clinicians, we would prefer the single systems where the manufacturer provides the dentist with a water-soluble try-in paste (e.g. Nexus2, Sybron-Kerr; Calibra, Dentsply) which allows us to check the final result prior to bonding the veneers in place permanently.

The Need for Bonding Ceramics

An inlay or a crown is frequently stressed similarly to a beam in a three-point bending test. If loaded from the occlusal surface, the inner surface of the ceramic restoration is subjected to tensile stress. Such situations are also possible with veneers.[67] Ceramic is a brittle material, and always contains micro cracks at the surface because of the finishing procedures. These micro cracks can propagate under load, even a moderate load, after fatigue of the biomaterial, with subsequent catastrophic failure (Fig 3-20a). There are two ways out of this problem: (1) improve the mechanical characteristics of the ceramic material, which leads to high strength ceramics (not suitable for veneers owing to their high opacity), or (2) eliminate/prevent the crack propagation at the inner surface of the restorations. This is done with adhesive techniques.

The question is: why are bonded ceramics more resistant to fractures? One can hypothesize that etching diminishes micro cracks, and after penetration of the surface with a resin-based material (composite) that is less brittle than ceramic, more stress at the inner surface is required to induce fractures (Fig 3-20b). This hypothesis is supported by several publications based on laboratory data. Fracture strength of ceramic beams is improved if the lower surfaces are carefully polished to a high gloss,[68] or strengthened (e.g. by ion addition[69,70] or by adhesively coating with composite resin).[71] There has also been clinical evidence for this behavior. Analysis of the survival rate of 1,444 Dicor complete crowns was performed using *Kaplan Meier* statistics by *Malament* and *Socransky*,[72,73] and they reported significantly better results for acid-etched and bonded restorations after fourteen years (Fig 3-21).

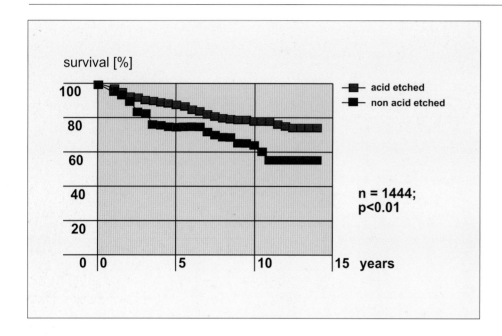

survival [%]

n = 1444;
p<0.01

Fig 3-21 Longevity of Dicor crowns (Kaplan-Meier statistics). Note that the bonded crowns show a superior longevity (*Malament, Socransky,* Survival of Dicor glass-ceramic).

The Benefit of Bonding for Veneers

Owing to the combination of excellent materials' characteristics and reliable bonding techniques, veneers are the optimal way to restore anterior teeth following the principle of minimal invasiveness. Finite element studies have clearly demonstrated that it is possible fully to restore the original strength of teeth with veneers.[67,74] We have confirmed this in a study.[75,76] Veneers were bonded with Variolink II (Vivadent) into more and more extensive veneer/crown preparations (Fig 3-22a-g). Afterwards they were loaded up to fracture. As can be seen in Fig 3-23, there were no statistical differences between natural teeth, which fractured at around 1,100 N, and all veneers and crown with finishing lines in enamel. The fracture analysis revealed that no tooth fractured at

the bonded interface. We found either cohesive fractures in the tooth (Fig 3-24a, b) or within the ceramic (Fig 3-24 c).

When veneers were placed on top of existing class III or class IV composite restorations,[77,78] the fracture load was in a range between 800 N and 1,000 N (median, Fig 3-25), which was only slightly less than the values obtained for the teeth restored with different veneers with finishing lines in enamel, and definitely better than the values for the teeth restored with veneers/crowns with finishing lines in dentin (see Fig 3-23). The use of composite repair materials had no influence on the fracture resistance of the veneers. However, the margin quality at the composite-composite interface was superior if composite repair materials were used.

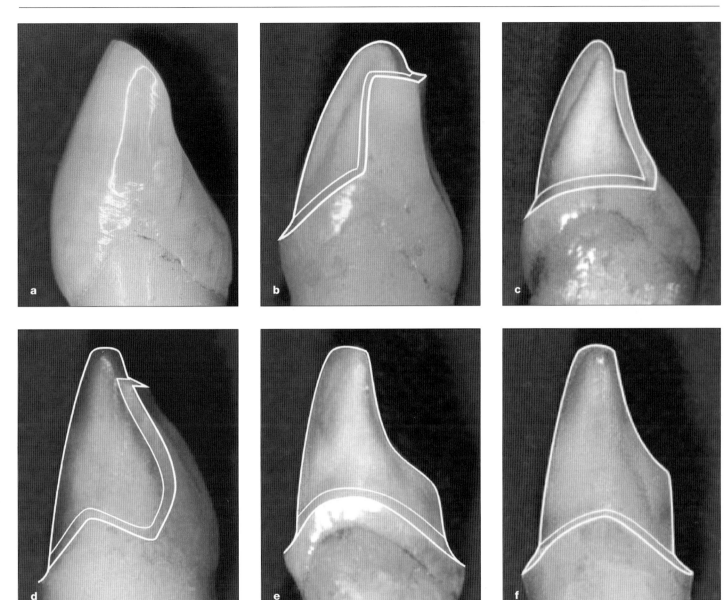

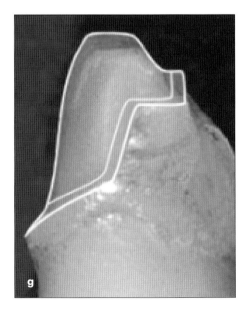

Fig 3-22a-g More and more extensive veneer/crown preparations on human central incisors seen proximally.

(a) Intact tooth.

(b) Preparation for veneer labial.

(c) Preparation for veneer proximal; finishing line cervical in enamel.

(d) Preparation for veneer proximal; finishing line cervical in dentin.

(e) Preparation for full crown, finishing line in enamel.

(f) Preparation for full crown, finishing line in dentin.

(g) Preparation for veneer on abraded tooth.

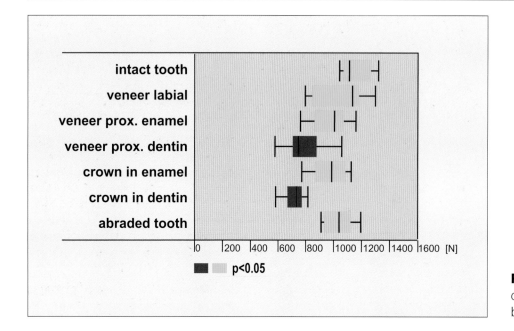

Fig 3-23 Fracture strength of human central incisors restored with veneers/ bonded ceramic crowns.

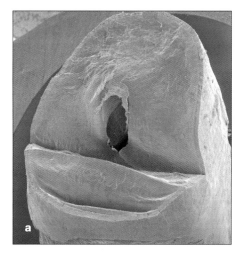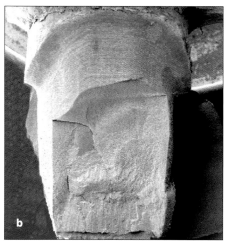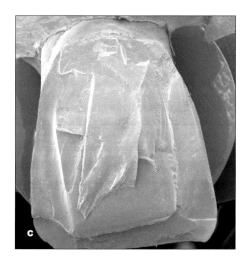

Fig 3-24a-c Tooth restored with veneer, fracture after loading up to failure. (a) Cohesive fracture at tooth neck. (b) Cohesive fracture in tooth, with small adhesive fracture portion. (c) Cohesive fracture in ceramic.

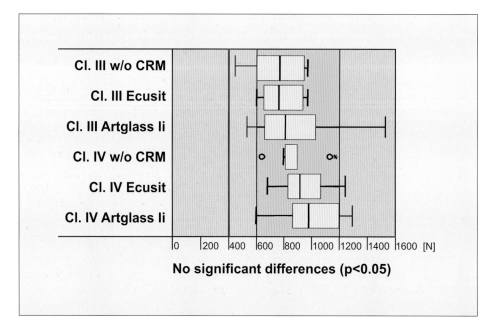

Fig 3-25 Fracture strength of human incisors restored with veneers placed on top of existing class III and class IV composite restorations.

w/o CRM = without composite repair material.

Artglass li and Ecusit = composite repair materials.

Conclusion

Veneers require reliable bonding mechanisms between ceramic and composite on one side and between tooth substance and composite on the other side to be feasible and successful. With the right selection of dental adhesive systems it is possible today permanently to bond veneers to anterior teeth and restore the original strength of the teeth. In the past, veneers were restricted to enamel as a substrate for bonding. Modern dental adhesives allow also bonding of veneers, if some portions of the preparation are in dentin. A meticulous adhesive technique with appropriate moisture control is a prerequisite for successful integration of veneers.

References

1. Roulet J-F, Degrange M. Adhesion. The Silent Revolution in Dentistry. Chicago: Quintessence, 1979.
2. Roulet J-F, Wilson NHF, Fuzzi M. Advances in Operartive Dentistry. Vol. 1. Chicago: Quintessence, 2001.
3. Wilson NHF, Roulet J-F, Fuzzi M. Advances in Operative Dentistry. Vol. 2. Chicago: Quintessence, 2001.
4. Brudevold F, Söremark R. Chemistry of the mineral phase of enamel. In: Miles AEW. ed. Structural and Chemical Organization of Teeth. Vol. 2. New York and London: Academic Press, 1967:247.
5. Angmar-Månsson B. Studies on the Distribution and Ultrastructure of the Main Components in Human Dental Enamel. Stockholm: Dr. Odont thesis, 1970.
6. Schröder HE. Orale Strukturbiologie. Stuttgart: Thieme, 1976:60-129.
7. Gwinnett AJ. The ultrastructure of the "prismless" enamel of deciduous teeth. Arch Oral Biol 1966;11:1109-1116.
8. Gwinnett AJ. The ultrastructure of the "prismless" enamel of permanent human teeth. Arch Oral Biol 1967;12:381-388.
9. Boyde A. The Structure of Developing Mammalian Dental Enamel. In: Stack MV, Fearnhead RW eds. Tooth Enamel. Bristol: John Wright and Sons Ltd., 1965:163-167.
10. Höhling HJ. Die Bauelemente von Zahnschmelz und Dentin aus morphologischer, chemischer und struktureller Sicht. Munich: Hanser, 1966.
11. Rönnholm E. An electron microscopic study of the amelogenesis in human teeth. II. The development of enamel chrystallites. J Ultrastruct Res 1962;6:249.
12. Frazier PD. Adult human enamel: An electron microscopic study of crystallite size and morphology. J Ultrastruct Res 1968;22:1-11.
13. Fosse G. The number of prism bases on the inner and outer surfaces of the enamel mantle of human teeth. J Dent Res 1964;43:57.
14. Fosse G. A quantitative analysis of the numerical density and the distributional pattern of prisms and ameloblasts in dental enamel and tooth germs. IV. The number of prisms per unit area on the outer surface of human permanent canines. Acta Odont Scand 1968;26:409; V. Prism density and pattern of the outer and inner surface of the enamel mantle of canines. Acta Odontol Scand 1968;26:501; VII. The numbers of cross-sectioned ameloblasts and prisms per unit area in tooth germs. Acta Odontol Scand 1968;26:573.
15. Eisenmann DR, Glick PL. Ultrastructure of initial crystal formation in dentine. J Ultrastruct Res 1972;41:18-28.
16. Takuma S. Ultrastructure of Dentinogenesis. In: Miles AEW. ed. Structural and Chemical Organization of Teeth. Vol. 1. New York and London: Academic Press, 1967.
17. Garberoglio R, Brännström M. Scanning electron microscopic investigation of human dentinal tubules. Archs Oral Biol 1976;21:355-362.
18. Ketterl W. Studie über das Dentin der permanenten Zähne des Menschen. Stoma 1961;17:148.

19. Frank RM. Ultrastructure of Human Dentine. In: Fleisch H, Blackwood JJJ, Owen M. eds. Calcified Tissues. Berlin: Springer, 1966.

20. Frank RM, Sauvage C, Frank P. Morphological basis of dental sensitivity. Int Dent J 1972;22:1-19.

21. Roane JB, Foreman DW, Melfi RC, Marshall FJ. An ultrastructural study of dentinal innervation in the adult human tooth. Oral Surg Oral Med Oral Pathol. 1973;35:94-104.

22. Brännström M. Sensitivity of dentine. Oral Surg 1966;21:517.

23. Bergmann G, Engfeldt B. Studies on mineralized dental tissues. VI. The distribution of mineral salts in the dentine with special reference to the dentinal tubules. Acta Odontol Scand 1955;13:1.

24. Ericsson SG. Quantitative microradiography of cementum and abraded dentine. A methodological and biological study. Acta Radiol Diagn (Stockh).1965;(Suppl.)246.

25. Tronstad L. Optical and microradiographic appearance of intact and worn human coronal dentine. Arch Oral Biol 1972;17:847-858.

26. Tronstad L. Scanning electron microscopy of attrited dentinal surfaces and subjacent dentine in human teeth. Scand J Dent Res 1973;81:112-122.

27. Mjör IA. Histologic studies of human coronal dentine following the insertion of various materials in experimentally prepared cavities. Arch Oral Biol 1967;12:441-452.

28. Mjör IA. Human coronal dentine: Structure and reactions. Oral Surg Oral Med Oral Pathol 1972;33:810.

29. Douglas WH. Clinical status of dentine bonding agents. J Dent 1989;17:209-215.

30. Eick JD, Wilko RA, Anderson CH, Sorensen SE. Scanning electron microscopy of cut tooth surfaces and identification of debris by use of the electron microprobe. J Dent Res 1970;49:1359-1368.

31. Gwinnett AJ. Smear layer: morphological considerations. Oper Dent Suppl 1984;3:3-12.

32. Tronstad L. Ultrastructural observations on human coronal dentin. Scand J Dent Res 1973;81:101-111.

33. Suzuki T, Finger WJ. Dentin adhesives: site of dentin vs. bonding of composite resins. Dent Mater 1988;4:379-383.

34. Pashley DH. Smear layer: overview of structure and function. Proc Finn Dent Soc 1992,88(Suppl 1):215-224.

35. Pashley DH. Dentin permeability and dentin sensitivity. Proc Finn Dent Soc 1992;88(Suppl 1):31-37.

36. Erickson RL, Glasspoole EA, Pashley DH. Dentin permeability changes from acidic dentin conditioners. J Dent Res 1991;70:378 (Abstr 903).

37. Vaidyanathan TK, Vaidyanathan J, Prasad A. Properties of a new dental porcelain. Scanning Microsc 1989;4:1023-1033.

38. Adair PJ. Glass ceramic dental products. US Patent No 4, 431 420, 1984.

39. Adair PJ, Grossman DG. The castable ceramic crown. Int J Periodontics Restorative Dent 1984;4:32-46.

40. Ludwig K, Kubick S. Vergleichende Untersuchungen zur Bruchfestigkeit von vollkeramischen Frontzahnbrücken. Dtsch Zahnärztl Z 1999;54:711-714.

41. Buonocore MG. A simple method of increasing the adhesion of acrylic filling materials to enamel surfaces. J Dent Res 1955;34:849-853.

42. Lutz F, Lüscher B, Ochsenbein H, Mühlemann HR. Adhäsive Zahnheilkunde. Zürich: Abteilung für Kariologie und Parodontologie, Zahnärztliches Institut, Universität Zürich (Selbstverlag);1976.

43. Noack MJ, Roulet J-F. Rasterelektronenmikroskopische Beurteilung der Ätzwirkung verschiedener Ätzgele auf Schmelz. Dtsch Zahnärztl Z 1987;42:953-959.

44. Nakabayashi N, Kojima K, Masuhara E. The promotion of adhesion by infiltration of monomers into tooth substrates. J Biomed Mater Res 1982;16:265-273.

45. Perdigao J, Lopes M. Dentin bonding. Questions for the new millennium. J Adhesive Dent 1999;1(3):191-209.

46. Peschke A, Blunck U, Roulet J-F. Influence of incorrect application of a water-based adhesive system on the marginal adaptation of class V restorations. Am J Dent 2000;13:239-244.

47. Tay FR, Gwinnett AJ, Wei SH. Micromorphological spectrum from overdrying to over wetting acid-conditioned dentin in water-free, acetone-based, single-bottle primer/adhesives. Dent Mater 1996;12:236-244.

48. Pashley DH, Tay FR. Aggressiveness of contemporary self-etching adhesives. Part II: Etching on unground enamel. Dent Mater 2001;17:430-444.

49. Hannig M, Reinhardt KJ, Bott B. Self-etching primer vs phosphoric acid: An alternative concept for composite-to-enamel bonding. Oper Dent 1999;24:172-180.

50. Bertschinger C, Paul SJ, Lüthy H, Schärer P. Dual application of two dentin bonding agents. J Dent Res 1996;75:257 (Abstr 1919).

51. Clotten S, Blunck U, Roulet J-F. The influence of a simplified application technique for ceramic inlays on the margin quality. J Dent Res 1998;77:942 (Abstr 2483).

52. Craig RG. Restorative Dental Materials. 8th ed. St Louis, MO: Mosby, 1989, 481-498.

53. Calamia JR. Etched porcelain facial veneers: A new treatment modality based on scientific and clinical evidence. NY J Dent 1983;53:255-259.

54. Calamia JR, Simonsen RJ. Effect of coupling agents on bond strength of etched porcelain. J Dent Res 1984;63:179.

55. Calamia JR, Vaidyanathan J, Vaidyanathan TK, Hirsch SM. Shear bond strength of etched porcelains. J Dent Res 1985;64:296 (Abstr 1086).

56. Plueddemann EP. Adhesion through silane-coupling agents. J Adhesion 1970;2:184-194.

57. Roulet J-F. Degradation of dental polymers. Basel: Karger, 1976.

58. Roulet J-F, Söderholm KJM, Longmate J. Effects of treatment and storage conditions on ceramic/composite bond strength. J Dent Res 1995;74:381-387.

59. Edelhoff D, Abuzayeda M, Yildirim M, Spiekermann H, Marx R. Adhäsion von Kompositen an hochfesten Strukturkeramiken nach unterschiedlicher Oberflächenbehandlung. Dtsch Zahnärztl Z 2000;55:617-623.

60. Göbel R, Luthardt R, Welker D. Experimentelle Untersuchungen zur Befestigung von Restaurationen aus Zirkonoxid und Titan. Dtsch Zahnärztl Z 1998;53:295-298.

61. Vogel K, Salz U. Factors influencing adhesion to Al_2O_3- and ZrO_2-ceramics. J Dent Res 1998;77:941 (Abstr 2475).

62. Wegner SM, Kern M. Long-term resin bond strength to zirconia ceramic. J Adhesive Dent 2000;2:139-147.

63. Musil R, Tiller H-J. Das Silicoater Verfahren nach fünfjähriger klinischer Bewährung. Zahnärztl Praxis 1989;4:124-128.

64. Musil R, Tiller H-J. Der Kunststoff-Metall-Verbund Silicoaterverfahren. Heidelberg: Hüthig, 1989.

65. Janda R, Roulet J-F, Wulf M, Tiller H-J. A new adhesive technology for all-ceramics. Dent Mater 2002 (submitted).

66. Kern M, Wegner SM. Bonding to zirconia ceramic: Adhesion methods and their durability. Dent Mater 1998;14:64-71.

67. Magne P, Belser U. Bonded Porcelain Restorations in the Anterior Dentition: A Biomimetic Approach. Chicago: Quintessence, 2002.

68. Fairhurst CW, Lockwood PE, Ringle RD, Thompson WO. The effect of glaze on porcelain strength. Dent Mater 1992;8(3):203-207.

69. Anusavice KJ, Shen C, Lee RB. Strengthening of feldspathic porcelain by ion exchange and tempering. J Dent Res 1992;71(5):1134-1138.

70. Anusavice KJ, Shen C, Vermost B, Chow B. Strengthening of porcelain by ion exchange subsequent to thermal tempering. Dent Mater 1992;8(3):149-152.

71. Rosenstiel SF, Gupta PK, Van der Sluys RA, Zimmerman MH. Strength of a dental glass-ceramic after surface coating. Dent Mater 1993;9(4):274-279.

72. Malament KA, Socransky SS. Survival of Dicor glass-ceramic dental restorations over 14 years. Part 1. Survival of Dicor complete coverage restorations and effect of internal surface acid etching, tooth position, gender, and age. J Prosthet Dent 1999;81:23-32.

73. Malament KA, Socransky SS. Survival of Dicor glass-ceramic dental restorations over 14 years. Part 2. Effect of thickness of Dicor material and design of tooth preparation. J Prosthet Dent 1999;81:662-667.

74. Magne P, Douglas WH. Additive contour of porcelain veneers: a key element in enamel preservation, adhesion, and esthetics for aging dentition. J Adhesive Dent 1999;1:81-92.

75. Raffelt C. Die Auswirkungen verschiedener Präparationsformen auf das Bruchverhalten menschlicher Frontzähne mit adhäsiv befestigten IPS Empress Veneers und Kronen. Thesis, Berlin: HU, 2002.

76. Roulet J-F, Raffelt C, Pfeiffer H, Blunck U, Chun Y-H. The strength of anterior teeth with bonded porcelain veneers and crowns. J Dent Res 2002;81 (Spec Iss A):A415 (Abstr 3357).

77. Pfeiffer H. Applikation von Veneers auf mit Kompositfüllungen versorgten Frontzähnen unter Berücksichtigung des Komposit- Komposit Verbundes. Thesis, Berlin: HU, 2002.

78. Chun Y-H, Pfeiffer H, Raffelt C, Blunck U, Roulet J-F. The quality of anterior veneers placed on composite restorations. J Dent Res 2002;81 (Spec Iss A):A250 (Abstr 1921).

4 Porcelain–Bonded Restoration and Function

Claude R. Rufenacht

Introduction

The field of function and occlusion has been widely investigated. We know today most of the parameters that contribute to good function. Unfortunately, in a modern general practice, where dentists concentrate their efforts mastering technically sensitive esthetic materials, little attention is paid to the application of these elements of knowledge. Emphasis is placed on the intrinsic beauty of a restoration, which all too often hides functional disturbances that insidiously develop in the oral cavity. Yet an appreciation of existing occlusal conditions and functional disturbances is critical when the restorative procedure involves porcelain-bonded restorations that neither wear nor show flexibility. In the constraining oral conditions, the esthetic finality of a restoration only makes sense when it is associated with its functional finality (Figs 4-1 and 4-2).

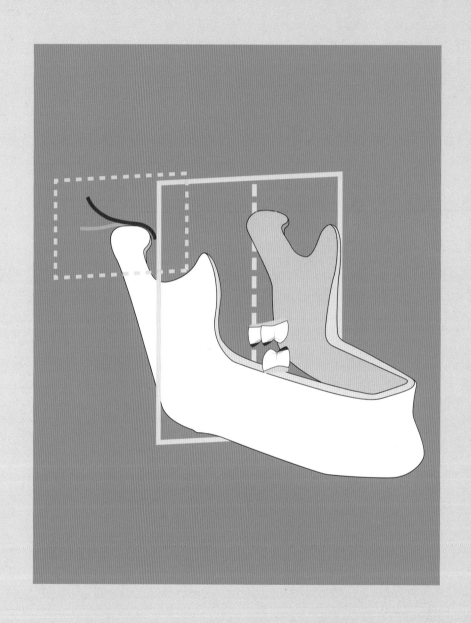

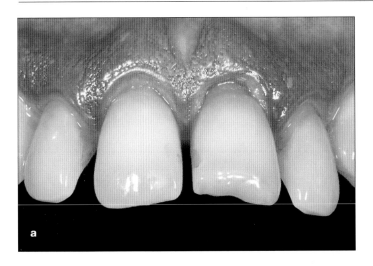
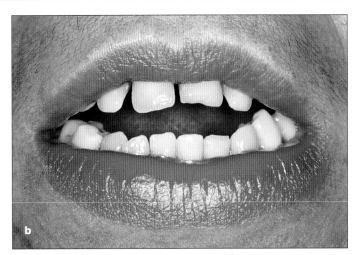
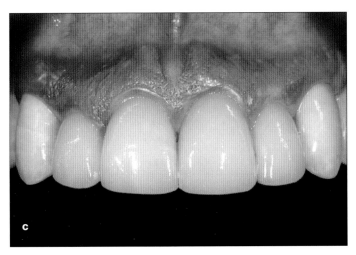
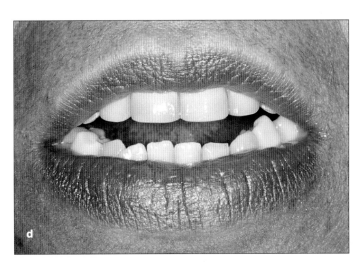

Fig 4-1a-d Migration of the whole anterior segment. (a) In occlusal relationships characterized by an anterior open-bite. (b) The restoration of this segment with porcelain-bonded restoration can certainly improve dental esthetic conditions but not tooth stability. (c) Long-term occlusal stability will require lifetime use of a removable acrylic night-guard, even if maxillary central incisors have been shortened to minimize tongue pressure.

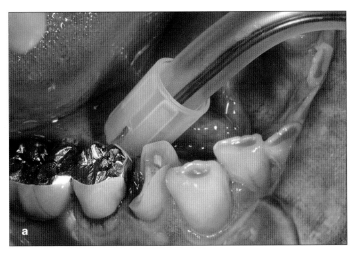
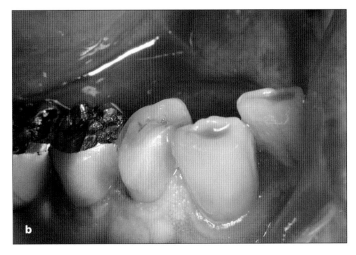

Fig 4-2a, b Such a porcelain-bonded restoration is designed to adapt or conform to antagonist or adjacent deformities. This design not only fools a basic principle of dental esthetics, which is the duplication of the morphologic reality, but its survival in such constraining occlusal conditions is limited. It broke seven years after insertion.

The Tooth-Porcelain-Bonded Restoration Complex

Enamel and dentin form a composite structure providing the natural tooth with unique characteristics which enable it to withstand for years the impact of masticatory forces and thermal variation. In this composite entity the hardness of the enamel seems to protect the soft underlying dentine, while the softness of the dentin and the presence of collagen fibers at the dentino-enamel junction provide the whole tooth with ideal biomechanical properties, and seem to compensate for the brittle nature of the enamel.[1] One can easily imagine that porcelain-adhesive material and remaining dental tissue could not only duplicate the original tooth structure but also reproduce the biomechanical properties of the original dentino-enamel complex.

Recent researches, however, have shown noticeable differences between these two entities. The strength of the tooth veneer complex was found to be greatly superior to that of the natural tooth in an in-vitro load-to-fracture test.[2,3] This has led to the hypothesis that the excess strength of the complex tooth porcelain-bonded restoration may lead to a stress transfer and failures at the level of the root, simulating the fractures affecting conventional restorations such as gold crowns or inlays, which are experienced in clinical practice.[4] To overcome these possibilities of fracture, attention has to be given to the proper design and adequate thickness of porcelain-bonded restorations[5–8] – elements that must be understood with the objectives of the most favorable load configuration or stress distribution,[9–11] or a search for a tooth porcelain-bonded restoration complex more compatible with the mechanical and biological properties of the original dental tissues.

Indeed, porcelain may well contribute to the recovery of crown biomechanical properties and compensate for structural tooth weakness following carious lesions, abrasion or erosion,[12] yet the advantages of increased strength remain questionable when flexibility is considered to be essential in the qualities of any structure to withstand the impact of a traumatic blow.[13] In this respect, the idea to modulate tooth resilience by the combination of composite resin and ceramics to reproduce the biomechanical characteristics of the original tooth deserves to be developed whenever such an approach is realistic.

We know that, whatever their design, all porcelain-bonded restorations increase tooth stiffness. Yet the restoration of the original tooth compliance can best be obtained with a large build-up of composite material replacing the fractured part of an incisor and covered with a thin facial layer of ceramics slightly overlapping lingually.[11] Clinically one has to point out that this type of restoration is loaded with the unfavorable high thermal expansion of the composite and may lead to marginal adaptation failures.

Fortunately, clinicians' inclinations have always clearly favored restoring fractured incisors with full ceramic restorations, for reasons including enamel-like thermal expansion, color stability and refined esthetics, unconsciously choosing increased tooth stiffness and low stress distribution versus flexibility. Thanks to research, these can be easily optimized by increasing ceramic thickness at the incisal level and reducing its overcontour.

Clinically it can be stated that, despite marked differences in biomechanical properties with the natural tooth, porcelain-bonded restorations have demonstrated their predictability in terms of fracture rate, microleakage or debonding during more than a decade of clinical practice and clinical studies.[14–19]

This has encouraged clinicians and researchers to extend the field of indications of porcelain-bonded restoration to substantial morphological modifications, extensive hard tissue fractures and even worn-out dentitions.[2,20–23] This supposes a full confidence in the nature and qualities of the adhesive systems relating the tooth to constraining occlusal conditions and the porcelain restoration even when submitted to the adverse conditions of a reduced hard tissue support. This reduced hard tissue support surface must be considered with attention as it not only could affect the maintenance of tooth vitality but question the reliability of the adhesion of the porcelain-bonded restoration.

Porcelain–Bonded Restoration and Pulpal Health

The combination of tooth fracture and tooth preparation may lead to excess dentin reduction that will affect not only the vitality of the tooth substrate but the integrity of pulpal tissue. We know that the closer one approaches to the pulp, the higher content of organic material is found in the smear layer as a result of a widening of odontoblast-containing tubuli, while intratubular dentin lessen. This increase of organic material in the oral environment faces high possibilities of deterioration.

Indeed, as the organic portion of the smear layer is lost, microchannels usually occur, allowing bacteria and by-products to gain access to dentinal tubuli.[24,25] This invariably creates a situation that leads to pulp inflammation. Therefore, control of the biodegradable smear layer becomes imperative to ascertain dentinal vitality, pulpal health and postoperative sensitivity.

The protection of the dentin must be considered as a key clinical step in porcelain-bonded restoration preparation, which in most systems available today consists in the cleaning of the dentin, usually by way of a removal of the smear layer, and the seal of the tubuli. The removal of the smear layer is carried out by etching, either by the application of a 10-3 solution (10% citric acid with 3% of ferric chloride) or a phosphoric acid solution (which has the advantage of providing a lower tensile strength to dentin, probably because of an increased denaturing of the collagen fibers).[26]

It remains to ascertain the biologic seal of dentinal tubuli, which can be achieved clinically by hybridization, a procedure consisting in the formation of hybrid layers of demineralized dentin combined with an adhesive chemical agent. This hybridization is the most currently accepted mechanism for dentin bonding, as research has shown that the hybrid layer obtained acts as a protection for ground dentin[27–29] and apparently succeeds in providing the maintenance of pulpal health.

Clinically, it remains to achieve a chemical bond between the adhesive coating layer and the resin luting cement in an association whose quality and biocompatibility are aimed at providing adhesive strength to the tooth-porcelain-bonded restoration entity to resist the constraining forces of the occlusion.

Occlusion

Occlusion refers to the act of closure and the state of being closed. It involves at the same time dynamic and static components. Static components will be first considered.

In a good occlusion, all the teeth in the mouth make simultaneous contacts. It is, however, acknowledged that in the anterior segment teeth should have lighter contacts, which clinically may mean: "anterior teeth do just not contact". Indeed, the perception of a fremitus at interocclusal contact can be detrimental to tooth stability and lead to interproximal separation.

The total tooth contact area, which includes the anterior and posterior teeth, averages 4 mm^2. Considering the number of interocclusal contacts (64 to 100 for the whole mouth), taking into account varying opinion and the type of occlusion,[30,31] each single contact area is estimated to be extremely small. The multiplication of posterior interocclusal contacts is mandatory for improving stress distribution, as studies have shown that in the posterior segment, muscle contraction develops at 100%, whether you have single or multiple contacts[32] (Fig 4-3).

In nature, cusp to ridge contacts are the rule and characterize class I occlusions. Cusp to fossa contacts are usually found in class II occlusions, while the tripodization of interocclusal contacts remains a dream, born from the imagination of dentists anxious to provide tooth stability.

A coincidental location of tooth interocclusal contact and porcelain-bonded restoration margin should be avoided, as alterations of the marginal seal of porcelain-bonded restoration can be more often stated than when the opposing contact is located elsewhere.[33]

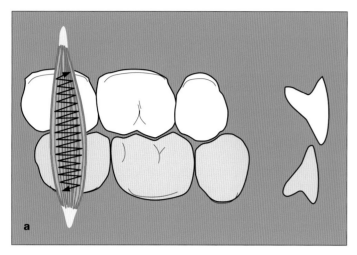
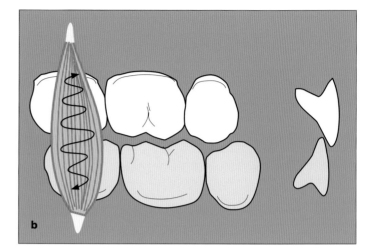

Fig 4-3a, b Research has shown (a) When only posterior teeth are allowed to contact, muscle contraction develops at 100%, whatever the number of interocclusal contacts. (b) When a single anterior tooth does contact in the absence of posterior contacts, muscle ability to contract is highly reduced but tends to increase proportionally with the number of anterior contacts.

Whenever this recommendation finds easy application in the anterior segment, clinical practice shows that the posterior segment appears as a privileged area where interocclusal contacts and PBR margins are coincidental by reason of posterior tooth morphology and the nature of interocclusal relationships. Observation shows also that it is in this area that the morphological design of the restoration is distorted to adapt to antagonist deformities, or inserted in a dental segment presenting various manifestations of abrasion (Fig 4-2). As a result, the possibilities of coincidental location of margin placement and enlarged interocclusal contacts increase. And with them the chances of altering the marginal seal resulting from porcelain microfractures under the load of occlusion. It can be assumed that further deteriorations of the marginal seal of porcelain-bonded restoration can take place under the impact of parafunctional habits such as clenching, when margin placement and interocclusal contacts are coincidental. This stresses the importance of tooth preparation for porcelain-bonded restorations that has not only to foresee interocclusal contact location but provide sufficient porcelain thickness to allow porcelain-bonded restoration to offer adequate resistance to constraining parafunctional conditions.

Function

Function takes place at the very moment teeth enter into action. This dynamic part of occlusion refers to the engagement of mandibular teeth towards centric, and to their disengagement. The spatial development of functional movements is dictated by condylar pathway, antagonist tooth morphology and tooth position. It displays at the registration a three-dimensional tracing delimiting an area defined as "the envelope of mandibular function" characterized by a droplet shape displaying, as a result of antagonist tooth morphology and position, infinite individual variations (Fig 4-4). This makes teeth the primary factors in tooth-closing patterns.[34–36] It has been established that tooth-closing patterns remain under neuro-muscular control – even if the exact nature of this phenomenon has always escaped scientific explanation.[37]

If we know most of the parameters that participate in function, the observation of unworn long-lasting dentitions clearly indicates the type of oral architecture that best integrates these parameters. These occlusions are characterized by similar parameters in the vertical and horizontal planes: that is to say in the overbite and overjet of incisors and canines. Frontal chewing patterns have an angle of about 70° from the horizontal for the canines and in eccentric occlusion we find a

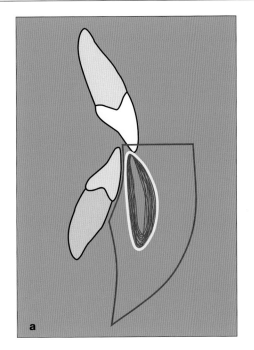
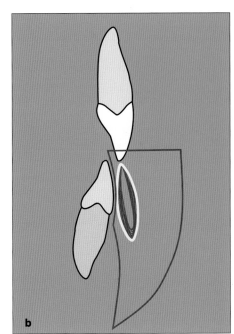
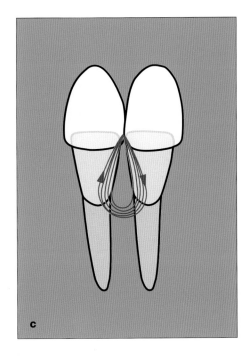
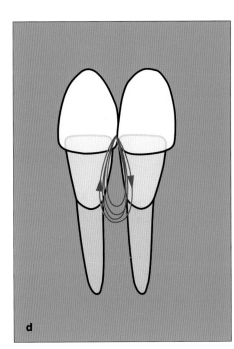

Fig 4-4a-d The "envelope of mandibular function" is, apparently, primarily dictated by antagonist tooth morphology and tooth position. It displays a characteristic droplet shape with noticeable individual differences in the sagittal (a, b) and frontal planes (c, d). Variations from those characteristic droplet shapes can be interpreted as the expression of a malocclusion.

tooth-to-tooth contact with a large posterior clearance (Fig 4-5). This tooth-to-tooth contact in eccentric occlusions can be considered as ideal, as it generates, according to research, a reduced muscular activity in comparison to group function and bi-balanced occlusion (Fig 4-3b).[38,39]

In these dentitions, morphologic integrity is the rule. The teeth can receive porcelain-bonded restorations without any specific restriction, but in respect of the environmental morphologic design: function follows forms. Functional integration will then be achieved by the control of simultaneous interocclusal contacts and the absence of interferences during tooth closure patterns.

In nature, however, oral architectural ideals are not the rule. Research has shown that in a selected population the occurrence rate of malocclusion, which includes open-bite, over-bite, class II and class III occlusions, averages 20%.[40] As a result, one in every five patients does not present an incisal pathway reflecting usual stan-

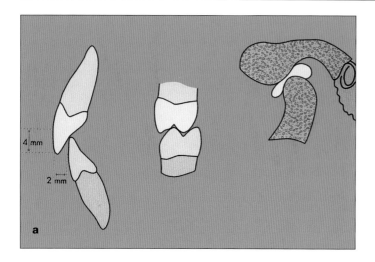

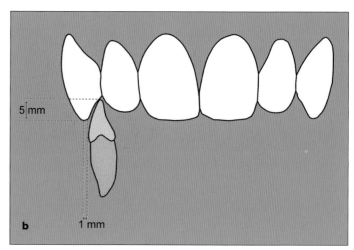

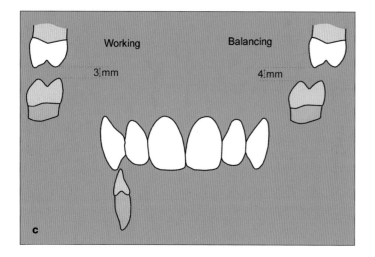

Fig 4-5a-c Long-lasting dentitions show similar characteristics: multiplication of interocclusal contacts for better stress distribution in centric occlusion and in eccentric occlusions, a tooth-to-tooth contact reducing muscle activity and preventing any possibility of posterior interference. A duplication of these parameters in reconstructions should ascertain long-term maintenance and occlusal stability. (a) Mean anterior relationships in the sagittal plane for the incisor. (b) Mean anterior relationships in the frontal plane for the canine. (c) Frontal relationships in right eccentric occlusion.

dards, which leads them to consider correction by way of orthodontics or orthopedic surgery. It also appears that out of the remaining 80% of class I occlusions; most occlusal schemes do not show anterior relationships, duplicating those displayed in long-lasting dentitions. Variations in the depth of the overbite, width of the overjet, and related incisal and canine guidance are unlimited, which justifies or imposes corrective measures necessary to prevent posterior interferences during function.

By deduction, it can be advanced that one of the challenges faced by restorative dentists in restoring a physiological occlusion is the changing of poorly related anterior relationships. The restoration of an anterior segment should never be envisaged from the viewpoint of minimal tooth preparation for veneer seating but from that of occlusal maintenance and functional excellence.

Occlusal maintenance involves the evaluation and correction of localized manifestations of wear affecting one anterior tooth or the whole anterior segment, concomitant with an appreciation of the degree of incisal or canine guidance necessary to prevent posterior interferences in eccentric occlusions. The achievement of these objectives requires an increase of the steepness of the disclusive angle which, depending on oral conditions, can be achieved either with an increase of vertical interocclusal relationships by way of a tooth elongation or with a reduction of horizontal relationships. A combination of these therapeutic measures is not unusual. Clinically, a modification of the palatal morphology of maxillary incisors and canines appears best suited to improve tooth guidance without compromising esthetics (Fig 4-6). The nature of this modification remains to be defined as long as it leaves open the question of the ideal steepness of the interocclusal angle

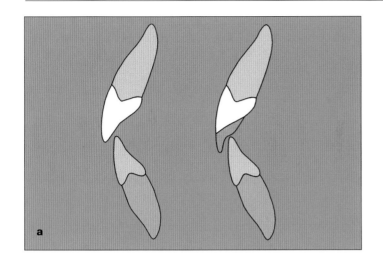

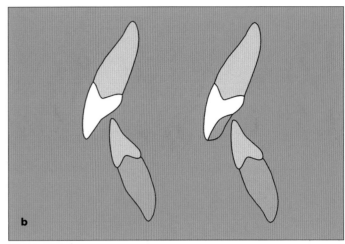

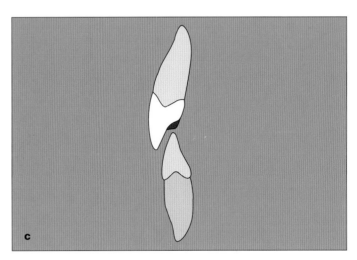

Fig 4-6a-c The improvement of anterior relationships for optimum guidance and occlusal maintenance may require a modification of maxillary anterior teeth morphology best achieved using porcelain-bonded restorations. (a) Palatal modification to correct insufficient horizontal parameters. (b) Incisal lengthening with palatal morphologic modification to correct insufficient vertical parameters following incisal wear. (c) Build-up of cingulum to prevent the eruption of antagonist mandibular incisors, correcting poor horizontal relationships.

(Fig 4-7). Mechanically, it appears that the deeper the angle the greater the likelihood of achieving tooth guidance and the greater the impossibility for posterior teeth contacting in eccentric occlusions. From a muscular point of view, the increase of the steepness of the disclusive angle may also produce a favorable result as it generates a proprioceptive inhibition that will shut down muscular activity thus reducing the load level in eccentric occlusions. This muscle inhibition has been explained by an increase of the torsional load affecting the teeth in their housing. This leads to a triggering effect on proprioceptive receptors[41,42] preventing muscles contacting harder through a feedback effect. However, careful attention must be paid, so that the increase in the disclusive angle does not cause the teeth, through their morphology or position, to interfere with neurological programmed tooth closure patterns. This will invariably lead to the abrasion of

antagonist anterior tooth surfaces, mandibular buccal or maxillary lingual surfaces (Fig 4-8). Damage of this type affecting antagonist surfaces is mainly generated by overcontoured porcelain-bonded restorations but may also be found in orthodontic and orthognathic cases.

In the absence of available clinical possibilities of tracing three-dimensional, programmed tooth closure patterns for want of an articulator programmed to register this information, it is left to the dentist's sensibility to prevent restorations impinging on the area of function. Despite these restrictions, there is no better restorative material today than porcelain-bonded restoration to achieve functional and esthetic excellence or to duplicate the conditions found in long-lasting dentitions. All that remains is to apply the appropriate treatment at an appropriate time.

The maintenance of occlusal stability requires the detection and treatment of early manifesta-

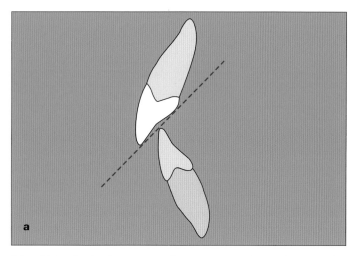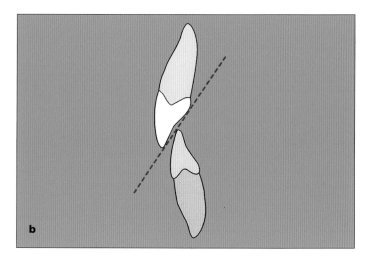

Fig 4-7a, b In the restorative process, the main remaining question is not the ideal interocclusal angle that should be given to anterior interocclusal relationships to ascertain tooth-to-tooth contact in eccentric occlusions but the individual limit allowed to the increase of the disclusive angle (a, b).

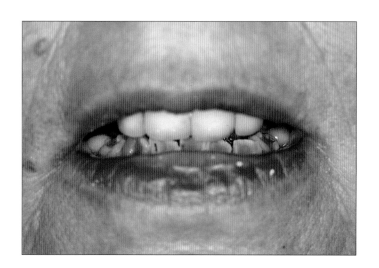

Fig 4-8 There is an individual limit to the increase of anterior interocclusal contact angle beyond which the tooth, through its morphology and position, may interfere with neurological programmed path of closure. The clinical consequences of this interference will abrade the facial surface of lower anterior teeth and/or lingual aspect of maxillary anterior teeth. An unfortunate design of the palatal aspect of maxillary porcelain-bonded restoration, including a probable increase of incisal width, is at the origin of antagonist hard-tissue destruction.

tions of wear affecting one anterior tooth or another (Fig 4-9). Given this opportunity of localized and restricted treatment, either the extension of occlusal degradation, labeled as occlusal disease, will invariably extend laterally to the lateral incisors and canines when affecting first the central incisors, or medially when canines have been first subjected to abrasion.

The period necessary for the spread of occlusal disease along the whole anterior segment offers many opportunities to motivate patients to restore anterior esthetics and function at the same time (Fig 4-10). But once buccal inclines of premolars and molars have been erased, the mesially inclined slopes of lower molars distalized or their

antagonist distally inclined slopes mesialized, when posterior tooth morphology has disappeared, nothing other than a full mouth restoration can be proposed to the negligent patient (Fig 4-11).

To satisfy a functional finality, this full mouth restoration involves the setting-up of anterior relationships generating the steepest possible anterior guidance capable of developing, over the long term, atraumatic tooth closure patterns during the functions of speech, deglutition and mastication.

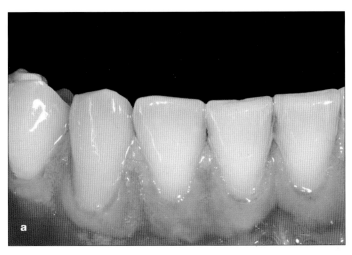 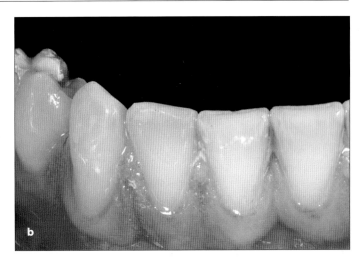

Fig 4-9a, b Initial manifestation of occlusal disease affecting the lower canine at a young age. (a) The porcelain-bonded restoration extending from lingual to incisal is expected to increase vertical relationships and disclusive angle (b) and prevent any possibility of interference in eccentric occlusions.

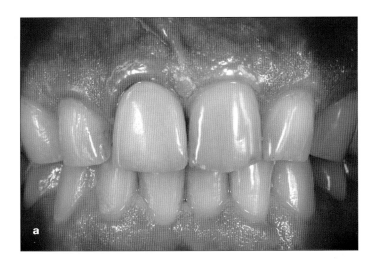 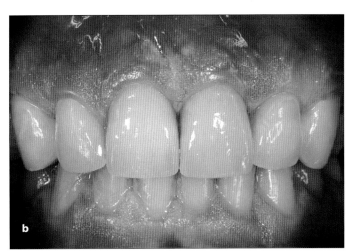

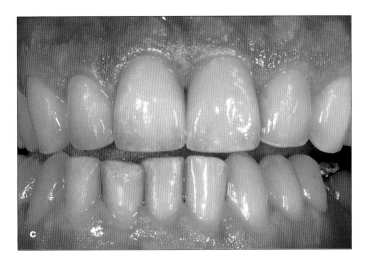

Fig 4-10a-c The extension of tooth wear patterns from canines to lateral and central incisors (a) offers a unique opportunity esthetically to restore the anterior segment and at the same time to ascertain long-term stability. Functional stability will then depend upon increasing anterior guidance through increased anterior relationships (b) to prevent any possibility of posterior contact during tooth closer patterns (c).

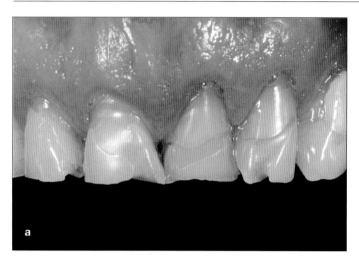 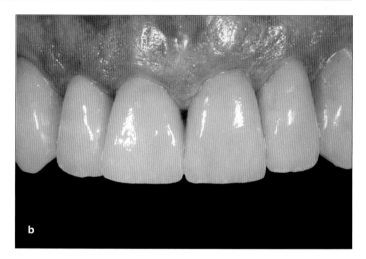

Fig 4-11a, b Once anterior and posterior segments have been erased (a) there remains no alternative for the restorative dentist other than proposing a full mouth reconstruction to restore esthetics and function (b).

Incising

Mastication starts with the incision of food, which is followed by a lateral chewing phase. This lateral chewing phase can be divided in an early tooth-closing phase and a late tooth-closing phase. Incising requires an initial mouth-opening necessary to introduce food followed by a closing movement of the mandible, which develops in the sagittal plane and places upper and lower incisors in a tip-to-tip position. This movement seems to load incisors along their long axis and bring both condyles in a forward and downward translation. With unworn incisors there is no more than 1mm of shearing load confined in the incisal edge of teeth. This shearing load will increase dramatically in the presence of worn-out incisal edges. As a result, the tip-to-tip incisal biting will gradually become a surface-to-surface biting, overloading incisors away from their long axis, allowing for the posterior confinement of condyles leading in turn to adverse neuro-muscular response. Finally, the incisal edges of the lower incisors will glide back along the lingual wall of maxillary incisors, a movement which develops atraumatically under neuromuscular control. Yet the presence of an increased incisal tip width affecting lower incisors will definitely overload the anterior teeth forcing lingually mandibular incisors (Fig 4-12).

It is therefore essential that porcelain-bonded restorations duplicate in their incisal design sharp unworn natural teeth and present in their whole configuration the most adequate compromise in terms of internal stress distribution and stress transfer following axial or horizontal loading.[6]

These mechanical requirements have to be considered when the presence of interproximal carious lesions, composite restorations, or tooth fractures impose a lingual extension of anterior maxillary porcelain-bonded restorations. In the same way, the palatal extension of porcelain-bonded restorations in the design of maxillary incisors and canines becomes unavoidable when functional finality demands:

- an improvement of anterior guidance to correct insufficient horizontal or vertical interocclusal relationships (Fig 4-6a)
- the design of cingulum and lateral palatal ridges to create punctiform centric interocclusal contacts and to prevent the eruption of lingually positioned antagonist lower incisors (Fig 4-6b).

To optimize the configuration of porcelain-bonded restorations one has to know that the area of the cingulum presents the lowest tensile strength of the whole palatal side at a tangential blow of 50 N directed against the incisal edge.[7] It can therefore be considered as an ideal location of porcelain-bonded restoration margin. Above all, a marginal location of porcelain-bonded restoration in this area of low tensile strength

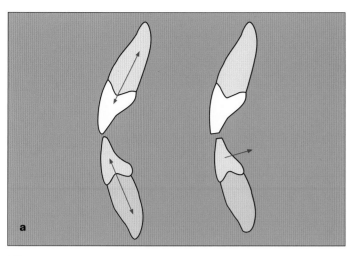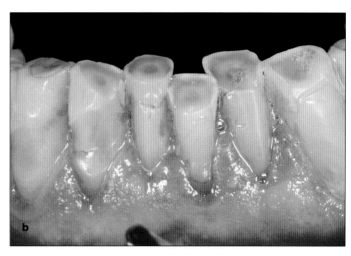

Fig 4-12a, b It is acknowledged that the incising function loads the teeth along their long axis (a). The evidence of an overload following the wear of the incisor edges can be clinically stated with the lingual migration of antagonist mandibular incisors (b).

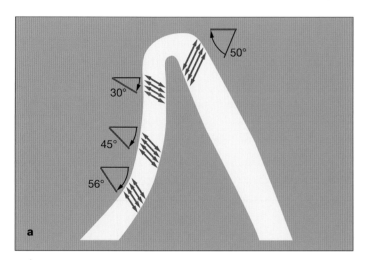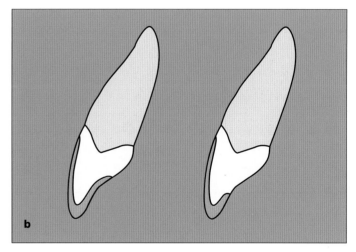

Fig 4-13a, b The direction of enamel rods varies from the incisal third to the palatal concavity and the cingulum. It presents an increasing angle to the horizontal from 30° to more than 50° (*Magne P, Douglas WH*).[6] (a) This imposes a specific design of porcelain-bonded restoration finish line according to its location. In the cingulum area a long chamfer cutting enamel rods at 90° is ideal for optimum adhesion, while a butt margin design remains perfectly valid. In the incisal third, the direction of the rods showing an angle at 30° from the horizontal, a mini-chamfer remains the best margin configuration. (b) The placement of the finish line at the lingual concavity should be avoided by reason of the extreme tensile stress experienced in this area following an incisal tangential blow.

reduces the importance of the design of the finish line: a butt margin cutting the enamel rods at an angle superior to 50° is perfectly acceptable while a long chamfer will reveal particularly resistant inasmuch it will cut the rods at 90°, allowing for an improved adhesion to enamel[43] (Fig 4-13).

Even if studies have shown that this type of porcelain-bonded restoration configuration presents the lowest relative compliance,[11] knowing that resilience is a key factor in fracture resistance,[13] fracture rate remains extremely low in clinical practice, maybe thanks to dentin bonds that have been proven to be a main determinant in the fracture mechanic.[44] As previously mentioned, the palatal extension of porcelain-bonded restoration is the rule each time functional conditions advocate an increase of anterior guidance to allow for sufficient posterior interocclusal clearance in eccentric occlusions.

The functional indication for palatal extension varnishes in functionally good occlusions where tissue preservation predominates. A limited incisal palatal overlap remains the most valuable configuration as long as it is located in an area displaying low tensile strength, allowing for a finish line design that can be either a butt joint or chamfer.

These porcelain-bonded restoration configurations, palatal overlap or palatal coverage present the qualities to perfectly resist the incising function or the tearing apart of food. Only a palatal extension of the porcelain-bonded restoration with a finish line ending up in the palatal concavity has to be avoided, as this thin extension of ceramic is precisely located in an area of high tensile strength.

Normal function not only implies the incision of food but the chewing of food.

Lateral Chewing

Lateral chewing starts with mouth opening, followed by a lateral movement of the mandible to the working or chewing side. The working condyle is brought in a retruded lateral position while the nonworking condyles move medially. The amount of this lateral shift varies, depending upon bone configuration of condyle and fossa, shape and conditions of disc and ligaments.

The shifting of the working condyle or *Bennet* shift[45] affects the mediolateral incline of the posterior cusps and conditions the direction of the buccal groove of lower molars whenever the occlusal scheme presents in eccentric occlusions a group function or a balanced occlusion (Fig 4-14).

In functionally good occlusal schemes, however, the importance of the *Bennet* shift is irrelevant. In the early closing phase of mastication, which sees both working canines starting to proprioceptively engage the closing movement, the importance of the mediolateral inclination of posterior cusps is irrelevant.

In the final closing phase, however, the approach to centric of opposing molar cusps can lead to interferences because the vertical guidance of the canine does not totally negate the path of the shifting condyle. As a result, interferences can occur in the mediolateral inclines of the second and first molars, especially when the condyle-fossa complex generates in the horizontal plane a shifting in lateroprotrusion (Fig 4-14) or a shifting in laterosurtrusion in the frontal plane (Fig 4-15).

The wear resulting from these interferences affects the mediolateral inclines of mandibular or maxillary molars predominantly in areas characterized by a cusp to fossa relationship such as the central groove of maxillary and mandibular molars. This is best visualized in natural unworn dentitions (Fig 4-16). In good occlusal schemes this occlusal wear is irrelevant but it may reach a pathological level with a decrease of the anterior interocclusal angle.

Under these conditions the introduction of a restoration in these areas may reveal itself detrimental to marginal material integrity as interocclusal contacts and margin location are often coincidental. The integrity of the porcelain-bonded restoration can even be compromised when mesial or distal transitional zones of tooth preparation present a too-abrupt angulation (Fig 4-17).

Clinical observation shows that porcelain-bonded restoration fracture rate increases precisely in the mesial part of maxillary molars and in the distal part of mandibular molars in occlusal schemes showing poor canine guidance. These elements need a configuration of posterior porcelain-bonded restoration with sufficient material thickness and suggest coverage of mediolateral cusps designed with a reduction of the inclination of the mediolateral slopes and a reduction of the MO or OD transitional angle.

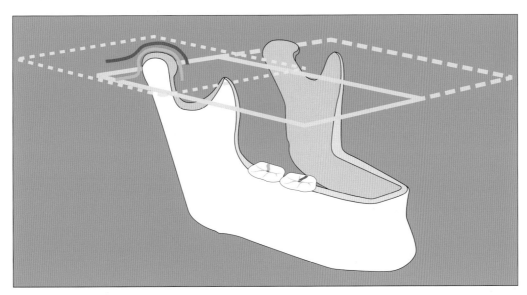

Fig 4-14 Pantographic tracing has demonstrated that in an occlusion provided with poor anterior relationships, the Bennet shift influences, in its horizontal tracing, the direction of the lingual groove of mandibular molars on the working side. However, in the late phase of closing patterns and in areas where cusp to fossa relationships can be found, a latero-protrusive Bennet pathway (green line) may generate the abrasion of the buccal incline of the lingual cusp of mandibular molar or lingual incline of maxillary buccal cusp due to the action of antagonist cusp. This suggests that porcelain-bonded restoration marginal integrity could be affected when placed in these locations and under these conditions. When good anterior relationships do exist, the influence of the Bennet shift on the horizontal plane is irrelevant.

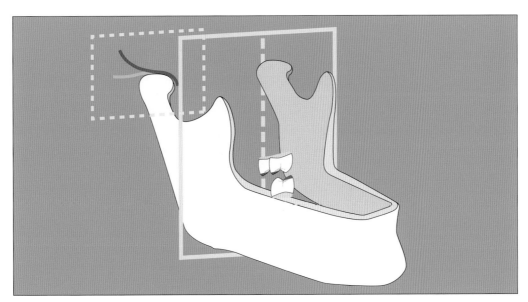

Fig 4-15 In the late phase of lateral chewing, to avoid the combined detrimental impacts of a Bennet shift showing not only a lateroprotrusion in the horizontal plane but also a laterosurtrusion in the frontal plane (red line), it could be helpful systematically to design the restoration with a more open mediolateral incline of maxillary buccal cusps or conversely mandibular lingual cusps, whatever the degree of guidance steepness. When applied to the maxillary posterior buccal cusps, this measure will highly improve the perception of the front-back progression.

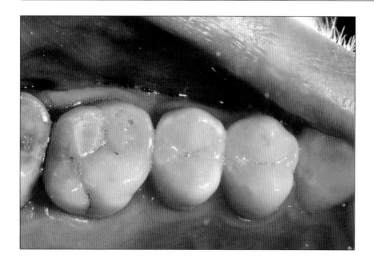

Fig 4-16 In functionally good occlusal schemes and in areas where cusp to fossa relationships do exist, wear-faceting affecting the mediolateral incline of maxillary buccal cusps, conversely mandibular lingual cusp, can be observed. It states that a steep vertical guidance cannot totally negate the path of the shifting condyle in the late phase of lateral chewing especially when it presents both a horizontal lateroprotrusion and a frontal laterosurtrusion.

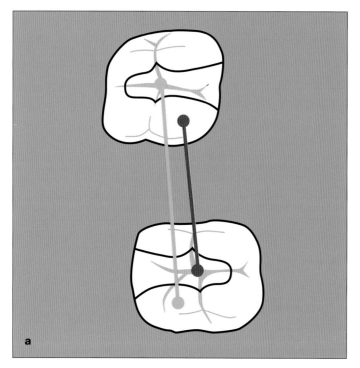

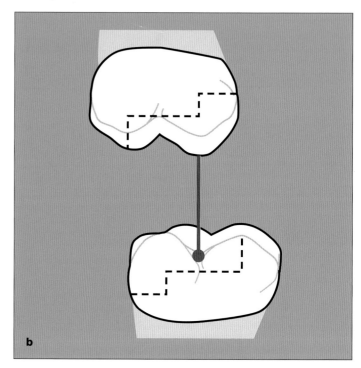

Fig 4-17a, b Constraining occlusal conditions such as poor anterior guidance cusp to fossa relationships. (a) Specific and individual TMJ morphology may affect the integrity porcelain-bonded inlays placed in strategic areas when weakened by too abrupt transitional zones. (b) Fracture rate seems to take place predominantly at the transitional zone of OD mandibular and MO maxillary inlays when placed on the first or second molar.

Dysfunction

The observation of unworn long-lasting dentitions has put in evidence harmonious relationships between skeletal and dental morphology and integrated function. It has long been speculated that abnormal function is mainly caused by abnormal tooth guidance. In turn, abnormal tooth guidance results from abnormal occlusal contact relationships.

We know that one out patient out of five does not have an incisal pathway reflecting an appropriate standard. Yet we can observe daily that out of the remaining patients reflecting appropriate standards in anterior pathways, few show or will show over the years an occlusal scheme free of wearing manifestations.

It can therefore be deduced from these observations that even appropriate standards in anterior pathways can display abnormal occlusal guid-

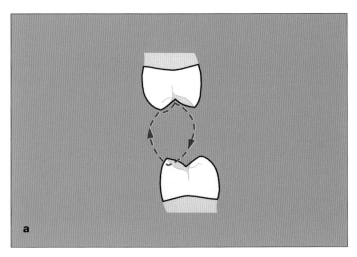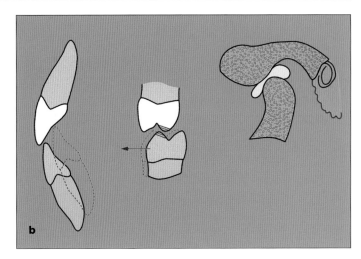

Fig 4-18a, b Frontal representation of a centric interference located in the mediolateral incline of a molar with lateral slide to centric. (a) Sagittal representation of interference leading to protrusive sliding during tooth closing patterns. (b) These types of interference can be easily eliminated by grinding.

ance. Submitted to registration these elements of abnormal guidance have been classified in a recent study in lack of guidance, poor guidance, overguidance, abnormal guidance, and interference.[46]

The presence of interferences in the development of tooth closure patterns has long been identified as the prime element of dysfunction. It has been even assumed that it could be at the origin of bruxism. There are two basic types of interferences:

- centric relation : anterior slide, lateral slide, protrusive-retrusive
- lateral border : non working and working side.

The elimination of centric interferences in the treatment of bruxism has always been controversial. In 1928, *Tischter* recommended occlusal adjustment in order to eliminate the so called "trigger contacts".[47] A large number of authors stress also the importance of eliminating these interferences in the treatment of bruxism,[48-50] while others deny any relationship between interferences and bruxism.[51] It appears, however, that clinically experienced practitioners never hesitate to proceed to occlusal correction before restorative procedure[52-60] by reason of the good results they obtained.

Dawson (1998) has written: "It is my experience that, when all occlusal interferences in centric relation and excursions have been eliminated on the posterior teeth, parafunctional movements resulting in anterior wear are eliminated or reduced to a point where they are of no clinical concern." His statement gives the restorative dentist the best reasons to proceed to occlusal controls, not only before restorative procedures but also following porcelain-bonded restoration placement, to eliminate the interferences that were either present or could have been introduced with new restorations.

This post bonding control is made necessary because of the great difficulty in appreciating before bonding porcelain-bonded restorations, the occlusal parameters because of the risks of fracture. Aside from interocclusal overcontacts in centric occlusion, centric interferences – lateral or anterior – can be found on posterior porcelain-bonded restorations (Fig 4-18), while protrusive-retrusive interferences are systematically present on anterior porcelain-bonded restorations, especially those showing a configuration with a palatal extension (Figs 4-7 and 4-8).

Clinical observation shows, however, that contrary to *Dawson's* statement, parafunctional habits can then be reduced to a point where they are of no clinical concern when both centric interferences have been eliminated and anterior guidance steepness has been concomitantly increased.

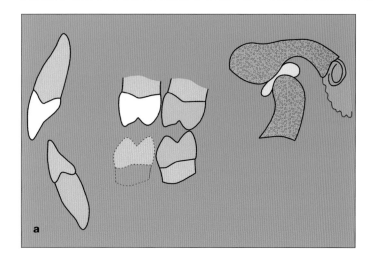

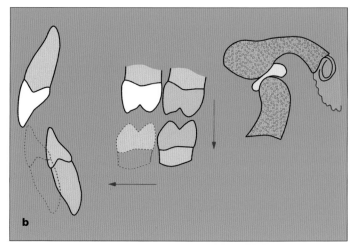

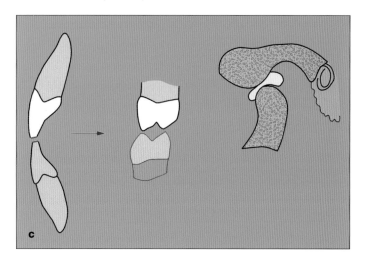

Fig 4-19a-c When an eccentric interference takes place in unusual mandibular positions (a). It generates a neuromuscular reflex action causing the mandible to avoid the prematurity with a pivoting movement, followed by a projection of the mandible against maxillary incisors (b). This back-and-forth movement progressively erases incisors or canines, reducing the posterior clearance in eccentric occlusion until wear progressively starts affecting posterior tooth morphology (c).

Indeed, nothing else but this increase of anterior guidance steepness can prevent possibilities of posterior eccentric interferences that may take place in the area of mandibular motion, clinically undetectable but made possible by increased muscle and ligament laxness, pillow or hang pressure. These interferences also can be the initiator of parafunctional movements.

Occlusal schemes showing moderate but apparently sufficient posterior clearance in eccentric occlusions must be looked at with suspicious eyes, especially those presenting deficiencies in tooth alignment. They open the possibility of unexpected eccentric contacts generator of avoidance patterns leading in an initial phase to the erosion of the elements of the anterior segment.

The rotation of the mandible around a posterior obstacle followed by a mandibular projection against the maxillary incisors has been observed in clinical tests, and the follow-up of muscles

participation clearly described[61,62] (Fig 4-18). It has even been demonstrated that parafunctional avoidance patterns could not only project the mandible against maxillary incisors but be moved outside the confine of the maxilla[63–66] – that is to say in a cross-over position. This uncontrolled back and forth movement will progressively erase antagonist anterior teeth whose progressive morphological reduction will finally permit posterior contact, and posterior wear faceting (Fig 4-19).

As a consequence, the set-up of veneers, that is to say porcelain-bonded restoration, covering the facial part of the tooth and provided with a reduced palatal overlap, is restricted to occlusal schemes showing a total absence of faceting (Fig 4-20). The presence of wear faceting in the occlusal scheme (it could be a simple chipping, a localized or generalized chevron-shape anterior wear), requires a modification of veneer configuration with the design of either an elongated

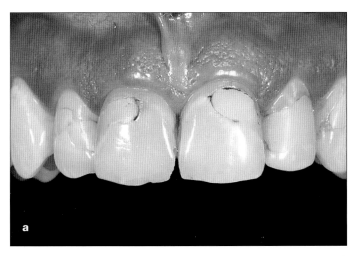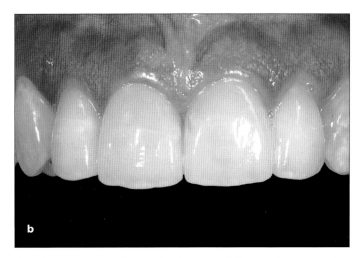

Fig 4-20a, b When porcelain-bonded restoration is only used to improve anterior esthetics, careful attention must be paid that the newly designed prosthesis does not interfere with neurologically programmed tooth-closure patterns. Initial situation (a) and following the restoration of maxillary incisors (b).

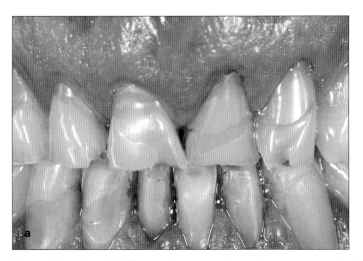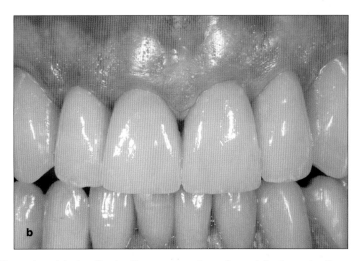

Fig 4-21a, b A full mouth restoration of a worn-out dentition should duplicate the parameters found in long-lasting unworn dentitions to ascertain occlusal maintenance and function. (a) Initial situation in centric occlusion. (b) Interocclusal relationships following restoration with porcelain-bonded restoration.

porcelain-bonded restoration or a porcelain-bonded restoration with a palatal extension, provided an increase of anterior guidance can be achieved to prevent any possibility of posterior interference in eccentric occlusions (Fig 4-21).

Conclusion

The predictability of any restorative process rests on the precise evaluation of oral and occlusal conditions. Porcelain veneer restorations can be considered as ideal restorations for the corrections of poor anterior relationships and anterio-guidance. Conversely, they can also be destructive for the dentition when occlusal conditions have been neglected or wrongly appraised.

References

1. Kreulen CM, Creugers NH, Meijring AC. Meta-analysis of anterior veneer restorations in clinical studies. J Dent 1998;26:345-353.

2. Andreasen FM, Flugger E. Daugaard-Jensen J, Munksgaard EC. Treatment of crown fractured incisors with laminate veneer restorations. An experimental study. Endod Dent Traumatol 1992;8:30-35.

3. Munksgaard EC, Hojtved L, Jorgensen EH, Andreasen JO, Andreasen FM. Enamel-dentin crown fractures bonded with various bonding agents Endod Den Traumatol 1991; 7:73-77.

4. Stokes AAN, Hood JAA. Impact fracture characteristics of intact and crowned human central incisors. J Oral Rehabil 1993;20:89-95.

5. Andreasen FM, Daugard-Jensen J, Munksgaard EC. Reinforcement of bonded crown fractured incisors with porcelain veneers. Endod Dent Traumatol 1991;7:78-83.

6. Magne P, Anthennis Versluis, Douglas WH. Rationalization of incisor shape: Experimental-numerical analysis. J Prosthetic Dent 1999;81:345-354.

7. Magne P, Douglas WH. Design opimization and evolution of bonded ceramics for the anterior dentition: A finite-element analysis. Quintessence Int. 1999;30:661-672.

8. Magne P. Douglas WH. Rationalization of esthetic restorative dentistry based on biomimetics. J Esthet Dent 1999;11:5-15.

9. Reek ES, Ross K. Tooth stiffness with composite veneer: A strain gauge and finite element evaluation. Dent Mater 1994;10:247-252.

10. Highton RM, Caputo AA, Matyas J. A protoelastic study of stress on porcelain laminate preparations. J Prosthetic Dent 1987;58:157-161.

11. Magne P, Douglas WH. Optimization and stress distribution in porcelain veneers for the treatment of crown-fractured incisors. Int J Periodontics Restorative Dent 1999;19: 543-553.

12. Magne P. Douglas WH. Additive contour of porcelain veneers: A key element in enamel preservation, adhesion and esthetics. J Adhesive Dent 1999;1:81-92.

13. Gordon JE. Strain energy and modern fracture mechanics. In: Gordon JE (Ed.). Structures or Why Things Don't Fall Down. New-York: Da Capo, 1978:70-89.

14. Fradeani M. Six years follow-up with Empress veneers. Int J Periodontics Restorative Dent 1998;18:216-225.

15. Peumans M, Van Meerbeek B, Lambrechts P, Vuylsteke-Wauters M, Vanherle G. Five-year clinical performance of porcelain veneers. Quintessence Int 1998;29:211-221.

16. Van Gogswaart DC, Van Thoor W, Lampert W. Clinical assessment of adhesively placed ceramic veneers after 9 years. (Abstract 1, 1978) J Dent Rest 1998;77:779.

17. Calamia JR. Clinical evaluation of etched porcelain veneers. Am J Dent 1989;2:9-15.

18. Calamia JR. The current states of etched porcelain veneers. J Ind Dent Assoc 1993;72:10-15.

19. Rucker ML, Richter W, Macentee M, Richardson A. Porcelain and resin veneers clinically evaluated: 2-years result. J Am Dent Assoc 1990;121:594-596.

20. Walls AW. The use of adhesively retained all porcelain veneers during the management of fractured and worn out anterior teeth. Part 1. Clinical technique. Br Dent J 1995;178:333-336.

21. Walls AW. The use of adhesively retained all porcelain veneers during the management of fractured and worn out anterior teeth. Part 2. Clinical results after 5 years of follow-up. Br. Dent J 1995;178:337-340.

22. Belser U, Magne P, Magne M. Ceramic laminate veneers: Continuous evolution of indications. J Esth Dent. 1997; 9:209-219.

23. Magne P, Magne M, Belser U. Natural and restorative oral esthetics. Part 2. Esthetic treatment modalities. J Esth Dent 1993;5:239-246.

24. Pashley DH, Pashley EL. Dentin permeability and restorative dentistry: A status report for the American Journal of Dentistry. Am J Dent 1991;4:5-9.

25. Pashley DH. Smear layer: Physiological considerations. Op. Dent Suppl 1984;3:13-29.

26. Britton GL, Moon PC, Barnes RF, Gunsolley JC. Effect of preparation cleaning procedures on crown retention. J Prosthetic. Dent 1988;59:145-148.

27. Mizusma T. Relationship between bond strength of resin to dentin and structural change of dentin collagen during etching. Influence of ferric chloride to structure of the collagen J Jpn Soc Dent Mater 1992;5:54-64.

28. Wang T, Nakabayashi N, Takarada, K. Effect of HEMA on bonding to dentin. Dent Mater 1992;8:125-130.

29. Nakabayashi N. Adhesive bonding with 4-META. Oper Dent 1992;Suppl. 5:125-130.

30. Lee R. Esthetics and its relationship to function. In: Rufenacht CR. Fundamentals of Esthetics. Chicago: Quintessence, 1990:137-210.

31. Castellani O. Elements of Occlusion. Bologna: Ed Martina, 2000.

32. MacDonald JWC, Hannan A. Relationships between occlusal contacts and jaw-closing muscle activity during tooth clenching. Part 1. J. Prosthetic Dent 1984;52:718-728.

33. Magne P, Perroud R, Hodges JS, Belser U. Clinical performance of Novel Design porcelain veneers for the recovery of coronal volume and length. Int J Periodontics Restorative Dent. 2000;20:441-457.

34. Graf H, Lander HA, Tooth contact patterns in mastication. J Prosthet Dent 1963;13:1055-1066.

35. Schärer P, Stalland RE. The use of multiple radio-transmitters in studies of tooth contact patterns. Periodontics 1965;3:5-9.

36. Parmejier JHN, Glickman I, Roeber FU. Intraoral occlusal telemetry. Part 2. Registration of tooth contacts in chewing and allowing. J Prosthetic Dent 1978;39:569-573.

37. Ramfjord S, Ash M. Occlusion. 2nd ed. Philadelphia: WB Saunders, 1971.

38. Manns A, Chan C, Miralles R. Interference of group function and canine guidance on electromyographic activity of elevators muscles. J Prosthetic Dent 1987;57:494-500.

39. Williamson EH, Lundquist DO. Anterior guidance: Its effects on electromyographic activity of the temporal and masseter muscles. J. Prosthet Dent 1983;47:816-823.

40. Kelly JE, Sanchez M, Van Kirk LE. An assessment of the occlusion of teeth of children. (Data from the National Health Survey: DHEW Publication No (HRA) 74-1612) National Center for Health Statistics: US Public Health Service, 1973.

41. Weinberg LA, Kruger BA. A comparison of implant/prosthesis loading with four clinical variables Int. J. Prosthodontic 1995;8:421-433.

42. Williams WN, Low SB, Cooper WR, et al. The effect of periodontal bone loss on bite force discrimination. J Periodontol 1987;58:236-239.

43. Munechika T, Suzuki K, Nishiyama M, Ohashi M, Horie A. A comparison of the tensile bond strenghts of composite resins to longitudinal and transverse sections of enamel prisms in human teeth. J Dent Res 1984;63:1079-1082.

44. Verluis A, Tantbirojn D, Douglas WH. Why do shear bond tests pull dentin. J Dent Rest 1997;76:1298-1307.

45. Bennet NG. A contribution to the study of the movements of the mandibule. Proc Roy Soc Med. 1908;1:79-95.

46. Mayurama T. Esthetics: Occlusion and function. J Esth. Dent 1994;6:296-299.

47. Tieshler B. Occlusal habit neuroses. The importance of eliminating these interferences in the treatment of bruxism. Dental Cosmos 1928;70:690.

48. Ramfjord SP. Bruxism. A clinical and electromyographic study. J. Am Dent Assoc 1961;62:21.

49. Jenkelson, B. Physiology of human dental occlusion. J am Dent Assoc 1955;50:664.

50. Dawson PE. Evaluation, diagnosis and treatment of occlusal problems. St Louis, MO: Mosby, 1974:103.

51. Robinson JE, Reding G. Zeplin H, Smith UH, Zimmerman SO. Noctural teeth grinding: A reassesment for dentistry. J Am Dent Assoc 1969;78:1308.

52. Krough-Poulson WG, Olson A. Management of the occlusion of the teeth. In: Schwartz L, Chayes CM (Eds.) Facial Pain and Mandibular Dysfunction. Philadelphia: WB Saunders, 1968.

53. Schuylen, CH. Correction of occlusal disharmony, natural and artificial. J Am Dent Assoc 1935;22:1193.

54. Sorin S. Traumatic occlusion. Its detection and correction. Dent Digest 1934:170.

55. Sorin S. Traumatic occlusal and occlusal equilibration. J Am Dent Assoc 1958;57:477.

56. McHorris, WH. Occlusal adjustment via selective cutting of natural teeth. Part 1. Int J Periodontics Rest Dent 1985; 5:9.

57. McHorris WH. Occlusal adjustment via selective cutting of nature teeth. Part 2. Int J Periodontics Rest. Dent 1985; 5:9.

58. Ross IF. Coronal Reshaping. Alpha Omega 1985;73:35.

59. Arnold NR, Frumker SC. Occlusal Treatment. Philadelphia, PA: Lea and Febiger, 1976:37-134.

60. Lauritzen AG. Function, prime object of restorative dentistry. A definite procedure to obtain it. J Am Dent Assoc 1951;42:523.

61. Assal J. Basculement mandibulaire provoqué par une surélévation des dents postérieures: Étude anatomique et électromyographique. Rev mens suisse odonto-stomatol 1998;98:459-464.

62. Assal J. Modification de la position de la mandibule chez l'adulte suite à une surélévation des dents postérieures. Rev mens suisse odonto-stomatol 1986;9:1022-1037.

63. Tanner. Personal communication 28 January 1999.

64. Wilson R. Harmonious anterior guidance in the crossover position. Presented at the Academy of Restorative Dentistry, Chicago, 25 February 1996.

65. Lytle JD. Occlusal disease revisited. Part 1. Function and parafunction Int J Periodontics Restorative Dent 2001; 21:265-271.

66. Lytle JD. Occlusal disease revisited : Part 2. Int J Periodontics Restorative Dent 2001;21:272-279.

5 Color

Stephen J. Chu

Introduction

Color is a language. Understanding color requires learning the language of color. It is frequently spoken, but often miscommunicated. Effectively to overcome the challenges associated with shade selection in esthetic restorative dentistry, it is essential to learn the science and art of color. It is a difficult task, because color is an abstract subject matter, intertwined with visual and scientific components. Compounding the dilemma is the inability of the human eye to perceive color in a clear, concise, and consistent manner. Individual differences in color perception may vary, since the eye is not the most reliable means for color analysis.

The inconsistent results in shade tab fabrication from a color control perspective were identified in the early 1900s, and the efforts of the clinicians are adequately presented in the literature.[1-10] Attention to this challenge was intensified in the 1980s[11-18] and has continued to the present time.[19-39] The emphasis has also been on close cooperation between the clinician and the laboratory technician and the development of new restorative materials[40-61] and dental adhesives.[62-68] Innovative restorative materials have enabled the clinician to enhance the vitality and translucency of dental restorations. Adhesive dentistry has maximized the strength of all-ceramic restorations while maintaining optimal color and translucency. A beautiful smile is no longer considered as a luxury but rather as an essential component in the current lifestyle.

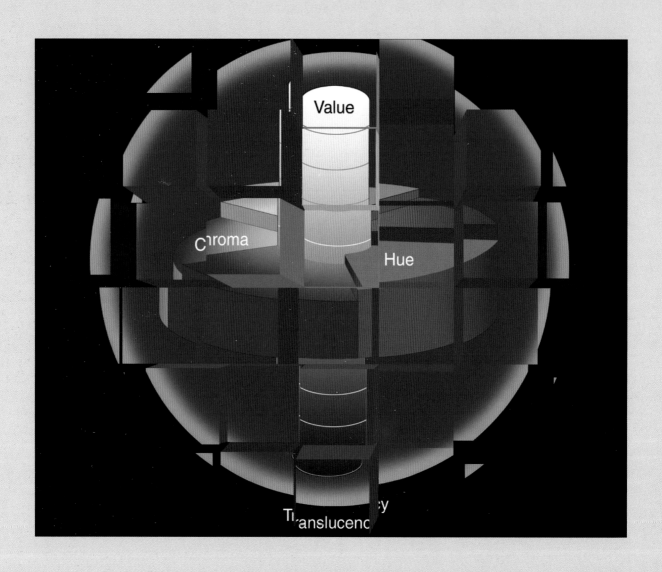

The ultimate test of an esthetically pleasing anterior restoration is the achievement of a natural visual appearance and function. The final results must satisfy the expectations of the clinician and the patient. Such results can be achieved only when the following prerequisites have been met:

1. The clinician has mastered the art and science of color treatment planning, including the correct color and shade selection for each patient.
2. The clinician has correctly communicated his treatment plan and shade selections to the dental laboratory.
3. The laboratory technician has correctly interpreted the received information and successfully combined materials in the fabrication process to produce an unobtrusive restoration with natural appearance.

The shade selection process, however, has become more complex, owing to the variations and differences in optical properties of the new generation of cosmetic restorative materials. The shade determination comprises five distinct parameters, which must be satisfied in order to achieve a predictable esthetic outcome:

1. analysis
2. communication
3. interpretation
4. fabrication
5. verification.

The challenges associated with shade selection in dentistry were first identified in 1931 by *Clark*, who described them in the literature.[1-3] *Preston* and *Bergen*[11] demonstrated the importance of selecting the appropriate quality and quantity of lighting for unbiased shade selection. They also identified the deficiencies in accuracy and consistency of shade tab fabrication. Subsequently, these efforts were further reinforced through the work of *Sproull*[4-7] and *Miller*,[15] who proved that discrepancies existed between the shades of natural dentition and the popular shade guide systems. Numerous other authors, including *Bergen*,[10] *Munsell*,[8] *Sorensen*,[58] *Yamamoto*,[14] and *Ubassy*[16] contributed to the literature on inadequacy of conventional shade selection systems owing to their subjectivity.

The latest innovative effort in the achievement of optimal shade selection has been the development of technology-based shade guide systems; several effective shade selection systems are currently available. A subjective or an objective approach to color treatment planning is now available to the clinician. The subjective approach – the use of shade tabs – is the most common practice and contains uncertainties owing to the human factors surrounding the perception of color. The objective approach – technology-based computer imaging and analysis – overcomes many of the human factors. It requires levels of skill and familiarity with the equipment that are not widespread in either prosthodontics or general dentistry. Additional challenges may arise if the practitioner has limited knowledge of materials and their properties or if the laboratory technician lacks experience in working directly with the patients.

The clinical importance of correct shade selection in esthetic dentistry cannot be overemphasized. Unless an appropriate shade is selected, the most careful attention to the material, structure, and other aspects of the restoration will not produce an optimal final result. The purpose of this chapter is to provide an overview of the key issues involved in achieving optimal results in color determination and shade matching for all types of restorations requiring color analysis.

Color

Dimensions of Color

Understanding color requires comprehension of the dimensions of color, i.e. its hue, chroma, value, and translucency. Translucency is not addressed in *Munsell's* color analysis (Fig 5-1),[8] but it may be the single most important factor in the ultimate result of an esthetic restoration. When restorations are labeled as too opaque, marble-like, or dead in appearance, the esthetic limitation is generally the result of inadequate reproduction of translucency. Translucency, in effect, is the three-dimensional spatial relationship or representation of value.

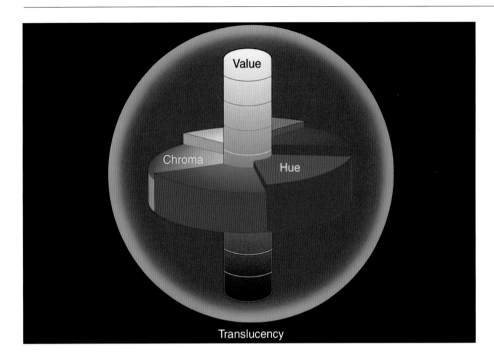

Fig 5-1 *Munsell's* color analysis modified (A Grammar of Color), identifying the four parameters: hue, chroma, value, and translucency.

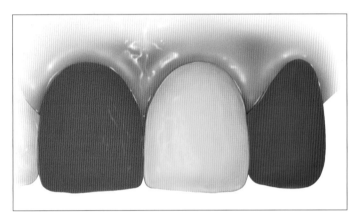

Fig 5-2 Hue is simply color tone, i.e. red, blue, yellow, etc.

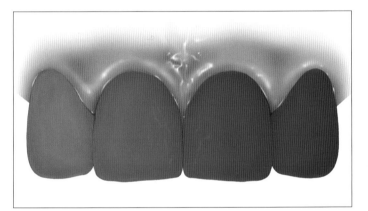

Fig 5-3 Chroma is the intensity or saturation of the color tone (hue), i.e. light blue, dark blue, etc. Chroma increases from tooth #7 (less chromatic) to tooth #10 (more chromatic).

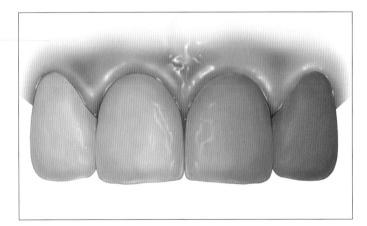

Fig 5-4 Value is the relative lightness (brightness) or darkness of the hue. Tooth #7 is higher in value (lighter); tooth #10 is lower in value (darker).

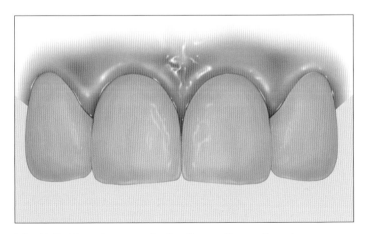

Fig 5-5 Translucency is the three-dimensional representation of value.

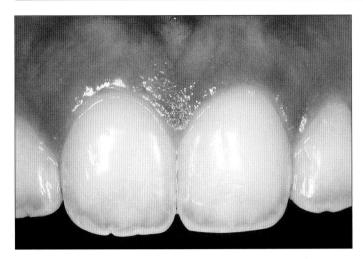

Fig 5-6 Highly translucent teeth tend to be lower in value, since they allow light to transmit through the tooth and pick up the shadows and darkness of the oral cavity and the surrounding environment.

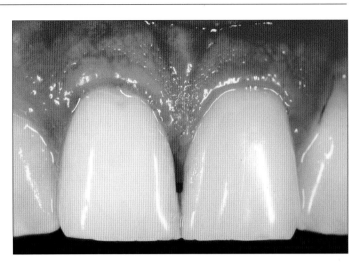

Fig 5-7 More opaque teeth allow less light transmittance; they are more reflective in nature and, therefore, appear brighter.

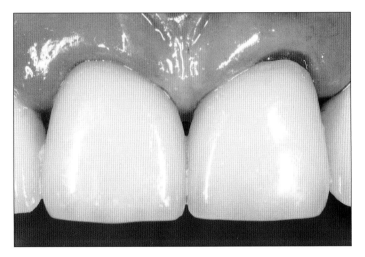

Fig 5-8 The opaque, dead appearance of a restoration should be avoided. Metal-ceramic crowns #8 and 9.

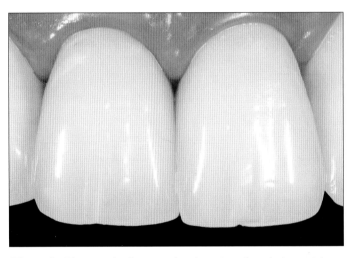

Fig 5-9 The goal of an optimal restoration is to achieve the natural appearance of the tooth. Metal ceramic crowns #8 and 9.

Hue is simply the color tone, i.e. red, blue, yellow, etc. (Fig 5-2). The term "hue" is synonymous with the term "color", and it is used to describe the color of a tooth or dental restoration. Chroma is the intensity or saturation of the color tone (hue), i.e. light blue or dark blue (Fig 5-3). It is used to describe, for instance, the orange or yellow hue of a tooth or a restoration. Value is the relative lightness (brightness) or darkness of the hue (Fig 5-4). Translucency is the three-dimensional representation of value (Fig 5-5). Translucency is abstract and intangible, and it is difficult to measure and standardize at the present time.

Translucency is best represented by value differences. Highly translucent teeth tend to be lower in value, since they allow light to transmit through the tooth (greater light absorption) and absorb the shadows and darkness of the oral cavity and surrounding environment (Fig 5-6). More opaque teeth allow less light transmittance; they are more reflective in nature and, therefore, appear brighter (Fig 5-7). The characteristic of translucency must also be present in the restorative materials in order to achieve a natural appearance and avoid the opaque, dead-in-appearance restorations (Figs 5-8 and 5-9). Translucency and value are the

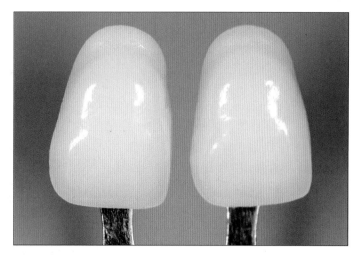

Fig 5-10 Translucency/value are the most important parameters in shade selection, since hue is not easily detectable and there is a lack of chroma in the lighter shades (A1 tab is on the left, B1 tab on the right).

Table 5-1 Dimension of Color

Dimension of Color	Terminology
Hue	Color Tone
Chroma	Intensity of Saturation
Value	Relative Lightness/Darkness

Table 5-2 Wavelengths of Light

White Light	Wavelength (0.000001 mm)
Red	800–650
Orange	640–590
Yellow	580–550
Green	530–490
Blue	480–460
Indigo	450–440
Violet	430–390

most important characteristics in shade selection, since hue is not easily detectable, and since there is a lack of chroma in the lighter shades (e.g. A1, B1, Fig 5-10).

Value differences are easier to identify, since there are more rods than cones in the anatomy of the human eye. There is an inverse relationship between chroma and value. With increasing chroma (greater intensity) there is decreasing value (increasing darkness, Table 5-1). For instance, A4 has a high chroma and low value shade; A1 has a low chroma and a high value shade.

Spectral Colors

Spectral colors are the colors of light in the visible light spectrum. Even though white light appears colorless and intangible, it is formed by distinct electromagnetic energy. When light passes through a prism (Sir *Isaac Newton*, 1676), it is refracted, and the light energy is dispersed into the various wavelengths of white light – hence the acronym ROY G BIV, i.e. red, orange, yellow, green, blue, indigo, violet (Fig 5-11). After a rain shower, we often see a rainbow, since the water droplets in the sky act as miniature natural prisms. The color of the sky also appears different at various times of the day (Fig 5-12). The cones of

the human eye can perceive only these wavelengths of light, hence the term "visible light spectrum". In physical terms, the wavelengths of visible light range from 390 to 800 microns (Table 5-2). Each hue is accurately defined by its wavelength or frequency (Fig 5-13).

Pigment Colors

In dentistry, we must understand pigment colors, since the restorative media (ceramics, composites, and acrylic resins) possess color. The interaction of colors has a role of critical importance in the esthetic continuum. A discussion of primary, secondary, and complementary colors is necessary in order to control and alter shades for a predictable esthetic restorative outcome (Table 5-3).

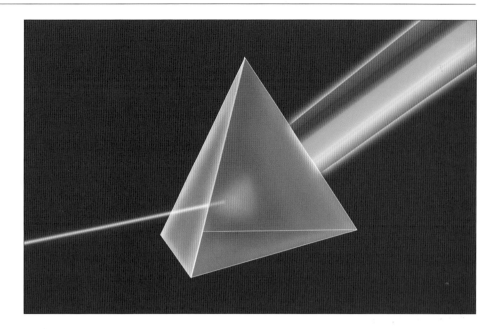

Fig 5-11 Light passing through a prism is refracted (Sir *Isaac Newton*), and the light energy is dispersed into various wavelengths of white light.

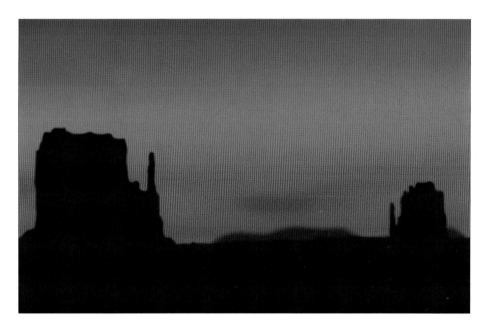

Fig 5-12 The color of the sky appears different at various times of the day.

Fig 5-13 The wavelengths of visible light range from 390 to 800 microns. Each hue is accurately defined by its wavelength or frequency.

Key:

IR = infrared light
UV = ultraviolet light
R = red
O = orange
Y = yellow
G = green
B = blue
I = indigo
V = violet

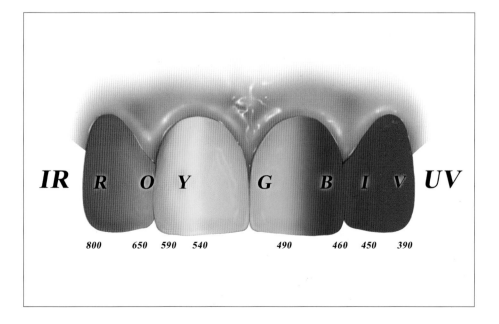

Table 5-3 Complementary Colors

Primary Color	Secondary Color	Complementary Color
Red	Orange	Red–Green
Yellow	Green	Yellow–Violet
Blue	Violet	Blue–Orange

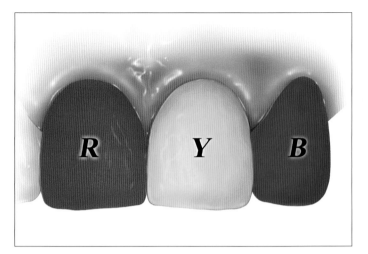

Fig 5-14 Primary colors: red, yellow, blue, occur naturally; they cannot be formed by mixing of other colors. Key: R=red; Y=yellow; B=blue.

Primary Colors

Primary colors – red, yellow, blue – are those that cannot be formed by mixing other colors; they occur naturally by themselves (Fig 5-14).

Secondary Colors

Secondary colors are formed by mixing primary colors: i.e. red + yellow = orange; yellow + blue = green; blue + red = violet (Fig 5-15).

Complementary Colors

Complementary colors look well together; they enhance the appearance of one another (Fig 5-16). When complementary colors are mixed together, they form the achromatic color gray (Fig 5-17).

The additive principle of complementary colors may be used to alter the value of restorations. For instance, if we want to lower the value (increase gray or darkness) of a restoration, the complementary color can be added to that hue (i.e. A3 shade contains: orange hue + blue stain = lower value). Adding gray stain to lower the value will only make the restoration look dull and unclean. Adding violet (purple) stain to a B shade (yellow hue) restoration will also appropriately lower the value. Therefore, adding the complementary color to a restoration will effectively alter the value. Conversely, raising the value of a restoration (increasing the brightness) cannot be managed with this modality.

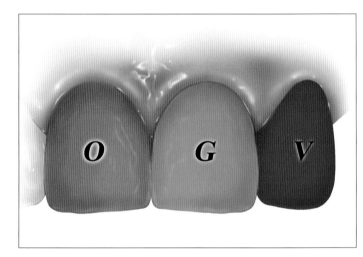

Fig 5-15 Secondary colors: orange, green, violet, are formed by mixing primary colors; for example, red + yellow = orange.

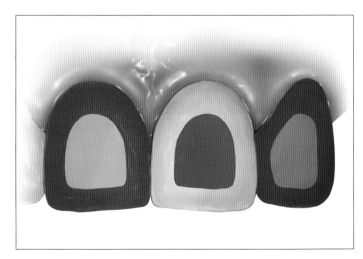

Fig 5-16 Complementary colors enhance the appearance of one another.

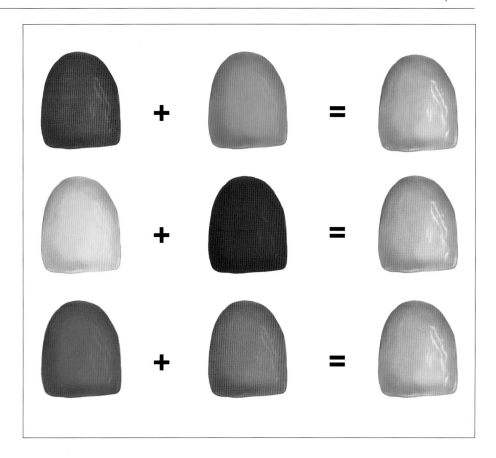

Fig 5-17 When complementary colors are mixed together, they neutralize one another, i.e. they form the achromatic color gray.

Color Perception

All objects exhibit color, such as white, black, red, purple, blue, yellow, etc. Color is perceived through absorption and reflection of the various wavelengths of visible light. For instance, a black object absorbs all the wavelengths of visible light completely (Fig 5-18), while a white object reflects all the wavelengths completely (Fig 5-19) A yellow object absorbs red, green, blue, indigo, and violet wavelengths of light and reflects orange (590-640 microns, Fig 5-20).

The light waves in themselves are not colored. Color arises in the human brain, with the cones in the eyes as the color receptors. Colors arise from qualitative differences in photosensitivity. The eye and the mind achieve distinct perception through comparison and contrast – a chromatic color (red, blue, green, etc.) may be determined by its relationship to an achromatic color (white, gray, and black, Figs 5-21 and 5-22). Color perception is the psychophysiological reality of color (Table 5-4).

Individual Differences in Color Perception

Even though an object may irradiate light with a consistent distribution spectrum, the perception of color may vary markedly between individuals. Table 5-5 presents the results of a study by *Nakagawa*, *Maruyama*, and *Shimofusa* (1975)[9,10] on individual color perception. Three dentists were asked to select a shade for a prosthesis and the adjacent natural teeth, using the conventional shade guide tabs. No dentists were in agreement 34% of the time; two dentists were in agreement 52% of the time, and only 14% of the time were all three dentists in agreement. Therefore, in 86% of the cases, all three dentists could not agree on the same shade. These figures clearly demonstrate a great divergence in visual shade selection with negative clinical predictability. Sources of error commonly originate from disparities in the shade selection environment, which influences color perception considerably. Shade determination under the same light source and positional relationship can eliminate such errors in individual color perception.

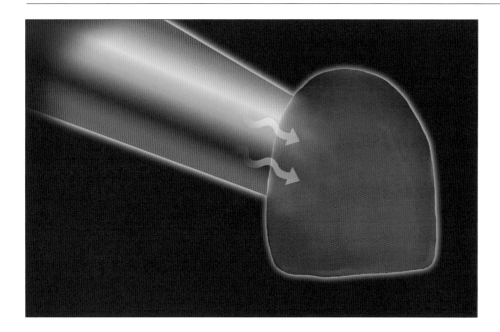

Fig 5-18 A black object or surface completely absorbs all the wavelengths of visible light.

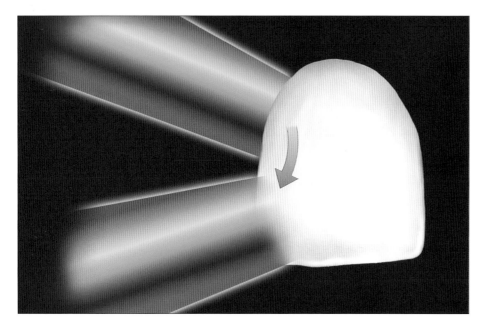

Fig 5-19 A white object or surface completely reflects all the wavelengths.

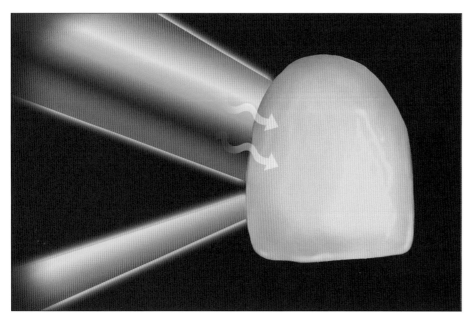

Fig 5-20 An orange object absorbs red, green, blue, indigo, and violet wavelengths of light, and reflects orange (590 to 640 microns).

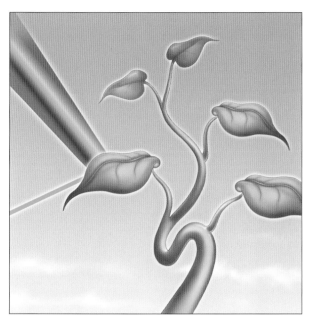

Fig 5-21 The perception of chromatic color by the eye and the brain.

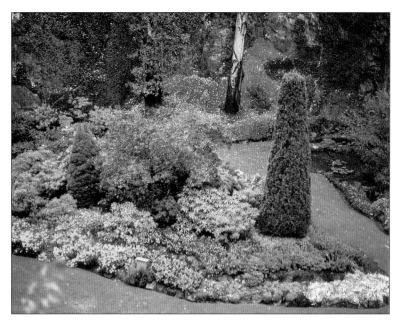

Fig 5-22 The perception of chromatic color by the eye and the brain, i.e. variations of green, based upon reflections of color green.

Table 5-4 Color Perception

Color Perception	Psychophysiological Reality
Physical	Wavelength of light
Psychophysical	Reception of wavelength of light by the eye
Psychological	Interpretation of wavelength of light by brain

Table 5-5 Individual Shade Selection Differences

Number of Dentists	Number of Prostheses	Number of Natural Teeth	Total
Same shade selected by 3 dentists	18 teeth (14%)	10 teeth (14.3%)	28 teeth (14%)
Same shade selected by 2 dentists	72 teeth (59.2%)	30 teeth (42.9%)	102 teeth (51.5%)
Same shade selected by 0 dentists	38 teeth (26.7%)	30 teeth (42.9%)	68 teeth (34.3%)

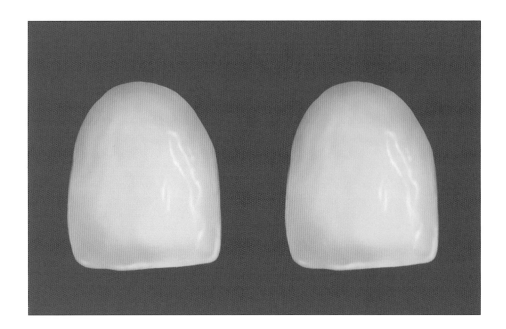

Fig 5-23 A diagrammatic presentation of an optic anomaly. When two objects of the same shape and color are arranged side by side, they may appear to be different, i.e. one seems slightly lighter than the other. It is a phenomenon where each eye perceives color slightly differently.

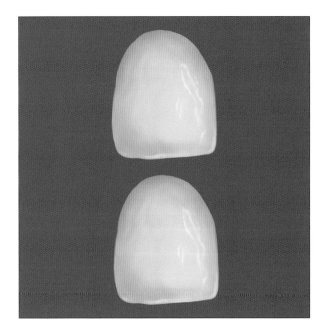

Fig 5-24 If the same two objects (as described in Fig 5-23) are placed on the same side, the effect is no longer evident.

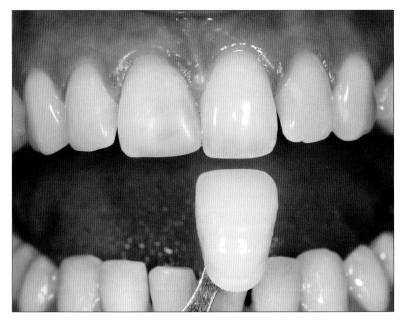

Fig 5-25 Binocular color differences may cause disharmony in shade selection. Placing shade tabs on the same side of the tooth to be matched will compensate for this effect and eliminate errors.

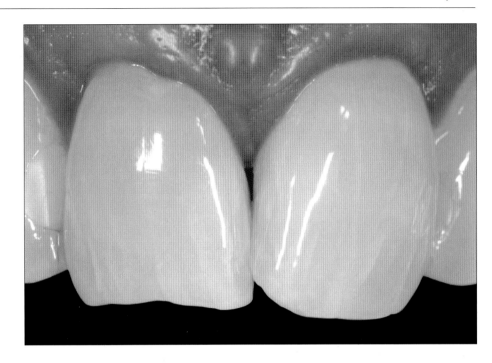

Fig 5-26 Owing to the increase in secondary dentine formation with age, teeth themselves become darker (increasing chroma and decreasing value).

Binocular Difference in Color Perception

Color perception differences between individuals are considerable as we have discussed. However, even in the same individual a color perception difference may be present. This phenomenon is known as binocular color perception – it is a perception variance between the right eye and the left eye. Such color perception disparity between the eyes of an individual is small; however, when it is present, there must be a compensation for it. When two objects of the same shape and color are juxtaposed (arranged side by side), they may appear to be different, i.e. one seems to be slightly lighter than the other. This effect holds true if the objects are reversed in order from left to right. A diagrammatic presentation of this anomaly is given (Fig 5-23).

There also seems to be a phenomenon where each eye perceives color slightly differently. Interestingly, if the two objects are placed on the same side, the effect is not evident (Fig 5-24). Binocular color differences cause disharmony in shade selection and color matching. Placing shade tabs on the same side of the tooth to be matched will help to eliminate error and compensate for this effect (Fig 5-25).

Chronological Age and Color Perception

There are two distinct effects that occur with increasing age. First, the teeth themselves become darker (increasing chroma), owing to the increase in secondary dentine formation (Fig 5-26). Second, the lens of the human eye becomes more yellowish-brown, thereby imparting a yellow-brown bias. Differentiation between white and yellow becomes increasingly more difficult. This process begins at age 30, becomes more noticeable after age 50, and has clinical significance after 60 years of age. This phenomenon may present a clinical problem for a clinician and color work should, therefore, be delegated to younger auxiliary personnel, between the ages of 20 to 30 years.

Fatigue and Color Perception

Adverse visual perception is the consequence of systemic, local, and/or mental fatigue. The inability accurately to distinguish hue and chroma is most noticeable at times of fatigue, and the color may be perceived as faded or bedazzled. Successive shade observations and improper lighting (too bright or dark) are the most common causes of fatigue.

Table 5-6 Effect of Chemicals on Color Perception

Drug	Effect
Alcohol/morphine	Long wavelengths = brighter (red, orange, yellow) Short wavelengths = darker (blue, green, purple)
Caffeine	Long wavelengths = darker Short wavelengths = brighter

Drugs and Color Perception

The abuse of drugs, alcohol, and caffeine may affect the ability to perceive color correctly. The effects are presented in Table 5-6.

Illumination

Color can be neither perceived nor correctly evaluated without correct lighting and illumination (Fig 5-27). The studies by *Nakagawa*, et al.[9,10] and *Preston*[11] clearly showed the importance of lighting in the treatment room. They also demonstrated the dramatic influence of inadequate quality and quantity on optimal shade perception. Shade tabs, viewed under different lighting conditions, look completely different in hue, chroma, and value (Figs 5-28 to 5-30).

Metamerism

Metamerism is a phenomenon where the color of an object appears different, depending upon the light source. When viewed together under the same light source, two objects may appear to have the same color; however, each appears to have a different color when viewed under different light sources. For instance, a crown may be matched under incandescent light; however, when the crown is viewed under color-corrected or fluorescent light, the crown will appear different in color. In dentistry, this phenomenon occurs predictably and frequently if the shade selection environment is not controlled and neutral. To avoid or minimize metamerism, it is of utmost importance to control the lighting conditions when shade is being determined.

Clinical Lighting Tips

1. If the clinician or the laboratory technician has access to a natural light source, it is best to take shades at 10 am or 2 pm on a clear, bright day, when the ideal color temperature of 5500 degrees K is present.
2. Color-corrected lighting tubes that burn at 5500 K should be installed when only artificial lighting is available (without natural light).
3. A lighting intensity of 175 + or – 25 foot-candles must be maintained (verified by color temperature meter).
4. A color temperature meter should be used periodically to verify that 5500 K is achieved in the shade taking area (treatment room or surgery).
5. Dust and dirt should be cleaned from lighting tubes and diffusers routinely, since the presence of dust may alter the quantity and quality of emitted light.

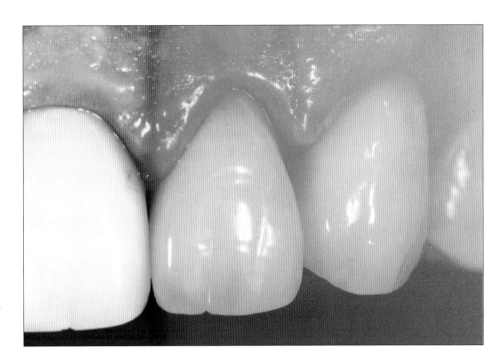

Fig 5-27 Optimal quantity and quality of lighting is required for accurate evaluation of the tooth color.

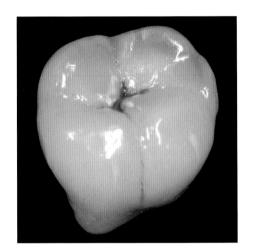

Fig 5-28 Shade under varied lighting conditions looks completely different in hue, chroma, and value. Here, the restoration is viewed under color-corrected light.

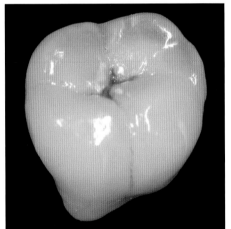

Fig 5-29 The same restoration as in Fig 5-28, now viewed under fluorescent light, looks completely different in hue, chroma, and value.

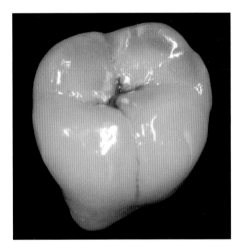

Fig 5-30 The same restoration tabs, viewed under incandescent light, looks completely different in hue, chroma, and value.

Contrast Effects

Optical Illusions

The phenomenon of contrast effect can alter the perception of color considerably, as well as the ability to evaluate color in a clear, concise, and objective way. The phenomenon is dramatically demonstrated in Fig 5-31. The purple-colored figures are all of equal length and size; however, owing to the optic illusion of converging lines, as our eyes move to the right side of the diagram, it appears that the far right figure is considerably larger than the far left figure.

Yamamoto described the various contrast effects in detail in his textbook on metal-ceramic restorations; it is a worthy reference.[19] In order to use colors effectively, it is essential to understand that value, chroma, and hue contrasts between an object and its background may severely influence color perception. There are four categories of contrast effects:
Simultaneous Contrast
When at least two objects are viewed at the same time
Areal Contrast
When the same colors are observed, appearing in different size areas
Spatial Contrast
When the same colors are observed in different positional relationships
Successive Contrast
When one color is observed after viewing another
The clinical significance of contrast effects is presented in Table 5-7.

Simultaneous Contrast

Simultaneous contrast is discerned when two objects are observed simultaneously. It may be further subcategorized as light/dark contrast and color contrast (hue and chroma).

Light/Dark Contrast

Visual judgement of brightness may not be dependable, since the relative brightness of an object is affected by the brightness of the contrasting background or surroundings. For example, if the surrounding background is dark, an object appears brighter; if the surrounding background is light, the object is perceived as less bright (Figs 5-32 to 5-34). The perceived brightness is inaccurate, even though the reflectivity of the object is constant. The retina is very sensitive to changes in light, and the phenomenon is the result of the interpretation of these changes by the brain.

A practical example of this phenomenon is inflamed gingival tissues. The redness of the gums – and consequently the background – act to distort our color perception abilities. The restoration invariably appears too bright when it actually is too dark. When the tissues heal, the crown is too low in value, since the perception indicated that the crown was of the correct shade (Figs 5-35 and 5-36).

Hue Contrast

When two chromatic colors are combined, the perceived hue varies closer to the complementary color than to that of the background (Figs 5-37). The perceived hue of the mock tooth against a red background takes on a green color tone (Fig 5-38 and 5-39); against a green background it takes on a red hue (Figs 5-40 and 5-41); against a yellow background its hue is purple (Figs 5-42 and 5-43); and against a purple background it appears to be yellow (Figs 5-44 and 5-45). Note how the same A3 Vitapan shade tab appears to be quite different in hue when imaged against a red versus a blue background (Figs 5-46 and 5-47). We use this phenomenon to our advantage when taking shades by preconditioning our eyes to see tooth shades more effectively. For instance, tooth shades fall predominantly into the orange hue family, and if we want to be able to see the orange tones more discriminately, we can precondition our eyes by first looking at a light blue background, i.e. immediately prior to the shade selection process. The closer the colors-to-be-combined are to the complementary colors, the more vibrant they appear, owing to mutual repulsion (Fig 5-48).

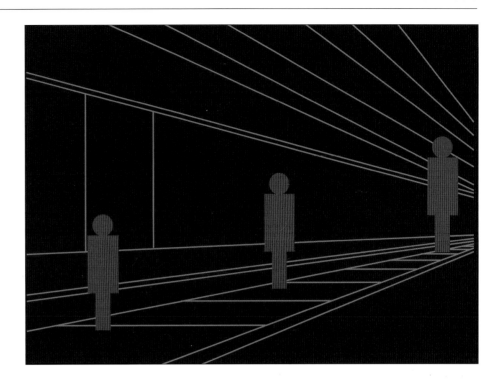

Fig 5-31 Perspective. The figures are all of equal length and size; however, owing to the optical illusion of converging lines, as our eyes move to the right side of the diagram, it appears that the far right figure is considerably larger.

Table 5-7 Clinical Significance of Contrast Effects

Contrast Effect	Clinical Effect	Clinical Application
Light/Dark	Can be correlated to surrounding environment, such as skin tone, hair and eye color, and the brightness of the adjacent (intra-arch) teeth. A darker environment tends to make an object brighter, as well as light.	Select brighter shades for light-toned patients and darker shades for pigment-toned patients, since the tendency is for the opposite contrast to occur – teeth will appear darker for lighter patients and lighter for darker patients. Error in value tendency of adjacent teeth (i.e., low value if dentition is dark; high value if teeth are the converse).
Hue	The complementary color of background or surrounding environment is more apparent.	Use a light blue or neutral gray background when selecting shades to precondition the eye for an improved perception of (complementary) color tones.
Areal	Large teeth tend to look brighter; bright teeth tend to look larger; dark teeth tend to look smaller.	Consider decreasing the value or increasing chroma by one-half the shade and lightening the shade of dark teeth by the application of bleaching/whitening procedures or ceramic laminate veneers.
Spatial	Tooth position may affect the perception of brightness.	Recessed teeth can be made brighter; protruding teeth can be made darker. Consider orthodontic therapeutic correction or ceramic laminate veneers.

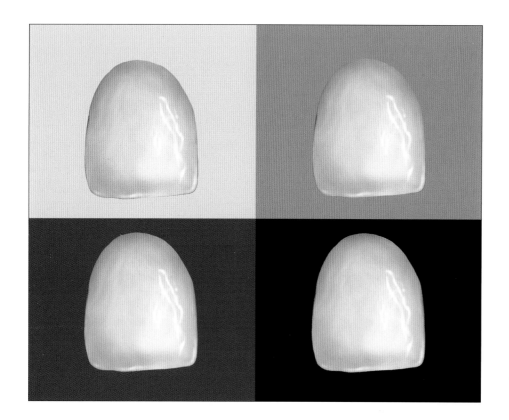

Fig 5-32 The relative brightness is affected by the contrasting background, owing to the light and dark contrasts. Even though the teeth represented are in the same light/darkness, the background influences the appearance (upper left is lighter; lower right is darker).

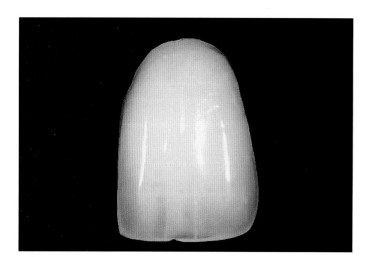

Fig 5-33 A ceramic crown against a dark background appears considerably lighter than against a light background.

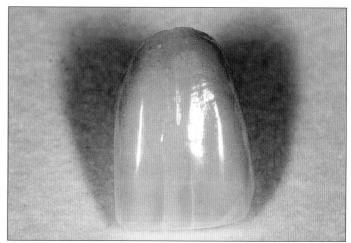

Fig 5-34 The same ceramic crown against a light background appears considerably darker.

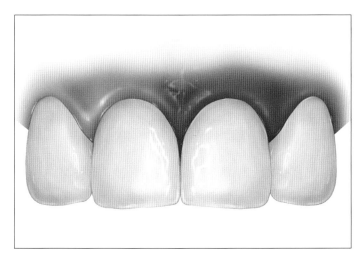

Fig 5-35 The redness of inflamed gingival tissue, for example, distorts our color perception. This phenomenon has a significant clinical importance: if the shade is taken while the gingival tissues are inflamed, the tooth will appear to be lighter, and the color selected will be too dark.

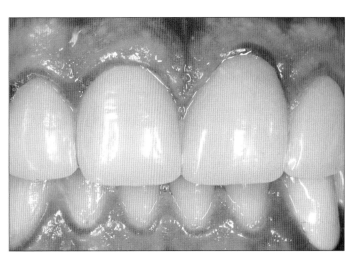

Fig 5-36 When the inflamed tissues heal, and the color returns to normal, the selected crown value may be too low (dark).

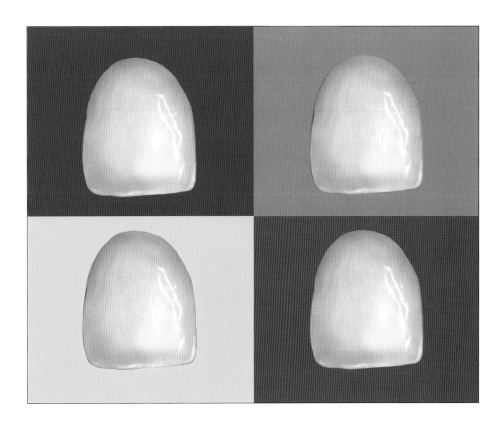

Fig 5-37 When two chromatic colors are combined, the perceived hue varies closer to the complementary color than to that of the background.

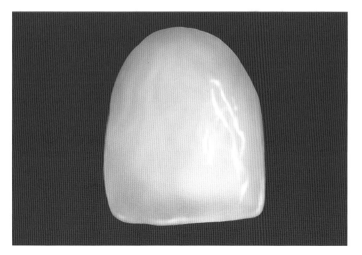

Fig 5-38 The perceived hue of a tooth against a blue background appears to be orange.

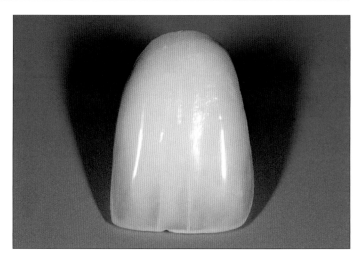

Fig 5-39 A metal-ceramic crown against a blue background appears to be orange in hue.

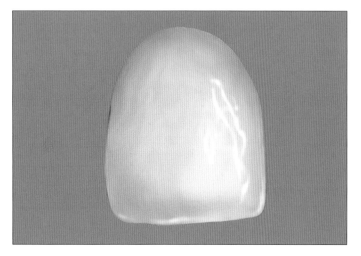

Fig 5-40 Placed against an orange background, a metal-ceramic tooth appears to be blue.

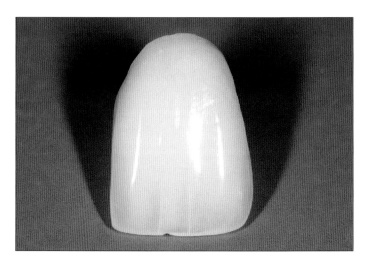

Fig 5-41 Placed against an orange background, a metal-ceramic tooth appears to be blue in hue.

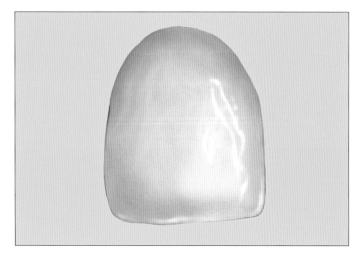

Fig 5-42 Placed against a yellow background, the tooth appears to be purple.

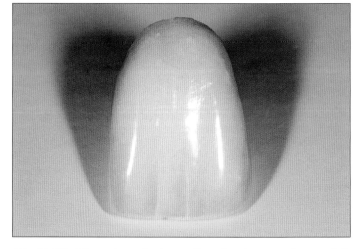

Fig 5-43 Placed against a yellow background, a metal-ceramic tooth appears to be purple.

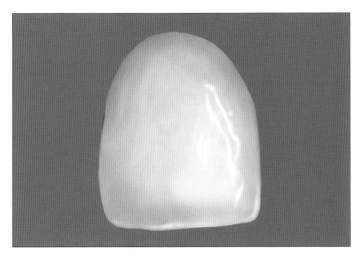

Fig 5-44 Placed against a purple background, the tooth appears to be yellow.

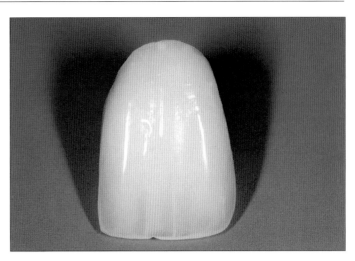

Fig 5-45 Placed against a purple background, a metal-ceramic crown appears to be yellow.

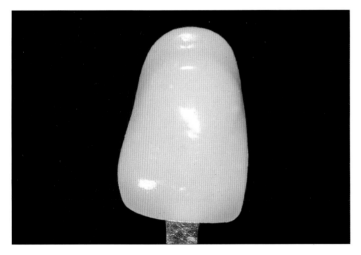

Fig 5-46 The hue of an A3 Vitapan shade tab against a black background takes on a brighter appearance.

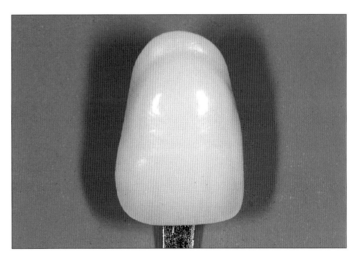

Fig 5-47 The same A3 Vitapan shade tab as in Fig 5-46 appears quite different when placed against a blue background – it takes on a darker, more orange hue.

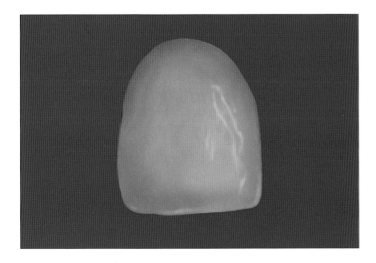

Fig 5-48 Mutual repulsion. The closer the colors to be combined are to the complementary colors, the more vibrant they appear.

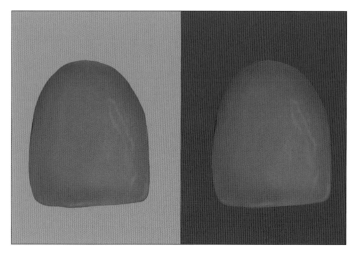

Fig 5-49 Chroma contrast. Clinical example: the color of the background is close to the color of the tooth, rendering the tooth color muted.

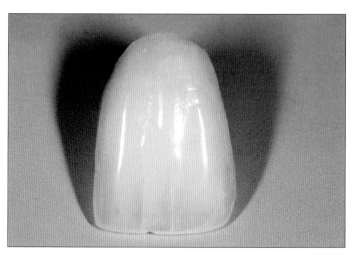

Fig 5-50 Chroma contrast. The closer the color of the orange tooth is to the orange background, the more muted it becomes. The effects are influenced by light/dark contrast and by hue contrast.

Chroma Contrast

This phenomenon follows the effects generated by light/dark contrast as well as hue. The image against the gray background appears brighter (light/dark contrast) since it is low in chroma. The image against the same hue background appears dull (light/dark contrast), owing to the increase in chroma of the background, as well as the slightly blue presence in tone (hue contrast) (Figs 5-49 and 5-50).

Areal Contrast

Visual color perception is also influenced by the size of the object. Optical illusion is present even though the object reflects the same wavelength of light in the visible spectrum. For instance, a large object will appear brighter, while one of a smaller size will appear darker, even though they both are of the same color (Figs 5-51 and 5-52).

Conversely, a brighter object will appear to be larger, while a darker object will appear smaller (Figs 5-53 and 5-54). Fig 5-55 shows a crown made for tooth #9, which is considerably lower in value than the natural tooth #8. Even though they are both of equal size and dimension, tooth #9 appears smaller because it is darker. (The fash-

ion industry employs the illusion of color perception as well. Dark clothes have a tendency to make an individual appear smaller and thinner, while white clothes tend to make the individual appear larger and heavier.)

Spatial Contrast

Spatial contrast can be equated to brightness and size as well. An object that is more recessed will appear to be smaller in size and not as bright; an object closer to the observer will appear larger and brighter (Fig 5-56). This phenomenon is frequently seen with rotated and overlapped teeth. The teeth that are recessed appear to be darker, and they tend to be more difficult to clean. However, once the stain is removed, the teeth will still appear darker, owing to the spatial contrast (Fig 5-57). Posterior teeth appear to be darker, since they are more recessed in the oral cavity. The shadows in the mouth further contribute to the darker appearance (Fig 5-58).

Successive Contrast

Successive contrast is a phenomenon that presents itself when one color is observed following the observation of another color. An afterimage

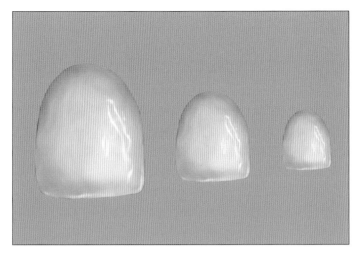

Fig 5-51 Area contrast. Visual color perception is also influenced by the size of the object: a large-size object will appear lighter, a small-size darker.

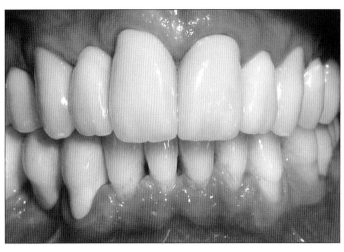

Fig 5-52 Example of area contrast as perceived in maxillary central (larger, brighter) and lateral (smaller, darker) incisors. Even though the crowns are the same (A2) shade, they appear much brighter since they are physically much larger.

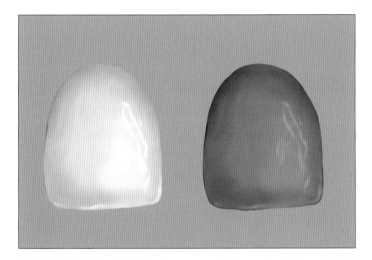

Fig 5-53 With objects of an equal size, a brighter object will appear larger.

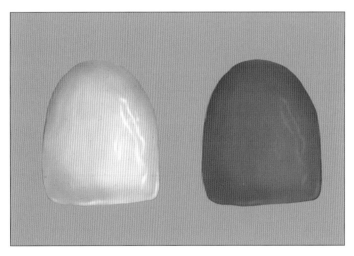

Fig 5-54 With objects of an equal size, a darker object will appear smaller.

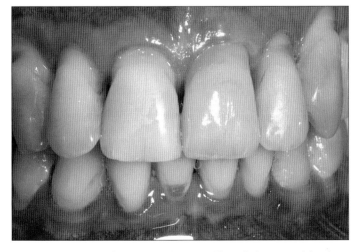

Fig 5-55 View of a crown for maxillary left central incisor that is considerably lower in value than the natural tooth #8 (right central incisor). They are of the same size and color, but the crown appears to be smaller because it is darker.

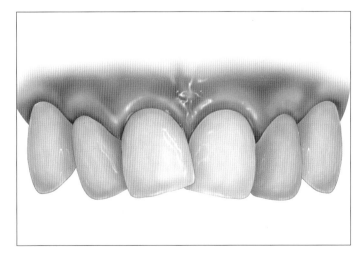

Fig 5-56 Spatial contrast. An object that is more recessed will appear to be smaller.

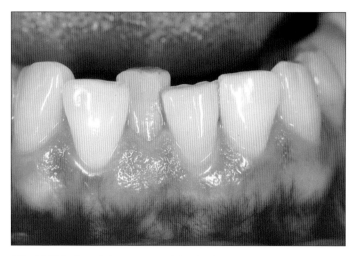

Fig 5-57 Spatial contrast. Teeth that are more recessed appear to be darker.

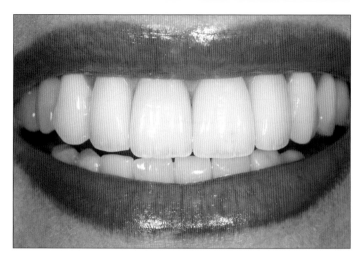

Fig 5-58 Posterior teeth appear to be darker because they are more recessed in the oral cavity.

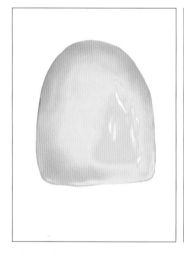
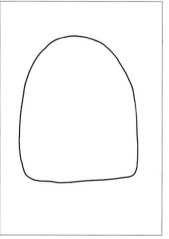

Fig 5-59 Afterimages. Positive after images occur after a short visual interaction and have the same color as the original perception. Negative after images occur after a long visual contact with an object and have the opposite or complementary color.

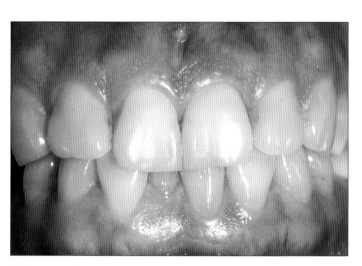

Fig 5-60 Preoperative view of a full maxillary arch to be restored with ceramic veneers.

(visual experience) is an example of successive contrast when the visual perception remains after the eye has left the object. Afterimages are categorized as positive (similar) or negative (different). Positive afterimages have the same color as the original perception; negative afterimages have the opposite or complementary color to the original perception. Positive afterimages occur following a short visual interaction, while negative afterimages occur after a long visual contact with an object (Fig 5-59). Figs 5-60 to 5-70 present the preoperative and postoperative views of a case of full maxillary arch ceramic restorations. Note how – by changing the background paper – the phenomenon of value, chroma, and hue contrast affects the appearance of the veneers of teeth #8 and #9 (Figs 5-63 to 5-70).

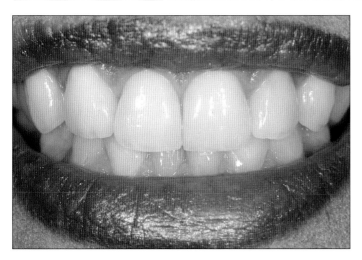

Fig 5-61 Postoperative facial view at a conversation distance.

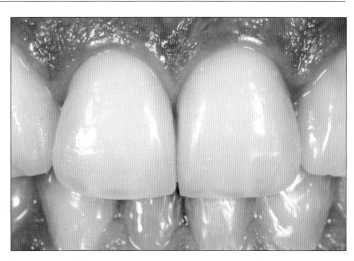

Fig 5-62 Postoperative close-up view of the maxillary central incisors, restored with ceramic veneers.

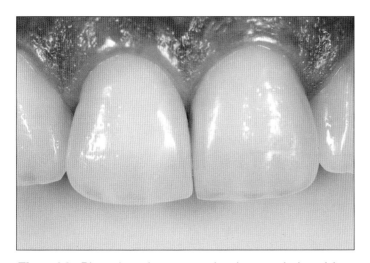

Fig 5-63 Placed against a gray background, the object will appear lighter in color.

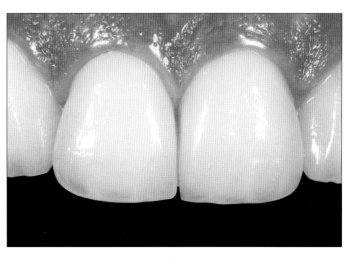

Fig 5-64 Clinical representation of the light/dark contrast. Postoperative view of the maxillary central incisors restored with ceramic veneers. Note the translucency of the incisal edges against dark background.

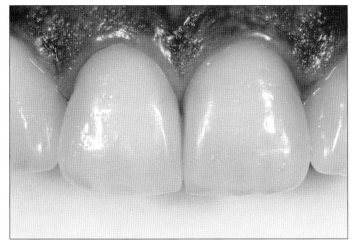

Fig 5-65 Placed against a white background, the maxillary central incisors restored with ceramic veneers. Note the difference of the incisal edges and the darker appearance of the teeth.

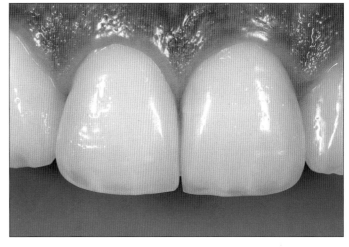

Fig 5-66 Placed against a blue background, the ceramic veneers take on orange appearance.

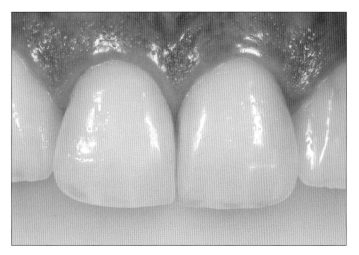

Fig 5-67 Placed against a yellow background, the ceramic veneers take on a purple appearance.

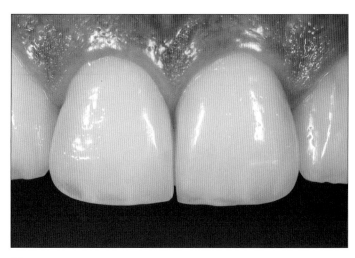

Fig 5-68 Placed against a purple background, the ceramic veneers take on a yellow appearance.

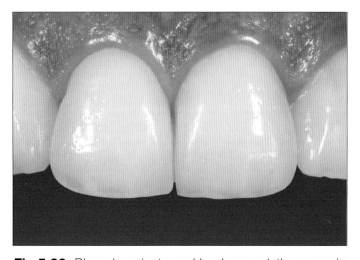

Fig 5-69 Placed against a red background, the ceramic veneers take on a green appearance.

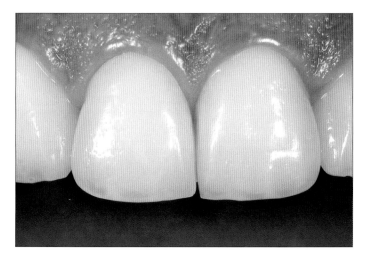

Fig 5-70 Placed against a green background, the ceramic veneers take on a red appearance.

Shade Guide Systems

Shade selection is a process of converting shade perception into shade communication – conversion of color into a terminology and language of the ceramic system and then communicating it to the laboratory technician for fabrication of the restoration. A technician with high color analysis acuity can look at a tooth and see the colors as they correlate to a porcelain system. Determining an accurate shade match is one of the most critically important procedures in esthetic restorative dentistry and has always been one of the greatest challenges in dentistry and a source of frustration. The dilemma lies in achieving accuracy, predictability, and consistency in shade selection.[2,26] Our dental schools do not provide adequate training of dental students in color education,[4,22] and most laboratory technicians have never had the opportunity to work directly with patients.

Shade guide systems may be divided into two categories: conventional, using shade tabs, and technology-based, using digital computer imaging and analysis.

Conventional Shade Guide Systems

Shade Tabs

Shade tabs are used as visual guides; they are only guides, not definitive answers. A neutral environment, maintenance of correct quantity and quality of light, and absence of eye fatigue are important prerequisites for achieving accurate shade selection. *Miller*[15,20,21] demonstrated that the Vita Classic shade guide was too low in chroma and too high in value when compared to the extracted natural tooth samples. Inherent inconsistencies in the fabrication of present conventional shade guide systems have also been described. For example, shade A3 Vita Laminate tabs may vary within and among several guides by the same manufacturer.

The Vitapan Classical, Ivoclar Chromascop, and Vitapan ED Shade Master are currently the most common and popular shade guides. In the Vitapan Classical shade guide, hue is categorized according to groups or families with letter notations:
A – Orange
B – Yellow
C – Yellow/Gray
D – Orange/Gray (Brown)

The Chromascop System uses numbers instead of letter to identify the shade:
100 – White
200 – Yellow
300 – Orange
400 – Gray
500 – Brown

The Vitapan 3D ShadeMaster is a unique departure from the conventional lettering/numbering categorization. It is based upon the pioneer work of *Miller*[15] and further developed by *McLaren*.[39]
L – denotes a tendency toward a yellow hue
R – denotes a tendency toward a red hue.

The Vitapan Classical and Ivoclar Chromascop Systems communicate chroma by a system of increasing numbers.

Vitapan Classical: 1 to 4 – 1 is the least chromatic, 4 is the most chromatic.
Chromascop: 10 to 40 – 10 is the last chromatic, 40 is the most chromatic.
3D ShadeMaster: 1 to 3 – 1 is the least chromatic, 3 is the most chromatic.

The Vitapan Classical and Ivoclar Chromascop Systems address value through chroma: 1 to 4 and 10 to 40 are not only increasing in chroma but also decreasing in value.

The 3D ShadeMaster addresses value first: 1 to 5-1 is the brightest (high value), 5 is the darkest (low value).

Value-based versus Hue-based Shade Guides

Value-based shade guides are a more accurate means of shade selection, as previously discussed, since our eyes are more sensitive to changes in lightness/darkness and chroma than subtle changes in hue. This is especially true for lighter shades (which are the current trend in cosmetic restorative dentistry). With lighter shades, there is very little saturation of hue (low chroma); therefore, hue is not apparent, nor is it a factor in the shade selection process. Value becomes the dominant parameter. Examining a B1 versus A1 shade tab, it would be difficult to assess which tab contains more yellow or orange; however, it is relatively easy to determine which tab is brighter (value). If value and chroma are correct, the restoration will be clinically acceptable, even if the hue is slightly off the optimal.

Clinical Need for Improved Systems of Shade Determination

In the conventional shade tab system, selection of the appropriate shade had always been left up to the subjective knowledge and skill of each practitioner. In such a system, great variability is inherent. The standard visual shade selection protocol has several inherent difficulties, already mentioned in the foregoing text. Metamerism, proper lighting, measured in foot-candles, illumination type (color-corrected versus fluorescent bulbs,

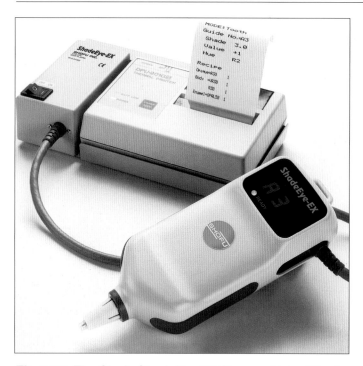

Fig 5-71 The Shofu ShadeEye-EX Chroma Meter (Shofu, Menlo Park, CA) uses a single point source spectrophotometer as the basis of shade analysis.

Technology-based Shade Guide Systems

The development of the Shofu ShadeEye-EX Chroma Meter (Shofu, Menlo Park, CA) in 1998, which uses a single point source spectrophotometer as the basis of shade analysis, marks the emergence of technology-based systems for determination of shade for fabrication of dental materials (Fig 5-71).

Goldstein first reported the Shofu chroma meter in the literature[69] followed by *Yamamoto*.[23] The system employs point source references of information to extrapolate color determination. The potential disadvantage of such a system is that it employs single point sources of information and subsequent extrapolation of that information. Teeth are polychromatic entities and, therefore, require multiple point sources of reference when using this system in order to achieve a more representative analysis of shade distribution. Correct interpretation of the information is of critical importance for a predictable and accurate result. An additional drawback of the Shofu chroma meter is its limitation of compatibility to the Shofu porcelain system. However, if the technology is employed properly, it provides sufficient and reliable information to fabricate well-matching restorations.

In 2000, *Robert*[37] reported the application of another technology-based system – ShadeScan (Cynovad, formerly Cortex Machina, Montreal, Canada) that used "artificial vision", i.e. computer-aided digital and video camera vision technology, to see and analyze tooth images and objectively infer their appearance properties based on color and translucency (Fig 5-72). The digital image is then cross-referenced with a database of shade tabs and guides from known manufacturers (e.g. Vita Lumin, Vita 3D Master, and Ivoclar Chromascop). Additional shade guides can be readily incorporated into the system by scanning them into the database. The advantage of such a system is the objective analysis of shade selection, mapped out in a clear concise manner. The report includes a translucency distribution map that identifies contrasting areas of translucency and opacity. Information concerning value, chroma, and hue differences between the original

color illusion, and color perception differences are merely some of the variables that contribute to the inconsistencies in shade selection).

Clinically, the development of new restorative materials with improved physical and optical properties became a major factor in highlighting the need for improved methods of shade selection. The improved characteristics of dental ceramic materials were primarily in material density with a direct influence on light transmission, i.e. opacity and translucency. Owing to the differences in molecular and crystalline structure of the new materials, changes took place in light reflection, absorption, refraction, and dispersion. The material science itself had become sophisticated and intrinsically involved in the optical aspects of the dental restorative processes.

As these clinical inadequacies in the conventional shade selection became identified, research was generated for the development of more accurate methods. A need for objective standards of shade selection became evident in the dental profession, which could virtually eliminate the wasted chair time consumed in repeated appointments and loss of productivity.

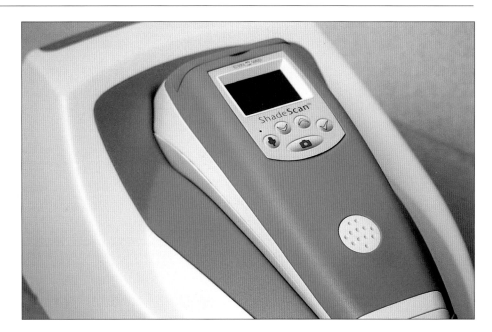

Fig 5-72 The ShadeScan System (Cynovad, formerly Cortex Machina, Montreal, Canada) uses computer-aided digital camera vision technology to analyze dental images and infer color and translucency.

tooth and the shade map is also presented in detail (Figs 5-73 to 5-79).

The optical device is easy to use. To capture an image, the device is held perpendicular to the tooth surface, and it can compensate for an angle deviation of up to 20 degrees. The halogen fiber optic light illuminates the tooth surface at a 45-degree angle to minimize surface reflectance that would cause image distortion. Image capture set-up takes approximately 5 seconds, and the actual capture takes less than 1 second. During the image capture, the patient should hold their breath so as not to fog the lens of the optical camera. Capture of the image is effortless for the anterior teeth; however, the head of the equipment may be too large to capture images of the posterior teeth in patients with smaller mouths. The key to the system is the consistent and constant level of light illumination, which standardizes the image capture and analysis. The output is internally calibrated to ensure constant intensity of illumination.

The SpectroShade System (MHT International, Newton, PA) is another technology-based shade matching system (Fig 5-80); it was described by *Cherkas* in 2001.[26] It differs from the Shade Scan system in that it employs spectrophotometric data (wavelengths of reflected light) for the analysis of shade, although it uses 300,000 points of reference, which are then computer reformatted. This process differs markedly from the ShadeEye-EX Chroma Meter, which measures only single-point sources of reference. Calibration is sensitive and requires 2 images for an exact match. Several reference images may be required before calibration is achieved. However, when calibrated, it provides a tremendous source of invaluable objective information to aid the dental technician in restoration fabrication (Fig 5-81).

The ShadeScan System differs from the other systems in that it uses RGB digital camera technology to infer color properties versus a spectrophotometer measuring wavelengths of reflected light and reformats the images based upon that information. Using a spectrophotometer in his study to measure the color of extracted teeth, *Miller*[15] identified the following provisions: reproducibility of the spectrophotometer was accurate to 1%; the spectrophotometer was sensitive to small shifts in location on a natural tooth; the high reflectance and translucency of natural teeth and porcelain restorations required making average measurements in the center areas of the tooth restoration; minor errors were created in translating spectrophotometer data into *Munsell's*[8] equivalents, since the ShadeScan technology is not governed by these conditions.

Using technology that responds to light in a similar manner to that of the human eye, the X-Rite ShadeVision System uses colorimetric data

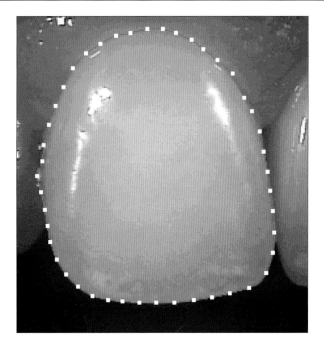

Fig 5-73 Clinical example of tooth #8. The ShadeScan system technology demonstrates the differences between the original tooth and the shade map. Tooth #9 to be restored with a PFG restoration.

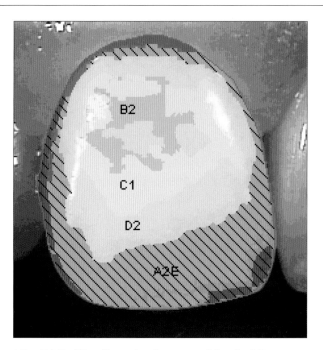

Fig 5-74 The fine shade map of tooth #8, correlated with Vita Classic shade guide tabs.

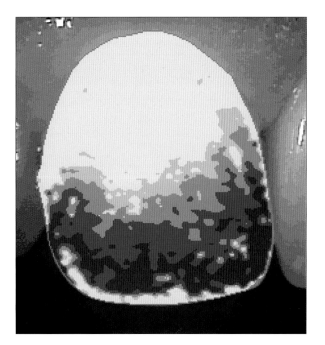

Fig 5-75 Inferred translucency map of tooth #8. The darker areas of blue imply greater translucency.

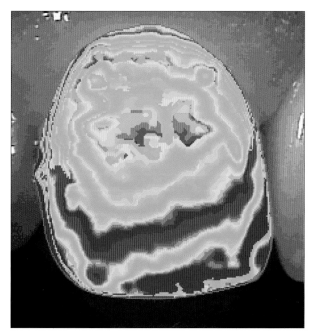

Fig 5-76 Value difference map of tooth #8. Note the change in low (blue), neutral (green), and high (red) value.

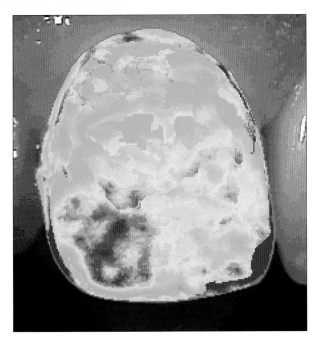

Fig 5-77 Chroma difference map of tooth #8. Note the color change: green is neutral.

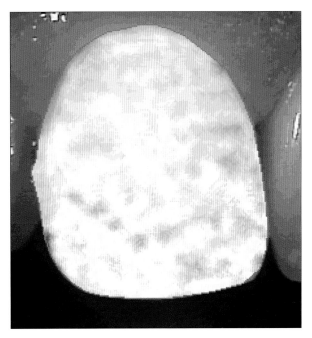

Fig 5-78 Hue difference map of tooth #8. Hue difference tendency is toward red or yellow.

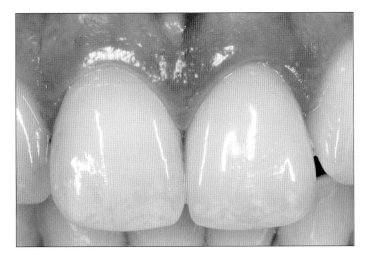

Fig 5-79 Final clinical photograph of tooth #8 and crown restoration #9. Note the imperceptible difference between tooth #8 (natural tooth) and tooth #9 (fabricated crown).

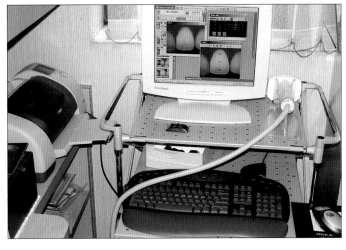

Fig 5-80 The SpectroShade System (MHT International, Newton, PA) uses spectrophotometric data for the analysis of shade with 300,000 points of reference, which is then formatted using computer imaging.

to provide consistent and accurate shade measurement technology (Fig 5-82). The cordless handheld instrument is an electronic shade-taking device that captures images of natural dentition and determines up to 22,000 individual measurements of hue, value, and chroma; these images are then uploaded into the computer via the docking station for analysis, processing and documenting. The information can be sent to the laboratory via an email, saved to media or printed (Fig 5-83). The lab uses the data for an accurate fabrication of the restoration using detailed color analysis of the tooth. The laboratory can also use the system to measure the restoration and compare with the original information supplied by the dentist without the presence of the patient. This is called the "virtual try-in" appointment where shade verification can be established.

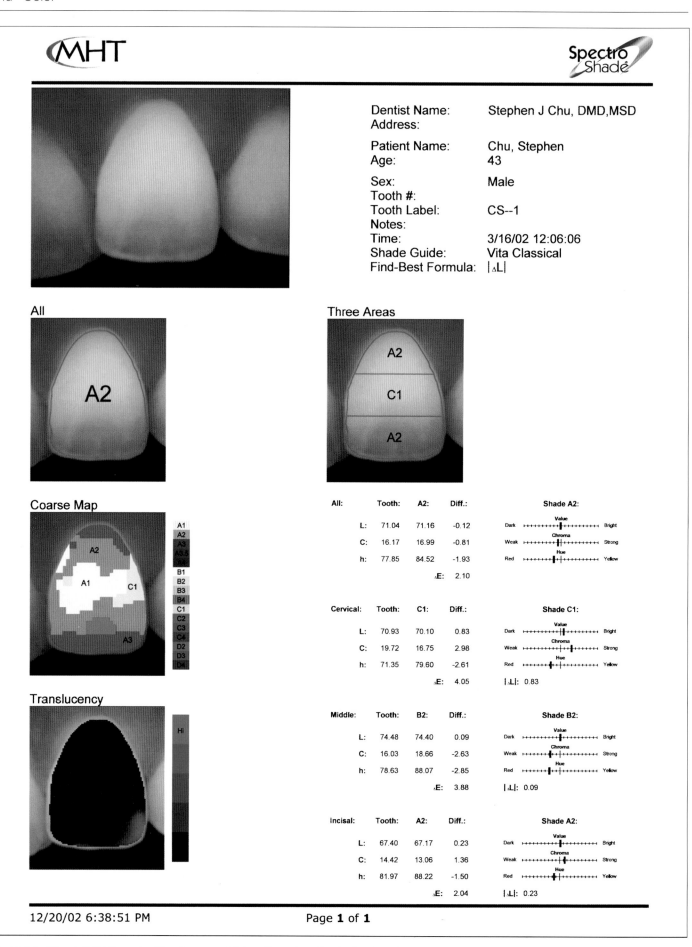

Fig 5-81 The MHT SpectroShade report identifies the shade broken into the gingival, body, and incisal areas, respectively. Information of shade is correlated to comparative ΔE values.

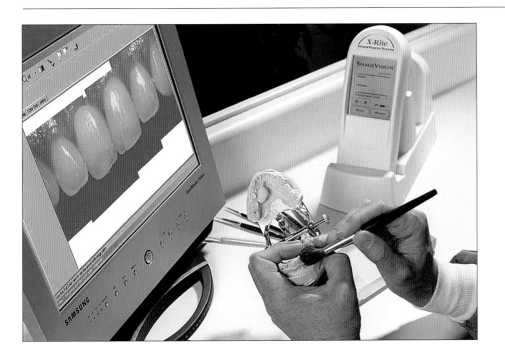

Fig 5-82 The Shade Vision System (X-Rite, Grand Rapids, MI). It uses colorimeter-based data for the analysis of shade with 22,000 measurement reference points. The image capture unit is cordless and portable allowing freedom between treatment rooms.

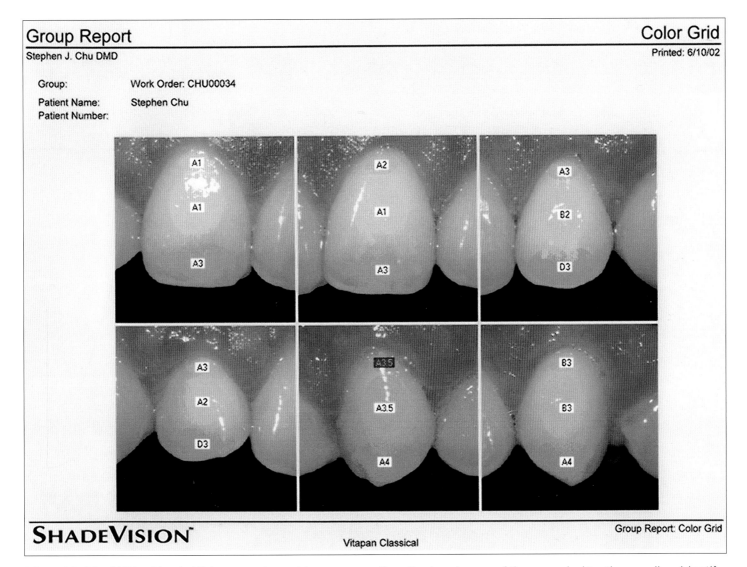

Fig 5-83 The X-Rite Shade Vision report provides an exceptionally clear image of the recorded teeth as well as identifying the respective gingival, body, and incisal shades. Up to eight images can be captured at a time.

189

Advantages and Disadvantages of the Technology-Based Systems

The technology-based shade guide systems have a distinct advantage over the conventional methodology. The reports are less subjective; the capture of an image takes less time, rendering the dehydration of a tooth a non-issue; and the shade of a restoration can be verified prior to the intraoral placement (Fig 5-84). In 2001, *Chu* and *Tarnow*[31] used a clinical case report to describe the subjective deficiencies in the conventional shade selection process and compared the method to computer-aided information with "artificial vision" technology. Shade determination is rapidly evolving towards a more objective standard.

The predominant current disadvantage of the technology-based systems is cost, owing to the expenditures incurred in research and development of these systems. Interpretation of the reports is still subjective, i.e. dependent upon the skill and knowledge of the technician fabricating the restoration. If shade determination can be divided into four critical areas – analysis, communication (of information to the laboratory), interpretation, and fabrication – technology-based systems address the issues of analysis and communication very well. Interpretation and fabrication of restorations are still inherently subjective. The advantages and disadvantages of the conventional and technology-based shade selection systems are summarized and compared in Table 5-8. As the efforts are proceeding in the direction of objective evaluation through unbiased technology-based information systems, the future in shade selection in the dental profession looks promising.

Impact of Materials and Material Science on Color

The importance of restorative materials and their effect on color shade cannot be overemphasized. With the esthetic dental industry driven by innovative materials, impressive strides in improvement have been made in material science and adhesive technology, offering improved physical and optical properties (Table 5-9). The major participants include Procera, Nobel Biocare, Yorba Linda; Creation AV, Jensen Industries; Empress I and II, Ivoclar-Vivadent; Cerpress SL, Leach and Dillon; In-Ceram; Omega 900, Vita Zahnfabrik; HeraCeram.

England's *McLean*[47,48,55] – one of the leaders and innovators in dental ceramic materials – developed a variety of present-day commercially available ceramics. The improved characteristics are primarily in material density, which correlates directly to light transmission (opacity and translucency). There are five categories of materials that have direct application as materials for fabrication of ceramic laminate veneers:

Sintered aluminum oxide ceramics
    (Procera)
Lithium-disilicate ceramics
    (IPS Empress 2 Eris)
Leucite-reinforced ceramics
    (Empress I, Cerpress SL)
Feldspathic ceramics
    (Creation, Ceramco 3, Finesse)
Synthetic low-fusing quartz glass ceramics
    (HeraCeram).

Sintered Aluminum Oxide

Full-coverage restorations using sintered aluminum oxide have achieved a new status in fixed prosthodontics. The excellent marginal adaptation that can be achieved, high resistance to fracture under compressive loading (690 MPa), and the ability to receive a variety of cosmetic veneering porcelains render these materials highly desirable. Their application in veneer restorations is just emerging. Preparation of the tooth is of critical importance in the fabrication process, since computer scanning is difficult and limited, owing to the inherent topography and irregularities in tooth preparation designs. The preparation must be able to resist distortion when the sprayed aluminum oxide powder is sintered onto the refractory die cast. If accurate copings can be made,

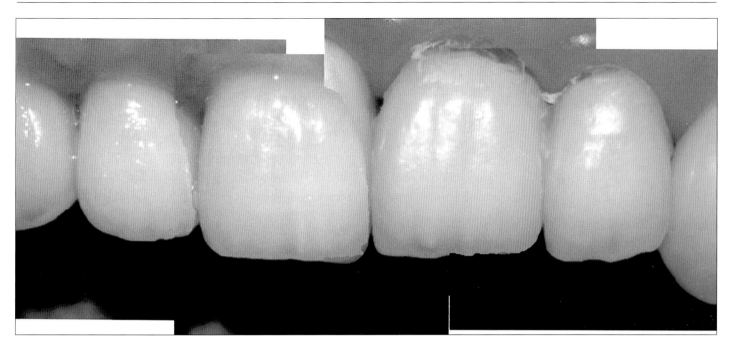

Fig 5-84 When using some technology-based systems (X-Rite, MHT International), the shade of a restoration can be verified prior to the intraoral placement. The Shade Vision system allows shade verification using a computer software program called the "Virtual Try-In Appointment". Laboratory images can be directly compared to clinical images on the same screen for visual approval without the presence of the patient.

Table 5-8 Advantages versus Disadvantages of Shade Selection Systems

System	Advantages	Disadvantages
Conventional	Cost	Subjectivity
	Ease of use	Inconsistency in fabrication by manufacturers
	Visual tool	Selection easily affected by surrounding environment and lighting conditions
	Transportable	
Technology-based	More objective	Increased cost
	Verification of restoration shade in the laboratory	Interpretation of the report is technician dependent
	Not influenced by surrounding environment and lighting conditions	Not easily transportable (Cynovad Shade Scan and MHT Spectro Shade Units)
	Increased productivity – less chairside time and fewer remakes	
	Tooth dehydration is a non-issue	

Table 5-9 Current Materials for Ceramic Laminate Veneer Restorations: Fracture Toughness and Relative Optical Properties

Material	Flexural Strength (MPa)	Opacity/ Translucency
Slip-Cast Alumina Ceramics		
(In-Ceram, Vita Zahnfabrik, Germany)	630	high/low
High-Alumina Reinforced (Sintered) Ceramics (Procera-Sandvik, Stockholm, Sweden)	600	high/low
Leucite-Reinforced Ceramics		
(Empress I, Ivoclar-Vivadent, Lichtenstein)	180	moderate/moderate
(Cerpress SL, Leach and Dillon, Cranston, RI)	180	variable (high/low)
Feldspathic Ceramics		
(Creation, Jensen Industries, New Haven, CT)	90	low/high
Synthetic Low-Fusing Quartz Glass Ceramics (HeraCeram, Heraeus-Kulzer-Jelenko, Armonk, NY)	120	very low/very high

cosmetic ceramic veneering can be applied predictably and confidently. Only the traditional facial/incisal preparation is indicated at this time. Interproximal preparation – which would be required if proximal caries and/or existing restorations were present – is not amenable to Procera scanning and fabrication.

Lithium-disilicate Ceramics

Lithium-disilicate material was developed in 1998 (IPS Empress 2).[61] It has 340 MPa fracture toughness, and it can be etched with hydrofluoric acid. It is pressed accurately, achieves excellent marginal adaptation, and is strong enough to provide superior marginal integrity. It is not as opaque in appearance as sintered aluminum oxide, yet it is more opaque than the conventional leucite-reinforced (Empress I) and feldspathic ceramics. This characteristic is esthetically beneficial for masking moderately advanced discoloration of dentition. Figs 5-85 to 5-94 present a clinical case of feldspathic ceramic veneer restorations, replaced with lithium disilicate pressed veneers. The difference in optical properties is quite evident between the two materials.

Leucite-reinforced Ceramics

Ivoclar developed leucite-reinforced ceramics in 1990 under the trade name IPS Empress 1, with clinical applications in full-coverage restorations. They have evolved to encompass veneer restorations, since they can be etched, possess ade-

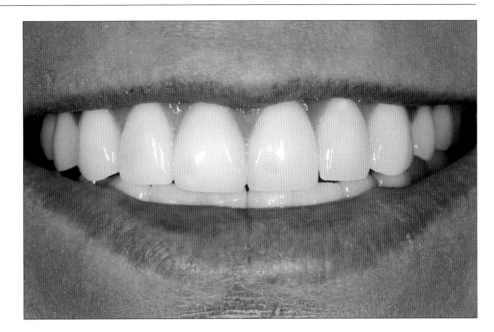

Fig 5-85 Case 1. Preoperative view of a clinical case, where the previous restorations of teeth #8 and #9 with feldspathic ceramic veneers are to be replaced with lithium disilicate pressed veneers.

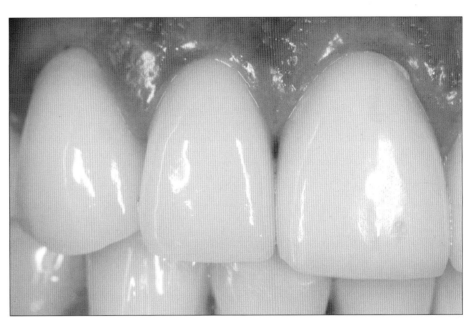

Fig 5-86 Preoperative clinical close-up view of teeth #6, #7, and #8.

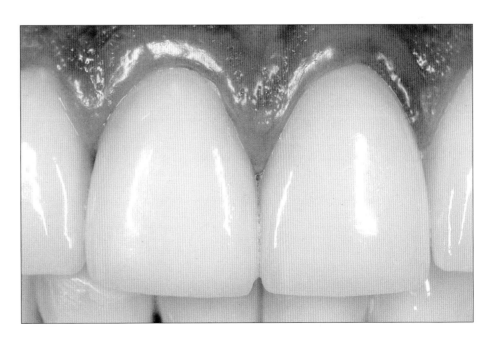

Fig 5-87 Preoperative close-up view of teeth #8 and #9 with existing feldspathic ceramic veneer restorations.

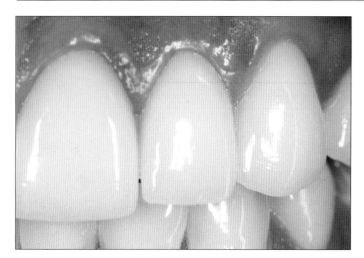

Fig 5-88 Preoperative close-up view of teeth #9, #10, and #11.

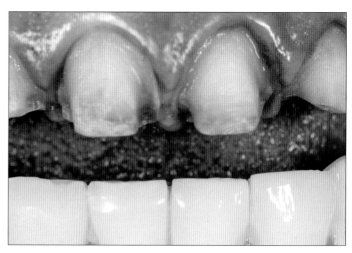

Fig 5-89 Intraoperative view of the prepared maxillary incisors. The existing veneers have been removed. Note the darkness of the stump shade. The dentition had previously been aggressively prepared.

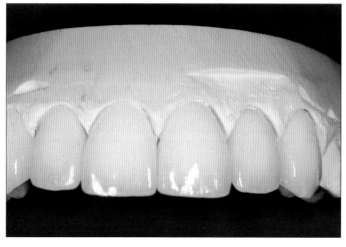

Fig 5-90 Laboratory view of the definitive lithium disilicate veneers for the 6 anterior maxillary teeth (#6 to #11)

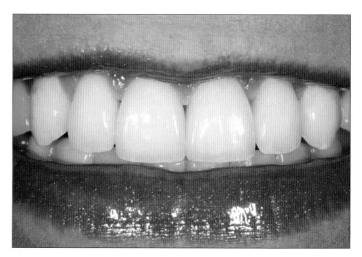

Fig 5-91 Postoperative view of the lithium disilicate veneer restorations, placed and cemented.

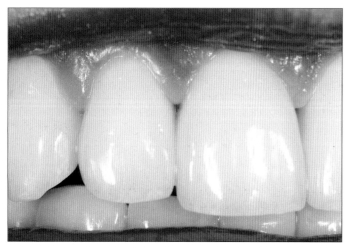

Fig 5-92 Right lateral postoperative view of the maxillary lithium disilicate veneer restorations, placed and cemented.

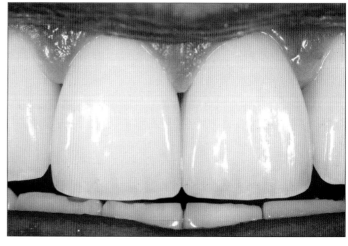

Fig 5-93 Anterior postoperative view of the maxillary lithium disilicate veneer restorations, placed and cemented.

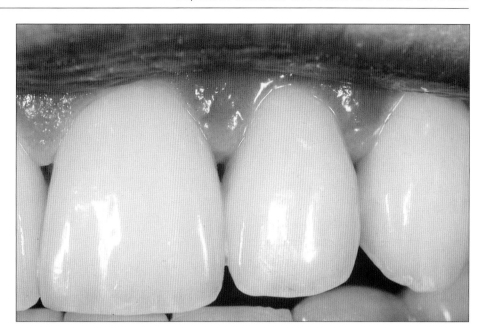

Fig 5-94 Left lateral postoperative view of the maxillary lithium disilicate veneer restorations, placed and cemented.

quate strength (180 MPa), and can be fabricated with varying forms of opacity, depending upon the manufacturer. Leach and Dillon manufactured pressed ceramic ingots in three types of opacity – high, medium, and translucent – depending upon the needs of the clinical circumstances. Excellent marginal fit and variable translucency render this material attractive.

Feldspathic Ceramics

Weinstein first described the use of feldspathic ceramics for metal ceramic restorations in the early 1960s.[43] The work of *Bowen*,[44] *Buonocore*,[65] *Calamia*,[62] *Calamia* and *Simonsen*,[63] and *Kanca*[66,67] dramatically changed the complexion of current dentistry and introduced a new generation of dental adhesives. Ceramic veneers – the thin fragile pieces of ceramics – can now be predictably adhered to the prepared tooth structure. The adhesive interface is no longer the weak link in the system. Feldspathic ceramics are the most commonly used material for veneer restorations at present. In their fabrication, they are highly versatile and can be produced using the platinum foil or refractory die techniques. They possess beautiful esthetic qualities, most importantly translucency, and have remained steady in clinical application – longer than any other ceramic laminate restorative material to date.[52]

Synthetic Low-fusing Quartz Glass Ceramics

In 1982, *Karino*[56] first described the use of low-fusing ceramics with metal ceramic restorations. In 1998, *McLaren*[57] discussed the development of a new low-fusing ceramic, also used with ceramometal restorations that fired at 100 degrees centigrade lower than feldspathic ceramics. In 2001, *Chu*[60] described the development of a completely synthetic glass ceramic material for metal ceramic restorations. This synthetic material is also applicable in laminate veneer restorations. The greatest benefit provided by these materials is kindness to the natural dentition, with less wear to the opposing natural teeth. Figs 5-95 to 5-104 present a case utilizing the same shade but two different restorative materials (feldspathic ceramic and synthetic low-fusing quartz glass ceramic) for the veneer restoration of teeth #8 and #9 and the color response to those materials. Note the differences in opacity/translucency of the restorations.

The above groups of ceramic materials present various and unique physical and optical properties, owing to the differences in molecular and crystalline structure. For instance, sintered aluminum oxide coping materials possess high strength yet greater opacity, while – on the other end of the spectrum – feldspathic ceramics have

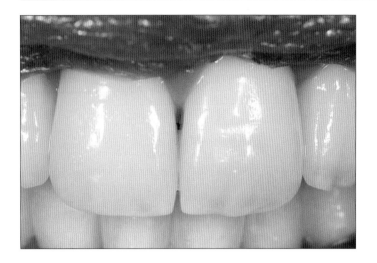

Fig 5-95 Case 2. Preoperative view of a clinical case, where both maxillary incisors are to be restored using the same shade but two different restorative materials (feldspathic ceramic and synthetic low-fusing quartz glass ceramic). Note the differences in opacity/translucency of the restorations (Figs 5-101 and 5-103).

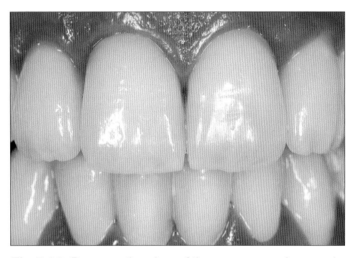

Fig 5-96 Preoperative view of the same case. An error in chroma and value is intolerable, while an error in hue is less noticeable.

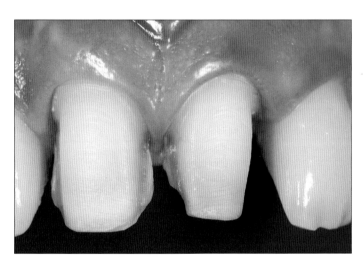

Fig 5-97 Intraoperative anterior view of both maxillary central incisors (teeth #8 and #9), prepared for restoration.

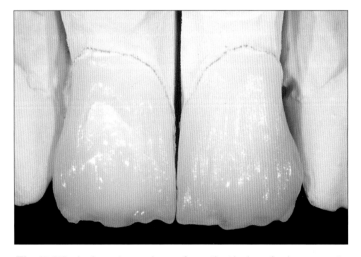

Fig 5-98 Laboratory view of synthetic low-fusing quartz glass ceramic veneer restorations for both maxillary incisors. Fired directly on to the refractory dies.

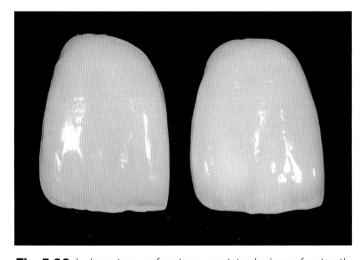

Fig 5-99 Laboratory refractory cast technique for tooth #8: feldspathic (left) and synthetic low-fusing quartz glass (right) ceramic veneer restorations. Note the difference in optical properties.

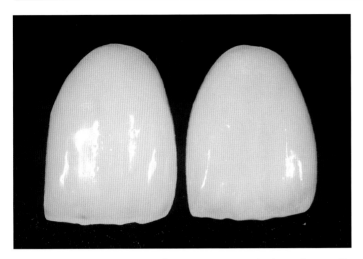

Fig 5-100 Laboratory refractory cast technique for tooth #9: feldspathic (left) and synthetic low-fusing quartz glass (right) ceramic veneer restorations. Note the difference in optical properties.

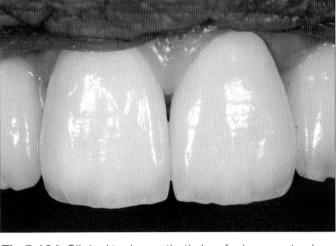

Fig 5-101 Clinical try-in: synthetic low-fusing quartz glass ceramic veneer restorations in place.

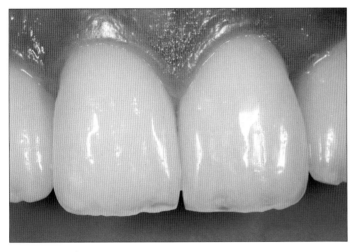

Fig 5-102 Clinical try-in: feldspathic ceramic veneer restorations in place.

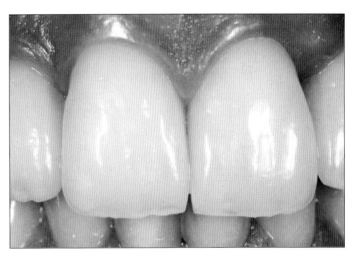

Fig 5-103 Definitive postoperative clinical anterior view: the feldspathic ceramic veneer restorations were selected, placed, and cemented. The feldspathic material better matched the adjacent lithium disilicate full coverage crowns.

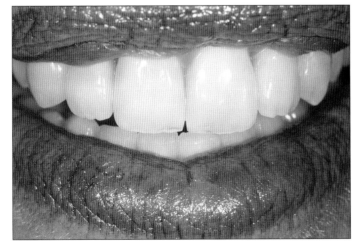

Fig 5-104 Postoperative natural view of the restorations at close conversational distance.

the lowest physical properties (690 MPa versus 90 MPa fracture toughness) but high translucency. Changes and differences in light reflection, absorption, refraction, and dispersion translate in the variations in optical effects perceived. There is a correlation between strength and opacity: high strength = high opacity; lower strength = high translucency.

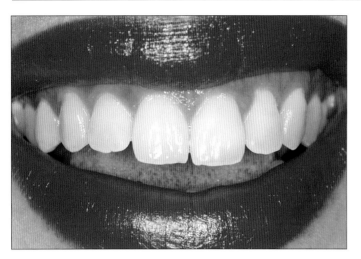

Fig 5-105 Example of a mild color variation often present in the natural dentition. The maxillary central incisors are the most esthetically dominant of the 6 maxillary teeth, the canines are usually the most dominant in hue and chroma.

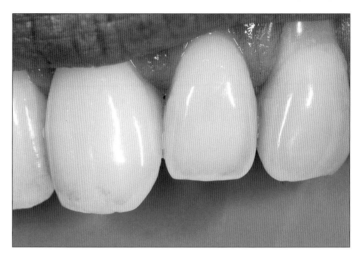

Fig 5-106 The hue of the canines is usually different from that of the central and lateral incisors, and their chroma is of greater intensity.

Clinical Applications – Ceramic Laminate Veneer Color Matching

The principles of translucency, value, chroma, and hue can be applied to either single or multiple unit ceramic veneer restorations. There is a considerable variability in shade within a given dental arch in the same patient. Slight variations are noticeable between the maxillary central incisors, lateral incisors, and the canines. Even though the central incisors are the most esthetically dominant of the six maxillary teeth, the canines are usually the most dominant in hue and chroma (Fig 5-105). The central incisors tend to be the brightest in the arch; the cuspids are the darkest. There may be slight variation of chroma and value between the central and the lateral incisors; the lateral ones are smaller and slightly lower in value. However, the hue is often the same. The hue of the canines is usually different from that of the central and lateral incisors, and their chroma is of greater intensity (Fig 5-106). The same holds true of the mandibular canines, yet the mandibular central and lateral incisors are equal in hue, chroma, and value when compared to the maxillary teeth. The posterior teeth – molars and premolars – match the central incisors more closely.

There is a stratification of color within each tooth. The enamel layer acts like a window, refracting and reflecting light waves. The enamel layer is linked more directly to value. True color (hue and chroma) arises from the dentine layer (Figs 5-107 to 5-112). This phenomenon is clearly evident when tetracycline-discolored teeth are prepared. As the enamel layer is stripped (made thinner), the tooth appears to be more chromatized (darker) (Figs 5-111 and 5-112), presenting a "Catch 22" situation. As we prepare the tooth structure to receive the veneer restoration, the discoloration increases – higher in chroma and lower in value (darker) – thereby making it more difficult to mask the discoloration.

Sulikowski and *Yoshida*[35] proposed that the depth of tooth preparation be based on the presentation level of discoloration. Greater depth of reduction is required to allow greater thickness of cosmetic restorative materials to mask the underlying tooth shade, even though this procedure is somewhat contradictory to nature, as previously mentioned. However, it is logical from a fabrication standpoint, since the technician has more layering options available to mask the discolored dentine.

Unlike metal ceramic restorations, where the shade can be controlled more predictably through the application of opaque porcelain over the metal framework, ceramic veneers rarely have that option – if they did, they would appear too bright and opaque. Often there is not enough

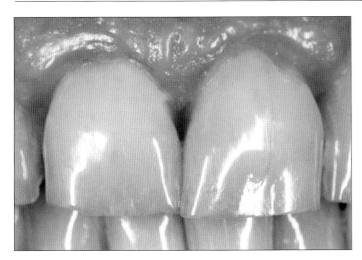

Fig 5-107 Preoperative view of unprepared anterior teeth for synthetic low-fusing quartz glass ceramic veneer restorations. True color (hue and chroma) arises from the dentine layer.

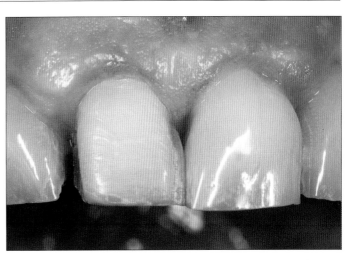

Fig 5-108 Preparation of tooth #8 (note moderate discoloration of dentine layer).

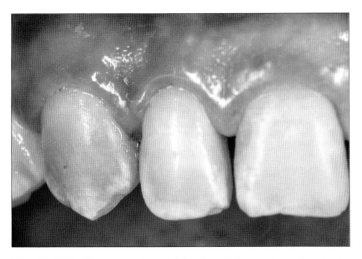

Fig 5-109 Preoperative right lateral view of moderate to advanced discoloration.

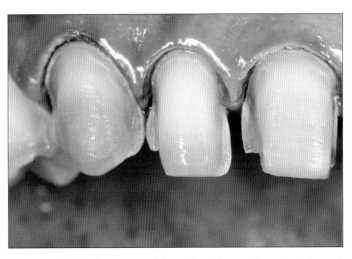

Fig 5-110 As the enamel layer is stripped (made thinner) the tooth appears to be more chromatized (darker) As the tooth is prepared to receive the restoration, the discoloration increases, making it more difficult to mask the discoloration.

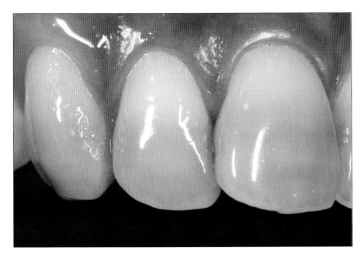

Fig 5-111 Preoperative right maxillary view of severe tetracycline discoloration.

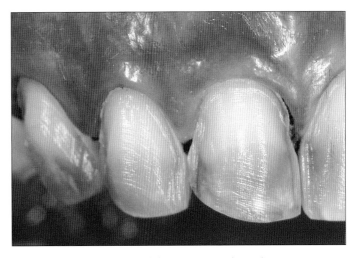

Fig 5-112 The underlying prepared tooth structure, or "stump", influences (affects) the background shade of the final cemented restoration. This is commonly known as the stump shade.

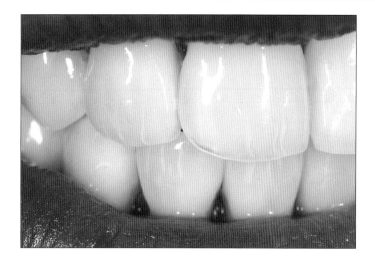

Fig 5-113 Postoperative view of the ceramic veneer restorations.

facial reduction to allow the opaque, dentine, and enamel porcelains to be layered while still maintaining vitality and translucency. Invariably, the underlying prepared tooth structure or "stump" acts as the background shade of the final cemented restoration. This is commonly known as the stump shade (Fig 5-113).

Ceramic veneers are a truly laminated structure: prepared tooth + cement + ceramic veneer. Hue, chroma, and value can be greatly influenced by the stump shade: color of the stump + color of the cement + color of the veneer = color of the final restoration. Value in the final restoration is the most notable dimension of color that the stump shade can influence. Hue and chroma are not often apparent in the lighter shades, since the saturation of hue is so low; therefore, value becomes the major variable in the esthetic effect. For example, patients cannot tell the difference in hue between A1 and B1 (orange versus yellow) because there is so little saturation of color in these shades. However, they can distinguish the difference in the brightness of the shade (value difference) more easily.

Alteration of hue is probably the most difficult characteristic to manage, since most composite

luting agents are value based – clear, light, dark, or white cements are frequently the only shades offered in the luting kits. Hue-based composite stain can be added to enhance color tone. An error in hue is less noticeable; however, error in chroma and value is intolerable (Fig 5-96). Fortunately, value of the final restoration is more easily altered and controlled by the luting agent.

Controlling value for a severely discolored dentition is best addressed using a lithium disilicate restorative material. The pressed core possesses adequate capacity to more effectively mask very dark, low value areas. Figs 5-114 to 5-123 present a laboratory case that demonstrates how black areas can be effectively masked using a lithium disilicate restorative material.

Shade selection and matching a single veneer restoration are best accomplished using a pressed ceramic restorative material (Figs 5 124 to 5-126). Base color is then controlled more easily, especially with variable opacity ingots (Cerpress SL, Leach and Dillon), and cosmetic veneer layering is accomplished in accordance with the conventional pressed ceramic build-up techniques.[33]

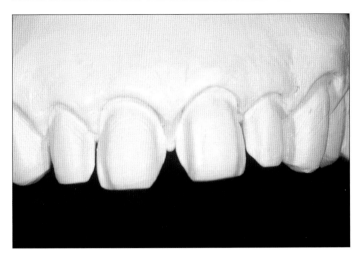

Fig 5-114 Case 3. A laboratory case that demonstrates how black areas can be effectively masked using a lithium disilicate restorative material.

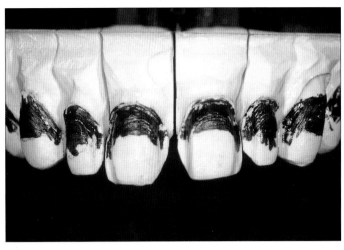

Fig 5-115 Cast after sectioning and trimming of the dyes. Dyes are trimmed and prepared. The cervical areas are marked black to identify areas of severe discoloration for masking.

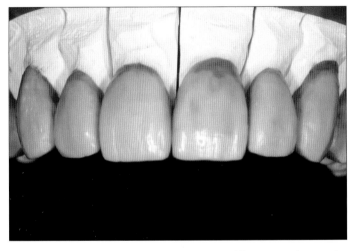

Fig 5-116 Wax-up of the pressed maxillary anterior teeth.

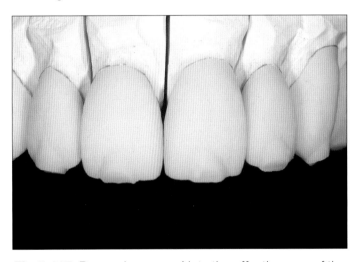

Fig 5-117 Pressed veneers. Note the effectiveness of the material in blocking out the discolorations.

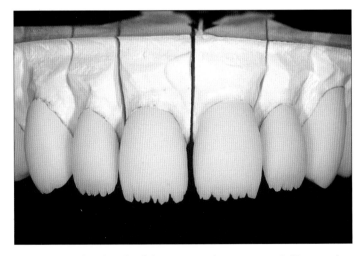

Fig 5-118 Cut-back of the pressed core material to receive veneering porcelain.

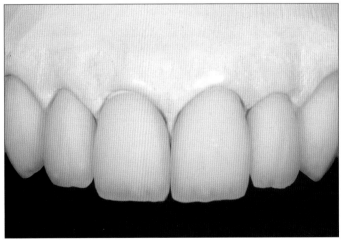

Fig 5-119 Veneer porcelain has been applied to the pressed cores.

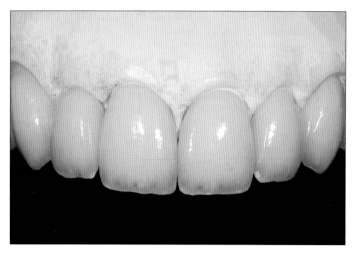

Fig 5-120 Veneers (teeth #5 to #12) are glazed and polished.

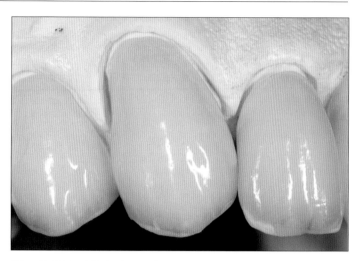

Fig 5-121 Right lateral laboratory view of the veneers for teeth #5, #6, and #7.

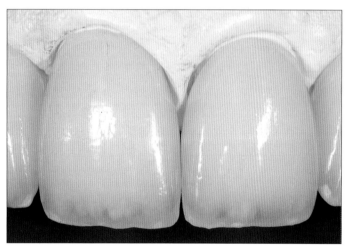

Fig 5-122 Anterior laboratory view of the veneers for teeth #8 and #9 – both maxillary incisors.

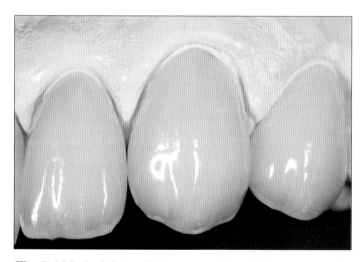

Fig 5-123 Left lateral laboratory view of the veneers for teeth #10, #11, and #12.

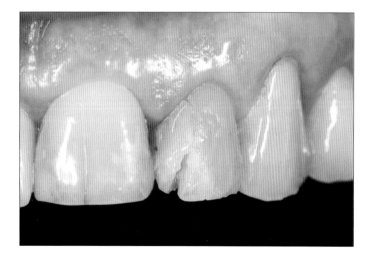

Fig 5-124 Case 4. Preoperative view of the maxillary left lateral incisor (tooth #10). Shade selection and matching a single veneer restoration was best accomplished using a pressed ceramic restorative material.

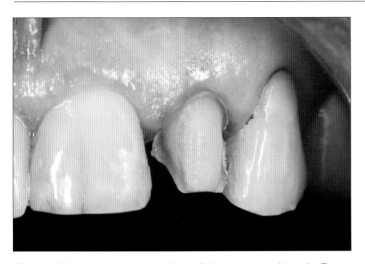

Fig 5-125 Intraoperative view of the prepared tooth. Base color is controlled with variable opacity ingots.

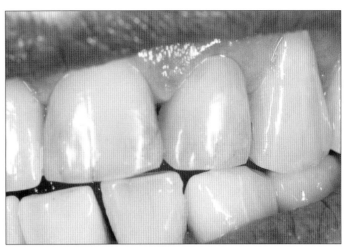

Fig 5-126 Postoperative view of the veneer on tooth #10 in place. Cosmetic veneer layering is accomplished in accordance with the conventional pressed ceramic buildup techniques by Aoshima and Mieleszko.

Clinical Tips for Ceramic Laminate Veneer Shade Selection

Multiple Units

1. Establish a properly lighted environment for shade selection.
2. Select the final shade of the veneers, based upon the patient's preference as well as the tone of hair, eyes, and skin.
3. Take a photograph of the selected shade tab adjacent to the unprepared tooth structure (Fig 5-25) as a reference shade for the technician (calibration interpretation of the color transference from slides or polaroids to clinical reality.
4. Select the original shade of the hydrated unprepared tooth structure as a reference point. The clinical significance is to identify the role of the enamel layer in reference to value. It is well to retain such documentation, since the patients quickly forget and lose perspective of the extent of discoloration of the preoperative dentition.
5. Select the stump shade after the final tooth preparation. Note that the stump shade can vary within each tooth as well as interproximally (between the teeth). This importance and clinical significance of this step cannot be overemphasized.

6. Take a reference stump shade photograph for the technician. (All these photographs will give the technician information and, therefore, an advantage in fabrication of the restorations, keeping in mind the influence the stump shade affords. In essence, the restorations must compensate for the darker, greater chroma stump shade and are frequently fabricated higher in value and lower in chroma in the correct hue.)
7. Always use a try-in or trial cement prior to the definitive luting in order to verify the final shade and acquire patient approval.

    Note that dual cure cements are prone to slight changes in value owing to degradation of benzoamines in the luting agent. The final color effect will be slightly lower in value (darker).

    The final shade is indicative of a laminate of materials as well as underlying tooth structure.

Single Units

Except for the deletion of Step 2, clinical shade selection tips for single units are the same as for multiple units.

Conclusion

This chapter has provided an overview of the current issues in achieving optimal results in color analysis and shade selection. Some aspects, however, are discussed in considerable detail for the dental practitioner and laboratory technician. The discussions of differences in color in color perception and the measures to recognize and compensate for these differences are extensive and include practical clinical advice on how to achieve optimal lighting in the surgery for shade selection. The recognition of contrast effects includes discussion of their impact in clinical practice and the measures for correction. Extensive illustrations, slides, charts and graphs are included to exemplify the concepts.

A historical review of the conventional shade guide system identifies the inadequacies that generated the current efforts in research and development of technology-based systems of color analysis and shade selection. The advantages and disadvantages of the conventional and the technology-based systems are juxtaposed and compared. The improvements in physical and optical characteristics of dental ceramics are outlined, along with the advantages of the new dental adhesives.

In a society where optimal achievement in esthetic restorations is expected from the clinician, the arrival of these new systems and materials is welcome. It is hoped that this chapter will contribute to the general efforts in providing improved dentistry for the patient.

References

1. Clark EB. Analysis of tooth color. J Am Dent Assoc 1931;18:2093-2103.

2. Clark EB. The color problems in dentistry. Dent Dig 1931;37:499-509.

3. Clark EB. Seventy-fourth annual session of the ADA. Buffalo, NY, 15 Sept 1932.

4. Sproull RC. A Survey of Color Education in the Dental Schools of the World. El Paso, TX: US Army Research Report, 1967.

5. Sproull RC. Color matching in dentistry. Part 1. J Prosthet Dent 1973;29:416-424.

6. Sproull RC. Color matching in dentistry. Part 2. J Prosthet Dent 1973;29:556-566.

7. Sproull RC. Color matching in dentistry. Part 3. J Prosthet Dent 1974;31:146-154.

8. Munsell AH. A Grammar of Color. New York: Van Nostrand Reinhold Company, 1969.

9. Nagakawa Y. Color analysis of shade guides. Shikai Tenbo 1976;48:1-9.

10. Nagakawa Y. Analysis of natural tooth color. Shikai Tenbo 1975;46:527-537.

11. Preston JD, Bergen SF. Color Science and Dental Art: A Self-Teaching Program. St Louis, MO: Mosby, 1980:42.

12. Bergen SF. Color in esthetics. NY State Dent J 1985;51: 470-471.

13. Preston JD. Current status of shade selection and color matching. Quintessence Int 1985;16:47-58.

14. Yamamoto M. Variations in color perception. In: Proceedings from Osaka Dental Technology Meeting (1980). Osaka, Japan.

15. Miller LL. A Scientific Approach to Shade Matching. Chicago: Quintessence, 1988.

16. Ubassy G. Shape and Color. Chicago: Quintessence, 1988.

17. Seghi RR. Spectrophotometric analysis of color differences between porcelain systems. J Prosthet Dent 1986;56: 35-40.

18. Seghi RR. Performance assessment of colorimetric devices on dental porcelains. J Restor Dent 1989;68:1755-1759.

19. Ishikawa-Nagai S. Using a computer color matching system in color reproduction of porcelain restorations. Part 1. Application of the CCM to the opaque layer. Int J Prosthodont 1992;5:495-502.

20. Miller LL. Shade matching. J Esthet Dent 1993;5:143-153.

21. Miller LL. Shade selection. J Esthet Dent 1994;6:47-60.

22. Pensler AV. What you were not taught about shade selection. Dent Econ 1995;85:80-81.

23. Yamamoto M. Development of the vintage halo computer color search system. QDT 1998;21:9-26.

24. Miyoshi Y, Sasaki J. Clinical application of the computer color search system and digital recording method of the buildup recipe: Use of the "Shade Eye File" database. QDT 1999;22:69-77.

25. Lichter JA. Shade selection: Communicating with the laboratory technician. NY State Dent J 2000;66:42-46.

26. Cherkas LA. Communicating precise color matching and cosmetic excellence. Dent Today 2001;4:52-57.

27. Ahmad I. Three-dimensional shade analysis: Perspectives of color. Part 1. Pract Periodont Aesthet Dent 1999;11: 789-796.

28. Ahmad II. Three-dimensional shade analysis: Perspectives of color. Part 2. Pract Periodont Aesthet Dent 2000;12: 557-564.

29. Priest G, Lindke L. Tooth color selection and characterization accomplished with optical mapping. Pract Periodont Aesthet Dent 2000;12:497-504.

30. Vanini L. Light and color in anterior composite restorations. Pract Periodont Aesthet Dent 1996;8:673-682.

31. Chu SJ, Tarnow DP. Digital shade analysis and verification: A case report and discussion. Pract Periodont Aesthet Dent 2001;13:129-136.

32. Chiazzari S. The Complete Book of Color. Boston: Element Books, 1999.

33. Aoshima H. Aesthetic all-ceramic restorations: The internal live stain technique. Pract Periodont Aesthet Dent 1997; 9:861-870.

34. Mieleszko AJ. The art of color mapping. i Magazine (Ivoclar Vivadent Inc.) 2001;5:6-7.

35. Sulikowski AV, Yoshida A. Clinical and laboratory protocol for porcelain laminate restorations on anterior teeth. QDT 2001; 24:8-22.

36. Heydecke G. In vitro color stability of double-layer veneers after accelerated aging. J Prosthet Dent 2001;85: 551-556.

37. Robert D. First contacts with the ShadeScan System. Canadian J Dent Technol 2000;4:52-60.

38. Preston JD. Digital tools for clinical dentistry. J Calif Dent Assoc. 1998;26:915-922.

39. McLaren EA. Provisionalization and the 3-D communication of shade and shape. Contemp Esthet Rest Pract 2000;5:48-60.

40. Bowen RL. Properties of silica-reinforced polymer for dental restorations. J Am Dent Assoc 1963;66:57-64.

41. Bertil H. Procera All-Ceram laminates: A clinical report. J Prosthet Dent 2001;85:231-232.

42. Seymour KG. Stresses within porcelain veneers and the composite lute using different preparation designs. J Prosthodont 2001;10:16-21.

43. Weinstein M, Katz S, Weinstein AB. Fused porcelain-to-metal teeth. US patent 3052,982 (1962).

44. Yamamoto N. Metal-Ceramics: Principles and Methods of Makoto Yamamoto. Chicago: Quintessence, 1985:219-305.

45. Preston JD. Perspectives in Dental Ceramics: Proceedings of the Fourth International Symposium on Ceramics (1985). Chicago: Quintessence, 1988.

46. Castelnuovo J, Tjan AH, Phillips K, Nicholls JI, Kois JC. Fracture load and mode of failure of ceramic veneers with different preparations. J Prosthet Dent 2000;83:171-180.

47. McLean JW. The science and art of dental ceramics. Bridge design and laboratory procedures in dental ceramics. Chicago: Quintessence, 1980:2.

48. McLean JW. Evolution of dental ceramics in the twentieth century. J Prosthet Dent 2001;85:61-66.

49. Spear FM. The metal-free practice: Myth? reality? desirable goal? J Esthet Rest Dent 2001;13:59-67.

50. Shoher I, Whiteman A. Captek ñ A new capillary casting technology for ceramometal restorations. QDT 1995;18: 9-20.

51. Shoher I. Vital tooth esthetics in Captek restorations. Dent Clin North Am 1998;42:713-718.

52. Garber D. Porcelain laminate veneers: Ten years later. Part 1. Tooth preparation. J Esthet Dent 1993;5:56-62.

53. Stewart RM. Electroforming as an alternative to full ceramic restorations and cast substructures. Trends Tech Contemp Dent Lab 1994;11:42-47.

54. McLean JW. The science and art of dental ceramics. Bridge design and laboratory procedures in dental ceramics. Chicago: Quintessence, 1980;2:189-209.

55. McLean JW, Sced IR. The gold/alloy porcelain bond. Trans Brit Ceram Soc 1973;5:235.

56. Karino S. A study of the development of low fusing porcelains for fusing to metals. D.Sc. thesis, 1982. Gifu University, Japan.

57. McLaren EA. Utilization of advanced metal-ceramic technology: Clinical and laboratory procedures for a lower-fusing porcelain. Pract Periodont Aesthet Dent 1998;10; 835-842.

58. Sorensen JA, Choi C, Fanuscu MI, Mito WT. IPS Empress crown system: Three-year clinical trial results. J Calif Dent Assoc 1998;26:130-136.

59. Jones W. Low-fusing porcelains. In: Preston JD. Perspectives in Dental Ceramics: Proceedings of the Fourth International Symposium on Ceramics (1985). Chicago: Quintessence, 1988:29-46.

60. Chu SJ. Use of a synthetic low-fusing quartz glass-ceramic material for the fabrication of metal-ceramic restorations. Pract Proced Aesthet Dent 2001;13:375-380.

61. Sorensen J, Cruz M, Mito W: Research evaluations of a lithium disilicate restorative system: IPS Empress 2. Signature 1998;5:4-10.

62. Calamia JR. Etched porcelain veneers: The current state of the art. Quintessence Int 1985;16:5-12.

63. Calamia JR, Simonsen RJ. Effect of coupling agents on bond strength of etched porcelain. J Dent Res. 1984;63: 162-362.

64. Kanca J 3rd, Gwinnett AJ. Successful marginal adaptation of a dentine-enamel bonding system in vitro and in vivo. J Esthet Dent 1994;6:286-294.

65. Buonocore MG. A simple method of increasing the adhesion of acrylic filling materials to enamel surfaces. J Dent Res 1955;34:849-853.

66. Kanca J 3rd. Effect of resin primer solvents and surface wetness on resin composite bond strength to dentin. Am J Dent 1992;5:213-215.

67. Kanca J 3rd. Improving bond strength through acid etching of dentin and bonding to wet dentin surfaces. J Am Dent Assoc 1992;123:35-43.

68. Roulet J-F, Degrange M. Prosthodontics of the future: Cementing or bonding? In: Adhesion: The Silent Revolution in Dentistry. Chicago: Quintessence, 2000.

69. Goldstein, GR, Schmitt, GW. Repeatability of a specially designed intraoral colorimeter. J Prosthet Dent 1993;69: 616-619.

6 Periodontal Considerations in Esthetic Treatment Planning

Korkud Demirel, Galip Gürel

Introduction

Esthetic dental treatment should not be limited to the technical skills and esthetic perspectives of the dentist and the dental technician; the patient's perceptions and her or his understanding of the problems and solutions are also important. Patients should be instructed that esthetic dental rehabilitation is a complex and complicated form of treatment and that she or he is a party to that treatment not merely a recipient of it. The patient needs to see treatment as a collaborative effort in particular because oral hygiene habits and periodontal status dictate the outcome and longevity of the esthetic result. The rehabilitation of a smile relies not only on restorative dental procedures, but also on a healthy and esthetic gingival appearance. Esthetic periodontal problems can only be tackled after efficient plaque control and proper initial periodontal therapy have been addressed. Soft tissue defects may become more apparent as gingival shrinkage occurs after the resolution of the inflammation.

The esthetic outcome of a case is determined by the relationship of the crown with the soft tissues, whether it is a natural tooth, a pontic, or an implant. A sound knowledge of the normal anatomy of the dentogingival unit may initially prevent violation of the basic principles and then one can understand the point where physiological tolerance may shift to inflammatory reaction.

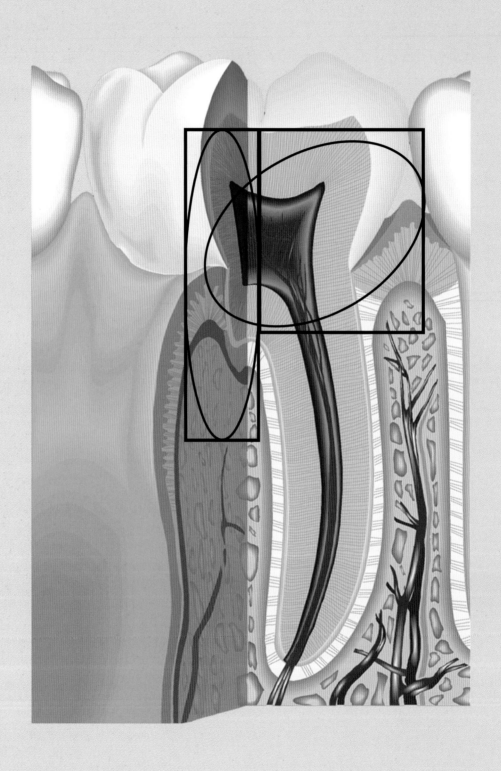

Periodontal Tissues in Health

The Dentogingival Unit and Biological Width

The dentogingival unit represents a unique anatomical feature concerned with attachment of gingiva to the tooth (Fig 6-1a). It is composed of epithelial and connective tissue compartments. Three types of anatomically distinct epithelia are associated with the dentogingival unit. The first, gingival epithelium, consists of stratified squamous keratinized epithelium which is continuous at the gingival crest with the second type, stratified nonkeratinized or parakeratinized epithelium. Sulcular epithelium relines the soft tissue wall of the gingival sulcus facing the tooth but not attaching to it and is continuous at the base of the sulcus with the junctional epithelium, or the epithelial attachment. The lack of keratinization of the sulcular epithelium is the result of inflammation in its supporting connective tissue. Junctional epithelium forms a collar around the tooth and the surface cells provide the actual attachment of gingiva to the tooth surface. In a study of autopsy material by *Gargiulo* et al.[1] it was determined that the average sulcus depth was 0.69 mm, and the average length of the junctional epithelium was 0.97 mm. A significant finding in that study was that the average depth of gingival sulcus was highly variable from tooth to tooth and around the same tooth.

Connective tissue compartment of the dentogingival unit presents fibrous attachment of the gingiva to the hard tissue wall and support to the epithelium of the dentogingival junction. Fibrous connective tissue attachment to the root surface is provided by a gingival collagen fiber system that also maintains the functional integrity of the teeth and its gingival collar. *Gargiulo* et al.[1] reported that the average length of the supracrestal periodontal fiber group was 1.07 mm and was constant at all locations around the teeth. The most important groups of fiber bundles that compose this gingival unit are dentogingival, alveologingival, dentoperiosteal, transseptal, circular/semicircular, and interpapillary fiber bundles[2,3] (Fig 6-1b).

The autopsy material reported by *Gargiulo* et al.[1] showed that the average length of the junctional epithelium was 0.97 mm, supracrestal collagen fiber group was 1.07 mm, and the average sulcus depth was 0.69 mm. Of these three tissue components the supracrestal connective fibrous attachment seems to exhibit the least variability, followed by the junctional epithelium and sulcus depth. In 1962, *Cohen*[4] defined the "biologic width" of supracrestal gingival tissue as those junctional epithelium and connective tissue elements of the dentogingival unit that occupy the space between the base of the gingival crevice and the alveolar crest, that the total dimension would be in the vicinity of 2.04 mm (Fig 6-2).

For practical reasons, as suggested by *Nevins* and *Skurow*,[5] the "biologic width" can be expressed as the sum of the supracrestal fibers, the junctional epithelium and the gingival sulcus. A better name that would prevent confusion could be "biologic zone" as used by *Kois*[6] (Fig 6-2). The minimum dimension of this space between the most coronal level of the alveolar bone to the most coronal level of gingival margin would be in the vicinity of 3 mm in a healthy and normal gingiva. This is the minimum space required for the tissues to maintain their continuity in a healthy status.

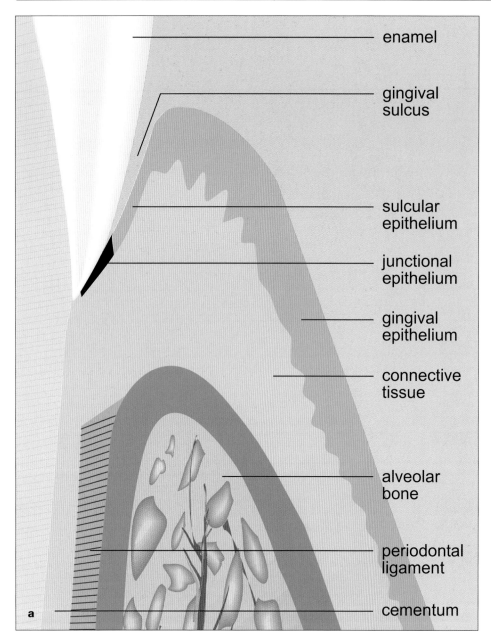

Fig 6-1a, b (a) Anatomical landmarks of the tooth-soft tissue interface. (b) Fibers of the gingival connective tissue. Dentogingival group: these are the most numerous fibers, extending from cementum to free and attached gingiva and they provide support to gingiva. Alveologingival group: these fibers radiate from the bone of the alveolar crest and splay into the attached gingiva. These fibers provide the attachment of gingiva to the underlying bone. Dentoperiostal group: running apically from the cementum over the periosteum of the outer cortical plates of the alveolar process. These fibers anchor tooth to bone and provide protection to periodontal ligament. Transseptal fiber system: these fibers run interdentally from the cementum just apical to the base of the junctional epithelium of one tooth over the alveolar crest and insert into a comparable region of the cementum of the adjacent tooth. These fibers maintain relationship of the adjacent teeth and protect interproximal bone. Circular and semicircular group: these are a small group of fibers that form a band around the neck of the tooth, interlacing with other groups of fibers in the free gingiva. They maintain the contour and position of free marginal gingiva. Interpupillary fibers: these are also a small group of fibers within interdental gingiva in an orofacial course. These fibers fix the vestibular papilla to the oral papilla and provide support for the interdental gingiva.

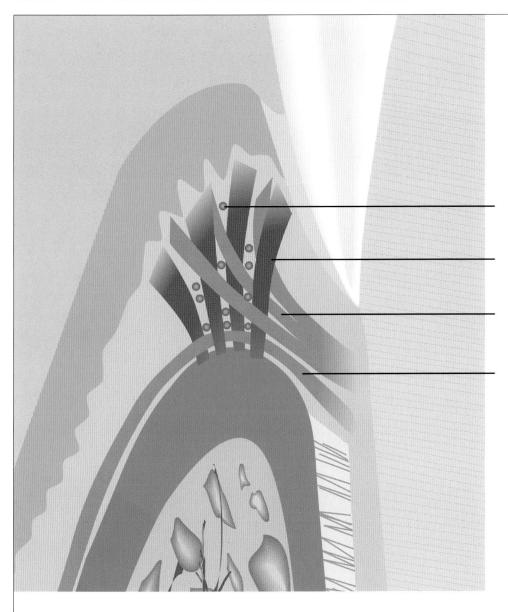

Circular group

Alveolo-gingival group

Dento-gingival group

Dento-periosteal group

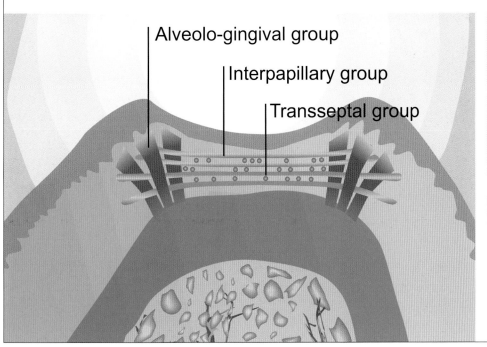

Alveolo-gingival group

Interpapillary group

Transseptal group

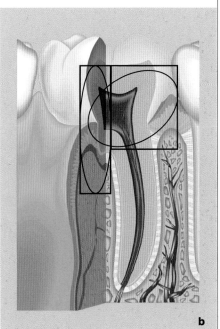

b

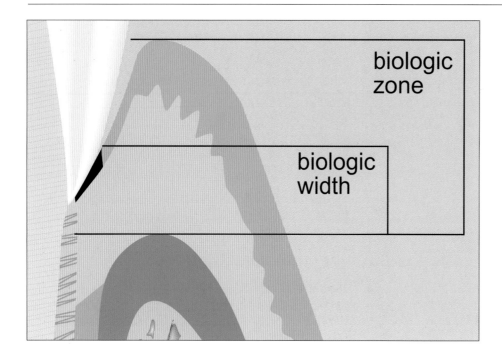

Fig 6-2 Biologic width and biologic zone refer to the minimum dimensions of the space between the most coronal level of the alveolar bone and the bottom of the gingival sulcus and the marginal gingiva respectively. This is the minimum space needed for the tissues to maintain their integrity in a healthy status. Violation of this space results in inflammation and eventually loss of periodontal support.

Clinical Features of Marginal Gingiva

Healthy gingiva could be characterized as the tissue having a coral pink color with varying degrees of pigmentation that embrace teeth in a collar-like fashion (Fig 6-3). The marginal gingiva follows a scalloped outline on the facial and lingual surfaces in a firm and resilient consistency that do not bleed on gentle probing. The clinical sulcus depth and bleeding on probing is clinically influenced by the status of gingival health, inflammation at the base of the sulcus, the diameter of the probe tip, the amount of probing force, probe angulation, and the location on the tooth.[7]

The contour of the gingiva varies considerably and is influenced by the shape of the teeth and their alignment in the arc, the location and the size of the area of proximal contact, and the thickness of the underlying alveolar bone (Fig 6-4). It forms a straight line along teeth with relatively flat surfaces. On teeth with pronounced mesio-distal convexity, or teeth in labial version, the scalloped contour is increased and the margin is thinned, and the gingiva is located farther apically. On teeth in lingual version, the gingiva is horizontal and thickened.

The level of gingival tissue normally mimics or follows the architecture of the underlying osseous crest (Fig 6-5). *Smukler* and *Chaibi*[8] report that the topography of the gingival margin was observed to relate to the underlying bone and to the surface anatomy of the teeth. In a healthy periodontium, the gingival margin was reported to be consistently parallel to the alveolar crest of bone, both labially and lingually. This parallel arrangement was also constant in the interdental concavities of tooth surfaces, where the tissues were seen to rise coronally, and on convex surfaces, where the tissues fell away apically. The accentuation of surface topography of teeth is reflected in the peaks and valleys of the osseous gingival continuum.

Thick, normal, and thin periodontal morphotypes can be defined according to the thickness of the gingiva and its bony component underneath (Fig 6-6). Thickness in the periodontal morphotype is a combination of factors such as the alveolar bone, gingival thickness, and the width of the tooth in the facial lingual plane. Subgingival margin placement should be avoided if possible in thin periodontal morphotypes since they are likely to recede even under minor chronic irritation or trauma.

Under ideal conditions at full smile the vermillion border of the upper lip is expected to correspond with the tangential line drawn between the facial gingival margin of maxillary central incisors and cuspids. The gingival margin of the lateral

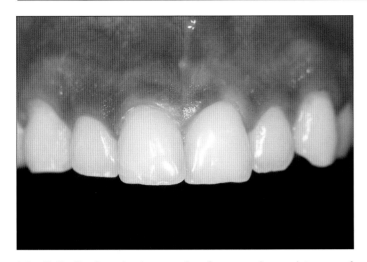

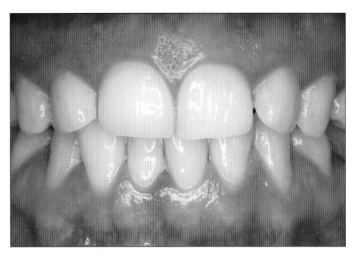

Fig 6-3 Surface texture, color, form and consistency of the gingiva correspond to the health status of the tissues. Stippling on the surface, coral pink color with varying degrees of pigmentation, scalloped outline that envelope teeth in a collar-like fashion are basic properties of healthy gingival tissues.

Fig 6-4 The contour of the gingiva is influenced by the shape of the teeth, their alignment in the arch and the thickness of the alveolar bone. The gingiva with scalloped contour is usually thinner and prone to recession with minor trauma. Thick gingival tissues display straight gingival contour, and are more resistant to trauma.

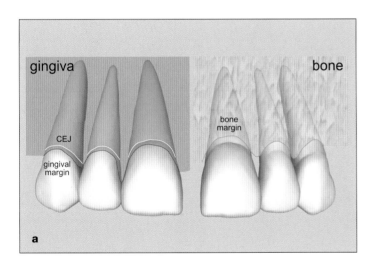

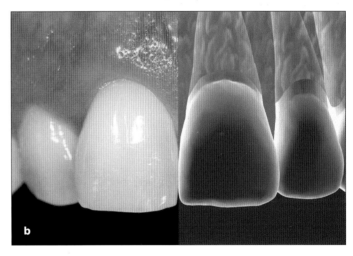

Fig 6-5a, b In healthy periodontium the gingival margin follows the architecture of the alveolar crest and the cementoenamel junction (CEJ).

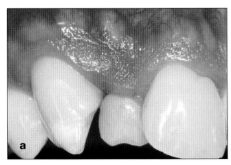

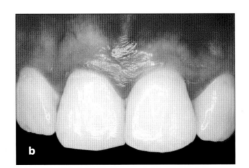

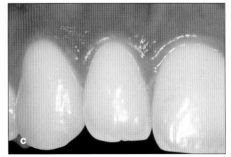

Fig 6-6a-c (a) Thick, (b) normal and (c) thin periodontal morphotypes. Thickness of the periodontal morphotype is a combination of factors such as the alveolar bone, gingival thickness and alignment of the teeth in the dental arch. Thickness of the gingiva can be modified by appropriate surgical techniques to achieve an ultimate esthetic result.

213

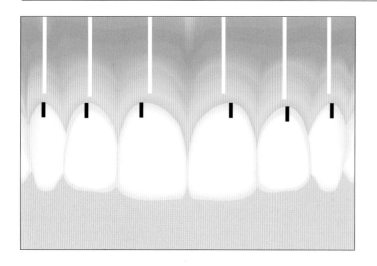

Fig 6-7 The most apical point of the marginal gingiva does not correspond with the midpoint at upper central and canines. The "zenith" is located at the distal line angles of those teeth. Lateral incisors have the zenith at the mid-facial. The "zenith" should be relocated by periodontal surgery in cases where diastema will be closed by restorative means.

incisors is usually located 1-2 mm more incisally, or at the same height of central incisor and cuspids. The height of the contour, or, as often called, the gingival zenith, is located at the distal line angle of the central incisors and cuspids (Fig 6-7). The maxillary lateral incisors have a symmetrical gingival height of contour with the gingival zenith at the midfacial tooth surface[9] (for detailed discussion of the ideal full smile see Chapter 2).

Clinical Features of Interdental Gingiva

The interdental gingiva occupies the space delineated within the area of tooth contact, interdental tip of the alveolar bone and tooth surfaces (Fig 6-8). The interdental gingiva can be pyramidal or have a "col" shape in the facial lingual direction. Increase in the facial-lingual diameters of teeth results in shift from pyramidial shape to col shape as observed in anterior to posterior regions. Where the shape of the interdental gingiva is pyramidal there is only one tip of the tissue which is immediately under the contact point. Cohen[10] was the first to describe the interdental papilla with two peaks, vestibularly and lingually, within a concave crest shaping the so-called col. The vestibular peak of the interdental papilla extends more coronally than the lingual one and the distance between those peaks increases from anterior to posterior (Fig 6-9).

The morphology of interdental gingiva is governed by the size, shape, and position of contact area between adjacent teeth and the level of underlying bone crest[11] (Fig 6-10). The interdental embrasure and the gingiva filling the space are narrow, mesiodistally, when the proximal surfaces of the teeth are relatively flat; buccolingually, the roots are close together, and the interdental bone is thin mesiodistally. Conversely, with proximal surfaces that flare away from the area of contact, the mesiodistal diameter of the interdental gingiva is broad. The location of the contact point is the result of the emergence profile and the line angle form of the maxillary incisors and cuspids.[12] Contact point between the maxillary central incisors is located in the incisal third of the labial aspect, between the central and lateral incisor in the middle, and between the lateral incisor and the canine in the apical third. The presence and the space occupied by the soft tissue is observed to be relevant to the distance from the contact to the crest of the alveolar bone. Tarnow, et al.[13] report that the papilla was present in all cases when the distance from the contact point to the crest of bone was 5 mm or less. A 1 mm increase in the distance from the contact point to the bone reduces the possibility of an intact papilla almost by half, in which papilla was present in 56% of the cases where the distance was 6 mm, and only 27% or less of the cases when this distance was 7 mm or more. Root angulation is another factor that affects interdental gingiva. Divergent angulation of the roots of two adjacent teeth creates a wider embrasure space and a contact point located incisally.

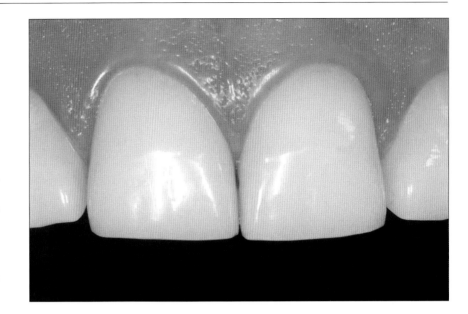

Fig 6-8 The base of the papilla corresponds to the line tangential to the gingival margins of adjacent teeth, while a healthy papilla reaches about half-way to the incisal edge, and shows a high degree of stippling. The papilla located between the central incisors is being the most challenging one by its location and volume.

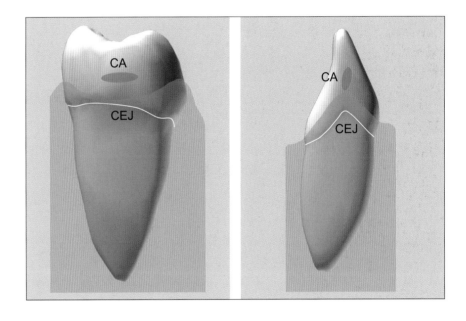

Fig 6-9 The interdental papilla has only one peak at the anterior teeth. The peak is located just apical to the contact area between two teeth. At the posterior teeth the papilla has two peaks and the concavity between two peaks is called the "col". The col is located just apical to the contact area and is not resistant to microbial irritation.

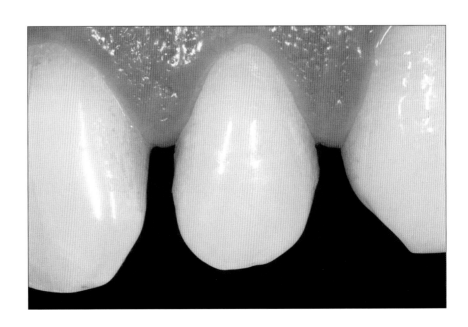

Fig 6-10 The interdental space is not filled with papilla in cases of diastemas. In such cases the interproximal gingival tissue shows a higher degree of keratinization.

Esthetic Periodontal Problems

Gingival Inflammation and Tissue Loss Owing to Periodontal Disease

Periodontal disease is the result of the accumulation of dental plaque at the gingival margin leading to inflammation of the periodontal tissues. Traditionally, periodontal disease has been divided into gingivitis and periodontitis, depending on whether destruction of the tooth-supporting tissues has occurred (Fig 6-11). Diagnosis and treatment of periodontal problems are based on clinical findings such as probing pocket depths, attachment loss, gingival bleeding, and radiographic evaluation of the alveolar crest. The objective of periodontal treatment can be summarized as the prevention of tooth loss, maintenance of periodontal support, repair, and regeneration of damaged tissues and their function. But when the etiology of the periodontal disease is considered, the main task seems to be the modification of patient habits in order to constitute an oral hygiene level that would prevent inflammation of periodontal tissues owing to plaque accumulation.

Gingival inflammation and associated periodontal destruction are leading factors that can reverse the esthetic outcome in the long term. Establishing definitive restorations when inflammatory periodontal problems are present not only restrains esthetic success, but also accelerates the rate of periodontal destruction. Elimination of gingival inflammation is mandatory before initiation of any restorative treatment. Initial periodontal therapy that consists of oral hygiene instruction, elimination of retentive factors, scaling and root planing will result in the resolution of inflammation. Patients with moderate to severe periodontitis may require advanced periodontal treatment that could consist of surgical procedures to eliminate residual periodontal pockets and regeneration of the lost periodontal tissues. Pocket elimination surgery usually results in long clinical crowns that may be esthetically unacceptable. In deep isolated angular periodontal defects, guided tissue regeneration offers good results to maintain the tooth and avoid an es-

thetic disaster. Alveolar ridge deformities are inevitable after the extraction of hopeless teeth when special attention was not paid to preserving the height and width of the ridge at the time of extraction.

Restorative Margins and Violation of Biological Principles

Preservation of the healthy status of periodontal tissues is the most significant factor in the long-term prognosis of a restored tooth. There are five major causes of plaque-related inflammatory periodontal disease associated with restorative procedures:

1. severe damage to the periodontal tissues during tooth preparation and impression making
2. failure to maintain emergence profile
3. inability to adequately finish and/or seal subgingival margins
4. placement of subgingival margins at sites with minimum to no attached gingiva
5. violation of the biologic width.

Teeth prepared without retraction cord which subsequently receive either retraction cord, electrosurgery, or rotary gingival curettage sustain various degrees of soft tissue damage, as reported by *Dragoo* and *Williams*.[14,15] Tooth preparations for restorative procedures should be accomplished atraumatically to avoid irreversible damage to the supracrestal connective tissue fibers and tissue loss.

The cervical one-third of the clinical crown is also referred to as the emergence profile of the tooth. This is the region where the crown emerges from the periodontium and its supra-subgingival contours should have a flat emergence profile, with the guidance of anatomic information in order to maintain an area that is cleanable with oral hygiene instruments and which has a good marginal seal of the restoration (Fig 6-12). There is a very strict relationship between marginal seal and emergence profile.[16] Poor adaptation and roughness of the restoration margin results in mechanical irritation of the sulcular epithelium and can harbor microbial flora.[17] Overhanging margins not only accumulate more plaque than

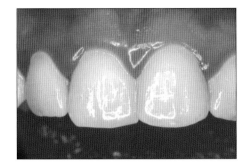

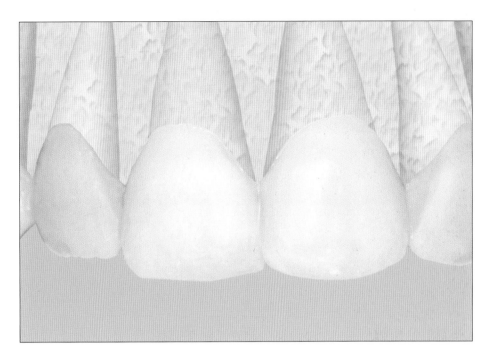

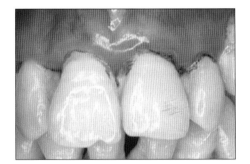

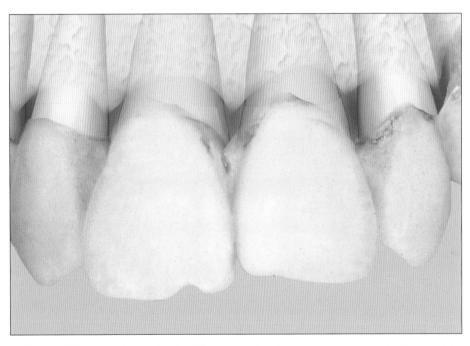

Fig 6-11 Chronic gingivitis is the inflammation of the marginal gingival tissue owing to plaque accumulation and is characterized clinically by redness, swelling and bleeding of the tissues. There is no destruction of the alveolar bone. Periodontitis, on the other hand, is the plaque-induced inflammation of the periodontal tissues that has resulted in destruction of the periodontal ligament and alveolar bone with apical migration of junctional epithelium.

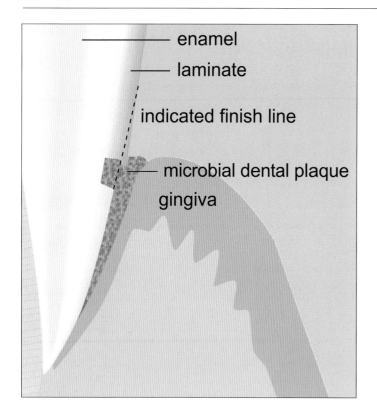

enamel

laminate

indicated finish line

microbial dental plaque

gingiva

Fig 6-12 The interface between the laminate and the tooth should not facilitate plaque retention and should always be cleanable with oral hygiene instruments. The restoration surface should be flush with the surface of the remaining tooth structure.

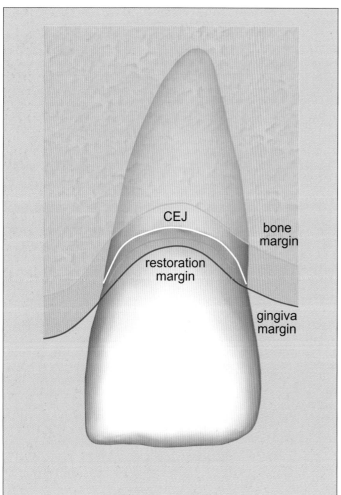

CEJ

bone margin

restoration margin

gingiva margin

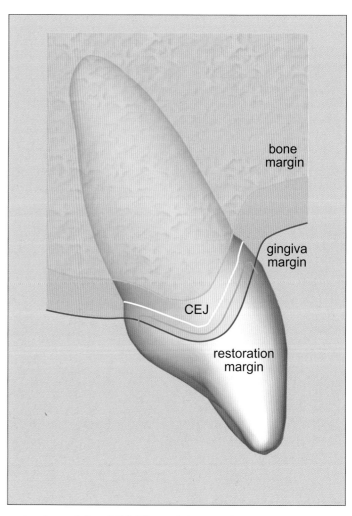

bone margin

gingiva margin

CEJ

restoration margin

Fig 6-13 The margin of the restoration should follow the accentuation of the CEJ. The minimum distance required to maintain periodontal health is 2.5 mm from the restoration margin. Violation of this principle results in inflammation of the junctional epithelium and connective tissue attachment, and eventually marginal bone loss.

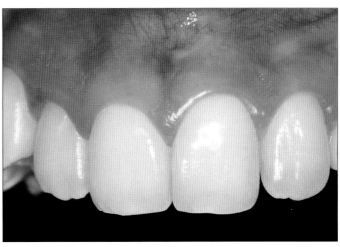

Fig 6-14 Maxillary central incisors require special attention since two teeth are adjacent and asymmetries could easily be detected. Lateral incisors, cuspids and bicuspids are also important but the distance between two identical teeth conceals minor asymmetries in most cases.

properly finished margins, but the plaque undergoes a shift in composition to that seen in association with destructive periodontitis.[18]

An adequate band of keratinized tissue is fundamental to successful restorative dentistry if the margins of the restorations are extended under free gingival margin.[17] Approximately 5 mm of keratinized tissue, composed of 2 mm of free gingiva and 3 mm of attached gingiva, is considered necessary to meet restorative objectives even in cases with ideal finishing and margin placement at the subgingival area.[17] Although no solid investigation is present to confirm this observation, augmentation of keratinized gingiva provides stability of the free gingival margin and surrounding gingival tissues so that the gingival health around the restoration can be maintained. Besides vertical dimension of the keratinized gingiva, the thickness of the tissue should be enough to tolerate intracrevicular restorations.

The gingival sulcus extends from the free gingival margin to the epithelial attachment. In health, its depth is in the vicinity of 0-3 mm,[1] and it is lined with thin sulcular epithelium. The depth of this sulcus may vary from tooth to tooth and from surface to surface on the same tooth. Compromising the apico-coronal width of the connective tissue attachment by placement of crown margins deep in to the sulcus initiates persistent and irreversible gingival inflammation owing to violation of the biologic width. Such violations sever the junctional epithelium and the supragingival connective tissue fibers. Apical

migration of the junctional epithelium encourages development of periodontal pockets and alveolar bone loss. The finish line of restorations should follow the contour of the cementoenamel junction and be always kept at least 2.5 mm away from the bone crest (Fig 6-13). A 2.5-mm difference means that although the biologic width is being respected, the finish line is located near the base of the crevice. A greater distance between the bone crest and finish line of the restoration is needed to ensure that margin of the restoration could be well reached by the plaque control instruments. The golden standard today is to prepare the finish lines of the restorations 0.5 mm below the marginal gingiva if the sulcus depth is 1 mm, 0.5 to 1 mm if the sulcus depth is exceeding 1.5 mm. This leaves enough distance for the junctional epithelium and supracrestal fibers, and is also close enough to the gingival margin to be reached by oral hygiene procedures. When the healthy sulcus depth is less than 1 mm, placement of the margin 0.5 mm subgingivaly could result in impinging upon the junctional epithelium. The margin in such cases should be terminated just at or above the gingival margin.

Gingival asymmetries and discrepancies

The esthetic appearance is considerably affected by the symmetry created by dental and facial midline (Fig 6-14). In the etiology of gingival asymmetries, altered passive eruption, different patterns of tooth wear, traumas that modify tooth

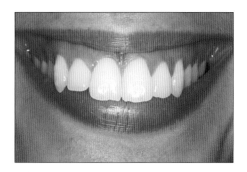 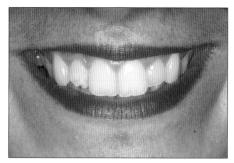 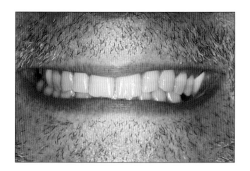

Fig 6-15 High, medium and low lip lines. Gingival margins of upper teeth and the vermilion border of the upper lip are the important landmarks in determining the level of the lip line. Esthetic treatment planning is complicated in patients with a high lip line.

eruption, tooth positioning in the dental arch, parafunctional habits and overzealous tooth brushing should be considered. The selection of an adequate method of treatment depends on adequacy of attached gingiva, tooth structure, vestibular depth, the distance from the gingival margin to the crest of the bone, root angulation and tooth positioning and interproximal level of the alveolar bone when recession is present. Correction of this disharmony requires surgical elongation or root coverage, orthodontic treatment and restorative procedures.

Excessive Gingival Display

"Gummy smile" can be considered as a significant esthetic problem by many patients. Ideally, the smile should expose minimal gingiva around the lateral incisors. The gingival margins of maxillary central incisors and cuspids should coincide with the vermillion border of the upper lip. The lip line, assessed when the patient is in full smile, is classified as high (gummy smile), medium (ideal), and low (maxillary lip covering a portion of maxillary teeth) (Fig 6-15). Aging leads to a decrease in the amount of anterior tooth display when smiling.[19] Maxillary overgrowth, insufficient upper lip, tooth malpositioning, and delayed apical migration of the gingival margin or a combination of more than one are among the most common reasons of "gummy smile".

Skeletal deformities that involve maxillary overgrowth can be diagnosed by evaluation of the proportions of the face and cephalometric analysis. In such cases the teeth's length-to-width ration usually remains constant – the ideal being approximately 10:8.[20] The ideally proportioned face is divided into three equal parts from the hairline to the eyebrow, from the eyebrow to the base of nasal process, and from the base of the nose to the chin. When the middle one-third of the face is longer than other two, "gummy smile" is diagnosed owing to maxillary overgrowth. In combined cases that maxillary overgrowth is superimposed with delayed passive eruption and the latter should be treated first. Treatment limited to periodontal surgery will be insufficient, since the level of the incisal edge to lip at rest position cannot be rebuilt. Minor maxillary overgrowth cases can be successfully treated with periodontics-orthodontics or periodontics-restorative combinations. Increase in the gingival and mucosal display necessitates complex treatment options that combine orthognathic-orthodontic procedures and perio-prostho treatment.

The normal length of the upper lip is between 18 and 21 mm, vertically. A shorter lip over a moderate dental arch could result in excessive gingival display. When the "gummy smile" is solely dependent on insufficient lip dimensions, a perio-restorative solution composed of surgical crown lengthening and restoring the teeth with laminates could be the choice of treatment.

A less frequent reason of excessive gingival display is the tooth malpositioning. Orthodontic repositioning and surgical correction are the treatment options in those cases.

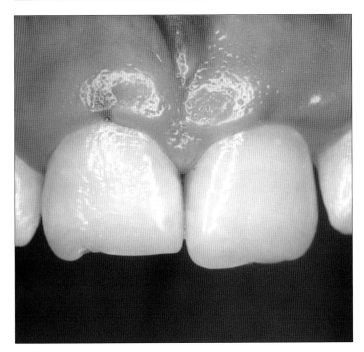
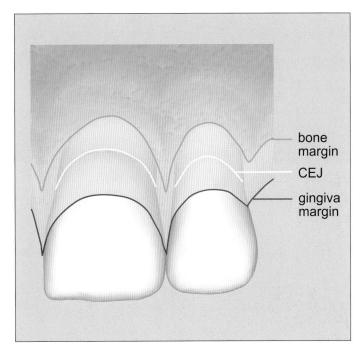

Fig 6-16 Square tooth form with thick and fibrotic gingival tissues indicates delayed passive eruption. Probing pocket depth measurements exceed 3 mm and the CEJ is at its base or underneath the bottom of the sulcus in such cases. The distance from the gingival margin to the crest of the bone is increased.

The last but not least reason for the excessive gingival display is the delayed passive eruption, or what some authors call "altered passive eruption". Passive eruption is the exposure of teeth by apical migration of the gingiva, whereas active eruption is the movement of teeth in the occlusal direction. When the teeth reach their functional antagonists, the gingival sulcus and junctional epithelium are still on the enamel, and the clinical crown is approximately two-thirds of the anatomic crown.[21] Delay in the apical migration of the marginal gingiva and the junctional epithelium results in a condition in adulthood in which the gingival margin is positioned incisally or occlusally on the anatomic crown and does not approximate the CEJ.

When the gingiva is not inflamed but thick and fibrotic, and displays a nominal degree of scallop to the free gingival margin resulting in a square tooth form, delayed passive eruption should be suspected (Fig 6-16). Diagnosis is made by probing the sulcus and sounding the alveolar bone margin to determine their relationship with CEJ. Clinical and anatomic crown length, width of the attached gingiva, tooth positioning and involve-ment of frenum are additional factors in diagnosis and treatment planning.

There are two types of delayed passive eruption, as proposed by *Coslet*, et al.[22] (see Table 6-1). In this classification, gingival/anatomic crown relationship is divided into two major groups. In type 1 cases, the gingival margin is located incisal or occlusal to the CEJ, with a wide zone of attached gingiva, and the mucogingival junction is usually apical to the alveolar crest (Fig 6-17). There is typically an excessive amount of gingiva as measured from the free gingival margin to the mucogingival junction. In type 2 cases the mucogingival junction is located at the level or near CEJ where the band of attached gingiva is in the normal range as measured from the free gingival margin to the mucogingival junction (Fig 6-18). The major distinction between two types is the location of the mucogingival junction, which also serves as a useful guideline in the treatment planning. A further subdivision evaluates the alveolar crest and CEJ relationships (Fig 6-19).

Treatment options of delayed passive eruption should be based on diagnosis of the type. A typical case of type IA delayed passive eruption

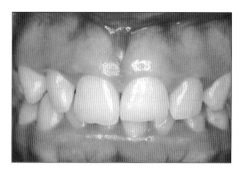 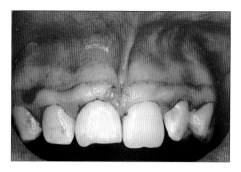 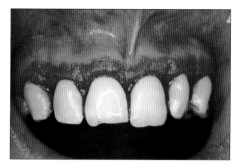

Fig 6-17 Delayed passive eruption type 1. Wide zone of attached gingiva. The case is treated with gingivectomy procedure since there is a wide band of attached gingiva.

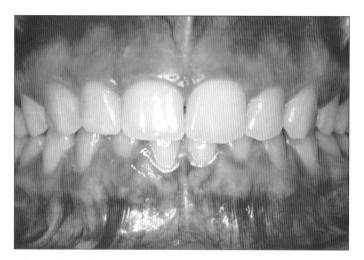 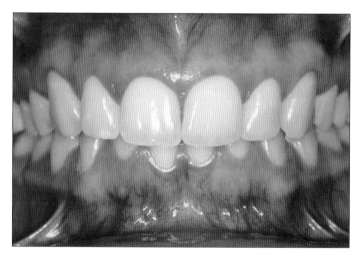

Fig 6-18 Delayed passive eruption type 2. Normal width of the attached gingiva. Normal width of the attached gingiva excludes the treatment choice of a gingivectomy procedure. An apically located flap procedure is needed to maintain the width of the attached gingiva.

Table 6-1   Classification of Delayed Passive Migration of the Gingival Margin

Type	A	B
1. Short clinical crowns with mucogingival junction being apical to the alveolar crest. Wide band of attached gingiva.	Alveolar crest to CEJ ≥ 2 mm	Alveolar crest to CEJ < 2 mm
2. Short clinical crowns with mucogingival junction being at the level or near CEJ. Normal band of attached gingiva.	Alveolar crest to CEJ ≥ 2 mm	Alveolar crest to CEJ < 2 mm

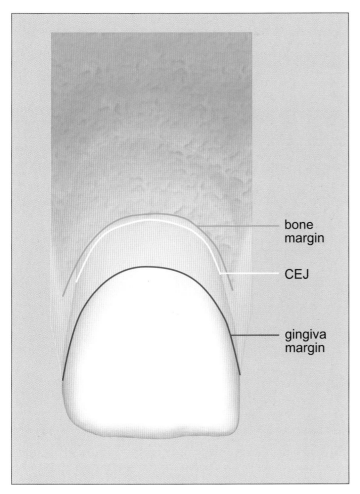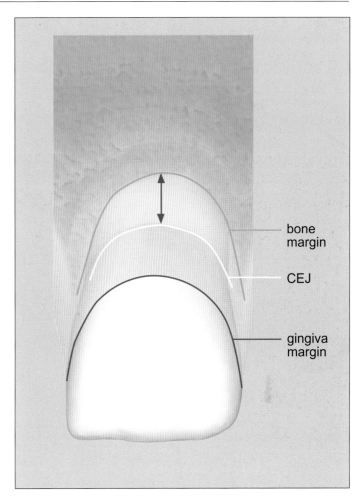

Fig 6-19 Alveolar crest-CEJ relationship in delayed passive eruption cases. In subgroup A, the distance from CEJ to the crest of the alveolar bone corresponds to the 2 mm distance, which is accepted as normal. In cases of subgroup B, the alveolar crest is almost at the level of CEJ.

exhibits short, square-looking teeth with a wide zone of attached gingiva and confirms the presence of sufficient space (biologic width) to maintain supracrestal fiber attachment on transgingival probing. A gingivectomy procedure performed by a scalpel, electrosurgery or CO_2 laser can remove the excess tissue (Fig 6-17). Tissue removal should be performed very carefully in order not to compromise interdental papilla and end up with some loss at the gingival tissue filling the embrasures. Removal of the tissue will result in more elliptical tooth form that restores the 10:8 length to width ratio. Initial wound healing takes place in the first couple of weeks where remodeling of the soft tissue continues for as long as 4 to 6 months.

Treatment options of type IB delayed passive eruption cases should create sufficient space for supracrestal fiber attachment to maintain the proper biologic width while eliminating the excess gingiva. In type IB cases there is an added dimension buccolingually to the osseous form.[23] This extra thickness of osseous structure allows for an apical angulation of the bone crest from the gingival aspect of the periodontal ligament side allowing for insertion of the connective tissue fibers just apical to the CEJ. Surgical correction of this reverse anatomy requires relocation of the alveolar crest, thinning of the alveolar margin, and securing enough space for development of proper biologic width (Fig 6-18). Since the level of gingival tissue normally follows the architecture of the underlying osseous crest, alveolar reduction should meticulously be performed in order to dictate the final gingival level and contour at the time of bony recontouring. The height of the interproximal bone should always be 3 to 4 mm coronal to the height of the newly created alveolar crest on the facial aspect in order to support the interproximal papilla. Surgical crown lengthening requires reflection of full thickness flaps and recontouring of the alveolar bone with chisels and burs. Surgical trauma owing to full thickness reflection of the access flap and bone recontouring results in resorption of the crestal alveolar bone approximately 0.63 mm.[24] This inevitable bone loss should be calculated at the time of surgical planning to prevent unexpected recessions, especially in cases with thin gingiva and facial alveolar plate where more bone loss is expected.

On the other hand, in a clinical study it was reported that a 3 mm biological zone was not routinely achieved after surgical crown lengthening procedure, and the amount of root surface was still short of the initially planned biologic width after healing.[25] A histometric study in monkeys demonstrated that healing following osseous crown lengthening procedure resulted in a junctional epithelium that extended to the apical level of root planing, reestablishing a reduced biologic width.[26] Scaling and rootplaning during crown lengthening was recommended to enable the surgeon accurately to determine the superior termination of the supracrestal connective tissue, since space for the supracrestal connective tissue fiber groups is created by crestal resorption of alveolar bone.[26] Initial wound healing takes around 10 days after surgery, and final remodeling usually continues for as long as 6 months, but the tissue reaches a stable position after 6 weeks. Gentle handling of the tissues and strict adherence to plastic surgery principles shortens healing and remodeling periods.

Treatment of type II cases requires relocation of the entire dentogingival complex to a more apical position without rendering loss of attached gingiva with or without removal of the bony margin. Loss of attached gingiva results in alveolar mucosa located at the gingival margin that jeopardizes maintenance of the marginal health, and unacceptable esthetics. Attached gingiva must be preserved at crown-lengthening procedures in such cases by reflection of full to split thickness flap and apical positioning of the mucogingival

complex. The healing pattern is similar to other crown-lengthening procedures.

Long-term stability of the gingival margin created by crown-lengthening procedures relies particularly on the respect paid for the biologic width. As previously mentioned, approximately 2 mm is needed between the base of the sulcus and the crest of the bone to provide space for the connective tissue attachment and junctional epithelium. Adding the depth of the sulcus to biologic width results in a minimum of 3 mm from the newly created gingival margin to the crest of the bone. Violations of this basic principle result in poor cosmetic results that require retreatment.

Gingival recessions

Chronic trauma caused by vigorous tooth brushing and plaque-induced periodontal inflammation is the major causative factor in the development of soft tissue recessions.[27,28] Beyond those two major causes, malpositioning of teeth,[29] dehiscence in vestibular alveolar plate,[30] high frenum,[31] and iatrogenic factors[32] contribute significantly in the etiology of recessions. Elimination of those factors is crucial in both prevention and treatment of recessions in a predictable long-term outcome. *Sullivan* and *Atkins*[33] made initial classification of the marginal tissue loss in two major vertical categories of shallow and deep recessions with horizontal subgroups as "narrow" and "wide". This classification was used until 1985 when *Miller*[34] presented an expanded classification (Fig 6-20). Based on this classification, the amount of root coverage can be determined presurgically. Total root coverage is expected in class I and II cases. In class III cases, the amount of root coverage can be estimated presurgically by placing a periodontal probe horizontally on an imaginary line connecting the tissue level on the mid-facial of the two teeth on either side of the tooth exhibiting recession. This is a very practical and important classification for the clinical decision-making process, because it allows the practitioner and the patient to have realistic expectations regarding the outcome of the case.

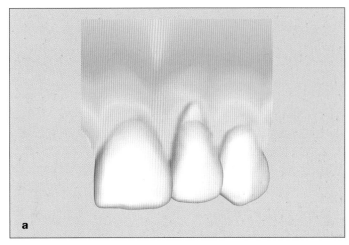

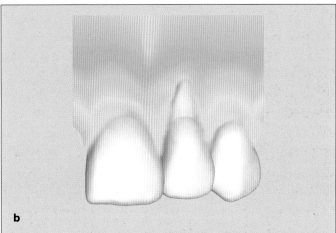

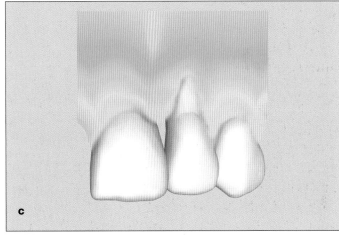

Fig 6-20a-d Classification of gingival recessions. (a) Class I: Marginal tissue recession that does not extend to the mucogingival junction. There is no periodontal loss (bone or soft tissue) in the interdental area, and 100% root coverage can be anticipated. (b) Class II: Marginal tissue recession that extends to or beyond the mucogingival junction. There is no periodontal loss (bone or soft tissue) in the interdental area, and 100% root coverage can be anticipated. (c) Class III: Marginal tissue recession that extends to or beyond the mucogingival junction. Bone or soft tissue loss in the interdental area is present, or there is malpositioning of the teeth that prevents the attempting of 100% root coverage. Partial root coverage can be anticipated. (d) Class IV: Marginal tissue recession that extends to or beyond the mucogingival junction. The bone or soft tissue loss in the interdental area and/or the malpositioning of the teeth is so severe that root coverage cannot be attempted.

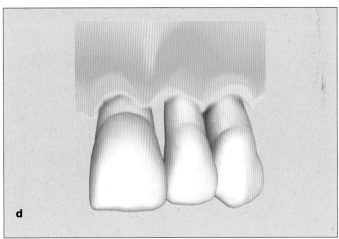

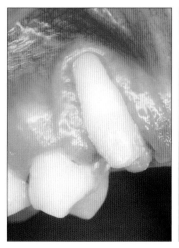 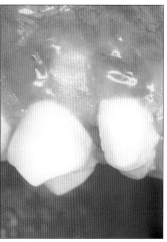

Fig 6-21 Laterally positioned pedicle flap procedure offers the advantage of single surgical site and a good supply of blood with an excellent color match. Good blood supply shortens the healing phase and minimizes the risk of complications. The major limitation is the lack of sufficient donor tissue lateral to the defect. Three weeks after surgery, as seen in the case, tissue has matured to a great extent despite the debris and poor plaque control.

Besides esthetic concerns owing to gingival recessions, increased root sensitivity and sensitivity related gingival inflammation and/or decay are major problems associated with exposed root surfaces. With the growing concern for cosmetic dentistry, and the subsequent need for periodontal procedures that would meet patient expectations, numerous techniques have been developed to cover the exposed root surfaces. Those techniques fall into the following four major categories.

Pedicle Flaps

Coronally[35] and laterally[36] positioned contiguous gingival grafts. The technique is used to treat shallow areas of recession (*Miller* class I) where 3 mm of keratinized tissue is present.[37] A modification of coronally positioned flaps by *Tarnow*[38] under the term "semilunar coronally repositioned flap" offers high predictability and superb color match to treat class I recessions. This procedure is limited with the height and thickness of the gingiva apical to the recession. Laterally positioned pedicle flap (called by some clinicians "rotational flap") received several modifications over the years but the fundamental principle is covering the exposed root surfaces by the gingival tissue lateral to the recession (Fig 6-21). This technique offers the advantages of good blood supply, excellent match of color, and a single surgical site. On the other hand, limitations like the necessity for adequate dimensions of gingiva lateral to the

site of recession, as well as its inability to treat multiple recessions and its requirement of deep vestibule, confines its application to cases of single recession with an adequate amount of neighboring attached gingiva.

Free Autogenous Soft Tissue Grafts

Free gingival[39] and subepithelial connective tissue[40] grafts have been reported to be predictable and successful ways of root coverage. Free gingival grafts are utilized to increase the zone of attached gingiva around teeth and implants, and to cover the exposed root surfaces. Having the palatal mucosa on the surface 1.5-2 mm thick, free gingival grafts heal in a lighter and more opaque color than the gingiva at the recipient site, and it increases the gingival thickness. Meta-analytic review of success rate of the free gingival grafts revealed a high predictability in classes I and II recessions with mean root coverage around 75%, and complete root coverage incidence 50%.[41] Subepithelial connective tissue graft is also used in root coverage surgery. The procedure takes advantage of a double blood supply from the recipient bed and the gingival flap that covers the graft. It generally results in a better color match, but increased thickness can compromise esthetics in the healing period until the remodeling process is completed within a year (Fig 6-22a and b). The major contraindication to this approach is the inability to harvest adequate thickness of donor material from the palate. Mean root

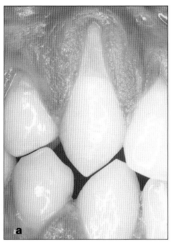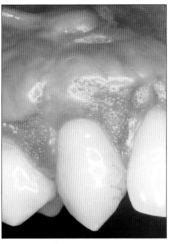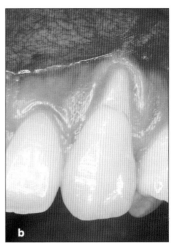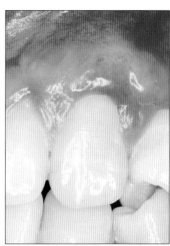

Fig 6-22a, b (a) Although full maturation of the thick subepithelial connective tissue grafts takes a long time, a thick and well-matched color can be obtained within a year. Thick gingival tissue is more important in cases where root prominence is evident. (b) The surface characteristics of thin grafted tissue mature in a shorter period of time. Color match is acceptable and the band of attached gingiva is increased.

coverage and total root coverage incidence is very high in classes I and II cases and reported to be 91% and 68% respectively.[41]

Combined Techniques

These are surgical procedures that combine more than one technique either in the same stage or at a second stage of surgery. Free gingival graft with a coronally positioned flap is a common example of this approach. Either a gingival graft is placed simultaneously with the coronally positioned flap, or following placement of a gingival graft the entire complex is moved coronally at a second surgical procedure. Another common combination is the root surface coverage with a subepithelial connective tissue graft and sliding the lateral two papillae over the grafted tissue. Other clinicians have suggested several more combinations to furnish the requirements of specific cases, but none has become popular and widely used.

Guided Tissue Regeneration

The technique is based on the principle to provide and maintain an adequate space to allow formation of a blood clot that is expected to transform into new cementum, new connective tissue attachment, and new bone. Results obtained by

resorbable and non-resorbable membranes to cover exposed root surfaces are comparable with subepithelial connective tissue grafts,[42] and can be used in the treatment of deep and wide (larger than 5 mm) facial recessions. No requirement for a donor site reduces patient discomfort during healing. Highly esthetic results can be provided since the color of the new tissue blends evenly with the adjacent sites. The main disadvantage is that the treatment is reserved for single tooth application. The specific use is limited to the cases that lacks donor tissue and attached gingiva until improved GTR devices and surgical methods are developed.

Open Interproximal Spaces

Reconstruction of the lost interdental papilla is one of the most challenging and least predictable problems in periodontal plastic surgery. Besides creating a black triangle at the maxillary anterior region, missing interdental papilla results in food impaction and phonetic problems. The presence and morphology of the interdental papilla is strictly dependent on the size and shape of interproximal contact, crest of alveolar bone, and shape of lateral tooth surfaces, as stated earlier.[11] Reconstruction of the lost interproximal tissues therefore requires techniques that reestablish

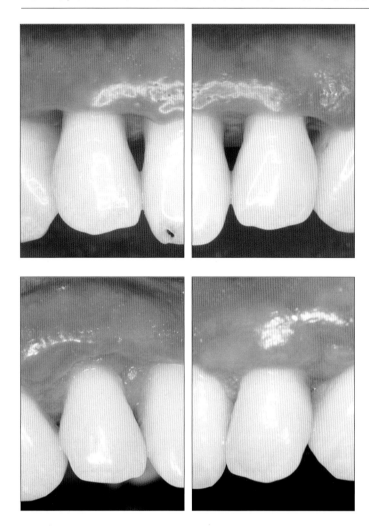

Fig 6-23 Subepithelial connective tissue grafts (especially thick ones) are a good alternative in creating papillae where interproximal bone loss is minimum. Primary good blood supply must be accomplished by choosing an atraumatic technique with the periosteum left intact.

the prerequisites of the presence of the papilla. Nonsurgical and prosthetic approaches may alter the contact point, lateral tooth structure and tooth angulation resulting in restoration of the lost interdental tissue. Surgical techniques that aim to increase the gingival soft tissue and bone content of the interproximal spaces are complicated with the anatomic limitations and the blood supply problem. Several surgical techniques have been suggested in case reports for reconstruction,[43-45] but none of them seems to be sufficient and predictable to restore the lost tissue. Limited success has been attained by soft tissue grafts (Fig 6-23). Regeneration of the interproximal alveolar bone seems to be the ultimate treatment method to achieve papilla reconstruction keeping in mind that the gingival contour follows the crestal alveolar bone and that the distance from the bone crest to the contact area dictates the interdental soft tissue level.

References

1. Gargiulo AW, Wentz FM, Orban B. Dimensions and relations of the dentogingival junction in humans. J Periodontol 1961;32:261-267.

2. Hassell TM. Tissues and cells of the periodontium. Periodontology 2000 1993;3:9-38.

3. Freeman E. Periodontium. In: Oral Histology: Development, Structure, and Function. 4th ed. Ten Cate, AR ed. St Louis, MO: Mosby, 1994:276-313.

4. Cohen DW. Periodontal preparation of the mouth for restorative dentistry. Presented at the Walter Reed Army Medical Center, Washington, DC, 1962. Cited from note 8.

5. Nevins M, Skurow H. The intracrevicular restorative margin, the biologic width, and the maintenance of the gingival margin. Int J Periodont Rest Dent 1984;4:30-49.

6. Kois JC. New paradigms for anterior tooth preparation: Rationale and technique. Contemp Esth Dent 1996;2:1-8.

7. Periodontal literature reviews: A su mmary of current knowledge. Chicago: American Academy of Periodontology, 1996:36-39.

8. Smukler H, Chaibi M. Periodontal and dental considerations in clinical crown extension: A rational basis for treatment. Int J Periodont Rest Dent 1997;17:465-477.

9. Allen EP. Surgical crown lengthening for function and esthetics. Dent Clin North Am. 1993;37:163-179.

10. Cohen B. Pathology of the interdental tissues. Dent Pract 1959;9:167-173.

11. Kohl JT, Zander HA. Morphology of interdental gingival tissues. Oral Surg Oral Med Oral Pathol 1961;60:287-295.

12. Miller PD, Allen EP. The development of periodontal plastic surgery. Periodontology 2000 1996;11:7-17.

13. Tarnow DP, Magner AW, Fletcher P. The effect of the distance from the contact point to the crest of bone on the presence or absence of the interproximal dental papilla. J Periodontol 1992;63:995-996.

14. Dragoo MR, Williams GB. Periodontal tissue reactions to restorative procedures. Part 1. Int J Periodont Rest Dent 1982;2:8-29.

15. Dragoo MR, Williams GB. Periodontal tissue reactions to restorative procedures. Part 2. Int J Periodont Rest Dent 1982;2:34-42.

16. Martignoni M, Schönenberger A. Precision fixed prosthodontics: Clinical and laboratory aspects. Chicago: Quintessence, 1990:255-258.

17. Maynard JG, Wilson RD. Physiologic dimensions of the periodontium significant to the restorative dentist. J Periodontol 1979;50:170-174.

18. Lang NP, Kiel RA, Anderhalden K. Clinical and microbiological effects of subgingival restorations with overhanging or clinically perfect margins. J Clin Periodont 1983; 10: 563-578.

19. Vig RG, Brundo GC. The kinetics of anterior tooth display. J Prosthet Dent 1978;39:502-504.

20. Borissavlievitch M. The Golden Number. London: Alec Tiranti, 1964.

21. Itoiz ME, Carranza FA. The gingiva. In: Carranza FA, Newman MG. Clinical Periodontology. 8th ed. Philadelphia: WB Saunders, 1996:12-29.

22. Coslet JG, Vanarsdall RL, Weisgold A. Diagnosis and classification of delayed passive eruption of the dentogingival junction in the adult. Alpha Omegan 1977;70:24-28.

23. Garber DA, Salama MA. The aesthetic smile: Diagnosis and treatment. Periodontol 2000 1996;11:18-28.

24. Pennel B, King K, Wilderman M, Barron J. Repair of the alveolar process following osseous surgery. J Periodontol 1967;38:426-431.

25. Herrero F, Scott JB, Maropis PS, Yukna RA. Clinical comparison of desired versus actual amount of surgical crown lengthening. J Periodontol 1995;66:568-571.

26. Oakley E, Rhyu IC, Karatzas S, Gandini-Santiago L, Nevins M, Caton J. Formation of the biological width following crown lengthening in nonhuman primates. Int J Periodont Rest Dent 1999;19:529-541.

27. Löe H, Anerud A, Boysen H. The natural history of periodontal disease in man: Prevalance, severity, and extent of gingival recession. J Periodontol 1992;63:489-495.

28. Khocht A, Simon G, Person P, Denepitiya JL. Gingival recession in relation to history of hard toothbrush use. J Periodontol 1993; 64: 900-905.

29. Kallestal C, Uhlin S. Buccal attachment loss in Swedish adolescents. J Clin Periodont 1992; 19: 485-491.

30. Löst C. Depth of alveolar bone dehiscences in relation to gingival recessions. J Clin Periodont 1984;11:583-589.

31. Mirko P, Miroslav S, Lubor M. Significance of the labial frenum attachment in periodontal disease in man. Part 1. Classification and epidemiology of the labial frenum attachment. J Periodontol 1974;45:891-894.

32. Stetler KJ, Bissada NF. Significance of the width of keratinized gingiva on the periodontal status of teeth with submarginal restorations. J Periodontol 1987;58:696-700.

33. Sullivan HC, Atkins JH. Free autogenous gingival grafts. 3. Utilization of grafts in the treatment of gingival recession. Periodontics 1968;6:152-160.

34. Miller PD. A classification of marginal tissue recession. Int J Periodont Rest Dent 1985;5:8-13.

35. Harland AW. Discussion of paper: Restoration of the gum tissue. Dent Cosmos 1907;49:591-598.

36. Grupe HE, Warren RF Jr. Repair of gingival defects by a sliding flap operation. J Periodontol 1956;27:290-295.

37. Allen EP, Miller PD Jr. Coronal positioning of existing gingiva: Short term results in the treatment of shallow marginal tissue recession. J Periodontol 1989; 60: 316-319.

38. Tarnow DP. Semilunar coronally repositioned flap. J Clin Periodontol 1986;13:182-185.

39. Miller PD Jr. Root coverage using a free soft tissue autograft following citric acid application. Part 1. Technique. Int J Periodont Rest Dent 1982; 2: 65-70.

40. Langer B, Langer L. Subepithelial connective tissue graft technique for root coverage. J Periodontol 1985;56:715-720.

41. Efeoglu A, Demirel K, Okan E. Dişeti çekilmelerinin tedavisinde kullanilan cerrahi yöntemelerin değerlendiril-mesi. Academic Dental 2001;3:20-26.

42. Ricci G, Silvestri M, Tinti C, Rasperini G. A clinical/statistical comparison between the subpedicle connective tissue graft method and the guided tissue regeneration technique in root coverage. Int J Periodont Rest Dent 1996;16: 539-545.

43. Han TJ, Takei HH. Progress in gingival papilla reconstruction. Periodontol 2000. 1996;11:65-68.

44. Blatz MB, Hürzeler MB, Strub JR. Reconstruction of the lost interproximal papilla. Presentation of surgical and nonsurgical approaches. Int J Periodont Rest Dent 1999;19:395-406.

45. Azzi R, Takei HH, Etienne D, Carranza FA. Root coverage and papilla reconstruction using autogenous and connective tissue grafts. Int J Periodont Rest Dent 2001;21:141-147.

7   Atlas of Porcelain Laminate Veneers

Galip Gürel

Determining the Essentials

In order to determine the optimal method of patient care, the patient's existing clinical condition must be accurately diagnosed and treatment objectives (biocompatibility, esthetics and long-term function) established accordingly. Once an analysis of the condition has been completed, the correct restorative procedure can be selected in order to address the complications presented by that particular patient. Comprehensive radiographic and clinical examinations (occlusal, muscular, joint) are integral components in the process of determining the preoperative status of the patient and, consequently, the evaluation of the possibility of achieving a successful rehabilitation.[1]

Dentistry continues to advance and present-day esthetic dentistry has evolved into effective functional biocompatible procedures that are appearance enhancing as well. However, esthetic dentistry can be a complex and demanding process. The dental profession has experienced a proliferation in the number of available choices in dental materials, prosthetic designs and laboratory techniques, especially in the last 10 years. The numerous choices now available increase the dentist's responsibilities, as it is not only diagnosis and treatment planning that are important but communication and performance as well.[2]

Various predetermining factors play important roles in the evaluation and decision-making process of the treatment planning of each case. In cases where PLVs are planned, many factors should be thoroughly determined before the actual treatment begins. These details must be carefully analyzed to minimize difficult situations that may arise during the actual treatment process and to avoid possible postoperative complications.[3]

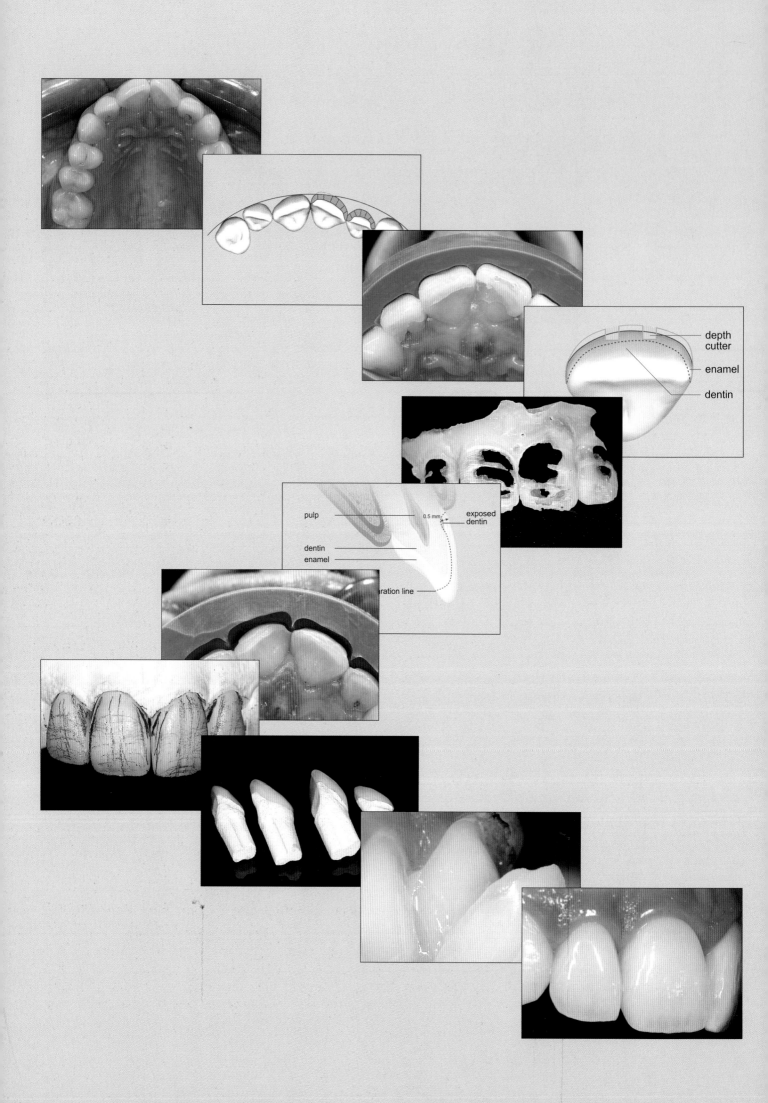

depth
cutter

enamel

dentin

pulp   0.5 mm   exposed
                                             dentin

dentin

enamel

aration line

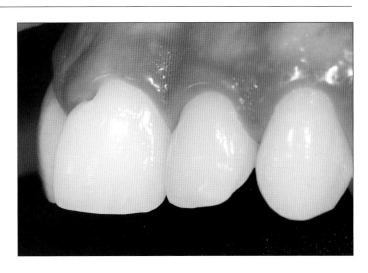

Fig 7-1 Protruded central #21(9) with irregular gingival architecture. Palatinally rotated mesial side of the lateral #22(10) results in a smaller mesial embrasure, whereas the distal torsion creates a larger embrasure than normal. Both the centrals and laterals are displaying shorter crown length and larger width.

Tooth Position

In-depth knowledge of the hard tissues of the mouth and the teeth is essential to the development of restorative procedures. Biomimetics, one of the new terms introduced to the dental glossary by *Magne*, et al.,[4] refers to the reproduction of the original performance of the intact tooth that is about to be restored. This is vitally important when restoring fractured, worn-out or aged teeth. In most cases, even if the teeth are intact, their improper alignment, rotation, lingual or labial position will play an important role in treatment planning (see aesthetic pre-recontouring), as the amount of sound tooth reduction is often related to the position of the teeth. For example, the extreme labial position of the tooth must be more aggressively prepared than the facial in order to keep the finished PLV level with the rest of the arch. Pulp status (for example, pulp size in a young patient) should be evaluated and, in lingually aligned teeth, care must be taken not to reduce unnecessarily the facial structure of the tooth (Fig 7-1).

Gingiva

The soft tissues and bone height in relation to adjacent teeth should always be taken into account to avoid gingival asymmetry and to maintain the height of the interdental papillae. If this is not carefully evaluated, the formation of black holes at the gingival embrasures will be unavoid-able, and in some cases may even be the cause of a variety of problems. This is especially true if it has not been discussed with the patient before the treatment begins. Poor dental hygiene, gingival inflammation and one or more gingival recession sites should all be treated. It is even more crucial that patients are observed for a period of time in order to determine the extent of the cooperation exhibited.

Gingival Margins

The cervical placement of the PLV margins is also an important issue to be taken into consideration. Although the laminate veneer's ideal margins are preferably located on the enamel and away from the gingiva, the condition of the teeth must always be apprised before deciding on any form of treatment. The extent of previous restorations and carious lesions, defective enamel or gingival recession and root exposure, especially in the case of a high lip-line, may necessitate the overextension of the preparation margins, and special care should be exercised in doing so.

The incisal edge position sets the starting point of the esthetic treatment planning, as discussed before. Therefore, to avoid unesthetic or unpredictable results, the crown length, incisal wear, and the extent of the lengthening of the incisal aspect should be carefully evaluated and only then should the extent of gingival alterations be decided.

Occlusion

Occlusal relations, heavy function or parafunction play vital roles in PLV applications. In some cases where the patient exhibits severe parafunctional habits or unfavorable occlusal relations, full ceramic or porcelain-fused-to-metal crowns may be considered the preferred choice for restoring these teeth.[3]

It is a well-known fact that cervical abfractions, specifically at the premolars, are due to tooth flexing under heavy occlusal forces. These are some of the clues to heavy occlusion that have to be very carefully evaluated before any definitive restorative treatment is undertaken. The relative fragility of PLV restorations requires an accurate analysis of the patient's occlusion, to ensure that the restorations do not extend into areas of occlusal stress. The results of this analysis may limit the opportunities for remodeling.[5]

PLVs can be widely used in incisally worn teeth if attention is paid to occlusion and anterior guidance. In other words, establishment of the correct protrusive anterior guidance, together with the canine-guided lateral excursions, are of vital importance. Occlusal relations such as horizontal and vertical overlap, or crowding of the mandibular dentition which may distort the protrusive relations, play important roles in setting the anterior guidance, and, if properly handled, should not affect the incisal lengthening of the incisor teeth.

Age

Aged or worn-out teeth exhibit different thicknesses of enamel and surface texture that are directly related to the extent and distribution of the occlusal interferences or external stimuli. While treating such cases with PLVs the most important issue is not the strength of the ceramic material, which has been proven to be three times stronger than the enamel in tensile strength, but the preservation of sufficient enamel and controlling the occlusal forces.[6] In the aged tooth, the enamel may be so thin that any extra preparation for PLV may lead to a loss of this existing precious enamel, while the loss of the surface area of etchable enamel may directly affect bonding. An even more critical issue, perhaps, is the loss of the thickness of this enamel that is so vitally related to the flexibility of the tooth. The thinner the enamel gets, the more flexible the teeth become. In order to avoid this and to maintain the natural strength of the tooth, preserving the already existing enamel is of prime importance, especially while working with the aged tooth. The strength of the bonded veneer, together with the preserved existing enamel, will minimize the tooth flex and thus create a strong bond between the PLV and the enamel.

The correct choice of treatment, and the sequence that is to be followed, must be thoroughly planned prior to the commencement of treatment. Each case should be carefully evaluated in advance, as there are numerous alternatives to the color, size, shape and position of a single tooth or a group of teeth within the arch. Attractive, predictable esthetic results can be obtained through the creative initiative of the dentist and coordinated with the ceramic skills of the laboratory technician.[7]

Pre-operative Evaluation (Analyzing the Smile)

To select the most appropriate option for each patient, the dentist must carefully evaluate each case, review all available options, and clearly define how that goal will be reached, along with what necessary steps must be followed in order to achieve the desired result. The dentist must first examine and evaluate each tooth and its surrounding tissues to ensure that they are functionally sufficient. Once this is established, careful attention to a functional diagnosis should be made, leading to the definition of reconstructive goals for both the dentist and his/her technical staff. Clear goals are essential to avoid any misunderstanding that could compromise the esthetic results, and when fully understood by all parties involved, the chances for success are greatly increased.[8]

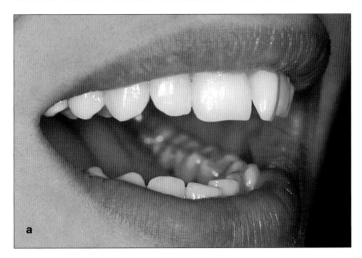
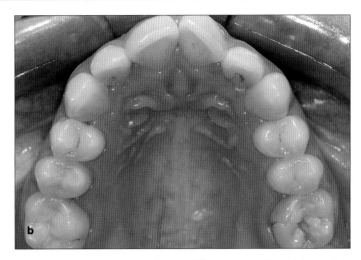

Fig 7-2a, b (a) The teeth, lips and smile should be observed and evaluated from different angles. Note the protruded left central and rotated right central and lateral. (b) These rotations can be best visualized from an occlusal view.

The Face

The initial impression when we first meet a person is not formed from focusing on a single tooth, but rather from taking in the person's face as a whole. In smile analysis, the dentist must consider and decide on what affects that person's appearance, directly or indirectly. Details such as the shape and color of the teeth, their harmony with other features, and perhaps even the character of that person, are what make up the whole appearance of that individual. Therefore, any variations in color and size will affect the way we perceive the finished product.[5]

Even though the shape of the individual tooth alone is important, the shape of an element becomes secondary to the shape of a series of these elements. The second important factor is the presence of a border, which binds the elements within into a separate, organized entity. In dentistry, the face and lips are provided for us by nature to serve that very purpose.[9]

The Lips

Being the frame of the smile, the lips and their size are also important factors. Full thick lips enable the dentist to use larger centrals and provides the dentist with a wider range of choice in relation to the proportion of the teeth.

While designing the smile, the extent of lip movement during function, and the visibility of the coronal portions of teeth, both natural and PLV, must be taken into account. Careful evaluation of the smile in a three-dimensional aspect is important and it must be observed from the front, both sides, and diagonally from different angles (Fig 7-2).[5]

The level of the upper lip-line must be evaluated while at rest, when talking and when smiling (see Chapter 2), as the level of gingival display and visible tooth surface are affected by these various positions. The incisal edge and lip-line must be in harmony. It is generally accepted that high lip-lines are less favorable because they display more gingival tissue. The cervical gingival line is also important in the case of a high lip-line and the resulting asymmetric problems need to be dealt with accordingly.

The Color

While these parameters play an important role in the spatial arrangement of the teeth, the importance of color should never be underestimated. The hue, value, chroma, translucency and texture should be carefully evaluated, as they directly affect the appearance of the teeth (see Chapter 5).

A thorough evaluation of the teeth, including all aspects of their color, shape, position and general condition should be completed before preparation, and this evaluation will be essential to the ultimate success. All characteristics of the teeth should be documented, taking special care to note any changes in color and value within each tooth from the gingival to the incisal. Any characteristic deemed undesirable by the patient should also be noted so that they can be neutralized by the final veneer.[10]

Photography and Videotaping

High-quality photographs, in addition to a full examination, are a must for the esthetic evaluation process. These photographs are not only important for communication with the laboratory, but also to help the dentist clearly to evaluate some of the details that might have been missed during the naked eye visual examination. However, these tools may not be sufficient for the in-depth evaluation of a smile. If the dentist wishes to go one step further, then the use of a video camera will enable him/her to record the patient's teeth and their relationship to the lips and face while smiling, talking, etc. To catch a natural smile in a photograph may be difficult or even forced, whereas, through the use of the video, the patient will eventually relax and allow these relations, and the range of facial expressions, to be observed in a more natural setting. With the introduction of digital video cameras, one can freeze any frame and easily print out the picture. This is a great communication tool, not only for the dentist and patient, but for the technician as well.

As mentioned in the first chapter of this book, understanding what you and the patient would like to accomplish will dictate the type of smile design and the veneer preparation to be used.

Treatment Planning

Defining our goals is as essential as the steps necessary to reach them.[11] In esthetic cases, the patient may help by clearly defining exactly what they would like to see at the end, which is a cru-

cial part of the treatment planning process. The worst scenario is when the patient does not know what they want and therefore constantly changes his/her mind. Once the esthetic needs are confirmed, the dentist should identify the potential difficulties. The patient's present clinical condition should be carefully evaluated and, in addition to esthetics, the biocompatibility and long-term function should be considered.[12] Only after a very thorough examination can a proper treatment plan for that particular patient be decided upon.

Checking Teeth Individually

Each patient's occlusal scheme will affect their smile design and the amount of compromise necessary for that particular individual to achieve an esthetic appearance while maintaining proper engineering.[13] Thorough radiographic and clinical examinations will help the dentist to determine the state of the patient's oral health and increase the chances for a successful treatment. For each site, the sulcus probing depths should be recorded, and, using a facebow transfer for the maxillary casts, the stone casts should be mounted in a semi-adjustable articulator. A diagnostic wax-up must be made, and the mandibular casts mounted in centric relation. In order to evaluate the patterns of occlusion, a mounting cast on the articulator should be used before defining an esthetic treatment plan. Careful evaluation provides clues to what the esthetic and functional results will be.[14]

This is especially true in the case of abfraction lesions that are commonly caused by grinding or bruxing, and which should be detected as they can be the cause of tooth flexure, necessitating an occlusal analysis of those teeth in question and a restorative treatment accordingly planned.[15] In order to be able to provide successful treatment, all factors relating to the final outcome must be carefully diagnosed prior to the commencement of treatment.[16]

Esthetic Integration

In the past, color matching was the main concern of both patient and dentist in esthetic restorations. However, in esthetic dentistry today, especially in the case of anterior restorations, color is only one of many factors to be considered in achieving a pleasant smile. It is not only a single tooth, or its adequate display, that are important, but also the gingiva in harmony with the tooth arrangement, as well as the lips and their integration into the facial characteristics (see Chapter 2). As the popularity of esthetic dentistry increases, the patient's expectations of a successful restoration increase as well and therefore nothing should be lacking in the quality of the color, contour, texture or shape. Good communication between the dentist, technician and patient, that begins before the actual treatment commences, is vital to the ultimate success.

Durability

In multiple-unit cases, the accuracy and durability of the final restorations are especially important, and a carefully planned occlusal scheme as well as an appropriate smile design should be well thought out.[17] The length and position of the anterior teeth are critical in the result and in the occlusal scheme for any dentition.[18,19] Perhaps an even more important factor to consider is the anterior guidance. When lengthening the incisor with PLV, a frequent mistake made is to shorten the anterior incisor's length instead of establishing proper anterior guidance.

Facial Analysis

The dentist should also evaluate the facial shape and categorize any irregularities. When evaluating the face, its symmetry and shape should be taken into consideration. The shape may vary from long to wide or average. As far as form, function and their relationship to the lips are concerned, the proportions between the anterior teeth will dictate the length of the central incisors as well as the lateral incisors in respect to the central incisors. Sometimes the lips may exhibit unusual characteristics such as an irregular upper lip-line, a high or low smile-line, or overly thick or thin lips. These characteristics must be evaluated and explained to the patient in accordance to the treatment plan that is to be undertaken.

Lip movements during function, and the amount of visible coronal portions of the teeth and the PLV, are very important in the planning stages for the PLV. Ideally, only a small portion of the incisal maxillary teeth should be seen when the lips are in rest position. As the mouth and therefore the lips move when in the process of function, the teeth will be more visible towards the apical direction depending on the maxillary incisor's incisal edge position. Accordingly, each esthetic plan should start with determining the position of the incisal edge. Once the incisal edge position of the incisor and the central incisor's facial curvature are determined, then it is possible to predict a successful result.[3]

Gingival Concerns

The length of the teeth and the incisal edge's position will determine the levels of the gingiva.[3] At times the gingival plane may not be parallel to the interpupillary line and therefore natural asymmetry is often exhibited or at times[3] asymmetry of the gingival tissues may exist. This is especially true if there is a case of high or medium lip-line, and so their alignment must be incorporated into the treatment planning. If the gingiva is visible when in full smile or during speech, the incisal and gingival planes must be harmonized with the face.[3]

Smile Architecture

An analysis of the shape of the teeth in relation to the patient's mouth, age and sex should be made.[9] Dominance is usually obtained by using a large central incisor that is capable of dominating the composition. The amount of this dominance or prominence in a smile depends on just how much of a youthful smile is desired.[20] Uniformity is achieved when the teeth harmonize with the age and sex of the patient. A natural variety of shading can be used to create an organic composition and gradation principles should be followed accordingly. When the PLV meets these requirements, and unity and harmony exist, then that individual's personality will be reflected in the final result.[9] The process of treating a patient and working it through to the final esthetic result is referred to as the process of "smile architecture".[21]

Smile architecture is directly related to the treatment plan. One of the most important elements in deciding on the new smile design is the individual patient. Their perceptions, expectations and feelings should never be underestimated. The parameters explained above and esthetic treatment planning will have no value unless they are discussed and shared with the patient. Although dentists are experts on defining the incisal edge position, tooth volume and altering the gingiva levels, problems can arise when the esthetic perceptions of the patient, the dentist and the dental technician differ. Sometimes the patient wants replication of an appearance they have become accustomed to, despite it not being esthetically ideal.[22]

Composite Mock-up

Additive wax-ups, silicon guides and corresponding diagnostic templates are very helpful in increasing the survival rate of restorations and patient satisfaction.[23] To get a better idea instantly of what the eventual outcome will be, utilization of the composite mock-up is wonderful as an aid.[24]

The neighboring tissues or teeth provide three-dimensional information that is necessary to give the restoration the correct volume and shape. A diagnostic "composite mock-up" which is the direct application of composite without surface preparation that perches itself on the teeth, is indicated when such elements are missing, or when an alteration of tooth forms is necessary.[25] A silicone key makes the final fix of the situation once it is programmed.[26] From the preparation to the PLV build-up and restoration finishing, the clinician is guided by these spatial references. The restorative steps will be facilitated by the visual inspection of the frontal, lateral and incisal planes.[27]

Determining the Incisal Edge Position

The composite mock-up is both diagnostic and informative. Especially in the case of diastemas, fractures, misshapen or malpositioned teeth, mock-ups can be extremely useful. It gives the patient an inexpensive preview of what the veneer will look like. Without these visual aids, it is difficult for even the most experienced dentist to predict the final outcome. It enables the dentist to establish the incisal length of the centrals as well as the buccal-lingual position of the incisal edge and the incisal edge plane. It is also helpful in establishing the lateral, central incisor relationship and their axial inclinations.

In addition, it will be a great visual aid for both the dentist and the patient to establish a favorable buccal corridor. On the functional side, it will give an indicative preview of the desired guidance schemes. In the more complex cases, where restoration with PLVs appears to be impossible, the use of these mock-ups often offers a chance for a good prognosis.[24]

Technique

Depending on the difficulty of the case, it takes from 5 to 20 minutes to prepare the new smile design with composite mock-ups for the whole upper arch. The easiest way of doing the mock-up is with the freehand carving method.[25] The composite is rolled between the fingers and applied over the dried tooth structure. It is shaped with the help of the fingers and special hand carving instruments and then light cured. The teeth can be lengthened or protruded, or the color can be altered for the patient to visualize. After placing the composite mock-up on the tooth, if any part is over exaggerated (in other words, if too much composite is applied and polymerized), it can be corrected with the help of a fissure diamond bur. However, careful attention should be given not to touch the intact tooth structure while doing so. Leaving a scratched enamel surface will be unfortunate if the patient does not accept the treatment.

Determining the Gingival Line

A trial that can be referred to as a "reverse mock-up" is also possible to make (see Chapters 12 and 13). If the dentist decides that the incisal edge positions of the teeth are in their correct place, but that the teeth still appear short, this may be an indication for alteration of the gingival levels. In such a case, instead of adding the composite material over the incisal edge, the material is added over the gingiva after it has been dried. This will appear a little overcontoured since the composite is being added over the original volume of the gingiva. However, it offers the patient a great chance to visualize and to formulate an idea about the appearance of the new smile and of the longer teeth that have been lengthened towards the apical direction. Once the patient is satisfied with the new appearance, an alginate impression can be made from this mock-up and sent to the lab together with Polaroid photo- graphs. After this, a transparent template can be built which can be used as a surgical stand, to dictate where the new gingiva should be located. This will serve as an indispensable communicative tool to the periodontologist who will be responsible for altering the gingival levels (see Chapter 13).

Interactive Patient Communication

These composite mock-ups can also be used to open a discussion with the patient as to how their smile can be modified. Here the finer details of the restoration, such as the nuances of color and all pertinent parameters – position, contour and proper communication – can be tested and given approval by the patient. For those who need complicated corrections, but who do not wish to experience a lengthy treatment or interdisciplinary procedures, such as orthodontic treatment, these mock-ups are indispensible.[28]

Short-term Provisionals

When the teeth need to be lengthened and/or protruded, some patients may complain that the pressure on the upper lip causes phonetic disturbances.[3] In such cases the mock-ups can be held in place for a longer period of time. Light retention can be provided by extending the composite over the gingival embrasures, or by other undercuts that can be incorporated into the composite build-up. The patient may then be dismissed with the mock-ups in their mouth for up to a period of a few hours in order better to evaluate the esthetic outcome. It is common for the patient's lips to adjust to the uncomfortable pressure from the mock-ups and it also enables the patient to get feedback from the people they trust the most, in terms of their opinion of the esthetic outcome. This is all done for the benefit of the patient and in respect to their desires for a functional esthetic goal.[29] The dentist should use the mock-up, if not for any other reason, just for the wonderful educational and enlightening experience it offers the patient.[30]

Laboratory Communication 1

It often happens that in some esthetic cases the laboratory results do not meet the expectations of the dentist or the patient. Discrepancies in tooth length, position, size proportion, color, function, phonetics and occlusion may cause disappointments. This negative impact on the outcome of an esthetic case can be eliminated when an efficient, well-informed and respectful relationship exists between the dentist and the technician and when both are capable of comprehending the desires of the patient.[2]

After the composite mock-up trial, a prosthetic solution should be prepared in the dental laboratory so that unrealistic patient expectations do not jeopardize a successful result. Solutions that are not prepared in this way are compromised, even though some acceptable results may develop in the course of ordinary prosthetic treatment. The harmonious integration of the new smile design, material selection and interdisciplinary communication must be implemented in order to deliver optimal treatment with PLV restorations.

In esthetic dentistry one of the main concerns and first priorities is the actual tooth preparation. Errors can be avoided through the diligent recording of any and all information useful to the patient, dentist and technician prior to the commencement of treatment.[5] All of the previous diagnostic studies should be carefully analyzed, thoroughly understood, and any changes necessary in tooth shape, size or color accepted by the patient. The question of whether or not a new smile design necessitates new esthetic conditions should be clarified.

Diagnostic Study Models

Study casts as a reference for use in the laboratory are a necessary requirement, whether for provisional or permanent prostheses. No matter if the patient wishes to preserve their original smile, to improve their tooth color or desires a new smile design, study casts are indispensable for conveying the pertinent information to the laboratory.[5] After a careful analysis of the existing problems and a consultation with the patient, these study models help to illustrate what must be changed and what can remain unchanged in their present state.

The use of mounted diagnostic casts and a diagnostic wax-up allows the dentist and laboratory technician to visualize the expected result. Although the esthetic outcome can be observed in the patient's mouth during the composite mock-up stage, it may be difficult completely to analyze the details and functional outcome while in the mouth. Therefore, diagnostic study casts have a very valuable place in determining these essential details and the problems that may arise during function. While preparing the mouth for an esthetic case, careful analysis of the ceramist's ability to create occlusal harmony may be affected by certain discrepancies. Effective use of study casts and double-checking will help to ensure that the desired occlusal plane is ultimately achieved even though there were irregularities in tooth position.[12]

Through the use of aids such as composite mock-ups, and after the dentist has clearly defined the desired esthetic appearance he/she is striving for they can now progress to the use of properly mounted diagnostic models. Before any preparation begins, an alginate impression of the arch should be made. Additional diagnostic cast alterations with white wax carving may be used to create any desired changes. Pink base plate wax can be used to simulate anticipated modifications in the soft tissues. The wax-ups made for both the hard and soft tissues can be used as a guide for treatment planning by both the periodontist and the dentist.[31]

Reference Points

Objective reference points are very important in the esthetic process and will be referred to throughout the treatment procedure, providing the dentist with a sense of security and a better chance of achieving success. It is also useful in their relationships with the patients and laboratory technicians. Dental technicians cannot make these decisions alone and must have input from the dentist. For example, the length of the teeth in relation to the upper lip, and other important parameters, cannot be verified by the dental technician alone. The reasonable way to transfer this information to the lab is via written explanations. The dentist can write down the patient's expectations in conjunction with his or her own personal ideas on improving the smile. In contrast, verbal communication concerning the length of the teeth or other details is subjective and not useful to the technician and hinders the chances of a successful restoration.

Transferring the Mock-ups

The author suggests that the best way to transfer this information to the lab is with an alginate or silicon impression made from the composite mock-up, which is simpler and self-explanatory. It is the ideal way of transferring the incisal edge's position and its inclination to the lab. As discussed before, the rest of the build-up will depend on this parameter. A model made from the composite

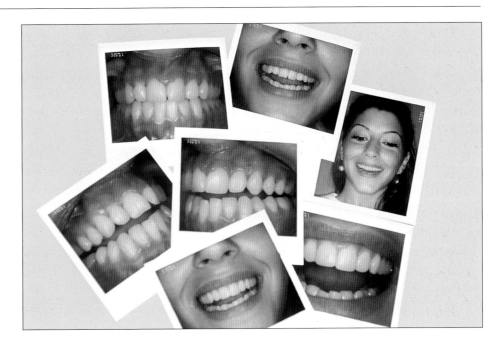

Fig 7-3 The pretreatment pictures are very useful guides to the dental technician in terms of reference points, color, shape and the texture of teeth.

mock-up of the new smile, that has been approved by the patient, and followed by an impression or the silicon index reflecting these changes in three dimensions, should be delivered for wax-up production together with the intra and extra oral pictures of the patient.

Photography

To isolate an object that is being scrutinized is impossible without also taking in its surroundings. It is not only the specific object we wish to observe but also the surrounding objects and how they relate to each other that create an image for the observer. For successful dental surgery, photographic equipment is vitally important, and very often pre-treatment slides can be a source of motivation for the patient.[5] Pre-operative photographs are useful in the evaluation of contour, texture, enamel cracks and amalgam restorations which can affect the color of the neighboring teeth. Variations in chroma and value that may be due to excessive attrition can easily be documented by photography.

Laboratory technicians who do not have much or any contact with the patient can benefit from full-face photos from different angles as well as intraoral close-up pictures, and each item is characterized in accordance to the other objects that are in the field of view (Fig 7-3).[9] Now that the technician has more solid information, at least about the esthetic outlines, he/she can check the functional compatibility of this mock-up on the articulator. For example, overlap on the original study cast or from the cast of provisional restorations determines the horizontal overlap in the laboratory.

Different casts that are commonly used are the reference, opposing and master casts. The master cast that is taken is of the original tooth shape and acts as a reference while also providing the dentist with pertinent information that is useful for the final restorations. The reference model that is the cast of the mock-ups remains the esthetic reference point, while the opposing cast is used for evaluating the functional relationship of the upcoming restorations with the opposing arch.

Silicone Index

The waxing-up of the veneers is aided by the use of a silicone index of the composite mock-up. The outline of the incisal edge is captured in the cast and enables freer esthetic design while maintaining sufficient porcelain thickness.[32] In order to achieve the proper esthetic orientation the cast of reference made from the mock-ups must be brought out with the opposing cast. The reference cast and the master cast are in fact interchangeable and share the same indexing. The wax-up's given dimensions can be precisely indicated with the silicone index that ensures the support of the porcelain and is vitally important for the thickness of the porcelain veneers. Proximal contact position can be created and optimal embrasures allowed.[3]

Esthetic Evaluation

The patient should be evaluated as an individual before any decisions about the size, color, shape or form are made. This lessens the chance of the laboratory making any esthetic errors, as the dentist is the one who actually sees the patient and should be the one to make all the final decisions. If it is necessary for the technician to make the wax-ups then he/she must first be provided with pictures, models, sketches and very detailed instructions indicating the desired tooth position.[33] In addition to all the communication tools explained above, the lab can also be provided with radiographs to enhance their understanding of the crown-root ratios and the support of the alveolar bone and help guide the lab technician in building up his/her occlusion. In PLV cases, the existing and desired tooth shape should be noted, and both intraoral and full-face photographs should be sent.

Realizing the Limitations

In this first stage, for each case the communication between the patient and dentist is as important as that between the dentist and the technician. There is no golden rule for effective communication. If it is excellence that the dentist strives for, precisely fitting restorations are a necessity. Attention to the details of color, shading and harmony with the surrounding teeth is of the utmost importance and only effective communication can assure this.[10] This will help to relate the esthetic needs to function.

After the first stage of laboratory communication, the dentist should be provided with preliminary wax-ups, silicon indexes and transparent templates that will play a crucial role in the esthetic pre-evaluation as well as in the actual tooth preparation.

Educating patients on the benefits and limitations of the veneer technique will save everyone involved time and money. After listening carefully to a patient's desires, an honest evaluation with feedback from the dentist and the dental technician must take place. At this point it must be determined whether the patient's needs and expectations can be satisfied with veneers, or if another type of restoration is more appropriate.[10]

After the initial communication with the laboratory, the esthetic and functional possibilities should be defined. Protrusive and lateral jaw movements should be controlled by the dentist and laboratory technician to determine if the space is sufficient for the restorations. This is especially true when the lengthening of the mandibular and maxillary teeth is in question. The cause of 75% of unsuccessful restorations is due to occlusal interference in the lateral or protrusive movements.[15] Requests for adjustments arising from such misunderstandings are familiar occurrences to dentists and technicians alike. When the dental technician is supplied with all pertinent information, he/she can start producing the wax-ups.

The diagnostic wax-up should be produced over the mounted casts. The study casts, which are the references for the preoperative condition, will be the foundation for the planned design of the wax-up. The technician at this stage should try to create a wax replica of the intended restoration.[2] The design and the production of the wax-ups are vitally important since the conservative preparation limits will be primarily based on these criteria. The provisionals will also be fabricated from the template that is an exact duplicate of the wax-ups. Therefore, the technician should very carefully design the wax-up. Some technicians even build up their wax-ups from different colored waxes in order to simulate the final look of the PLVs they will be producing They should not only be esthetically pleasing but functional as well (see Chapter 10).

Wax-up for Tooth Preparation

One of the very crucial issues in the production of PLVs is to keep the maximum existing enamel of

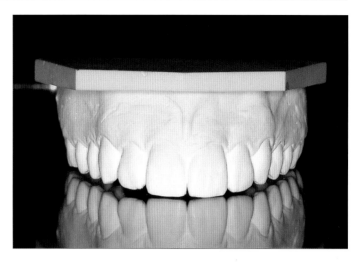

Fig 7-4 The models have to be waxed–up in order to visualize the final outcome in terms of both esthetics and function. Then a stone model is duplicated from this wax-up in order to prepare the silicon index, transparent template, etc.

the tooth structure. Before the dentist even starts the treatment planning, and especially when treating the aged tooth with PLV, the amount of remaining enamel and the final volume of the PLV should be very carefully analyzed.

The amount of tooth reduction should never be made according to the existing tooth surface but rather to the final volume of the restoration. The spatial orientation and architectural dimensions of the wax-up will be used to predesign and validate the intended preparations for the teeth involved. This illustrates the importance of using correct wax-up techniques in creating the exact tooth shape desired. In PLV treatment the most important element in the process is the wax-up (Fig 7-4).[34] In order to transfer these data to the clinic, the dentist should be supplied with transparent templates and silicon indexes by the laboratory technician (see Chapter 10).

Aesthetic Pre-recontouring (APR)

The final esthetic and functional form determines the actual tooth preparation and entire PLV build-up we seek to achieve. In the restoration process, factors like occlusion, function, interproximal position of the adjacent teeth and their contact zone, the size of the pulp and the hard and soft tissues, along with the age of the patient, are all very important. Smile design and the artistic arrangement of

the teeth can only be dealt with in relation to these various factors. When necessary, these parameters can be manipulated into the desired position in order to achieve the finest esthetic results. Tooth preparation that has been done without prior evaluation and planning is doomed negatively to affect the final result.[35]

Chairside Evaluation

It is important to identify the primary anatomic structures before the preparation phase begins. There are numerous components that make up the linguoincisal anatomic form and incisal edge survey form that interact with each other to create physiologic and bioesthetic harmony in the natural dentition. These components are: the cementoenamel junction, the cervical ridge contour, points of concavity, longitudinal developmental lobes, proximal concave lines and the mesial and distal line angles.[36]

The varying components of the normal human body are proportionally related to each other,[37] each contributing towards the body esthetics as a whole. The proportions of the teeth are an important factor in the beauty of a smile. The beauty of any smile depends on the proportion between the length and width of the teeth, their distribution in the arch, the shape of the arch and the smile configuration. When two teeth are the same width but different lengths, the longer tooth seems narrower. Consequently, the width length relationship of each tooth to the adjacent teeth has a significant effect on the visual appearance of the ensemble.[37]

Teeth are single objects that are part of a whole – the dental arch. The visibility of the teeth decreases from the dental mid-line to the posterior area of the arch. The frontal view only allows a certain amount of visibility, but the important issue here is the interchange between the visible and invisible aspects which determines the invisible aspect of morphology.[38] When a lateral incisor is viewed from the front, the tooth can be seen near the mesial margin. However, the mesial line angle is in the middle of the line in view.[38]

Position of Teeth

The position and alignment of teeth in the arch can significantly affect the appearance and balance of a smile. Rotated lingually or facially positioned or aligned tooth or teeth will disrupt the total harmony and balance (see Fig 7-2). A smile is more pleasant when the teeth are adequately positioned and aligned. Poorly positioned or rotated teeth not only distort the shape of the arch but they also interfere with their apparent relative proportion. Anterior esthetics necessitates the contouring and shaping of the teeth in order to create an illusion that gives the perception of pretty teeth and an attractive smile. The ability of the dentist to reshape the tooth to conform to or enhance nature's given contours is truly an art form that is essential to esthetics.[39] One of the most important avenues that requires this artistic procedure is (a)esthetic pre-recontouring (APR). In order to dictate the final outcome of a pleasant smile and to obtain an adequately equal tooth reduction for the technician for his/her PLV build-up, an APR should be considered before the actual material preparation.

APR

When the individual tooth position or their alignment need to be altered, the basic principle of APR is to put the partially protruding axially misaligned or rotated teeth into proper alignment on the arch, having the imaginary finished PLV designs in the dentist's mind before starting the actual material preparation. Therefore the dentist should first have a solid understanding of that particular individual's tooth form and the alignment of their teeth in order to improve their APR technique. This is especially important in morphological correction and in the related preparation for PLV. The ability to trim and shape the tooth is as important as being able correctly to perceive and to interpret the teeth and their alignment and to fabricate the individual PLVs.

Teeth that are to be treated with PLVs may exhibit positions on the dental arch different from what is considered to be pleasing. For example, when the distal of the lateral is too bulky or in labial version (protruded), the view of the mesial aspect of the canine may be blocked. Teeth may have mesially or distally tilted positions; exaggerated lingual or facial inclinations; rotations around themselves and malformations—or the mid-line may be canted.

In the actual material preparation (AMP) the required amount of enamel, and sometimes dentin, must be removed to provide enough space for PLV build-up. However, before doing so, any minor or major problems must be evaluated and misalignments corrected. In other words, an APR has to be made in order to put these things into order and to obtain a pleasing symmetry and balance in the arch. This will depend on how many teeth are to be restored for the new smile design and should definitely be decided before the actual material preparation starts. Unfortunately, this field of pre-recontouring tends to get far less attention than is necessary.

Incisal Edge Position and the Mid-line

To start preparing the teeth for the esthetic improvement of the arch, the dentist must first decide on the position of the incisal edge and the mid-line. These two parameters will set the starting point of the whole treatment. APR should start by adjusting the incisal edge position, and then should be followed by redirecting the angle of the mid-line perpendicular to the incisal edge and the infraorbital line, if necessary. The angulation of the

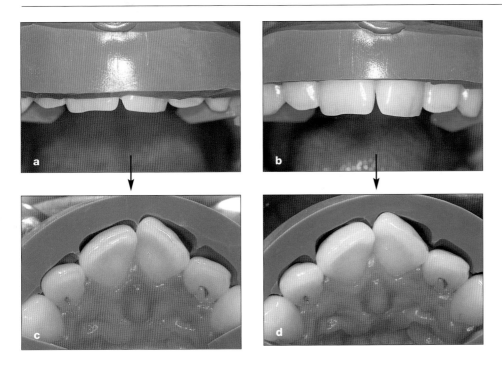

Fig 7-5a-d (a, b) If the dentist has hesitations on exacting the facial contour during the APR phase, the most accurate way to analyze this is via a silicone index. It is better to prepare the silicone index in slices to observe different depths. However, two indexes can also be prepared instead of a sliced index. (c and d) Once the silicone index is produced on the duplicate model of the wax-up it is seated over the arch, and the facially protruding portions will come in contact with it, sometimes creating problems with its proper seating. Note tooth #21(9) touching the silicone index and the distance between the centrals and the silicone index. Comparing slides c and d it is possible to observe that the middle 1/3rd of the tooth #21(9) (d) is protruding more than its incisal 1/3rd (c).

mid-line is extremely important when focusing on the symmetry and balance of the max arch. A misalignment of the angle of the mid-line, or, in other words, if the mid-line is not perpendicular to the horizon or the pupillary line, all symmetry will be distorted. It will be very difficult for the dental technician to correct the mid-line with the PLVs if the mid-line is not aligned properly and teeth are not prepared enough to supply the space to adjust to it. Correcting such a problem during the APR stage will make life easier for both the dentist and the dental technician. It will not only ease the technician's problems, but also help the dentist better to visualize what he/she will be preparing afterwards.

Facial Contours

The dentist should also be careful to relate the teeth to each other as well as to their original existing positions. In cases where it is not possible to use homologous teeth as a reference, teeth from other groups, such as the canines or incisors that are on the opposite side of the same arch and which are properly placed, can supply information as to tooth shape and position.

If, for example, the facial inclination and/or rotation are not corrected before treatment, and the prep is done according to the existing position, the final preparation will also result in a facial inclination or rotation that will be very difficult to correct with PLV that has a maximum thickness of 0.3-0.5 mm.

Exacting the Contours

However, if a dentist has difficulties in trying to perceive where and how the teeth should be aligned from the start, the simplest method to overcome this problem is to use a simple silicon index that is prepared from the diagnostic wax-up. By placing this customized index over the teeth, the dentist can visualize the teeth or a portion of a tooth that creates the disharmony, either by a facial protrusion or unnatural axial inclination (Fig 7-5). The dentist can now trim down the protruding incisal edges, marginal ridges or axial inclinations until they can easily fit into the silicon index. By doing so, overextended teeth towards the facial, or those that tend to stay out of the expected arch line, will be brought into their esthetically pleasing positions both vertically and horizontally (see Chapters 9 and 10). In this way, the facial limits of the PLVs will be well defined even before beginning the actual preparation stage (Fig 7-6).

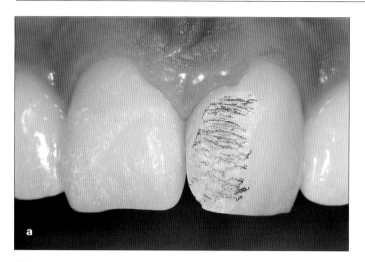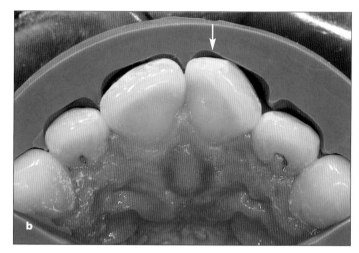

Fig 7-6a, b In order to achieve a natural-looking smile, with teeth proportionally aligned on the maxillary arch, the teeth exhibiting different positions can be brought back to where they should actually appear. This has to be done before the actuel material preparation. (a) The facially protruded central is trimmed down with a fissure diamond bur. (b) The new position is achieved before the actual material preparation. Once the protruding areas are trimmed down (white arrow), the silicone index can passively sit on the unprepared teeth.

APR of Gingiva

The APR in some cases is not limited to the hard teeth tissue. It can also be applied to minor gingival alterations. Biologic parameters permitting (see Chapter 6), gingival contouring to achieve proper height can be accomplished with a diode laser (see Chapter 13). While doing that, the zenith points can also be changed, especially in the diastema cases. When minor gingival tissue remodelling is done with the diode laser surgery, no post-op apical migration of the tissue is witnessed. For the post-op comfort of the patient, gels including Oxyfresh can be prescribed to be applied to the gingival tissue 3-4 times a day.[40]

Aesthetic Pre-evaluative Temporaries (APTs)

Lingually Positioned Teeth

Aesthetic pre-recontouring (APR) refers to the necessary mean reduction of the tooth surface that protrudes out before the actual material preparation. However, in some certain cases, the tooth or teeth may be lingually positioned in the

arch. For those teeth that are extremely lingually inclined, orthodontic intervention is a must. On the other hand, for the patients who do not want to receive orthodontic treatment with teeth that are only slightly inclined to the lingual, PLV treatment is possible. On such occasions the most important issue is to be able to visualize the final outcome (see Fig 7-7).

Preserving the Sound Enamel

In order to preserve the maximum amount of tooth enamel, the final tooth reduction should be designed according to the expected final outcome. If not, the reduction of dental structures will not be the same within the space requirements for porcelain veneers, which vary from 0.3-0.9 mm. One example of this is the misalignment caused by the lingually misplaced tooth in the arch.[41]

Composite Mock-ups

In order to fill the esthetically missing volume, materials such as composite mock-ups can be added to the facial surfaces of these lingually positioned teeth. This will help to create the correct esthetic placement of the tooth surface on the dental arch. This is a very simple way of visualiz-

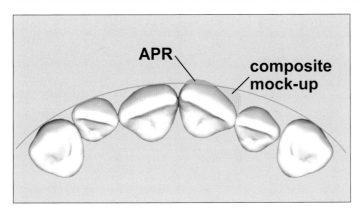
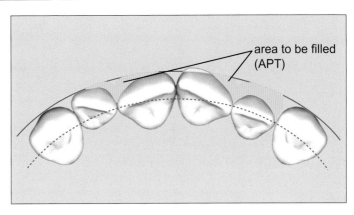

Fig 7-7a, b (a) The buccaly produced portions of the teeth are trimmed down to achive a better esthetic layout (APR). If the preparation is limited to one or two teeth, then the lingualy positioned teeth can be buccaly contoured with composite mock-up. (b) However when multiple teeth are involved a flowable composite can be placed on the teeth with the help of a transparent template or silicon impression, thus creating the APT.

ing their positions in the new smile design. This is done not only to perceive how the new smile will look, but also to evaluate its occlusal compatibility.[42] When the position of the tooth is corrected with the composite mock-up, before the actual material preparation, excessive healthy tooth reduction can be avoided and a thicker layer of porcelain built up over the unnecessarily over-prepared tooth (which can compromise the natural value and chroma) that will result in a restoration with an artificial appearance is prevented.[42]

Depth Cutters

As we all know, the first step for the actual material prep is to obtain a sufficient depth with the help of depth cutters. However, the depth cutters always reduce the same amount of tooth that their grid depth indicates. In other words, no matter what the position of the tooth is, or whether they are lingually or buccally inclined, the depth cutter will always remove the same amount of tooth structure that will not necessarily dictate the true depth of the restoration. For the inexperienced dentist, who religiously follows systematic preparation techniques for PLVs, the improper application of these depth cutters can be extremely destructive.

Technique (Gürel Technique)

A simple technique, which has great value for controlling the depth of the preparation in such special cases, can be easily used. This technique using a composite resin can simply be added to the facial surfaces of lingually positioned teeth with spot etching and bonding up to where the tooth needs to be buccally reoriented or filled by volume (Fig 7-7). This is especially very efficient when dealing with a single tooth or up to 2 to 4 teeth. It mimics the final outcome that we aim to restore with the PLVs. When the composite mock-up is still on the tooth, it is logical to use the depth cutter over that composite build-up, so that the true depth will be reached when the depth cutter is used and thus preserve the maximum enamel on the tooth surface. By doing this, we limit our depth cutter to go only as deep as our smile design dictates, resulting in an even more conservative tooth reduction.

For example, let us assume that the tooth is tilted 0.2 mm lingually. If we do not use the technique explained above, then when we use the depth cutter of 0.3 mm we will end up with a 0.5 mm space that the PLV must fill. However, if we add the composite mock-up, and use the depth cutter over that volume, we will end up with the necessary reduction of only 0.1 mm, which will still provide the 0.3 mm of thickness for the final PLV. This way the enamel is being preserved

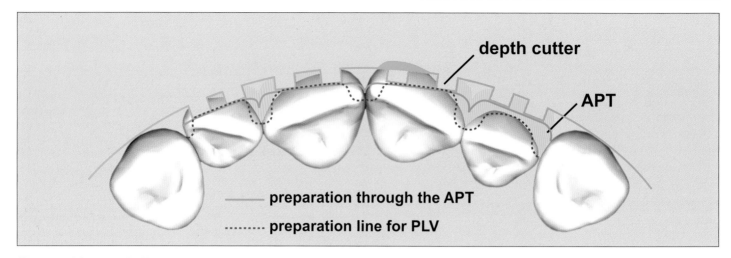

depth cutter

APT

—— **preparation through the APT**

········· **preparation line for PLV**

Fig 7-8 After the APR, the composite mock-up or the APT is placed over the teeth. The APT is a duplicate of the exact final out come, In order to save maximum sound tooth structure, thus to be minimaly invasive; the depth cutter is used through the APT. This way the depth cutter can only go as deep as the APT allows (green line). It will be surprising to see that in most of the cases the necessary material removal will not even reach the enamel surface. In such instances, the APT should be removed and the surface of the untouched enamel be roughened, to remove the surface luster for improved bonding (red dots).

whenever possible and the geometric principles of tooth preparation for porcelain veneers are followed to maximize their strength.[43]

Sometimes the lingual inclination of the tooth can be more than the depth of our depth cutter. Therefore, the amount of mock-up composite added to that surface properly to align its position over the dental arch might be thicker than our intended reduction (e.g. more than 0.5 mm). In such cases, after we prep the tooth with our pre-decided depth cutter, we will still see some composite over the tooth. In this situation, the area that was prepped with the depth cutter relative to where the facial surface of the PLV will be is actually in a position deeper than the grid depth of the bur. This is why we should still see the composite from underneath the prepped area of the depth cutter (Fig 7-8). If this is the case, and the dentist wants the finished PLV to have maximum contact with the enamel surface, he/she should go ahead and remove the remaining composite mock-up from the surface and slightly roughen the enamel surface to remove the surface luster for improved bonding,[44-46] even though the result will be a veneer displaying greater thickness. This should be discussed with the lab, informing them that the thickness of the veneer will be thicker in that area.

New Smile Design

Proper tooth form should be developed and evaluated throughout the restorative process. In order to facilitate this analysis, and especially when designing the new smile, diagnostic information, impressions and wax-ups are all essential. More specifically, this has to be precisely applied and transferred to the mouth before any unnecessary reduction is made.

Even though the final outcome can be predicted with the provisionals that are prepared after the actual tooth prep is finished, the question is, what if the expectations of both the patient and the dentist are not met after all the teeth have been prepped? Or what if the dentist realizes that they have already removed far too much sound tooth tissue than was necessary?[47]

(A)esthetic Pre-evaluative Temporaries for Visualizing the Final Outcome

The author, after years of experience, has discovered that the best way to overcome this unpleasant surprise is to prepare what he terms "aesthetic pre-evaluative temporaries" (APTs) even be- fore preparing the teeth.

To further explain this technique: a wax-up and a transparent template should be provided by the

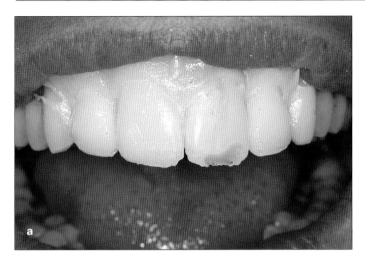 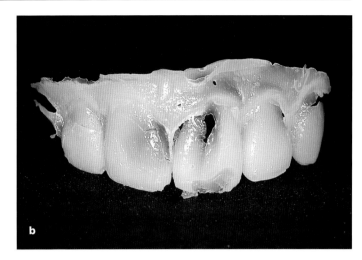

Fig 7-9a, b APT can be produced over the teeth to be prepared for a veneer construction. A transparent template or a translucent silicone impression is made from the wax-up. It is filled with a flowable composite (Luxatemp), seated on the unprepared teeth and light cured. (a) Note the show-through spots especially at the middle 1/3rd due to the position of the tooth and the thin wax-up for that area. (b) The APT removed from the mouth and showing the different depths of the existing tooth structure, in relation to the final outcome.

technician before the actual tooth prep appointment (see Chapter 9). If the dentist is not provided with a template, a translucent silicon impression of the waxed-up model can also serve the same purpose. The dentist should first finalize the APR, and eliminate all the protruding parts of the existing natural teeth that are about to be veneered, so that this template can be easily placed over the unprepared teeth (see Fig 7-6). Once the template is easily seated over the teeth, it will be filled with a flowable resin and placed over the teeth again and followed by light curing, just as if the provisionals are being made. After the composite is polymerized, the template is removed. With the help of the APTs, which duplicate the neatly prepared wax-ups exactly, the final outcome can now be easily visualized by both the patient and the dentist in terms of form, shape, length and even color (Fig 7-9). It is at this stage that phonetics, lip support, smile-line and function can be partially determined to decide what proper form and esthetic result will be achieved through the procedure. As this will be done prior to anesthesia, since the lips are not numb, the above parameters can easily be evaluated by both the patient and the dentist, using the lips as references to the new teeth position and thus smile design.

Esthetic Adjustment on APT

If for some reason the new smile design has to be modified, then minor corrections can be made over the APT. When the shape of a tooth is altered, the direction of light striking that tooth also changes. Flatter, smoother surfaces reflect a greater amount of light directly towards the observer, so that they tend to look wider, enlarged and closer to the observer. On the other hand, rounded and irregular surfaces reflect light sideward, reducing the amount of light directly reflected towards the observer. They appear to be narrower, smaller and further away. This can also be adjusted during the APR together with the application of APT, if necessary. If the tooth needs to appear narrower at the final stage, the exact space for that can be provided by rounding the mesial or distal line angles of the APT before the actual prep is made. An evenly executed reduction over this preliminary preparation will give the technician the exact space needed to build up the PLV, which will look narrower. The opposite can also be done by flattening the middle portion of the tooth in advance in order eventually to achieve a wider-looking, flatter PLV surface.

However, if major alterations are to be done on the APT, in order to ensure accuracy on the

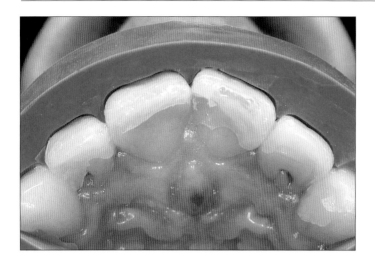

Fig 7-10 The exact facial thickness of the APT, and so of the final outcome, can be double checked with the help of the silicone index. Note that there is no gap between the silicone index and APT.

actual material preparation a quick impression should be made from the new design. A new silicon index should be prepared chairside with a heavy body silicone to be used for the final preparation, together with a new template which will be the foundation of the provisionals.

APT For Exact Facial Reduction

The major advantage of using the APT is to ensure the final outcome is accepted by both the dentist and patient. The exact facial thickness can be double checked with the help of a silicone index (Fig 7-10). As the APT now mimics the final outcome, the teeth can be prepared very precisely through the use of APT being that they represent the final contours of the actual PLVs. The APT's facial thickness and the use of depth cutters through them will dictate the necessary facial reduction. In doing so, the dentist will avoid the unnecessary loss of enamel associated with excessive tooth preparation and be able to supply the ideal preparation depth and volume for the PLV production (Fig 7-9b). When talking about the ultimate esthetic dental approach, one should never forget that the most important factor concerning the nature of the PLV is that it cannot be thinned down or shortened without seriously affecting the outer surface, incisal edge or the general esthetics of the restoration.[5]

APR and APT for Rotated Tooth

The rotated tooth may need both APR and APT in advance. When discussing such a condition, it is possible that the mesial portion of the tooth may be buccally rotated whereas the distal portion is lingually positioned. If a combination of the rules mentioned earlier is applied, it will be very easy to visualize the tilt that will transform the tooth into its normal position as it should be in a pleasant smile (see Fig 7-7). It is obviously necessary to make a thorough, deeper preparation of the protruding prominent area so that the restoration can be made with the proper physiologic contour.[48] This can be accomplished by first contouring any of the surfaces that extend buccally.[49] The buccally positioned mesial part must be ground down enabling the dentist to visualize whether the necessary preliminary reduction has been achieved or not, by using a silicone index made from the wax-up model. Once the silicone index is properly seated over the facially reduced teeth, it confirms that the APR is successfully finished. Once this is established, the transparent template, which has actually been prepared to build up our provisionals, can easily be seated into its original position without touching the reduced, facial surface of the tooth, which was protruding before. When this is achieved, the teeth are spot etched and an adhesive is applied to the surface area and light cured.

Then the template is loaded with a small portion of the flowable composite or acrylic resin and

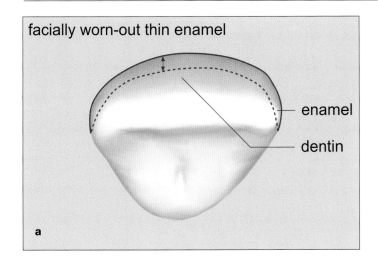

facially worn-out thin enamel

— enamel

— dentin

a

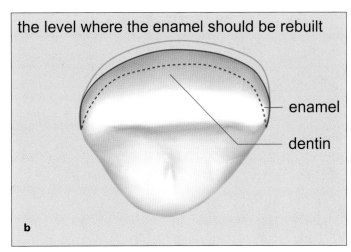

the level where the enamel should be rebuilt

— enamel

— dentin

b

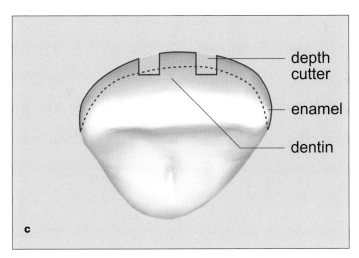

— depth cutter

— enamel

— dentin

c

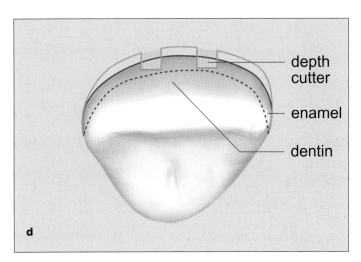

— depth cutter

— enamel

— dentin

d

Fig 7-11a-d (a) Aged or facially worn–out central. (b) The level of where the enamel should be. That can easily be seen after a composite mock-up, or APT which is duplicating the wax-up. (c) The preparation without the APT. Note the invasion to dentin. (d) The preparation with and through APT. Note that the maximum amount of enamel is preserved, without entering the dentin.

seated over the teeth, and light cured. This way the APT is firmly seated on the teeth that are about to be prepared. This now resembles the finished surface and volume of the PLV. The two advantages of this application are that the patient will immediately see the final outcome even before we start treating the case, and because the preparation will be executed through the partially bonded temporaries it will be a very conservative preparation with no removal of unnecessary enamel with the depth cutter (see Facial Prep).

APT on Aged Teeth

This has been an aspect of veneer preparation often ignored or overlooked until now, but it becomes an important issue when this application is performed over facially eroded or aged teeth. These teeth, owing to the thinning of the existing enamel surface, have already lost their original facial volume and have become weakened. If this is not taken into account, the ignorant application of the depth cutter will be extremely destructive, resulting in the total loss of the existing thin enamel surface (Fig 7-11).[42]

It is vitally important to respect the thickness of enamel that remains during the tooth's preparation as well as the biomimetic recovery of the crown and the original enamel thickness.[29] The pre-diagnosis and the material preparation of the tooth have been covered in recent research and have been found to be vitally important. When these principles are followed, the healthy tooth structure is preserved while the flex factor of the tooth is decreased.[29]

The final forms and contours of the teeth can also be accomplished during the provisionalization phase. This is possible in terms of evaluating the outcome, however, in the case of tooth prep; if the teeth are over prepared nothing can replace the unnecessarily lost healthy tooth structure resulting in the loss of the enamel which is the source of the strength of the teeth.[24]

This has always created a problem during the preparation of aged teeth for PLV. During the natural aging process, the enamel thickness of the aged teeth gets thinner and thinner, gradually losing its original volume. The thinner the enamel the more flexible the tooth becomes and therefore the dentist must try his/her hardest to preserve as much of the existing enamel as possible. However, if the tooth prep is executed without correctly estimating the special condition of the aged or worn-out teeth, almost all the existing enamel surface and thus its support will be lost. This is one of the most important situations where the APT must definitely be utilized. If the APT is not used, at least a silicon index prepared over the wax-up should be utilized (see Fig 7-5c, d). It will dictate the final volume and hence inform the dentist about the depth already lost to facial erosion. In this way, the maximum conservation of the enamel will be achieved which in turn will enhance the strength of the final outcome helping to minimize crack propagation.

On the other hand, if a solid reference such as a silicone index is not used, the extreme preservation of enamel thickness during tooth preparation often leads to overcontouring of the final restorations.[23,50]

APT For Incisal Preparation

The use of APT is not limited to preserving and exacting the final facial volume but is also used to determine the exact incisal length and the nec-

essary amount of reduction of the incisal edge. Reduction during the preparation should also be done through the APT to exact the prepared incisal edge position (see Chapter 9).

In the restoration process, it is important that the functional incisal edge has been properly contoured. When restoring the lingually inclined tooth, an overly thick incisal edge must be avoided. In order to reduce the faciolingual dimension of the incisal part of the tooth, the enamel must be prepared to the lingual edge of the incisal surface, if permitted by the occlusion. If the lingual areas take part in the functional contacts while engaging in protrusive movements, then no alteration can be introduced. However, if slight reductions of the incisal edge on the lingual surface of the tooth will not affect the anterior guidance, then this portion can be slightly modified within the limits of the enamel to prevent excessive thickness of the final incisal outcome.

Conclusion

If this needs to be summarized, it can be said that it will be beneficial to bring these "off-the-arch" positioned teeth into a favorable position on the arch. This can be accomplished with a combination of the APR followed by filling the negative spaces, as in the case of lingually positioned worn out teeth or teeth that need to be incisally lengthened with the APT. Then one can proceed with the actual material preparation in order to finish the PLV with its proper physiological contour by establishing the teeth's new facial volume and creating the required amount of thickness all over instead of trying to duplicate the existing morphology.

Even though utilizing the APR and APT sounds like a long and time-consuming procedure, it is not—and it is extremely beneficial to the final outcome. By utilizing these procedures, nothing is left to chance. Everything is controlled and the dentist very accurately dictates the result.

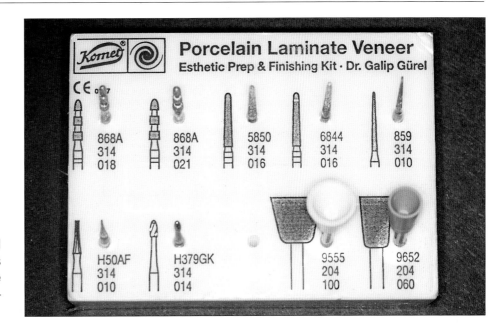

Fig 7-12 Specifically designed PLV preparation and finishing kits ease the whole procedure, since the chosen burs can be used in step-by-step techniques

Actual Material Preparation (AMP)

Instruments do not create beauty, people do.[7] PLVs provide us with a unique tool to restore function and recapture exceptional esthetics through a procedure that is not only conservative but also highly predictable. Dentists, however, may still experience problems and complications which are often related to post-bonding cracks that are mostly due to bad preparation design, insufficient space for the ceramic, and inadequate bonding techniques.[34]

When PLVs were first being utilized, there was little or no tooth preparation recommended[51-53] and therefore there was a considerable increase in tooth thickness and also gingival and proximal overcontouring. The actual tooth preparation for laminate veneers has experienced many advancements and changes, especially in the last 10-15 years,[52,54-57] and all techniques believe in some form of removal of varying amounts of tooth structure.[54,58-63] Most dentists accept the importance of tooth preparation in increasing the longevity of a procedure. The enamel should be reduced by 0.3-0.5 mm in a conservative intraenamel preparation with the finish line as close to the gingiva as possible. However, no matter what the condition is, cervical preparation is essential to display the laminate's normal emergence and to prevent overcontouring.

In order to maximize esthetics, improve fracture resistance, optimize laboratory artistry and maintain soft tissue health, meticulous tooth preparation is required for the PLVs.[64] Although PLVs can be applied with very little tooth preparation, this should not be misinterpreted as being a simple procedure and, in fact, actually requires great skill. Various kinds of PLV preparation and finishing kits have been designed which can help the dentist to achieve success through systematic procedures (Fig 7-12).

Enamel Removal

To ensure the bond strength of the resin composite to the tooth surface it is necessary to reduce the enamel.[44-46] Due to its poor retention capacity, the aprismatic top surface of mature teeth that have not been prepared must be removed. Careful attention is of the utmost importance in order to obtain successful results and solid bonding.[65] As the anatomy and the shade of the restoration are directly affected by the preparation design, very precise planning is necessary.[66] The ceramic material allows for the reproduction of natural light transmission (i.e. refraction, reflection, translucency) and an esthetic result can be hindered by insufficient tooth preparation in relation to the soft tissue parameters and the restoration.[67] The shape of the preparations also influ-

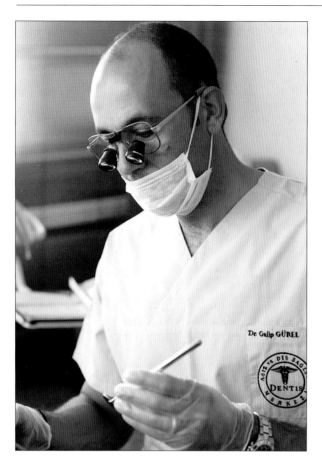

Fig 7-13 The loops widen the working area. It is one of the indispensable armamentariums for delicate esthetic preparations.

ences the appearance and longevity of a restoration. In order to manipulate light and to establish a depth of translucency and space for the incisal effects, a minimum ceramic thickness of 0.3 to 0.9 mm is desired.[67]

Delicate Preparation

When this proves impossible, it can cause misunderstandings between the dentist and technician. In such cases, to avoid frustration, the use of available materials, space and the methods at hand will be the best solution.[66] Preparations for laminate veneers do, in fact, require great stringency and a great deal of training, as no rectification can be made once the procedure is completed.[5] Experience is required for mastery of 0.3-0.5 mm reductions.

Tooth preparation for the PLVs is exacting (Fig 7-13). Using magnification loupes to facilitate careful preparation is tremendously helpful for

accomplishing this step. It also helps to preserve as much enamel as possible[15] as the bond strength of porcelain bonded to enamel is still superior when compared with the bond strength of porcelain bonded to dentin.[68,69] Some studies have demonstrated that porcelain veneers restore the mechanical behavior and microstructure of the intact tooth in vitro even when they are bonded to an extensive dentin surface, using an optimized application mode of dentine adhesives.[70] Recent research showed that if the periphery of the preparation can be kept on intact enamel, larger areas of dentin can be incorporated in the PLV restoration, such as is the case in traumatized or broken teeth.[41]

Relieving the Stress

A facial reduction of 0.5 mm with chamfered margins and 1.0 mm of incisal reduction are preferable considering the conservative nature of PLV preparation.[62,71] It is not difficult to ensure the adequate uniform thickness that is necessary for structural integrity when under stress, when there is emphasis on conservative tooth reduction in this preparation phase.[72] A ceramic and luting composite thickness ratio of above three for crack propensity will provide the restoration with a pleasant form when an adequate even thickness of ceramic and a minimum thickness of luting composite exist.[73] Stress distribution in the porcelain laminates appears to be influenced by this ratio. Higher stress at the surface and interface of the restoration may occur when a restoration is too thin or has a poor internal fit (Fig 7-14).[74]

Precision

The tooth that is about to be prepared may be intact or damaged (broken, endodontically treated, etc.). In the case of preparing the intact tooth structure, many variables affect the preparation form and depth. The position of the tooth on the dental arch needs a different approach and different preparation depths so that an adequate amount of tooth reduction is provided for an evenly distributed PLV thickness. Protruding teeth or facially slanted teeth, even without color alter-

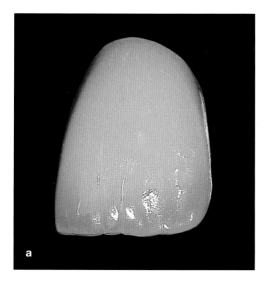 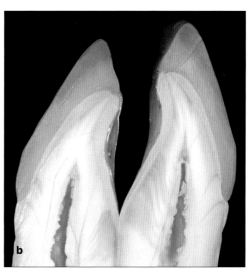 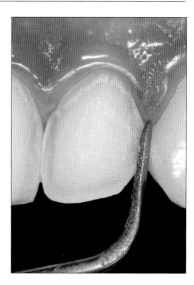

Fig 7-14a, b The thickness of the luting cement should be at least three times less than the thickness of porcelain. (a) The veneer and the tooth before bonding. (b) The cross section of the PLV bonded tooth. Note the minimal thickness of the luting resin at the tooth-porcelain bonding interface.

Fig 7-15 All the line angles should be rounded to minimize microcracks and prevent crack propagation

ations, must be reduced more to allow adequate space, so that the finished PLV will not be over-bulked. Occasionally with the tooth in linguo-version, very little preparation is necessary. Most of the time, preparation of the lingually tilted tooth may be limited to creating a finish line on the proximal and the gingival regions and/or the removal of surface luster on the facial enamel. This strategy is especially indicated to improve the appearance of cone-shaped lateral incisors.

The previously explained APR and APT techniques enable these treatments to be accomplished with very little effort and the utmost precision. The slanted position of these teeth, no matter if they are lingual or facial, affects the dimensions on the location of the proximal contours. The size and shape of the facial embrasures can also affect this area. Interproximal preparation should be extended as far as the facial aspect of the contact area to ensure that the margin between the veneer and the tooth is not visible.[75]

Rounded Transitions

In order to obtain successful results, clear logic and precision are of vital importance. The most demanding of all anterior preparations is that of the PLV. In order to minimize the microcracks that sometimes occur during the firing of porcelain on the refractory die, a uniform thickness of porcelain is needed (Fig 7-15).

Fractures along these microcracks can grow when static fatigue occurs due to the moist environment,[76] which will result in an ultimately unsuccessful restoration. The formation of microcracks will increase during the firing procedures if there are no smooth, rounded line angles between preparation surfaces produced and, instead, acute line angles between the proximal, occlusal and lingual (palatal) preparation surfaces created. To prevent crack propagation related to time-dependent stress or so-called station fatigue, rounded transitions between preparation surfaces is suggested.[77]

Dynamics of Color

The etiology and dynamics of color are important in the proper estimation of the depth of tooth reduction. The tooth enamel tends to be thicker in the incisal region and thinner in the cervical region, with a mean thickness of 1.0 mm on the incisal 2/3rds regions. Shallow, well-defined limits with chamfered finishing lines are used to prepare teeth that do not need color alteration.

Preparation depth for these teeth with slight discoloration must be approximately 0.3 mm in the cervical area and 0.5 mm at the middle third and incisal areas The aim should be to preserve as much enamel as possible—however, it should not jeopardize the restoration planned by minimizing the preparation. In other words, the dentist should keep in mind that the exaggerated preservation of enamel thickness during tooth preparation often leads to the overcontouring of the final restoration.[50] In general, the preparation should provide a reduction of approximately 0.5 mm.[54,78,79]

In order to produce veneers with minimal overcontouring and overextension, we must use preparations with distinct margins that offer bulk as well as clear boundaries to work from. To provide the space for a thickness capable of masking a dark background color without making an excessively thick restoration should be the main aim of any restoration's preparation (see Chapter 10). There is no need for an exaggerated contour if necessary facial reduction is used and therefore there should not be any problems with the care of the teeth at the margins.[49]

The same general principles are followed with the preparations for the PLVs of discolored teeth and of those with little or no alteration. In the case of severely discolored teeth, the important difference is the extent of the preparation, as it is not only the severely discolored teeth's facial surface, but also the gingival and interproximal as well that requires a deeper preparation. To form the finish line, a slight chamfer should be placed in the enamel slightly subgingival or at the level of the gingival crest.[70]

Intrinsic shading of the porcelain is demanding, time-consuming and requires experience, but it gives the best esthetic rendition with the proper depth of color and adequate tooth reduction. Although it is time-consuming and is a skill that requires a great deal of expertise, interior shading is vital to achieve the best esthetic result that will include adequate tooth reduction as well as proper depth of color.[80] Approximately 0.5 mm of enamel removal for the majority of PLV restorations allows for the minimal thickness of porcelain. Some believe that the best enamel removal is 0.75 mm,[81] but, no matter what the depth is, the required uniform reduction can be achieved by following an orderly progression of steps.

Patient Communication

Besides the physiological conditions of the tooth, understanding what you and the patient would like to accomplish will often dictate the type of veneer preparation to be used. This is particularly true in patients who wish to have their esthetic appearances changed or improved. On the surface of the anterior teeth the enamel on the gingival half of the labial surface is quite thin. Especially in the cases of discolored teeth, where the gingival margin needs to be hidden by means of extending the preparation line subgingivally, the dentist should evaluate the smile-line and the position of the cementoenamel junction.

Although it may be necessary to hide the discoloration at the gingival margin, in the cases of patients with a low lip-line, it should be discussed with the patient. The positive and negative aspects of placing the PLVs subgingivally must be explained, and in such cases the patient's esthetic concerns and desires will be definitive. If it is decided that the margin will be extended apically, then the cementoenamel junction should be properly identified. Usually in the case of gingival recession, this junction may be level or supragingival with the soft tissue level that means the preparation should be placed over the cementum or dentin.[49] The results of the newest generation of dentin adhesive systems are very promising.[68,69] However, when cervical margins are bonded to dentin or cementum, the longevity of the restoration is questionable due to the leakage at the margins. Ideally, cervical margins should be located in the enamel.[50,70] If this is not possible, the patient should be informed that this is not an ideal indication for the procedure.[82]

Deeper Preparations

Preparation of crowded teeth also needs a pre-planned, delicate approach, especially if the mandibular incisors are of concern. Since some special cases need more aggressive preparation depths, such as in the case of the discolored or facially misaligned teeth, reduction of the facial surface on the teeth that suffer from severe discoloration must not be limited to the enamel (see

Chapter 10). The preparation will have to be deeper, even if it exposes the dentin. Whenever it is feasible, increasing the depth of reduction to 0.5 mm in the cervical region and 0.7 mm in the middle third and incisal areas is recommended.

Proper Preparation

Lengthening the tooth requires special attention during the preparation stage. The occlusion, especially the anterior guidance, should be very carefully evaluated. If the anterior guidance needs to be altered with the help of the PLVs, then palatally finishing preparation lines can be applied and in doing so the facial-palatal thickness of the incisors should be taken into consideration.

Rigidity in the tooth is due to the amount of enamel thickness and thus the more enamel that is removed the more the tooth flexes. Throughout our lifetime the teeth change in color, volume and flexibility. Sometimes teeth that are facially eroded or deficient in enamel should therefore be minimally prepped with very little or no reduction other than the definition of the margins. Preservation of this valuable existing enamel can only be sufficiently achieved when APT and/or silicon index are used during the preparation (see Chapter 9).[83] In the actual tooth preparation there should be control of the contour, emergence angle, margin, facial profile and the color. Influence over the margin placements, veneer seating, placement and bonding are also important for both the dentist and the technician. Some of the advantages of proper tooth preparation include careful management of porcelain bulk for occlusal loading, preservation of the glaze in the finishing procedures, tooth recontouring for misalignment and enamel etch by removing the fluoride-rich layer.[61]

Surface Roughness

Dental literature has often argued about the final surface roughness of the preparation. Some studies have shown that there is greater retention when the tooth is prepared with diamond stones.[84,85] In contrast, other studies have found little difference between rough and smooth preparations as far as retention is concerned.[84,86,87] A recent study reports that the level of efficiency in cutting does not increase when coarser grits are used as opposed to medium (100 micrometer) grits.[88] The author believes in using a medium coarse diamond to create a more retentive surface for better bonding. The bur selected for the "esthetic preparation and finish kit" (Komet #5850 314 016) number perfectly fulfills this purpose. In addition, the extra-fine round-end tip provides a very smooth chamfer margin at both the gingival and interproximal margins.

Acquiring a smooth surface requires light pressure of the hand piece during preparation as excessive force can result in pulpal damage. There is little improvement in the cutting efficiency if the hand piece load is increased beyond the clinical range of 50 to 150g. Degradation and debris accumulation of the bur are more important and both have an affect on efficiency.[89]

Hand Pieces

Magnification, illumination and other technical improvements (e.g. electric hand pieces) are of the utmost importance in producing precise natural restorations. Certain hand pieces differ from the traditional air-turbine, and operate more concentrically, allowing enhanced speed control, such as in the use of a high-torque low-speed electric hand piece. These tools enable the dentist to develop their tactile sense, which is reflected in their work. Caution must be observed when the high-speed tooth preparation is done with ultra-coarse diamonds that can induce thermal damage in the pulp tissues.[90] Plenteous irrigation with the low-speed electric hand piece may help to prevent thermal damage to the pulp and deserves further enquiry. Oscillating hand pieces (KaVo) can also be used, while preparing an incisor, adjacent to another unprepared teeth.

Facial Preparation

Facial Convexity

Today restorative dentistry means the production of biocompatible restorations that exhibit a very natural appearance. If tooth preparation is not properly preformed it is difficult, if not impossible, to copy the natural dentition with the manipulation of light that today's ceramics are capable of.[35]

During the preparation of the buccal plane the facial of the incisors, which are convex, should be addressed in the incisal, middle 1/3rd and cervical aspects.[3] Different characteristics are apparent when viewed from the mesial and distal aspects.[91] The maxillary central incisor's vertical mesial line angle profiles are basically the same, and the cervical, middle and incisal portions of the central display proportions of 1 to 2 to 3 respectively, when viewed from the mesial prospective. However, individual variations of the vertical distal line angle of the maxillary centrals exist. The variations in length (according to each developmental lobe) of the cervical, middle and incisal aspects of the buccal plane add diversity and character to the anterior teeth.[91] Preparation according to the length of these three aspects of the buccal surface enables the dentist to preserve character in the veneer restoration.

Depth Cutters

Accurate judgement of size, depth and angle is required in the practice of restorative dentistry. Most assessments are made simply by visual examination, and are therefore often subjective. The limitation of visual perception renders such judgements inaccurate and subject to variation. Ceramic laminate veneers have become synonymous with controlled enamel preparation. It is a substitute enamel that closely resembles the natural tooth enamel with its optical, mechanical and biological properties.[5]

The use of standardized objects to allow size or angle judgement by direct comparison improves accuracy, and their routine use may improve the quality of the restorative treatment.

Two different-sized depth cutters (Komet # 868A.314.018 and # 868A.314.021) control the depth of the facial tooth preparation. They enable the dentist to guide, visualize and quantify enamel reduction. Due to the rounded tip, margins can be plotted if deemed necessary. When the color changes are two shades or less,[61] as in more than 90% of the cases, 0.3 mm and 0.5 mm depth cutters are used. Without a depth guide, it can be dangerous to gauge reduction in enamel depth between 0.3 mm and 0.5 mm.[5] However, if the pre-operative evaluation is not done properly, these depth cutters can be very destructive in terms of unnecessary sound tooth structure loss, and thus weaken the intact tooth structure (see APR and APT).

Necessary Depth

PLV restorations can at times fail to meet the expectations of the dentist and patient owing to dissatisfaction with the tooth color. This is often due to the relative thinness of the PLV and the light that they allow to pass through making the background color of the tooth and mouth somewhat visible. To overcome this, the dentist must increase the PLV thickness by deepening the preparation to minimize the effect on the restoration.[48] In other words, greater reduction is required to provide the necessary thickness for the proper optical properties in the veneer in order to block or change tooth color.[15] The color and position of the existing teeth will determine the technique to be used in order to achieve a desirable result. The facial preparation should reduce an adequate amount of tooth structure to facilitate the placement of the PLV. Depending on the severity of the tooth discoloration, additional reduction of the facial enamel may be required at the expense of dentin exposure to generate adequate space for the PLV to hide the discoloration. When preparing an individual treatment plan, three different preparation depths, "minimal", "medium" and "deep", should be considered.[16,92]

In the "minimal" preparation, the teeth that are about to be restored are no more than one shade different from the proposed final PLV restoration

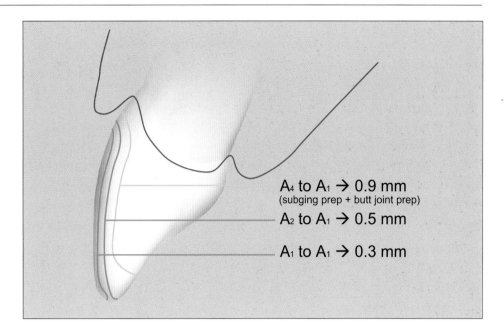

A₄ to A₁ → 0.9 mm
(subging prep + butt joint prep)

A₂ to A₁ → 0.5 mm

A₁ to A₁ → 0.3 mm

Fig 7-16 Generally speaking, a depth of 0.2 mm is needed to change the hue of the tooth by one shade.

color, and therefore only a 0.3 mm reduction is required from the proposed contours. The background color will provide a natural look and the margin location will be supragingival.

In the "medium" preparation, the shade variation with the original tooth color is up to two or three shades in comparison with the proposed PLV color. More attention to the modification of the background shades will be necessary in these cases in order to acquire the desired level. Approximately 0.6 mm space from the proposed contours is required for tooth preparation, with the margin location at the gingival crest. When the tooth is dark and a shallow preparation must be done, a different technique can be used to achieve the final desired color with a relatively thin PLV. The resulting shade can then be a combination of the existing tooth shade and a thin PLV lighter than the shade that it is expected will be achieved through the restoration. To create an A2 shade when the background is A3.5, the technician will use A1 shade in order to achieve the desired effect.

In the "deep" preparation we are dealing with three or more shade differences between the desired shade and the original teeth. When a considerable difference in color exists, masking is required. Masking provides the desired color by hiding the unwanted discoloration. Subgingival margin location will frequently be necessary.[16] In

general, the underlying hue can be modified by one shade for every 0.2mm of tooth reduction (Fig 7-16).[93]

Enamel Thickness

Enamel has different thicknesses at the gingival, middle and incisal 1/3rds of the facial surface of the tooth. They can be 0.3-0.5 mm at the facial gingival third, up to 0.6-1.0 mm at the middle third and 1.0-2.1 mm at the incisal third.[94]

This indicates that having these variables both on the surface texture (i.e. convexity) and using a special diamond instrument at different angles, designed specifically for the task, can better facilitate enamel thickness tooth preparation. Diamond depth cutters (originaly designed by Dr. *Tuoti*) (models 868 A.314.018 and 868A.314.021 Brasseler, Germany) have different cutting depths within themselves, relative to the enamel thicknesses of the facial surface of the incisors. The self-limiting depth cutter is designed so that it can cut to a depth limited to the radius of the wheel (Fig 7-17). The wheels are limited to penetrating the enamel until the shaft is flush with the tooth surface. Course diamond wheels with different diameters mounted on a 1 mm-diameter noncutting shaft create the correct depth – orientation grooves on the facial surface of the incisors. Once again, the wheels cut through the enamel until the

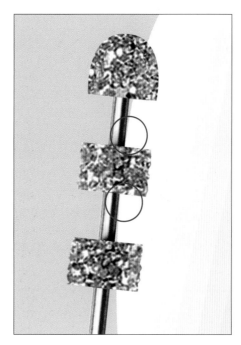

Fig 7-17 The depth cutter can only penetrate until the noncutting shaft is flush with the tooth surface.

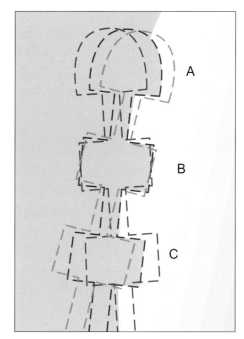

Fig 7-18 The surface after the depth cutter is used in only one angle. Note that the only true depth is gained in the area of B (middle 1/3rd, black dots). To reach the necessary depth on points A (gingival 1/3rd, green dots) and C (incisal 1/3rd, red dots), the bur should be used in three different angulations.

shaft is flush with the surface, and 0.3 to 0.5 mm deep grooves are created. The most important issue here is to hold the depth cutter at three different angles so that all the diamond wheels will be able to reach the necessary depths.

Technique

At the beginning of each preparation horizontal grooves are traced. Labial surface striations are apart from the margin. Especially in the case of the lower premolars and the canines, the three striations are very rarely allowed on the natural curve of the facial surface.[5] When the bur is held parallel to the surface of the tooth, only the middle (Fig 7-18) section of the three-tiered deep-cutting bur penetrates into its entire depth, which is due to the convex labial surface of the tooth.[95] Under-preparation of the cervical or incisal area can be avoided by positioning the bur at three different angulations to ensure its penetration.[96] However, if an APT is not used, extreme care should be taken to prevent over-preparation of the tooth, especially in cases of malpositioning or

loss of enamel volume due to aging. As the tooth preparation is developed from calibrated depth cuts, the incisal 1/3rd of the preparation will assume a correct position as the facial convexity of the tooth about to be prepared serves as a reference.[3]

Painting the Surface

Once the desired depths are achieved and horizontal groves are prepared, the remaining part of the APT can be removed (Fig 7-19). To further remove the remaining tooth structure found between the depth-orientation grooves, and to acquire the desired depths, a tapered round-ended fissure diamond bur (originaly designed by Dr. *Goldstein* (model 5850.314.016 Brasseler, Germany) is used. Painting of the facial surface of the tooth with waterproof paint enhances the contrast between the prepared and unprepared teeth, and is a useful method for inexperienced eyes (Fig 7-20). The horizontal grooves will remain painted until the desired depth is acquired through the use of the round-ended fissure diamond bur (Fig

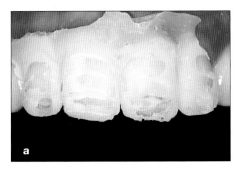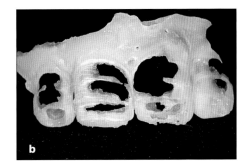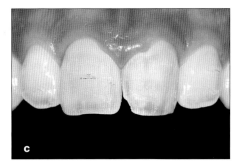

Fig 7-19a-c (a) The depth cutters are used through the APT. This will provide the dentist with the minimal invasive preparation. (b) The APT after the depth cutter is used. Note that remaining parts would have been uselessly prepared if the APT was not used. (c) The horizontal grooves produced through APT. Note how shallow the grooves are.

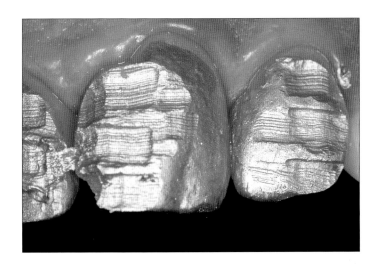

Fig 7-20 Coating the surface of the tooth with a water insoluble tint allows the depths of the horizontal grooves to be more easily perceived. Note the horizontal grooves hardly reach to the distal of the central and mesial of the lateral. Any unnecessary entry is prevented by the preparation done through the APT.

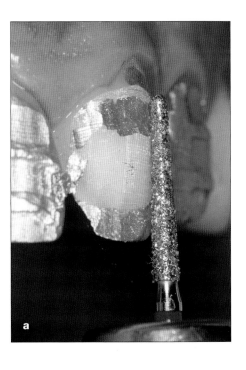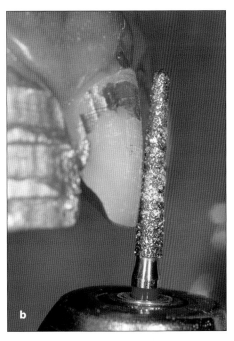

Fig 7-21a, b (a, b) The round ended fissure diamond bur is used in three different planes until all the color at the surfaces of the bottom of the grooves disappears. This will indicate that the true actual material preparation depth is fully achieved.

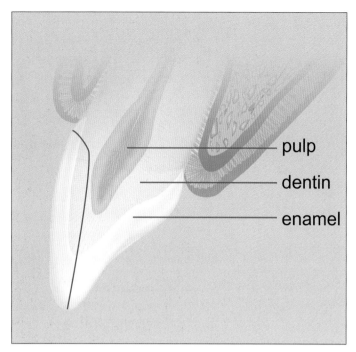

Fig 7-22 Tooth preparation without respecting the facial convexity. Such straight preparations can result in irreversible pulp damage.

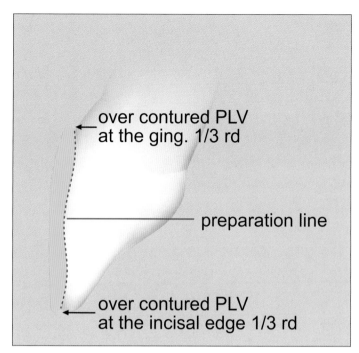

Fig 7-23 If the incisal or cervical 1/3rd is not prepared deeply enough, the final PLV may be overcontoured in this area.

7-21).[91] To provide a natural healthy look for the incisor that mimics its true convex nature, a uniform removal of substrate is essential and can be achieved through the use of the bur, keeping it at three different angles. Otherwise, one plane facial reduction may come too close to the pulp (Fig 7-22).[97] When thediamond is swept in the mesiodistal direction, a gentle convex surface in the gingival and incisal 1/3rds is obtained.[15] The facial reduction is complete once the paint becomes invisible on the facial side, and to complete the final reduction, the horizontal labial depth grooves are connected.[91]

Preparing the Incisal 1/3rd

A common error is to place the incisal 1/3rd too far labially in the final restoration.[98] This is frequently due to insufficient tooth reduction (Fig 7-23). The preparation must reproduce the natural convexity of a maxillary central incisor and provide for a minimum reduction thickness of 0.7 at the junction of the middle and incisal thirds of the tooth.[99,100] Insufficient tooth reduction, in terms of leaving a sharp line angle and not rounding off the incisal labial area, is the leading cause

of an overtapered preparation, or produces opaque show through, or overcontouring of the incisal third of the restoration. This will not only influence the external facial form of the tooth, but the light reflection as well. Light reflects off the tooth and travels through it at the incisal. If the edge has a rounded surface at the incisal-labial, that reflected light is being diffused and yields an ideal transition of the shade from incisal color to body color (see Fig 7-38).

Silicone Index

Using a silicone index is a controlled way of prepping the remaining portion of this side and can frequently determine sufficient tissue reduction during the preparation of the tooth.[5] This can be prepared by the dental technician from the initial wax-up model. When viewed from the incisal preparation depths, cutting the silicone index into horizontal slides can follow different vertical levels of the facial surface.[101] The middle or gingival 1/3rd can be visualized when the slides are moved once the incisal 1/3rd has been checked. The desired homogenous depth can be completed in this accurate way (see Fig 7-5).

Gingival Preparation

The fabrication of the PLV is directly affected by the placement of the finishing line. Smooth margins that are fully exposed and readily cleansable generally provide the best results.[102] Consequently, the essential key here is for the dentist to place the finishing line where the margins of the restoration can be kept clean by the patient and properly finished by the dentist. In addition, finish lines must be placed so that they can be duplicated by the impression, without tearing or deforming the impression when it is removed past them.

Unlike circumferential preparations, and like the metal ceramic crowns that have their margins buried into the sulcus, the thin porcelain and the resulting chameleon effect on the cervical margin enables the dentist to place the gingival margins of the PLV supragingivally. With no cement line or metal margin visible, the porcelain blends in with the underlying composite resin in a harmonious finish. Whenever possible, the finish lines should be placed in the enamel following the contour of the soft tissue from mesioproximal to distoproximal.

Kourkouta, et al.[103] demonstrated that after the placement of the PLVs there was noticeable plaque index reduction and plaque bacteria vitality. For those patients who have problems with oral hygiene, PLVs are the restorations that cause the least problems.[29] In comparison to gold, resin or hard tooth structures, dental porcelain is less likely to accumulate bacterial plaque and therefore the periodontal response is favorable.[104,105]

Supragingival Margins

Placement of the gingival margin supragingivally or coronally frees the gingival margin. This has many advantages such as: eliminating the chances of injury to the gingival tissue, cutting down on the risks of undue exposure of the dentin in the cervical region and obtaining crisp clear margins, as impressions are easier to make with supragingival preparations compared to subgingival preparations. It also increases the likelihood that the restoration will end on enamel and this increased area of enamel is extremely important for stronger adhesion and less microleakage in the future.[48]

Microleakage

Finishing the gingival margins supragingivally also has other positive aspects. During the try-in and bonding stages, proper isolation of the operative field is easier, so moisture control and the chances of contamination during adhesive procedures are reduced. It also offers easier access for the finishing and polishing stages with easily accessible margins. Postoperatively it eliminates the possibility of impingement on biological widths by an inadvertent overextension of the preparation, making it possible for the patient to perform meticulous hygiene in this critical region and allowing the dentist to evaluate marginal integrity during the follow-up and maintenance visits.[48] Restrictions to enamel[106,107] are a necessity for marginal tooth preparations and bonded restorations, including ceramic veneers, as exposure of the dentin margins may reduce bond strengths and increase the chance of microleakage.[94,108] When the preparation margins are completely located in the enamel, microleakage is minimal or none at the tooth/luting composite interface[50,70,82,109,110] and negligible in the luting composite/porcelain interface.[50,70,82]

Enamel in the cervical region has a prismatic configuration.[111,112] The poor marginal sealing that is often reported in the porcelain veneers in vitro at the cervical margins may be due to the fact that aprismatic enamel is generally located in this region where the veneer preparations end.[50,82,110] In spite of this, it is always better to finish the cervical margin on enamel since more microleakage has been found at the luting composite/tooth interface when the cervical preparation margin was located in the dentin.[280]

Subgingival Margin

The reaction of the gingival tissues largely depends on the cervical extension of the restoration in regard to the location to the gingival margin.[113] Generally speaking, the major etiological factor in periodontitis is the subgingival placement of a restoration.[114,115]

On the other hand, it is reported that PLVs typically show less gingival reaction than metal ceramic restorations as the extension comes closer to or below the gingival margin. In a majority of the cases, the subgingival margin preparation of the intracrevicular margins should be placed at about half the width of the crevice depth. To create a buffer zone between the epithelial attachment and the bur, it is best to place the margins half way in the crevice to leave enough space for the gingival cord placement.

Sometimes the preparation may be deeper than the desired depth. If the objective is to place the margin at half the depth of the sulcus, there will be some leeway preventing encroaching of the epithelial attachment of the biologic width. The deeper the restoration margin resides in the gingival sulcus, the greater the chance of inflammatory response[116,117] and that such tissues can bleed upon probing.[118,119]

Although some studies reported that no differences between subgingival and supragingival margins were seen, it is still recommended that the placement be supragingival whenever possible.[102,120]

Another aspect is the difficulty of visually following the cervical margins so that even the experienced restorative dentist can miss marginal defects as great as 120 micrometer when the margins are subgingival.[121] On the other hand, placing the veneer preparations slightly subgingivally allows the technician to preserve the existing height of the papilla as well as to make certain that all interproximal spaces and/or diastemas will be closed while permitting control over the emergence profiles.[122]

In non or minor tooth color changes (such as one or two shades lighter), there is no need to prep the tooth subgingivally. In other words, once the teeth are free from discoloration or presenting "discreet color alteration", the gingival margin must not be placed in the gingival sulcus.

It is not only the color but the nature of the lip-line as well that determines whether the PLV marginal placement will be supragingival, equigingival or subgingival. Supra or equigingival placement is preferred for the patient with a high lip-line. If there is gingival exposure while smiling, subgingival placement may be necessary in order to achieve desirable esthetic results, but to a certain extent it depends on the esthetic expectations of the patient.[123]

Chamfer Preparation

It is almost impossible to finish an accurately fitting PLV without being overcontoured over a knife-edge preparation at the cervical area (Fig 7-23). Therefore, irrespective of its placement (sub or supragingivally), a chamfer is preferred for all the gingival margins. A study was conducted using finite element analysis to gauge the total strain on porcelain stresses on 90- and 120-degree shoulders and chamfer preparations, with the chamfer showing the most resilience.[124] In comparison with the 90-degree shoulder, the chamfer finish preserves more natural tooth. Owing to the gradual color transition between restoration and tooth substrate, thereby avoiding the sudden delineation between tooth and crown, it is also a better option esthetically.

In order to obtain a very distinct and visible finish line, removal of the serrated, overhanging enamel prisms is essential.[123] To avoid periodontal inflammatory responses and future gingival recession, improving gingival architecture, survey lines and points of concavity with a chamfered margin while carefully controlling the anatomical contours in the cervical third, is of the utmost importance.[124] The rounded tip of the fissure diamond bur will enable the cervical margin to be initiated slightly above the gingival level.

Enamel Thickness

One of the major concerns the dentist should be aware of is that the thickness of the enamel decreases in this area, especially when moved apically. This becomes more obvious towards the cementoenamel junction. Consequently, the preparation of this area should be kept to a minimum and ideally should not exceed the depth of

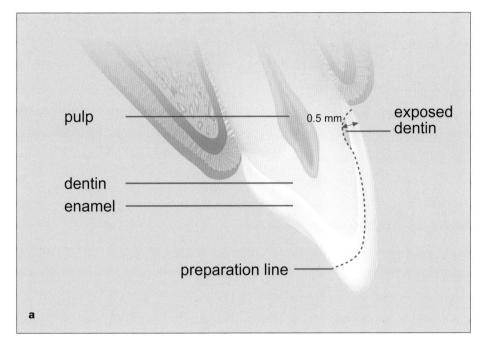
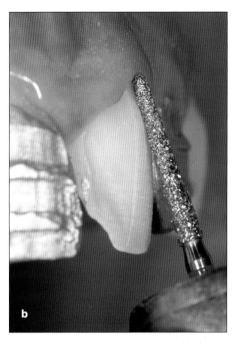

pulp

0.5 mm

exposed dentin

dentin

enamel

preparation line

a

b

Fig 7-24a, b The round-ended fissure diamond bur is held almost parallel to the facial inclination of the cervical 1/3rd to prepare the cervical margin. In most of the cases a preparation depth of 0.3-0.5 mm ends up in exposing the dentin in the cervical area.

0.3 mm labio-lingually, which is the minimum recommended thickness for the PLV during fabrication.

However, primarily due to the extent and thickness of the enamel, a reduction of 0.3-0.5 mm in the gingival area of the anterior teeth is not possible without interfering with the dentine.[94] The mean thickness of enamel at the gingival third is 0.4 mm on the maxillary central incisors and only 0.3 mm on the maxillary lateral incisor.[94] In actual daily practice in the majority of cases where the dentist has used a freehand preparation technique, not only is the dentine exposed but the proximal and cervical enamel is reduced to more than 0.5 mm (Fig 7-24).[125]

Gingival Displacement

Supragingival preparations do not need special attention. However, if the preparation is subgingival, it necessitates the displacement of the gingiva, to avoid injury. During preparation, gingival displacement is achieved by delicately inserting the braided retraction cords into the sulcus so as to avoid any bleeding. It may also be beneficial to use non-medicated deflection cords instead of the medicated ones as they may be the cause of

secondary gingival recession. While doing this, the coronal preparation limit of the gingival contour of the tooth can be recorded, before the gingival displacement. If the dentist wants to be certain of the exact placement of the cervical margin in order not to make a deeper preparation than is necessary, he/she should draw a line at the present location of the gingival cavo surface margin with a sharpened pencil or a water insoluble pen before placing the tissue displacement cords into the sulcus (see Chapter 10).

Dentin Exposure on the Margin

In the majority of cases, the placement of the gingival margins for the PLV is open to subjective criteria. However, there will be some situations where subgingival margins are unavoidable, such as in the case of caries or old fillings that extend under the gingiva (Fig 7-25).[126-130]

Patches of dentin exposure are no longer a problem during the preparation as long as the margins are kept on the enamel. However, in most of the abnormal situations, such as extensive caries lesions in the gingival areas, placement of the subgingival margin can go as deep as to be placed on the dentin. Therefore, in order to stop,

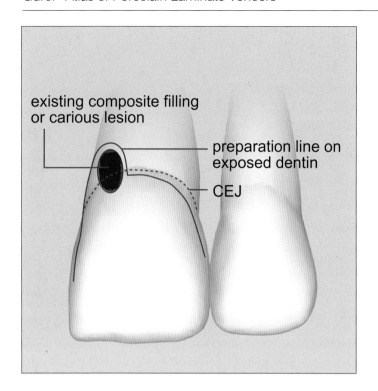

existing composite filling
or carious lesion

preparation line on
exposed dentin

CEJ

Fig 7-25 Cavities that extend over the cementum may be the reason for an extended marginal preparation line towards the apex, leaving the margins with exposed dentin or cementum.

Fig 7-26 It is important to control the depth of the preparation in relation to the radius of the round-ended diamond bur to avoid the formation of a reverse margin.

or minimize, the possible marginal leakage, the dentist should very carefully identify the condition of the existing dentin. Thus, obtaining a successful bond to dentin with a perfect marginal seal that will not exhibit discoloration[131-133] has became a much larger problem that has occupied many researchers over the past four decades.[134]

When dealing with the depth of the preparation, the dentist must be aware that the dentin has a mean thickness of 2.3-3.0 mm[135] In all age groups, the most critical area of bonding at the level of the cementoenamel junction is the superficial and middle-deep dentin, which consists primarily of intertubular dentin. It is not the tag formation into the tubuli, but the interlocking of the bonding agent to the collagen network of the intertubular dentin that seems to be responsible for the adhesion of composites to the dentin.[136] The age of the dentin has only a minor influence on the bond strengths and sealing capacity of the dentin bonding agents.

Sclerotic Dentin

Bonding to and preparing the sclerotic dentin is slightly different from normal dentin preparation and may necessitate further attention. When there

is a sclerotic area in the cervically exposed dentin in the gingival margin, there is a morphologic differentiation to the unaffected normal dentin. Numerous tubules obstructed by highly mineralized peritubular dentin are characteristic of this.[137] The sclerotic surface zone is removed during preparation and/or decalcified by extending the application time of the etching gels, so that adhesion to this altered dental material can be achieved.[137-141]

Abfractions

Abfraction is another interesting feature of the condition of the cervical area, due to occlusal disturbances especially in the premolar areas. If the problem is not solved, however, this PLV system will eventually result in failure, as it appears not to be capable of preventing occlusal load from causing accumulated fatigue damage in vital dentin and enamel.[142] Interfacial debonding of the enamel and dentin may be due to highly stressed regions of the dentoenamel junction and the gingival third of the crowns.[143-145] Unsuccessful retention of the restoration may cause gap formation at the cervical margin.[146,147] Therefore, in

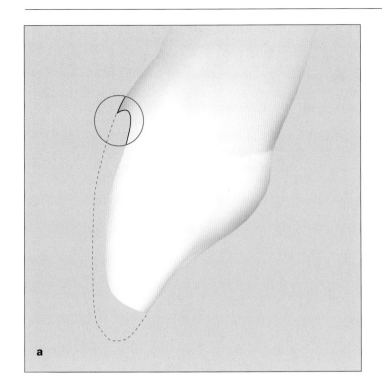

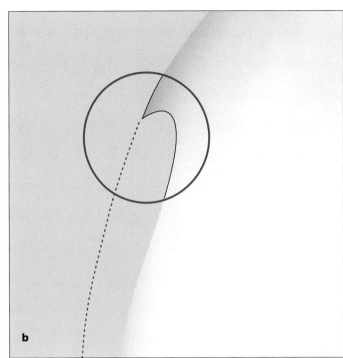

order to achieve success in such cases, occlusal disturbances have to be corrected before starting the preparation.

Technique

After finishing the preparation of the labial surface, the round end of the fissure diamond bur (model 5850.314.016 Brasseler, Germany) is held almost parallel to the inclination of the cervical 1/3rd of the labial preparation surface and moved from the apical end of the distal proximal surface towards the apical end of the mesial interproximal surface, delicately following the gingival contour. This gingival contour should already have been esthetically shaped and the gingiva must be in optimum condition. To improve the health of the tissue or for esthetic recontouring, if any periodontal surgery need be performed, a minimum of 6-8 weeks should be given for the tissue to heal completely and settle into place, thereby eliminating the chances of tissue displacement.

The physical properties of the fine diamond particles located at the tip of a two-grit diamond bur give us the chance of removing and finishing the cervical margin, while at the same time refining it to a very smooth finishing edge. Coarser dia-

monds should be used sparingly as they may cause cracks at the preparation margins that can reduce enamel toughness. In time, this will lessen the resistance to crack propagation within the enamel. Diamond tips with progressively finer grits and reciprocating handpieces[148] remove the median-type cracks and microcracks between and within the enamel rods, and result in the smoothest of finish lines. Resultant preparation margins become stronger with fewer cracks through the use of this method.[149]

The final cervical margin will take on the profile of a mini chamfer, measuring an average of 0.3 mm, and matching the tip of the diamond instrument. It is also important to pay attention and not to exceed the cementoenamel junction, which if violated during the preparation may be a reason for microleakage at this junction in the future.[150]

When the chamfer margin preparation is deeper than one-half of the width of the bur, a thin shell of reverse margin is occasionally left (Fig 7-26).[151] This reverse margin is difficult to impress and is subject to fracture in the lab by distorting the marginal fit or on the tooth leaving a marginal gap between the PLV and the tooth. If deeper chamfer preparations need to be placed at the gingival margin, the appropriate fine-grit round-ended fissure diamond burs of a larger diameter should be used.

This is an ideal margin for a PLV. This chamfer enables us to reproduce a natural visible tooth profile while avoiding overcontouring of the PLV in the cervical zone. This accurate finish line will be easy to record, identify and reproduce in the laboratory. Ideal continuation of the emergence profile, without any ledge at the junction of the veneer and enamel, can only be achieved through such a chamfer preparation. Additionally, it allows the veneers to be more easily inserted at try-in, and during the final placement it provides a higher fracture resistance and avoidance of fractures at the edges of the PLV.[5]

A natural transparent precise PLV restoration is dependent on the fabrication and delivery of this technique. Laboratory technicians maximize the use of their contemporary ceramic systems with the space and margins provided by the finishing process. The health of the tissues and the restoration itself may be in danger if this process decreases the potential by infringing on the biological width. If the restoration is to be harmoniously integrated with the natural teeth, this process is vital to the definitive restoration that it necessitates.[67]

Proximal Preparation

Prior to the facial preparation and the creation of the gingival margin, the preparation for the proximal surfaces must be thoroughly planned. The aim must be to place the margins beyond the visible area and to preserve the contact area.

Esthetics should be carefully considered when placing the proximal "stop-line", providing that the teeth are free of proximal restorations. It is very important to go beyond the visible area that can be viewed from the front or side, especially when tooth color is very different from that of the laminate veneers.

Destroying the contact areas in order to create the margins is unnecessary, but, in some cases, the preparation margin may be extended further

in a lingual direction. The margin can be drawn back even more in the lingual direction if the natural contact area has already been lost due to a diastema, restoring a broken angle or to encompass a proximal composite.[5]

An ordinary viewer's attention usually focuses on the facial surface of the teeth, whereas the dentist tends to look straight at the central incisors while interpreting the depth and the proximal surfaces. The ordinary viewer actually sees the incisors without any contour.[38] In order to be accurate and to achieve the best results esthetically and functionally, the dentist should always be able to visualize the three-dimensional form. For PLVs' biologic integration into the area, one should have a better understanding of the placement and design of the proximal finishing line.

It is useful to study this surface in two regions: the gingivoproximal area, which extends gingivally from the interdental contact area, and the direct proximal contact area, which is located in the incisal 2/3rd of the proximal surface.[48]

Gingivoproximal Preparation

A segregate esthetic factor that assures harmony in the dental composition is the interdental embrasure that is formed from the cervical point of contact, the interdental papilla and the proximal wall of the adjacent teeth.[7] Interproximal embrasures and interdental papilla are vital areas in our PLV procedures and a solid understanding of their anatomy is essential.

The tooth form, related bone and gingival relation differ as we proceed from the centrals towards the molars. At the gingival margin, when viewing the gingiva from a mesial aspect, there is a concavity almost following the form of the enamel (Fig 7-27) that is deeper towards the incisal at the anterior and gets shallower towards the posterior of the mouth. This actually refers to the shape of the cementoenamel junction that is related to the form of the tooth and the intercrestal bone morphology. The deeper the cementoenamel junction at the proximal, the higher the intercrestal bone should be so that the papilla will fill that space.

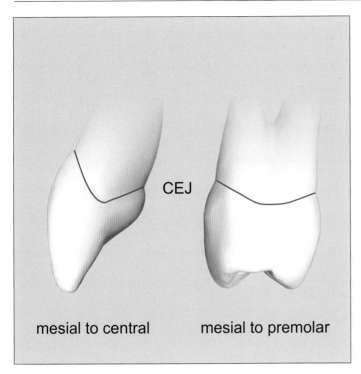

Fig 7-27 The cementoenamel junction gets flatter as one proceeds to posterior.

In the image: CEJ, mesial to central, mesial to premolar

Papilla

It is acknowledged that bone is the foundation of the soft tissues. The shape of the bone is followed by the interdental gingiva and according to its location the shape varies. Although flatter in the posterior region, the anterior area appears convex, with a knife-shaped edge that is reduced in width. The general rule is that the interproximal tissues become higher and more convex as the roots get closer. If the roots are further apart, the interdental tissues will be that much flatter. In the anterior, where the roots are the closest, the length of the papilla is a solid 5.0 mm when measured from the crest of the interproximal bone (see Chapter 6).

This increases the importance of the delicacy of the gingivoproximal preparation, especially in the anterior region and more specifically between the centrals, laterals and canines. The dentist should be aware of the fact that he/she will be dealing with a delicate papilla, prone to change if not handled properly. When preparing the area for PLVs, the prognosis of the papilla, periodontal tissues and its marginal integrity is directly pro-

portional to careful planning and delicate preparation, with a true understanding of all the anatomical structures involved.

Esthetics and Hygiene

It has been mentioned that a decrease in esthetics increases the accessibility for oral hygiene. Oral hygiene is more easily accomplished when there are open embrasures in the posterior area that leave room for the gingiva.[152-158] However, phonetic and esthetic requirements are not compatible with the maintenance of wide-open embrasures in the anterior area. Furthermore, there is a very delicate balance in the anterior region. Hygiene should be properly maintained with naturally placed crisp triangular-shaped papilla without the formation of any black holes.

When normal tooth structure exists with an adequate interproximal root proximity and a sound periodontal state, the maintenance of the embrasure space depends directly on the delicacy of preparation and margin placement, the proper fit of the restoration, the emergence profile, the interproximal tooth design and the location and the width of the gingivoproximal area. Consequently, regardless of the patient's oral hygiene, maintenance of a healthy embrasure is entirely dependent on the ability and capability of the restorative dentist.

Maintenance of Gingival Embrasure

In PLV preparation, maintenance of the gingival embrasure space is only possible when sufficient tooth preparation has been done. Sometimes overpreparation of the tooth may be indicated to avoid any overcontouring. Tooth preparation and tissue protection are as important as the systematic, accurate approach they necessitate. Esthetics and oral hygiene will dictate the amount of enlargement of the embrasure space involved in the preparation and final stages of the restorations.[7]

Although it is generally underestimated, the interproximal tooth structure which is gingival to the contact area of the adjacent tooth, is very important. This area is not visible from a direct

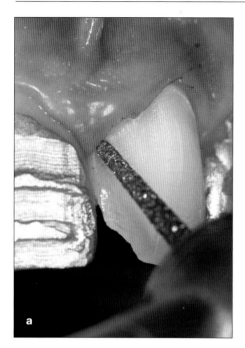
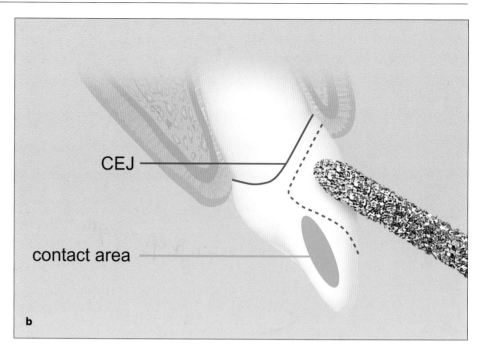

Fig 7-28a, b (a) Care must be taken to avoid penetration into the dentogingival complex as well as the cementoenamel junction. (b) The bur is held almost 60 degrees to the axial inclination and gently pushed towards the palate to create a dogleg gingivoproximal extension.

frontal view and so it is left either underprepared or totally unprepared. However, when observed from obliquely, it is visible and it is therefore essential that this area be meticulously prepared.[159] This is even more critical in cases where the unprepared tooth structure and the final restoration differ significantly in terms of color.[160]

Technique

Gingivoproximal margin preparation should begin after the gingival preparation is finished. The round-end tapered fissure diamond (Fig 7-28) (model 5850.314.016 Brasseler, Germany) is held at an almost 60-degree angle, and follows the gingival prep towards the palatinal, from both the mesial and then the distal. When viewed from the mesiofacial aspect, a concavity is created with the ultra-fine tip of the bur in the shape of an interproximal elbow or dogleg form.[15] Depending on the facial convexity of the incisors, their depth can alter. It is usually kept supragingival.

Depth of Chamfer

As mentioned previously, the type of margin is preferably a chamfer form in this particular area. The question can be, "what kind of chamfer should be used?" or, in other words, "what should be the depth of that margin?" (Fig 7-29). Adjusting the color of PLV with the help of different-colored composite luting resins, at the time of bonding, is not suggested. However, in real life, these problems may occur owing to a lack of proper color communication with the lab. If the chamfer is kept too deep then the replacing porcelain will be thicker than it should be and the thicker porcelain will allow less of a color change. Therefore, color-adjustment options will be limited when a heavy chamfer is used. Any attempt to alter the color with the help of a composite luting agent will be unsuccessful.

Although thin chamfer may produce improved color control, it is impractical because its thin porcelain margin makes it vulnerable in the dental laboratory or even in the dentist's chair. Light chamfer without internal line angles allows preservation of the enamel and thereby prevents marginal microleakage.[70] However, the author prefers medium chamfer that allows color adjust-

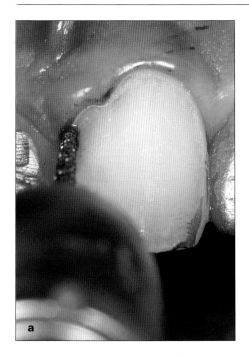

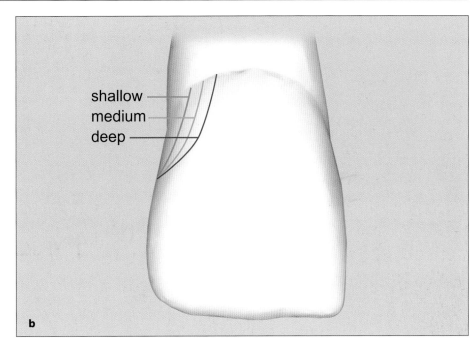

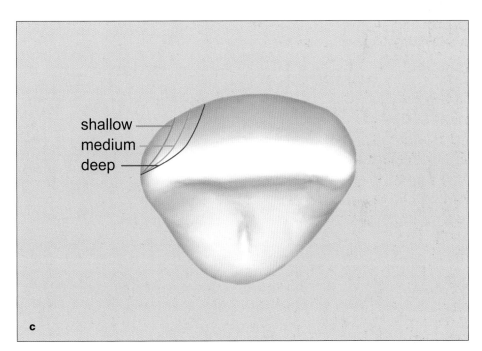

Fig 7-29a-c The horizontal depth of the gingivoproximal preparation will affect the thickness of the porcelain in that area.

ments and yet has a porcelain margin of adequate thickness. Especially in cases of dark discoloration and thick gingiva, the margins will still be placed on enamel.[7] They can be placed subgingivally and more palatally in cases that display severe discoloration or diastema closure, or in cases where it is followed by a reduction of the gingival level, or when periodontal disease or perio surgery has taken place.

The visual area of the labial embrasure influences the viewer's perspective. Shadows that are cast from the surrounding structures are particu-larly influential as well as other important factors such as the lips, the adjacent teeth's contours, gingival architecture, contour, shade and the position of the teeth.[161]

Depth of Extension

When significant shading differences exist between the tooth and the restoration, and distinct color alteration is necessary, in order to prevent the margin from being visible, the proximal margin must be extended palatally and halfway

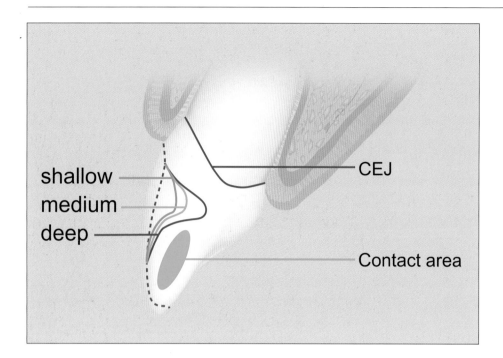

Fig 7-30 The palatinal extension of the gingivoproximal area is related to the required color change and the visibility of the area. Usually distinct color changes necessitate deeper preparations towards the palate. If the color does not need to be changed, the preparation margin can be kept shallow.

into the faciolingual dimension of the contact area. It is possible to extend the proximal margin palatally in the gingivoproximal area until the unprepared tooth surface is no longer visible (Fig 7-30). In this way the esthetics is not harmed by unsightly tooth angles that remain visible. The color and visibility of the teeth in that area will determine the amount of palatal extension in the gingivoproximal area.

It is important to consider the visibility from different angles in order to determine the margin finish line in the gingivoproximal area.[48] After the preparation is completed, esthetic problems may arise if the gingivoproximal area of the tooth structure is visible from any angle. For those teeth with slight color alteration or even those with none, the preparation must be extended palatally to include 0.2 mm of the gingivoproximal area.[48] Throughout the placement of the proximal margin, the dentist must continually check for any portion of darkened tooth structure beyond the preparation that will still be visible after the restoration is complete, by frequently checking from different viewpoints.[48]

Gingival Response

In addition to its importance in improving the final esthetic result, this space is very important because it is a favorite location for microorgan-

isms that cause caries and inflammatory tissue problems. Interdental tissue can be vulnerable, as is observed in daily practice. It is known that the spread of this inflammatory process to the interdental papilla through to the transeptal fibers can follow the blood vessels directly into the dental canals of the osseous septum (see Chapter 6).[7]

There are various studies being conducted to try to determine gingival reactions to bonded porcelain margins. Porcelain is the material closest to natural tooth enamel and it is also the most esthetic and biocompatible material available. Studies have shown that it also retains less plaque than even natural enamel,[29,117,162,163] and that the plaque is more easily removed with less bacterial plaque vitality.[164] Glazed porcelain's low surface roughness is the vital key to this phenomenon.[165] Short-term[166,167] and medium-term[113,168,169] clinical studies suggest a positive reaction of the marginal gingival tissues to porcelain veneers as well as a decrease in plaque accumulation on the restorations.[170] It has been found that, although both are porcelain materials, PLV shows much less gingival inflammation when compared to PFM restorations. While plaque index and plaque bacteria vitality decrease considerably, the volume of gingival crevicular fluid increases.[167,171] However, one should never forget that all these studies are produced under

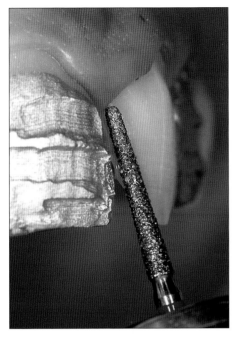

Fig 7-31 After the gingivoproximal preparation is finished, the fissure diamond bur is uprighted vertically to make the interproximal preparation

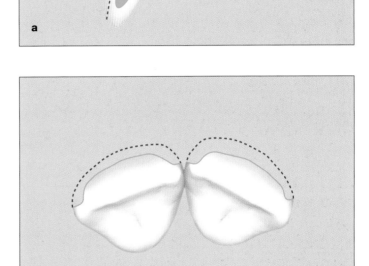

Fig 7-32a, b Preferably, the interproximal margin should stay short of the contact area.

circumstances where there were relatively excellent marginal fits. If the principles explained above for the gingivoproximal area preparation are not applied properly, and if marginal gaps or uncontrolled overbulked porcelain margins are created, these statements will have no value. Periodontal problems can be expected in the case of improperly placed gingivoproximal margins.

Interproximal Preparation

Technique

Proximal reduction is simply an extension of facial reduction. Using the same round-end tapered fissure diamond bur, the gingivoproximal reduction is continued by uprighting the angle of the bur vertically (Fig 7-31) into the proximal area, making sure to maintain adequate reduction, especially at the line angle. To correct an uneven finish line, ensure that the diamond is parallel with the long axis of the tooth and parallel to the mid-line. Even though this seems to be a minor detail, it is a vitally important one. It not only helps the dental technician to have enough space for PLV build-up, but guides him/her to the correct esthetic incisal line by mounting the cast into the articulator (see Chapter 13), perpendicular to the correctly placed mid-line.

Under normal circumstances this preparation should stop just short of breaking the contact (Fig 7-32).[172] The proximal margin on teeth that are free from color alteration or with "discreet discoloration" should be hidden by the preparation made far enough into the contact area so that the proximal wall will end 0.25 mm facial to the actual contact area.[48]

In some instances, the dentist may only be preparing a single tooth or two teeth and must

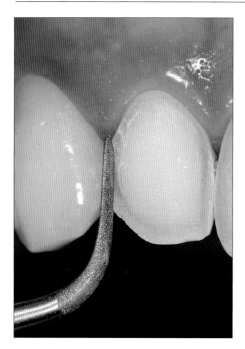

Fig 7-33 Oscillating instruments work the best on the interproximal areas that are being prepared next to an intact adjacent tooth.

100% of the perfect margins without enamel defects are obtained with working tips of 40-micrometer grits.[176] During the interproximal preparation of the anterior teeth, the "half-torpedo" working end can be used to avoid scratching the adjacent tooth that will not be prepared (Fig 7-33).

Interproximal Contact Area

It is no longer necessary to split the models with the modern techniques available. There are numerous factors that determine how deep to prepare the contact area. Whenever possible, it is best to preserve the contact area, as it is an anatomical feature that is difficult to reproduce. When the actual treatment is in progress and the teeth are not periodontally stable, then it becomes a challenge to keep them intact and to prevent displacement of the teeth between the preparation and placement sessions. Consequently, the try-in procedures are simplified and save clinical adjustments of the contact areas where the fine ceramics are intricately placed. Bonding and finishing procedures are thereby simplified and easier toothbrushing and dental flossing is made possible.[15]

therefore pay extra attention not to scratch the tooth next to it, which will stay intact. One of the ways of protecting the proximal surface of the adjacent tooth is to place a metal matrix band in between. However, sometimes, poor placement of this metal band may injure the papilla.

Oscillating Instruments

Rotary instrumentation with fine-grit diamond points most often leads to injury of the adjacent tooth if proper precautions are not taken.[173] In addition, they may produce uneven margins with enamel fractures next to areas that are untouched.[174,175] The safest way of preparing the interproximal area as an alternative preparation method, is to make use of oscillating instruments. They have differently shaped tips and the beauty of the system is that one side has a noncutting flat surface that cannot cut or scratch the adjacent tooth while the other side perfectly prepares the interproximal area.[173,174] Oscillating working tips that are diamond-coated on one side, allow very precise apposition of the instrument to the surface to be worked on, while the uncoated side can be exposed to the adjacent tooth surface without damaging it. It is reported that an overall 79% to

Breaking the Contact

Certain clinical circumstances, such as closing a diastema or changing the shape or position of a group of teeth, may require some specific preparation of the interproximal area[5] in order to allow the technician greater freedom in alteration of the form or position.[177] Another reason for designing specific preparations at the contact area is the existence of caries, defects or preexisting composite fillings. In such cases it is important that after thorough elimination of carious dentin, the weakened residual enamel thickness be evaluated. A compromise must be made between saving the tooth structure and mechanical principles that govern support and stability for an indirect restoration.[27]

At times it may be necessary to full-slice through the contact to open a diastema (Fig 7-34). The esthetic and functional demands of the

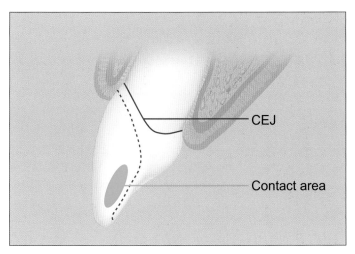
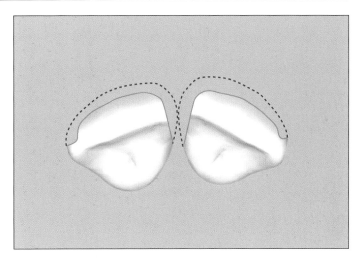

Fig 7-34 Sometimes the contact area can be sliced from the facial to palatinal, to open a diastema and to give freedom to the dental technician.

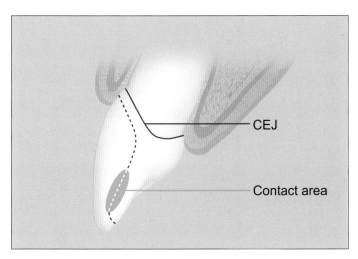
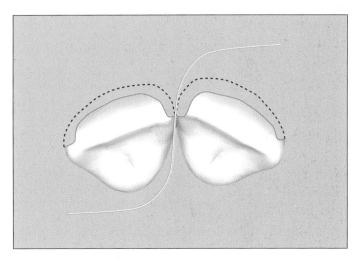

Fig 7-35 However, if the interproximal margin has to be placed on the interproximal contact area, a diamond strip should be used to create a definite, crisp marginal edge.

specific tooth involved will determine the design of the preparation of the proximal walls.[15] However, if for some reason the preparation must finish on the proximal contact area,[178] instead of extending the preparation more palatinally, which will cause the loss of intact enamel in the contact area, it can be stripped to achieve a clear interproximal margin (Fig 7-35).

Eliminating Existing Restorations

At the restoration dentin interface, the connection of resin cement to dentin may be the weakest link. Bonding PLVs onto a composite filling considerably increases the risk of failure.[179] When the preparation margin is located within an existing filling, numerous failures have been reported.[180,181] The author believes in the incorporation of all the existing composite fillings and caries cavities into the PLV preparation (Fig 7-36). However, in some instances, the removal of the composite, which may be too palatally located, can prevent the insertion of the PLV unless sound tooth structure is removed. These are the conditions where the dentist must use his/her common sense for removing the composite to the extent that the intact tooth structure allows, leaving the rest of the composite as it is and finishing the PLV line over the remaining composite filling. In doing so, the old composite filling should be thoroughly

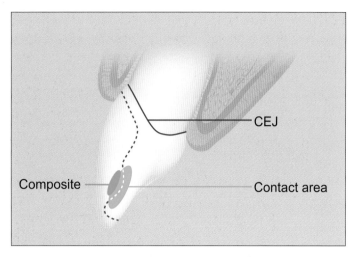

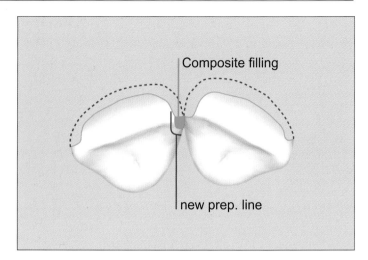

Fig 7-36 The already existing cavities or composite fillings are usually removed and incorporated into the PLV preparation.

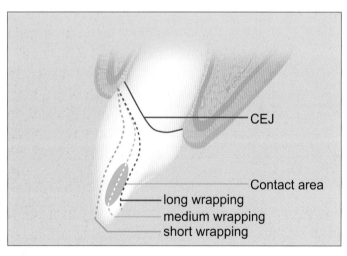

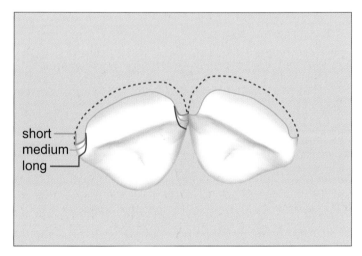

Fig 7-37 The depth of the interproximal preparation can be classified as short, medium and long wrapping (*Magne*).

checked, and if any secondary caries or defects are suspected, or if marginal discrepancies are seen, they should be redone before the actual PLV preparation takes place. Nevertheless, in order to initiate the shaping of the preparation, a definitive chamfer finish line must be clearly established.[67]

Palatinal Extensions

If needed, the preparation may go as deep as possible towards the palatinal, in order to break the interdental contacts. There are three different degrees of interdental preparation depending on how deep the preparation line extends towards

the palatinal (Fig 7-37). *Magne* and *Douglas*[41] classified the penetration depths of the interproximal preparation as "short wrapping" (the veneer to extend only to the facial margin of the tooth), "medium wrapping" (the veneer that extends into the bulk of the mesial or distal marginal ridge by penetrating 50% of the interdental area) and "long wrapping" (the veneer which entails covering the entire interdental area).

In their studies, it appeared that "medium wrapping" was the preferred choice. In conclusion, this interesting study found that during an extension of the veneer to the interdental area the use of wraparound laminates can provide improved stress distribution within the restoration when it is subjected to incisal loading[41] The safety and innocuousness of interdental wrapping can be supported by other investigators who indicate that the most important mechanical events in incisors appear within the buccolingual plane.[182]

Thermal Changes

Extreme thermal changes, curing contraction of the luting composite and mechanical loading are all sources of stress. Cracks can be initiated in porcelain veneers through the harmful stress that thermal changes can create.[6,74] Short-wrap veneer, when compared to the other veneers, showed higher risk failure due to thermal changes and shrinkage. This veneer technique is facial to the contact and conservative in nature.

On the other hand, owing to difficulties in their fabrication and application arising from the problems in handling both the extension of ceramic and the delicate margin definition and insertion axis, long-wrap veneers are also quite impracticable. Consequently, it should only be used in cases where major changes are necessary, as in the closure of diastemas (or interdental triangles), which necessitate adequate margins (marked chamfer) and ceramic thickness. Partial wrap (medium wrap) is a suitable compromise between clinical practicality and stress distribution when restoring class III composites.[183] The margin can be hidden, and extending the preparations into the contact area can provide a better, more stable seat for cementation.[177]

Incisal Preparation

There are two basic techniques for the placement of the incisal finish line. The first terminates the prepared facial surface at the incisal edge. There is no incisal reduction or prep of the lingual surface and it can be in the form of a window or intra-enamel preparation or the feathered incisal preparation. In the second technique, the incisal edge is slightly reduced and the porcelain overlaps the incisal edge, terminating on the lingual surface. In a retrospective clinical evaluation the two techniques were used equally and both provided clinically acceptable results.[184]

After two and a half years of clinical functioning, porcelain veneers have shown no relation between survival rates due to incisal preparation design (no incisal overlap versus incisal overlap).[185] Many different techniques—such as the overlapped incisal edge tooth preparation, the feathered incisal edge tooth preparation, the incisal 0.5-1 mm bevel preparation and the intraenamel or "window" tooth preparation in which 1.0mm of incisal edge is preserved—are presently being used.[142,186]

Incisal Overlap

Whether or not the incisal edge of the tooth should be included in the preparation of the PLV is still a matter of debate. Several authors favor the overlapped incisal preparation.[60,61,81] Some authors believe[182,187,188] that full coverage is vitally important in order to improve the mechanical resistance of the veneer, despite the fact that to accomplish this, 0.5-2 mm of intact incisal edge may have to be removed thereby placing the vulnerable cavosurface margin in an area of opposing tooth contact. It is better to incorporate an incisal overlap in the preparation as the porcelain is stronger and produces a positive seat during the cementation process. The proper seating of the veneer is made possible by the vertical stop that the slight incisal overlap provides.[54]

The esthetic characteristics of the porcelain veneer are more easily handled and controlled by the dental technician with this type of incisal preparation. To improve the translucency of the veneer, a 1 mm incisal reduction is suggested with rounded line angles (Fig 7-38),[60] even though a two-dimensional photo-elastic stress analysis confirms that such preparations increase the resilience to incisal fractures.[182] This preparation reduces stress concentration within the veneer by distributing the occlusal load over a wider surface.

It is also emphasized that only when occlusal or esthetic requirements necessitate should the incisal edge be incorporated into the preparation.[62,184,189,190]

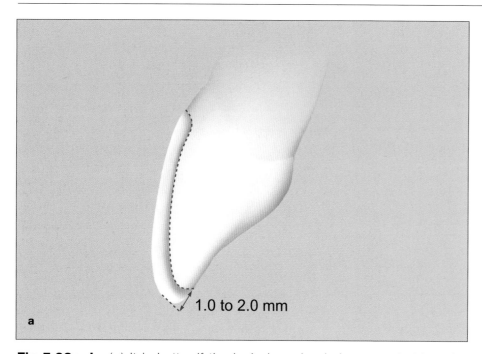
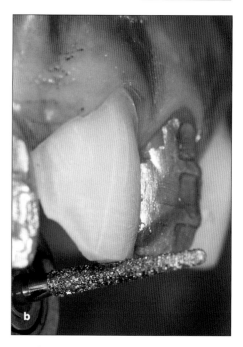

Fig 7-38a, b (a) It is better if the incisal overlap is incorporated into the preparation. It will not only improve the esthetic effects such as translucencies, but also improve the mechanical resistance of the veneer. (b) The bur is held 90 degrees to the incisal edge and the necessary preparation is done.

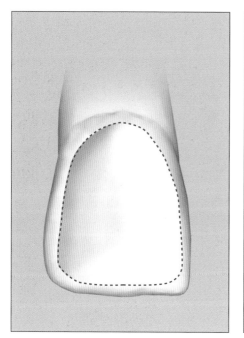
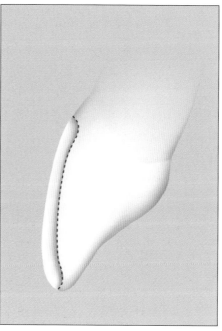

Fig 7-39 Window preparation is the most conservative preparation design.

Window Design

On the contrary, an in-vitro increased risk of cohesive fracture due to the maximum stress placed on the veneer caused by an overlap in the PLV design was demonstrated.[186,191] This study showed that a window design prepared entirely into the enamel was resistant to axial stress. It concluded that the most conservative type of veneer or window preparation was the treatment of choice when strength was the first priority (Fig 7-39).

Points of Reference

The incisal edge of the preparation assumes a precise position whether the aim of the treatment is occlusal, esthetic or for retention requirements. The dentist needs a reference for the incisal edge and must therefore use the adjacent teeth. This is especially convenient if that tooth is not part of the preparation itself, as the tooth about to be prepared can simply be aligned to the adjacent tooth of reference. If the reference tooth is to be part of the preparation, it should be prepared last so that it can serve as a reference point during the earlier stages of treatment.[3] In cases where no reference point exists, the best way of estimating where the finished PLV margin will be is to use the APT in conjunction with the silicon index.

Cohesive Fractures

Due to the greater stress at the incisal edge of the veneer, clinical cohesive ceramic fractures can occur.[192] Chamfer was believed to be required to strengthen the veneers.[58] Photo-elastic studies have shown that by providing a wide vertical stop to resist loads by covering the incisal edge lessens the stress concentration in them.[182] The author prefers reducing the incisal edge from 1.5-2.0 mm shorter than the final incisal edge of the PLV. This will not only enhance the mechanical resistance but the esthetics as well. The gradation effect of translucency can only be obtained if the incisal edge is prepared like this and the esthetic outcome through the coverage of the incisal edge is usually the most desirable method for patients.

Butt Joint

Instead of a chamfer margin that may weaken the final restoration (see lingual preparation), a flat shoulder should be used at the incisal edge.[108] However, if the tooth exhibits the length desired for the PLV, a 1.0-1.5 mm reduction will be required which will establish a thickness of 2.0 mm in the buccal palatinal direction of the incisal margin. Sub-sequently, a flat incisal surface that emerges perpendicular to the angle of the final emergence profile in the PLV restoration should create the

delicate incisal edge configuration where the incisal edge grooves are connected.[91] This will place the margin finish line 2.00-2.5 mm down from the incisal on the lingual, away from the incisal edge while creating a pleasing length, form and incisal characterization, allowing the ceramist much more flexibility.

Another important aspect to be aware of is the condition of the palatal surface of the tooth that is about to be prepared. The finish line on the lingual aspect of the restoration should not end on a wear facet and it is also preferable not to place the finish line on the central contact points. In the case of a worn incisal a 2.0-2.5 mm reduction from the desired length of the finished veneer is required.[10] If the already existing tooth length is 1.5 mm shorter than the expected final outcome, than in order to achieve a 2.0 mm incisal reduction, only 0.5 mm of preparation will be sufficient. In any of these cases, the fracture potential of the final restoration can be avoided by the rounding of the incisal line angles that reduce the internal stress.[182]

Adhesive Bonding

In adhesive dentistry, all ceramic restorations are dependent on the macro mechanical retention from geometric form that is not very important when it comes to bonded ceramics. The butt joint preparation is simpler and consumes less time than the tooth preparation with palatal chamfer, and the master cast can be used for a precise palatal finish line. However, the only true mechanical indications of a butt joint are the cases where the proximal preps are extended all the way to the palatinal. In these long-wrapping PLV preparations the path of insertion is from the facial. Therefore, only butt joint incisal preparations will allow such a buccal-palatal path of insertion.

Porcelain Support

As it is preformed on the facial surface with adequate support for ceramic veneers, it makes it easier for the dental technician to fabricate the PLV. Buccal, palatal and incisal cervical directions should be followed in the insertion of these

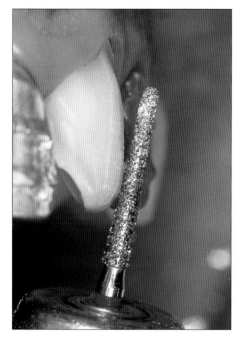

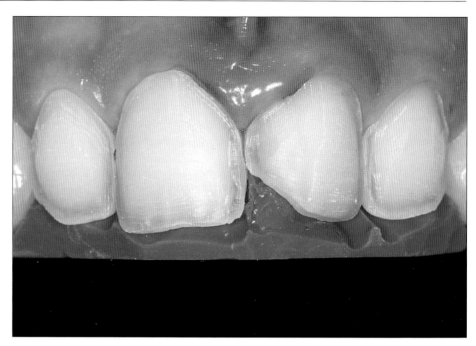

Fig 7-40 The sharp horizontal edge that is created at the incisal 1/3rd is rounded with a fine fissure diamond bur.

Fig 7-41 The incisal depth should be double checked to finalize the preparation.

restorations. This design makes it easier to control the risk of fracture for these thin unsupported palatal ledges. A favorable ceramic/luting composite ratio at the palatal surface, which reduces the risk of post-insertion palatal cracks caused by shrinkage of the composite cement during polymerization and by natural thermal changes in the oral environment, is also provided by a joint butt design. A peripheral enamel layer around all margins is preserved by this butt joint incisal configuration. Microleakage at the palatal tooth reduction interface can be eliminated by the presence of enamel, which is also critical to counteract shear stress.[58,108]

Overcontouring

The pronounced facial curvature of the natural maxillary incisor with its various reflection patterns has a pleasing affect. In poorly countered crowns, convexity in a direct profile is commonly evident.[98] The greatest difficulty in correcting the incisal profile is to preserve a comfortable and unrestricted anterior guidance while pushing the incisal edge to its original esthetic appearance.

In order to detect the gross overcontouring of the incisal third, measurements of the buccolingual thickness of PLV with the tooth crown at the junction of the middle and incisal third should be made. The natural central incisor's thickness ranges from 2.5 mm for a rather thin tooth to 3.3 mm for a thick tooth. When the PLVs thickness together with the tooth exceeds 3.5 mm, over contouring may be suspected.[3]

Rounding the edges

To reduce the number of weak points in the ceramic, all angles and corners should be rounded off. In order not to detract from the bonding, red-banded diamond instruments are used for finishing (Fig 7-40).[5] The use of abrasive paper discs can help to achieve a finish line on the vertical flare without rest to polish.[193] Rounding this horizontal sharp line angle not only improves the strength of the PLV, but also reduces the internal restoration stresses, and the esthetic acceptance of it. If this line remains sharp, it will stand out when the PLV is inserted unless the technician built overbulked porcelain on the incisal 1/3rd, which will not appear esthetic as well.

Ideal Preparation

If the ideal preparation was accomplished when viewed from the labial, the incisal outline of the proposed final restoration should be identical to the incisal outline of the tooth except for the 1-2 mm incisal reduction. In this way, an even thickness of porcelain is achievable.[96]

Even if all the details explained above are considered to be ideal, in certain cases the size of a defect will dictate the extent of preparation. Numerous factors must also be taken into consideration as far as the anatomic and internal topographic structure of the anterior teeth. Relative size and extent of the pulp as compared to the position of the anterior teeth in the dental arch are also important while making extensive preparations.[194]

Tensile Forces

If the ceramic is exposed to tensile loads it is more susceptible to failure.[192] In a study of veneers with 2 mm of unsupported incisal ceramic and butt joint configuration, it was found that the incidence of fractured ceramic veneers was reduced to zero.[108] This will also optimize the luting composite to veneer thickness ratio of which the ideal ceramic thickness should be three times greater than the luting composite.[6]

The strongest veneers that remain intact for the longest period of time are those with 2.0 mm of unsupported incisal ceramic and butt joint ceramic veneers. Placing a palatal chamfer does not increase the PLV strength. Ease of tooth preparation, PLV fabrication, insertion and bonding are some of the clinical advantages of a butt joint preparation.[108] The final depth should be double checked with the help of a silicone index (Fig 7-41).

Lingual Preparation

The special nature of the palatal side of the anterior teeth plays an extremely important role. It is of prime importance to be careful during the preparation stage thus increasing the longevity of the porcelain veneer or the bonded ceramic restoration.

Although applied in practice by the majority of clinicians some researchers have only minimally explored the systematic creation of an incisal overlap scientifically in relation to the biomechanical integration of the veneers.[4] Excessive care should be applied to the concavities as well as the convexities since the impact of the stresses will change depending on the nature of the surface. Palatal concavity that provides the incisor with its sharp incisal edge and cutting ability, proved to be an area of stress concentration. This shortcoming can be compensated for by the cingulum and the marginal ridges that feature thick enamel (Fig 7-42).[6] In their research, *Magne* et al showed that when a horizontal force is applied to the tip of the anterior teeth from the palatal aspect, the recorded strains were always higher in the concavity when compared with the cingulum whereas at the same time the entire facial surface was submitted to compressive forces. It became more dramatic in the absence of facial enamel and tensile stresses measured in the palatal concavity when they reached the elevated and potentially harmful level of 272 Mpa.[4] However, smooth and convex surfaces with local enamel bulk such as the cingulum, the marginal ridges, and the facial cervical third of the anatomic crown showed the lowest stress level. The modified natural tooth that exhibited thick palatal enamel and a mostly convex palatal surface gave the optimal configuration with regard to the stress pattern.[4]

Margin Placement

If a lingual preparation is to be done, this raises the important issue of where to finish the palatinal margins and how deep to prepare the lingual surface of the maxillary anteriors. Logically, the preparation should preferably not finish at the

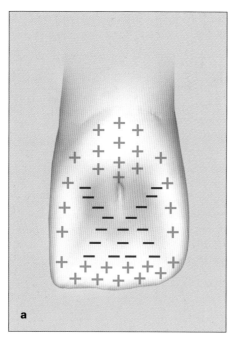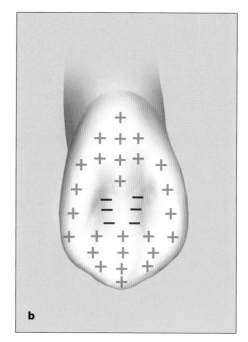

Fig 7-42a, b (a) Palatinal view of central areas. Red (–) markings correspond to concavities that are proven to be the area of stress concentration. (b) The palatinal view of a canine. Due to the thick nature of the enamel and the longer cingulum, there is less stress concentration on the canine. Green (+) markings correspond to the conuexities where the palatinal preparation margin can be located.

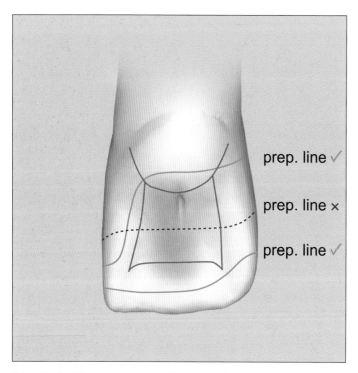

Fig 7-43 The preparation lines on the lingual should not be located on the palatinal concavity.

concavity but rather it should be placed either above the concavity or below on the smooth convex area of the cingulum so that they will be subject to low tensile forces (Fig 7-43). The vertical palatinal marginal ridges also support the strength of the anteriors and therefore care should be given to keep them intact.

Incisal Notch

Placement of the lingual finish line for a laminate veneer will also depend on the thickness of the tooth and the patient's occlusion. If the preparation needs to be extended palatinaly over the incisal edge, the remaining part towards the incisal should have enough thickness to prevent breakage. When the teeth are thinner than 1.5 mm labiolingually at the incisal 1/3rd; reducing the labial and the lingual incisally by 0.5 mm, the preparation leaves us with a thin sliver tooth structure that cannot be rounded off and is susceptible to breaking. These areas are sometimes kept so thin that they even break at the laboratory while the technician tries to take the refractory dies out of the impression, or at the time of the provisional's removal. This situation may cause another

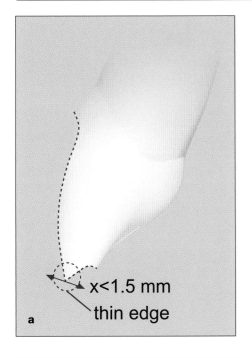

x<1.5 mm

thin edge

a

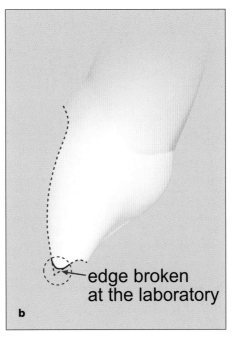

edge broken
at the laboratory

b

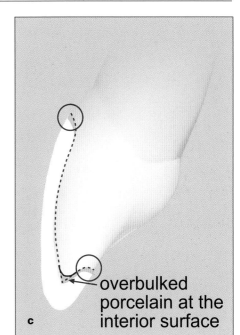

overbulked
porcelain at the
interior surface

c

Fig 7-44a-c (a) If a very thin notch is left at the incisal edge (b) it may break at the lab. (c) The extra porcelain that is fired into that area will prohibit the natural seating of the final PLV.

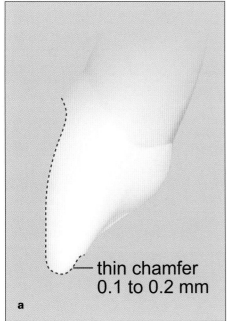

thin chamfer
0.1 to 0.2 mm

a

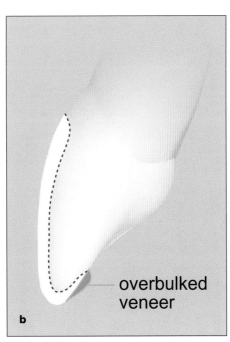

overbulked
veneer

b

Fig 7-45a, b If the palatinal chamfer is prepared thinner than it should be, the result is an overbulked lingual extension. It will cause discomfort to the patient's tongue, and, if it is to be thinned, then the porcelain in this area will be prone to microcracks.

serious problem if the tip of the stone model coincides with the very thin portion and is broken during the lab procedures, resulting in a PLV with extra porcelain in that area. When that PLV is seated on the tooth, care must be taken to avoid mistakes due to the overbulked interior surface of the incisal edge which will make it impossible to seat the veneer properly and result in an inaccurate fit at the cervical margin (Fig 7-44).

Overbulked Porcelain

Accordingly, in a situation where a lingual chamfer is to be prepared without preplanning, the tendency is to under reduce the depth of the lingual chamfer to 0.1-0.2 mm instead of the minimum of 0.5 mm. As the porcelain can not be made as thin as 0.1 or 0.2 mm, the end result will be a joint with a ledge of porcelain beyond the normal contour of the tooth (Fig 7-45). After being bonded, the first feedback will be in the form of a complaint from the patient due to the uncomfortable feeling

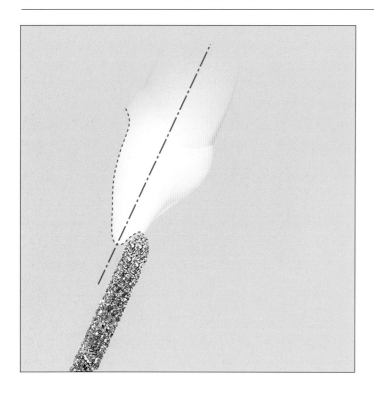

Fig 7-46 The round-ended fissure diamond bur should be held parallel to the long axis of the tooth while preparing the lingual side.

Fig 7-47a, b (a) Sometimes a sharp notch is created on the proximal. (b) This should be rounded to facilitate impression-making, try-in, bonding, etc.

of their tongue. To comfort the patient this ledge must be thinned down to the lingual contour of the tooth with a rotary instrument, leaving the remaining 0.1 or 0.2 mm thick porcelain prone to cracks in the near future. Having this in mind, it is always better to keep the distance from the tip of the prepared incisal edge to the edge of the palatinal wrap around shorter than the distance between the prepared tip of the tooth to the expected incisal edge of the PLV.

A palatally extended preparation should make use of a round-end tapered diamond that will make it easier to create the lingual finish line. Its end should form a slight chamfer, 0.5 mm deep with the instrument held parallel to the lingual surface (Fig 7-46). The finish line should preferably be about one-fourth the way down the lingual surface about 1.0mm from the centric contacts while connecting two proximal finish lines. Care should be given not to locate this finishing line on the palatal concavity. The creation of the lingual finish line often produces a notch (Fig 7-47) at the mesial and distal incisal corners.[172] These corners are often not taken into consideration and left sharp. This kind of a preparation will cause a lot of problems during impression making, try-in and bonding, therefore weakening the bonding

strength of the porcelain. Once the palatinal finishing line is placed, these sharp mesial and distal corners should be gently rounded as in interproximal and incisal overlap which will ease the placement of the final restoration. They will not only be stable at the time of insertion, but an improved esthetic definition of the PLVs will be obtained in the incisal zone.

Orientation of Enamel Rods

In order to produce more effective enamel etching the prismatic and interprismatic mineral crystals must be removed.[195] Therefore it is advisable to expose the cross sections of the palatal enamel rods versus their sides while developing a margin, which will enhance the etchant contact with the interprismatic enamel.[108] As they are placed at an angle of 30° to the tooth axis, the orientation of enamel prisms appears to be critical in the incisopalatinal area.[183] A minichamfer can be prepared to overcome this situation since it will section enamel rods at an angle close to 90° and yet still be distant from the concavity. The orientation of the enamel rods change towards greater angulations of approximately 50°, if the palatinal preparation line is to be placed away from the

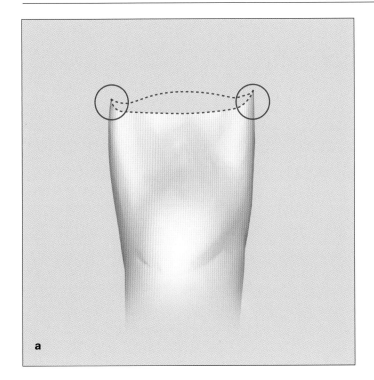

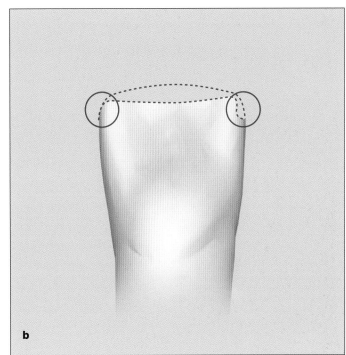

incisal, more towards the middle 1/3rd. A butt margin should be the choice of preparation as such a position is sufficient for strong bonding, when preparing a fractured tooth to receive a PLV (see Fig 4-13).[183]

Finishing the Preparation

After all the steps that have been explained for tooth preparation have been finished, a thorough examination of the prepared teeth is necessary. Especially at the junction of the incisal angle and the lingual reduction, the dentist must be careful to remove any sharp angles that might serve as a focal point for stress concentration. At the point where the facial, proximal and lingual planes of reduction meet, other sharp features that may have formed in the final preparation should be avoided and there should not be any sharp angles.[172]

The dentist must always strive for the most natural pleasing effect and in order to do so, they must check to see if the incisal embrasures are

opened, rounded and of varying depths. The dentist must also check if the embrassures are sufficiently deepened and if the gingival embrasures are carved to create a healthy gingival papilla.[31]

Checking the Prepared Surfaces

The author recommends that all the margins be checked with magnification systems in order to avoid any scratches on the under prepared areas. Another great way to visualize these defects is to take a picture of the prepped teeth. Looking through the lens with 1:1 magnification; will most often surprise the dentist as many minor defects that would otherwise never be seen with naked eye, will be observed.

If everything is under control up until that point, then one final check should be made with the previously prepared silicone index from both the occlusal view and from the lateral view. This will ensure that the necessary reduction of the facial surface is done properly (Fig 7-48). Once the final adjustments are made, dentin sealing, impression and the provisionals can now be prepared. If there is no dentin exposed, than the next step is to make the shade selection. However, if there is any dentin

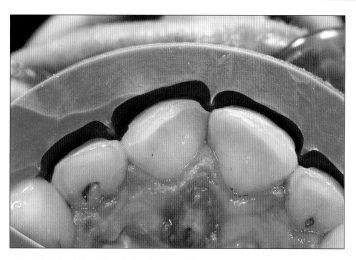

Fig 7-48 The final facial and interproximal reduction is checked with two silicone indexes at different levels.

exposure, the author believes in sealing the freshly cut dentin, just after preparation and before impression making.

Pre-sealing the Exposed Dentin

An important aspect is the sealing of the dentin tubules of the freshly prepared dentin. To prevent post-operative sensitivity and bacterial invasion of the exposed dentin, protection for the period between preparation and final cementation is important.[196,197] It is only possible to partially seal the surface with the temporary materials (resin composite or acrylic resin) that are presently available.[198,199] It is recommended that right after the completion of the tooth preparation, etching and a dentin bonding agent should be applied immediately, before the final impression is taken as it's potential for superior bonding is best when applied to the freshly prepared dentin.[200,201]

After the dentin is etched for 15 seconds, a primer, which is a hydrophilic reactive monomer in an organic solvent, can be more effectively used to prime the exposed dentin.[202,203] If the exposed dentin surface area is adequately retreated at the appointment prior to the actual cementation, then the primers or desensitizers that are used after the preparation do not seem to deteriorate the adhesion to the dentin.[204]

The frequent problem of bacterial leakage and dentin sensitivity experienced during the tempo-

rary phase, can be avoided through the use of a bonding agent. Application of this technique has been found to improve the bond strength in vitro. The recovery of crown stiffness has improved due to the more efficient bonding to dentin techniques.[205]

Indirect Preparation Desensitization

On the dentin, waterproofing, resistance to debonding similar to natural enamel and especially in the field of bonded ceramics is possible to obtain with fourth and fifth generation adhesives.[206] The superficial layer of the etched dentin can be penetrated intertubularly and peritubularly by the modern dentin bonding systems that contain hydrophilic primers. Bond strength in the dental operatory has increased due to a better understanding of the results of etching dentin and the more recent developments in this field. A hybrid layer is important to the micromechanical retention of resin composite to dentin.[207] The dentin's surface must first be demineralized followed by penetration of adhesive hydrophilic monomers.[206]

Exposed Dentin

When the preparation is finished, the surface of the tooth is carefully examined in order to find the exposed dentin areas. Under normal circumstances they will usually appear on the gingival 1/3rd of the tooth. However in cases of facially protruded tooth, the dentin can even be exposed on the incisal area, due to the aggressive nature of the teeth preparation. It is better to immediately etch and seal these areas.

Etching

Many details have to be considered to be able to accurately assess the effect of acid etching on dentin[208] such as, the time of etching, the remaining dentinal thickness and the ability of the restorative materials to seal the etched dentin, along with the type of acid as well as its pKa an pH and the applied concentration (Fig 7-49).

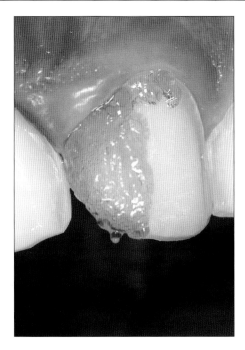

Fig 7-49 The freshly exposed dentin is acid etched with 37% phosphoric acid.

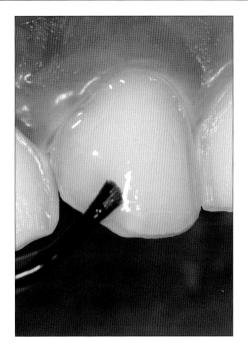

Fig 7-50 Primer is applied only on the blot-dried dentin. Precaution should be taken to limit the application on the dentin avoiding too much spreading over the enamel.

In clinical practice, the most important factor with today's etching agents is that the dentist should not exceed the recommended time of application that is usually less than 15 seconds. Longer applications will cause the collagen to collapse and negatively affect the bonding.

If etching is properly done, the smear layer should be removed to permit bonding to the dentin matrix. It will also cause the demineralization of the matrix dentin, uncovering both the intertubular and peritubular dentin, to permit resin infiltration. It will also clean the dentinal surface free of any biofilms.[208]

Primer and Adhesive Application

Then the etch surface is washed thoroughly, but not dried. It should only be blot-dried with the help of a cotton pellet. The dentin itself has a wet character, which does not necessarily interfere with proper bonding. In fact, fourth generation bonding systems can be used effectively on wet dentin[150,209] and it is inadvisable to demineralize dentin on purpose as it may draw more fluid up from the pulp to the surface, resulting in collapse and shrinkage of the dentinal surface. This phenomena forms the basis for the so

called wet-bonding technique advocated by *Kanca.*[210,211] There should be no misunderstanding about the term wetness, as it is not a technique that allows saliva, blood or gingival fluid to contaminate the etched dentin as they contain proteins that coat the surface of the conditioned dentin and the spaces between the collagen fibers through which the resin must diffuse. While the dentin is reasonably wet, the primer should be applied (Fig 7-50) and left there for a minimum of 30 seconds. It can then be gently warm-air dried from a distance, so that it's carrier weather alcohol, water or acetone will evaporate. At the end of this stage a shiny, stable surface should be visible.

Now the adhesive can be applied over the primer. The resin tags can penetrate into the intertubular dentin to a depth of 6 microns.[212] This micromechanical bond can be better achieved if the bonding agent is cured directly after application.[213] It should be kept in mind that an oxygen inhibited layer of 40 microns will exist over the polymerized adhesive. Therefore high filler content adhesives should be used and covered with a barrier (DeoX-Ultradent) to prevent this layer forming during light curing. It is better if a highly filled adhesive like Optibond FL. (Kerr) is used. It

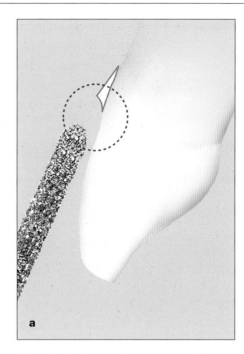
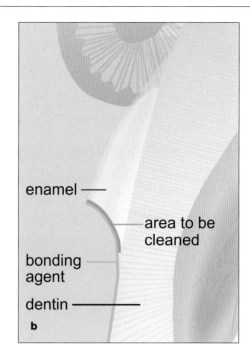

enamel

area to be cleaned

bonding agent

dentin

Fig 7-51a, b The adhesive that may have covered the cervical margin should be cleaned with a round-ended, tapered, extra-fine diamond fissure bur.

has a thickness of 80 microns. This automatically resists the 40-micron oxygen inhibited layer and if sealed with oxygen barrier (Deox Ultradent) a true thickness of 80 microns can be obtained.

Cervical Marginal Check

A popular way to avoid the use of local anesthesia at the seating appointment and to keep people comfortable during the provisionalization period, is to seal the freshly cut dentin of the preparations at the preparation appointment prior to taking the impression, as explained above. However, the existence of this 80-micron thick adhesive may stay on the gingival-enamel margin. Therefore, the last thing to do in the tooth preparation is to delicately go over the gingival margin with an ultra fine, round-ended fissure bur, to create a crisp clear fine enamel margin for the impression (Fig 7-51).

Due to the use of a highly filled adhesive, a similar stress breaker effect may occur. This filler content of low viscosity acts as an intermediate resin and has exhibited improved strength.[214,215] and less leakage[216] than other systems.

As the dentin is hybridized at the preparation appointment, it is fully protected. To prevent the provisional from totally bonding to, or from damaging the area, the hybridized area must be scrubbed with Vaseline after taking the impression and prior to provisional cementation.[24]

Shade Selection

The dentist and the laboratory technician often have difficulties in communicating when it comes to the sensitive area of shade selection for the anterior indirect restorations. There has been a conscious effort to develop techniques to overcome this problem, including pictures, drawing diagrams, and the use of multiple porcelain shade guides (see Chapter 5). However, there are many dentists who have not kept up with the progress that has been made in this field and are only familiar with their already less contemporary techniques from dental school, and so remain unaware of the superior methods that are available to them and their patients.

Color Selection

To achieve a natural appearance details such as color, surface texture, luster, translucency and contour all play important roles in the creation of the ceramic restoration.[217] The range of tooth color that exists in nature is far more than the colors available on shade guides.[218-221] In comparison to the thin veneer ceramic restorations, the guides are made of a much thicker porcelain and therefore the porcelain used for the shade tab is quite different from the porcelain used for fabricating the restorations.[222] A commercial color guide with 16 selections cannot possibly cover the variations exhibited in natural teeth.[172] Subsequently, any treatment must begin with first determining the color. The entire process of reconstruction and its success is directly related to the correct shade selection. Therefore, the technician must have all the related details to be able to make the precise and necessary adjustments. The enamel and body shades are selected in the same way. To do this effectively, an experienced dentist and technician must evaluate a thorough understanding of the various shade combination possibilities. In order to select the base color, custom shade tabs and resin shade rings can be utilized.[8]

Color Vision Deficiency

Color vision deficiency may exist in the form of not being able to distinguish certain colors and although more common in men, it can also exist in women as well. One recent study found 9.3% of the men to be color deficient as opposed to 0.1 of the women.[223] Individuals with a red green deficiency showed lower color vision scores in the yellow region of the visible light spectrum.[224] This can be a serious concern for a dentist and therefore a dentist must be aware of any such condition, and if severe, they must use their assistant's or technician's trained eye to match the shades for them.[225]

Importance of Light Source

In any successful esthetic restoration the dentist must not only consider the artistic side of the procedure but also the scientific side. Color is actually a phenomenon of light and a matter of visual perception that allows us to differentiate between similar objects. The perception of color depends on the object, the observer and the light source[226] and our perception of a particular color may change when any one of these factors is altered.

The light that falls on an object, reflecting, absorbing, transmitting and refracting part or all of the light energy will produce color. Even a single object can exhibit varying amounts of light or color variations. Scattered or reflected light from walls, furniture or other objects may influence our perception of an object.[225] Perception of color is primarily influenced by light and so environmental light is very important. Gray is an excellent color for the environment in order to accurately evaluate the shade of the restorations, as it is a combination of primary and secondary colors and does not have a contrasting complementary color.[227] An interior shade room should be a part of any good dental office or laboratory and should be painted in neutral gray and be well light with color corrected fluorescent bulbs. The patient should not be wearing lipstick and their clothes must be covered with a gray bib. Only after these conditions have been met can the shade selection process begin.

The ideal situation will exist if both the dental office and the lab have the same illumination sources as well as wall colors. This is especially important to minimize the metameric confusion (see Color Chapter).

Timing

The shade selection should be done even before the tooth preparation begins. This will avoid any value alteration during the preparation period (i.e. dehydration). In order to attempt to match the shade, the dentist must first be certain that the patient's teeth are perfectly clean and unstained. Accordingly, just before the shade is to be

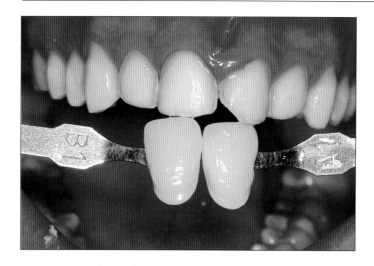

Fig 7-52 Stump shade is very important since the technician prepares a very thin layer of porcelain according to the color of the prepared teeth.

matched, that area of the mouth must have a quick rubber cup and paste prophylaxis done, followed by a thorough rinsing of the paste in that area.

In any examination the patient's teeth suffer from dehydration, therefore shade taking should be done as the first step of the process. In fact, it can take up to two hours for the dehydrated tooth's shade to return to normal if white calcification occurs due to dehydration.[228] Consequently, it is very important to take the necessary photographs as quickly as possible, as even the simple procedure of using a cheek retractor for more than a minute is a cause for dehydration.[16]

Stump Shade

One of the most important procedures in communication with the technician is the transfer of the stump shade, which refers to all the shades of the prepared teeth after the reduction. Since the PLV is a very thin piece of ceramic, the technician should definitely know the color of the underlying structure in order to compensate for this underlying discoloration and achieve the desired shade of the final PLV (Fig 7-52).

A common mistake during this procedure, that is made by most dentists, is to dry the prepared tooth surface before taking the stump shade. However, due to the phenomenon of dehydration, the color of the remaining tooth surface will appear lighter than when they are wet. Consequently, when it comes to the try-in and bonding stage, all of a sudden the tooth and therefore

the PLV will appear darker than it is expected to be. This is a point that should be seriously considered so as not to face unpleasant surprises at the final stage.

Low Value versus High Value

Even though it is not recommended; while talking about a perfect color match, if a dentist cannot decide between two colors; it is beneficial to choose the lighter shade. It is always safer to go along with the lighter shade, as it is easier to darken PLV than to lighten it. (lower the value and increase the chroma) Therefore, whenever in doubt, opting for the lighter color alternative is more logical.[96] In such cases the dentist should also remind the technician to place a double or triple spacer, in order to open some space for the bonding composite that is effective in the color change. The average spacer has a thickness of 3 to 10 microns upon single coating. A composite that is squeezed into such a thin area, during bonding, may not suffice to change the color of the final PLV result.

Character of the Tooth

There are numerous factors to consider in the complicated issue of shade matching. The three most influential factors are illuminant, observer and object. Careful recognition of these factors which include metamerism, gloss, translucency and fluorescence, will help to improve the result of the match. One of the keys to good matching is to recognize the tooth's original form, whether opaque, translucent, dull, or highly reflective. No matter if the porcelain restoration is brilliantly done or if the shade has been correctly chosen, if the surrounding teeth are dull, a high, glossy glaze will be incompatible.[31]

Ocular Fatigue

It can be difficult for the observer to distinguish between colors if ocular fatigue sets in.[229] In order to prevent retinal fatigue (retinal adaptation) concentrated short 5 second intervals will be more useful in detecting the difference in shades.[31] The perception of color is determined by cone cells on the surface of the retina that send a signal to the brain.[230] If a color is viewed for an extended period of time, these cells become fatigued and the signals to the brain thus decrease in accuracy of their perception of the object being observed. Since blue fatigue accentuates yellow sensitivity, the dentist should glance at a blue object (wall, drape, card, etc.).[172]

The cone cells correct the inaccurate shade perception by recharging the sensation of orange when observing the complimentary blue shade of the bib. The aged teeth need additional consideration, as their glossy surface tends to absorb any color close to them and thus distort the perception.

Impression Making

After the tooth preparation is completely finished and the exposed dentin areas are sealed with the bonding agent, it is now time to make the final impression. Each time, and even if it is only to be a single tooth veneer preparation, the impression of the whole arch should be made with a polyvinyl siloxane impression material. This will help the technician to accurately relate the two arches to each other and have more control on occlusion. The full impression of the opposing arch should also be made. However, a precise alginate impression will suffice for that.

In order to properly handle the impression materials, one should have some knowledge of the mechanical properties of the most frequently used impression materials for PLV cases in order to make a restoration that can fit precisely, an accurate undistorted impression of the prepared tooth must be made.[172]

Impressions need careful handling until poured into the gypsum product. Impression making is an area of restorative dentistry where much abuse of materials occurs, and improper handling or untoward delays between removal from the mouth and pouring have distorted many an impression.[172]

With a successful impression the dentist and the technician should be certain of the location and configuration of the finish line. In order to do so they should make an exact duplication of the prepared tooth that includes all the preparation and enough undercut tooth surface beyond the preparation to allow for this. Preserving the health of the gingiva is the key to successful impressions. The first priority is a healthy, stable, non-traumatized gingival sulcus.[7] After this, all considerations are secondary. To accomplish proper articulation of the cast and contouring of the restoration, the adjacent teeth and tissue must be accurately reproduced. The occlusal surfaces of the other teeth in the arch and especially in the area of the finish line must be free of bubbles.[172]

It is the operator's choice to choose from any number of the fine materials available. Today's impression materials are so stable and accurate, that under normal circumstances, all dentists should be able to easily obtain an excellent impression of the teeth they plan to prepare for the PLVs.

It has even been shown in a scanning electron microscopy study[231] that, the molecular structure of the material (usually gypsum or an epoxy resin) used for the master model determines the quality of the reproduction and not the impression material.[136]

Hydrophilic-Hydrophobic

When choosing an impression material it is important that the dentist and their team find the characteristics that they work best with, as each impression material has different handling techniques. Impression materials can be classified as hydrophilic and hydrophobic.

Hydrophilic materials are the easiest to pour, as in irreversible hydrocolloid (alliginate), reversible hydrocolloid and polyether. Polyvinyl siloxanes and condensation reaction silicones are the most hydrophobic, as can be observed in their high contact angle. Hemorrhage and moisture in the gingival sulcus may more easily repel them. However these findings certainly do not contraindicate the use of polyvinyl siloxanes.

Viscosity

According to the type of material, the viscosities for impression materials vary. The least viscous are the light bodied polysulfide and condensation silicones.[232] Viscosity will also increase as time elapses after the start of mixing.[234] Cast restorations need accuracy and there are several types of impression material with the necessary adequacy. Many factors may affect the choice, from simply personal preference to the ability to manipulate, to economics. However, there is no clinical evidence to show any differences between these materials as far as accuracy is concerned.[172] The most frequently used impression materials today are polyvinyl-siloxanes and polyethers.

Polivinyl Siloxane

The author prefers the polyvinyl siloxane and irreversible hydrocolloid, to the other available materials, for PLV cases. Polyvinyl siloxane silicone is also commonly called addition silicone. Addition silicones represent advancements in accuracy over condensation silicones. This has been achieved by a change in polymerization reactions to an addition type, and the elimination of an alcohol by-product that evaporates, causing shrinkage. These materials are available as two-paste systems in four viscosities and a range of colors, allowing the dentist to monitor the degree of mixing.[235] One paste contains silicone with terminal silane hydrogen groups and inert filler. The other paste is made up of a silicone with terminal vinyl groups, chloroplatinic acid catalyst and a filler.[233]

Packing

The two pastes usually come packaged in separate tubes, or for those that are used with a dispenser gun, a twin barreled cartridge. A mixing tip with multiple varies or baffles mix the materials together. As this method eliminates the spatula and mixing pad by mixing the material, these mixing guns have become the most popular method of dispensing. There are great advantages to this system as there is no air entrapment and contamination is prevented by ensuring a constant ratio of catalyst and base.[236]

Chemistry

Upon mixing equal quantities of the two materials, there is an addition of silane hydrogen groups across vinyl double bonds with the formation of no by-products.[237] As no volatile by-products are produced in the reaction, addition silicones have a much greater dimensional stability,[233,237,238] than condensation silicones. The pastes are available in light, medium, heavy and putty viscosities. Some manufacturers include a retarder for extending the working and setting times.[235] The result is an exceptionally stable material. The working time and setting times of addition silicones are faster than polysulfides and a retarder is often supplied to extend the working time.

Storage

They have excellent elasticity and show very low dimensional shrinkage upon storage.[235,239] and it is still accurate, even when poured 1 week after removal from the mouth.[240] Therefore, addition silicones can be safely poured up later or sent to a dental laboratory.[235] It has been demonstrated that the storage of unpoured polyvinyl siloxane and polyether impressions in the temperature range of 4°C to 40°C do not affect the accuracy of the master model.[241] It is easy to imagine, however, that the temperature in a car or airplane that the impression is being transported in from the office to the technician can easily surpass this range of temperatures. Studies of the effect of storage conditions in the range of −10°C to 66°C, revealed significant distortions in the materials following an extended period of storage at 66°C.[242] Therefore, the dentists working with advanced laboratories overseas should especially consider this interesting research when sending their impressions. Special boxes that are insolated and that are not affected by temperature changes should be used to prevent temperature related distortions.

Impression Making with Polyvinyl Siloxane

The casts should be made from articulated full arch impressions, as PLVs will play a role in providing protrusive or lateral guidance. High viscosity polyvinyl siloxane putty is the most rigid impression material and is therefore never used alone but with the low polyvinyl siloxane (wash), with low rigidity.[243]

Before the impression is made, the impression tray should be coated with its special adhesive at least 15 minutes in advance. Most of the time the gingival margins of the prepared teeth are left supragingival and in such cases, there will be no need to place a retraction cord into the sulcus.

Retraction Cords

However, if the margin is placed subgingivally, or the technician needs to be supplied with detailed information on the emergence profile for some reason, retraction cords can be used. If there is too much tissue fluid coming out of the sulcus, and if it is suspected that this may distort the impression, than a double cord technique can be used. A thin (2.0) silk surgical suture is gently placed into the sulcus. Care should be given when it is placed, so that the two ends do not overlap each other. In other words, they should come edge to edge. Then a braided retraction cord is placed over the silk cord. The dentist should not

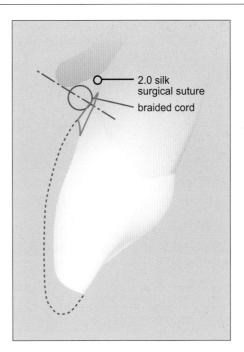

Fig 7-53 If the cervical margin is located subgingivally, a retraction cord can be use for better impressions. A 2.0 silk suture cord is placed into the sulcus in order to stop tissue fluids coming out. On top of that a braided retraction cord is placed in order to deflect the sulcus. It should not be buried into the sulcus. Its thickest part should be leveled with the sulcus tip.

push the second cord excessively (Fig 7-53) and remember that, the aim of using the second cord is only for "displacement" and consequently it should be pushed only half way, to keep the largest part of its diameter level with the sulcus tip. The cord is left in the sulcus for a couple of minutes and then gently removed, keeping the first one in the sulcus, which will help to stop the tissue fluid flow. The impression should be made as soon as possible, before the deflected gingival margin collapses back to its original position. In addition, if there are big undercuts at the palatinal surface or if larger gingival embrasures exist, it may be beneficial to block these sites out before making the impression, as the material will most likely tear away from these areas and at times distort the impression.

Avoiding Cross Contamination

If a tube-dispensed material is used in a double-mix technique, the assistant and operator start

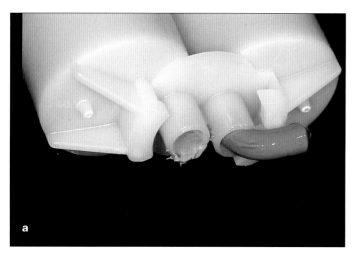
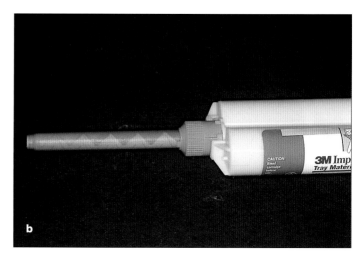

Fig 7-54a, b (a) If not properly managed, the end of the barrels can get cross-contaminated and become blocked through polymerization. (b) The best way to prevent this from happening is to keep the used mixing tip on the cartridge untill the next time it is used.

mixing material at about the same time. Removing the cap opens the cartridge and a small quantity of the material from the tip of both barrels is squeezed out. It is possible that the end of the barrels may have been cross-contaminated from the previous application, and thus, the reason for the polymerized plugs at the nozzle (Fig 7-54). If the nozzle is not carefully inspected before the impression is made, the dispenser may jam, causing an unexpected delay, as the dentist struggles to get the impression material out of the barrels by over powering the jammed dispenser. The easiest way to overcome this problem is to leave the used mixing tip on the cartridge as a cap. This way, the next time the dentist is ready to make a new impression, removing the already used mixing tip will provide a very clean area in the exit region of the barrels.

Fig 7-55 If the true gingival displacement is obtained with the retraction cords, the impression material should display all the details in the cervical area.

Technique

Once this is achieved, the dentist starts applying the light bodied material with the syringe, which should have a relatively thin mixing tip nozzle, right over the gingival margins of the preparation. However it should be kept in mind that if unmodified additional silicones are used, these hydrophobic materials cannot displace any moisture or hemorrhage that is not removed prior to placement of the impression material.[235] Therefore, even though they may be hydrophilic, the area should be kept clean of saliva, hemorrhage and sulcular fluids. The aim should be, to try to place the material in between the gingival margin and the sulcus (Fig 7-55). The most predictable way of achieving this is to start from one point and keep on going in the same direction, with a gentle touch of the nozzle over the area, without any interruption, to avoid the formation of any bubbles. At the same time, the assistant loads the tray with the medium or heavy-bodied material.

Once the application of the light-bodied impression material is finished, than the medium body loaded tray is seated (over the light body material) firmly in the mouth and it is held in place for seven minutes from the start of mixing. As the material does not stain and has both pleasant scents and colors, they can be used with stock or custom trays while the patient is reclining.[235] The temperature can affect the working and setting time of the impression materials. The components of two different systems cannot be mixed together as they are not compatible and the material will not set if addition silicones are combined with condensation silicones. Caution must be exercised as temperature increases will decrease the working and setting times.[335] Once set impression must be removed as quickly and as straight as possible to prevent distortion. Addition silicones exhibit excellent recovery from deformation and they are very accurate and have high dimensional stability after setting. Then the impression is rinsed, blowed, dried, and then inspected. It should be placed in a disinfectant solution before pouring it.[235]

Disinfection of Impressions

Prior to disinfection it has been found that fewer microorganisms are retained on the surface of polyvinyl siloxane impressions than on any of the other materials.[244] Polyvinyl siloxanes generally display excellent tolerance to immersion in sodium hypochlorite,[245,246] glutaraldehyde[247-250] iodophor[239,248,251] and phenols.[237,252,253]

Reaction to Latex

No matter how precise the dentist makes the impression, in some cases, at the time of the inspection, there remains some still soft, unpolymerized spots or larger areas that can be detected. This is due to one of the points that is often ignored, the polymerization retardation of the polyvinyl siloxanes, which is due to their reaction to latex. The use of latex gloves while mixing or dispensing the putty will interfere with the setting

process. The sulfur derivatives in the latex are probably responsible for the polymerization retardation.[254] If it is not automix putty and mixed putty,[255] it is more susceptible to contamination. However, only some brands of impression material, in combination with some brands of gloves, cause restarted setting.[256] Other latex items such as a rubber dam that is used to seal the area may cause problems when they come in contact. The contact does not even have to be made directly. Even if the impression material comes in contact with a tooth that has been touched by a latex glove (not even directly the glove itself), it may cause polymerization retardation. To avoid this vinyl gloves can be used during impression making while handling the impression material.[257]

Pouring Time

Another important aspect is the pouring time of the impressions. Usually the impressions are sent to the labs and poured there. However, if the dentist wants to pour it himself or herself for some reason, he/she must be careful not to do it too quickly after making the impression, because as explained before, these materials may release hydrogen gas on setting. That will cause surface porosity and voids on the stone cast. Even though their formula has been improved by the addition of palladium to absorb the hydrogen that has minimized this problem, pouring should be delayed for a short time of 15 to 30 minutes.[225] Therefore careful study of the available materials and the ability to interpret the information is essential. The dentist must be fully aware of how long to wait before pouring the impression, since it will determine the dimensional stability (Fig 7-56).[235]

Irreversible Hydrocolloid

Irreversible hydrocolloid can be used to make the preliminary study cast impressions as well as the opposing arch impression however the most widely used impression materials in dentistry today are the alginates.[235]

Alginates are supplied as a powder containing sodium or potassium alginate (12% to 15%) and calcium sulfate dihydrate (8% to 12%) as reac-

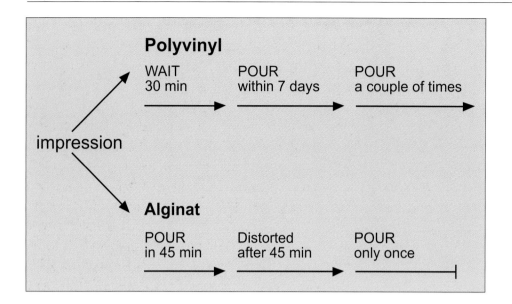

Polyvinyl

WAIT	POUR	POUR
30 min	within 7 days	a couple of times

impression

Alginat

POUR	Distorted	POUR
in 45 min	after 45 min	only once

Fig 7-56 The dentist must be fully aware of how long to wait before pouring the impression

tants; sodium phosphate (2%) as a retarder; a reinforcing filler (70%),such as diatomaceous earth, to control the stiffness of the set gel; potassium sulfate or alkali zinc fluorides(10%) to provide good surfaces on gypsum dies; and coloring and flavoring agents (traces) for esthetics. The sodium phosphate content is adjusted by the manufacturer to produce either regular-or fast-set alginates.[235] A dustless version, where the powder is coated with glycol, has been introduced to avoid the inhalation of alginate dust. This powder is mixed to obtain a paste.

Advantages

Alginate impression materials are pleasant tasting, easy to manipulate, easily poured into stone, hydrophilic, inexpensive and capable of displacing blood and body fluids. As alginates have a tendency to tear easily, they must be poured immediately after removal. They can be used with stock trays and also have limited detail reproduction, and as they are dimensionally unstable they can only be used for single casts. Therefore, they cannot be used, if the dentist does not have a pouring access in the clinic, and if the alginate impression has to be sent to a laboratory far away from where the dental office is located. In order to achieve proper disinfection, the manufacturers recommendations must be followed carefully. Immersion in iodphors or sodium hypochlorite can be used to disinfect the alginate hydrocolloids.

Facebow Transfer

A commonly overlooked aspect of communication between dentist and ceramist is the correct orientation of the master model. The ceramist must be able to visualize the patient, just as the dentist does from the frontal view, by utilizing the master model. The ceramist can only estimate horizontal and vertical alignment of the working cast from landmarks taken from the cast itself, unless precise information has been transferred to them from the laboratory. Especially in the case of multiple anterior preparations where there is always the potential for misalignment due to poor communication between dentist and ceramist, it is unwise to leave judgement to pure chance.

The best way to evaluate the inclination of the incisal plane is to face the patient directly to view their face as a whole. In order to make a final appraisal, it is necessary to examine the direction of the dental mid-line and gingival plane from one canine to the other. The incisal plane may be observed to be slightly to moderately canted or parallel to the pupillary line. Although not frequently seen, severe canting may exist. A canted incisal plane frequently exists with the dental midline perpendicular to it when there are deficient crowns. Incorrect orientation of the working cast can cause a different inclination of the incisal plane of the teeth in the mouth, in comparison to the articulator. A slightly canted incisal plane requires either no correction at all, or only minor incisal reshaping of the incisal edge. Before any prosthetic reconstruction takes place, a partial or full correction of the incisal plane is required when there is a moderately canted incisal plane. The key to success in a partial correction of a moderate cant is to make certain that the gingival margins of the incisors are also parallel to the pupillary line. Even with misalignment of the canines, a moderately canted plane can be made esthetically pleasing as long as the gingival margins of the maxillary incisors are aligned on a horizontal plane and the incisors are restored and aligned with the interpupillary line. A unilateral surgical elongation of the incisor on the lower aspect is indicated if the orientation of the gingival plane follows the cant of the maxilla and appears oblique in relation to the interpupillary line.[258]

A divergence between the interpupillary line and the intercondylar axis may occur due to natural asymmetries of the head leading to unnatural canting of the maxillary cast due to the facebow record transfer converts and the asymmetrical axis locations to the horizontal symmetrical axis of the articulator (see Chapter 13).[259] The dental laboratory technician may not recognize this problem on the bench surface, and improperly canted incisal and occlusal planes of the crown restorations may ensue at try-in.[259,260]

Bite Registration

In most of anterior PLV cases (unless the occlusion has to be improved or changed, or if the patient is having some TMJ pain or discomfort) a simple "centric occlusion" registration will be sufficient. It is always preferable to have registration material that is as stiff as possible. It should be very soft when introduced into the mouth to prevent the patient from biting with force and forming different closing positions than normal. It is a common phenomenon that when biting on a harder material, a patient will apply some force and unconsciously their bite will be considerably different than it normally is.

It is also wise to use a minimum amount of material in order to prevent the material flow into the undercut areas beyond the equatorial limits of the posterior teeth since the technician will have difficulties when seating the stone models on the bite-registration material and relating the upper and the lower stone models to each other. In most cases, if only the maxillary anterior teeth are to be treated with the PLVs, due to the reduction limited to the facial surfaces of these teeth; almost all the teeth will be in contact when the 2 stone models are brought into contact.

However, if the mandibular teeth are also being prepared for PLVs it is easier to place an anterior jig after the centrals and laterals are prepared in order to stabilize the arches into position. The occlusal-registration can then be made more accurately after the jig is seated over the lower incisors.

Provisionals

In PLV cases, the ultimate goal of provisionals is to master the function and esthetics of the final restorations. This makes it an integral part of the treatment, providing proper communication with the patient and laboratory, which directly enhances and positively affects the smile design process.

Provisionalization is a practical means of obtaining feedback, on the esthetic parameters, from not only the patients, but the dentist and technician as well, since the subjectivity of a smile design can never be overemphasized.[261] This will eliminate most of the guesswork which may be the cause of an imperfect esthetic and functional outcome.

The dentist is able to create and develop facial esthetics,[262] smile design.[7,258] tooth form and contour or occlusion and function.[263,264] as well as marginal integrity and emergence profiles[115] through the use of diagnostic wax-up and provisional restoration. With the aid of provisionalization, verification of esthetic modifications and biological compatibility of the proposed restoration is made possible for the restorative team.

As was previously explained, the APT is produced prior to tooth preparation, and gives a better idea of what can be expected in the final outcome. This is especially important if the original position of the anterior teeth has been lost through disease or trauma, or if significant changes are to be made for the sake of creating a new smile design. The new form, position and length of teeth can easily be visualized using the provisionals.

Patient Communication

Although it is ultimately the dentist's responsibility to decide on the type of treatment that will work best for each patient, the patient also has the opportunity to express what is esthetic, comfortable and functional for them. The closer the temporaries are to the desired result, the less surprises will be incurred on the day of delivery. Even though the APT can help most of the patients finalize their visual expectations, some patients are strongly influenced by comments made by colleagues, family and friends once they leave the dentist's office. This kind of patient can voice their final approval in a few days after the provisional is inserted and if any changes are to be made, final touch-ups can be done. Well-established communication between the dentist and the laboratory is necessary. Despite this communication, the technician can still occasionally misjudge the incisal edge position and length due to the absence of the lips on a stone model.

Incisal Edge Position

The position of the incisal edge and the length/ width ratio of the central incisors are two of the important factors that the dentist must decide on. The position and width/length ratio of the incisors is dictated by the two central incisors, Therefore, it is not only the color of the tooth that must be precisely described to the ceramist, but the entire smile as a whole.[3]

The original incisal position should be tested with provisional restorations that have been fabricated from a diagnostic wax-up. However, a common error is to drastically alter the original position before doing so. If a significant alteration in the incisal edge position is planned with new PLVs, the patient should first demonstrate functional adaptation to the new position in the provisional restorations.[265] Functional disturbances such as mobility, pain, or discomfort, which prove difficult for the patient to adapt to, can occasionally be caused by retraction of the protruded incisal edge position toward the lingual. Thinning of the palatinal portion of incisal edges of the provisional restorations may be necessary to attain a comfortable guidance. However, this thinning of the incisal may result in the final incisal edge position being further labial than anticipated from the diagnostic waxing. Significant esthetic alterations necessitate very careful planning and simultaneous restoration of both esthetics and function.

Phonetics, Function and Esthetics

Functional and phonetic parameters are an intrinsic part of esthetic results. To truly test the function, phonation, position of the lips and vertical dimension, these prostheses must be used.

Real life tryouts must be done to avoid situations that may jeopardize the ceramic preparations. The length, protrusion and position must all be "tried out" in the patient's mouth. The dentist and the patient must work together to find the esthetic and functional components they can agree on. A precise adjustment is necessary once they are cemented. The patient must be asked to perform protrusive, lateral and excursive movements while checking the anterior and canine guidance, so that the occlusion and function can be verified. The new smile should not affect speech or lip closure[2] if the overbite and over-jet relationship are balanced.

The final position and appearance of the central incisors will be dictated by the dentist's knowledge of smile design and the patient's guidance through functional movements and speech. When the dentist and patient are satisfied with the function and esthetics of the provisional restorations, an impression of the approved provisional is taken and sent to the laboratory. This is one of the most important communication tools along with the photographs, study models, and the incisal index.

Blueprint for the Ceramist

The approved provisionals act as a blueprint of what the ceramist will create. A well-fabricated temporary will dictate a proper occlusal scheme and esthetic form. Carefully designed provisional restorations, which fulfill the esthetic, biologic and functional criteria, will provide a constructive foundation for the long-term restoration.[261] The time spent at the delivery or final visit will decrease when more time is spent during the temporization phase. An approved point of reference gives the ceramist confidence to successfully complete the final product. The success of this visit is very important and the dentist's ability to gain the patient's confidence is reflected in the success of the final restoration.

Pulp Protection

Provisionals traditional indication, have been to protect the prepared tooth structure. Provisional restorations are essential for ensuring health and esthetics until the definitive restorations are fabricated, during the time between the preparation of the tooth and the placement of the final restoration.[172]

Minimal invasive techniques are used for the PLV cases. However, in cases of altering very dark discolorations or incorporating the existing cavities or the worn out composite filling into the PLV restoration, deeper preparation of the tooth may be necessary. Prolonged exposure of the dentin permits microbial penetration and increases the potential thermal and chemical trauma.[266] Due to tooth sensitivity, the patient will also practise inadequate oral hygiene, which will cause gingival inflammation. In such cases, the provisional will be protecting the pulp, as well as decreasing post-operative sensitivity. In order to achieve this, the provisional must be fabricated from a material that will prevent the conduction of temperature extremes.

In today's dentistry, all materials used for fabricating the provisionals for PLV cases fulfill these criteria. However, care should be given to the adaptation of the margins to prevent microleakage, and thus bacterial invasion, which is considered the most important cause of post-op sensitivity. The sensitivity will be minimal or non-existent if the exposed dentin surfaces are sealed with the bonding agent just after the preparation and before impression making and provisionals.

Provisionals should also help maintain the periodontal health and tooth position. In cases where there is mobility of the teeth due to periodontal problems, the provisionals will also supply positional stability. However, while trying to achieve this and by connecting the provisionals together, the contours and the gingival embrasures should be delicately designed so that the area can easily be cleaned throughout the provisionalization period.

Even though most of the PLV margins are prepared supragingivally, in special cases where the margins are placed subgingivally, it is of the utmost importance that the margins of the provisional restoration do not impinge on the gingival tissues.[267-270] The resulting inflammation may not only cause gingival proliferation or recession, but hemorrhaging during the final bonding, which will severely affect the longevity of the PLVs.

Various techniques such as spot etching and luting with a composite,[271-273] eugenol-free temporary cement[274] or the use of dental adhesives[275] have been suggested for the bonding of provisional restorations.

Technique

The fabrication of the provisionals can be classified into two groups, as direct (intraorally) or indirect (extra oral) prefabricated provisionals.

The latter is prepared at the laboratory on a plaster, stone or epoxy model before or after the teeth are prepped. The technician approximately prepares the stone model and builds up the provisional mostly from acrylic. After preparing the teeth, the dentist tries to adjust the interior surface of the acrylic veneers for an easy fit over the teeth. Once the provisional can be easily placed, then the inside of it is filled with a flowable composite and temporarily bonded.

However, the author prefers the intraoral provisional fabricating techniques. There are various approaches for the different techniques.

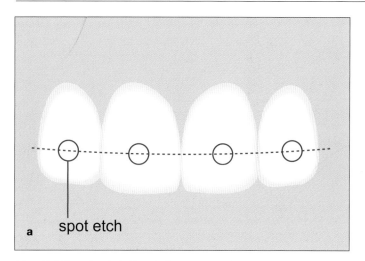

spot etch

a

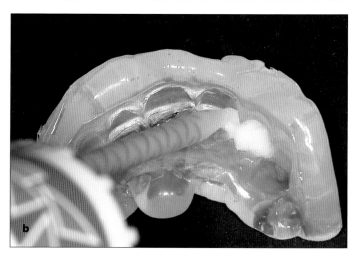

b

Fig 7-57a, b (a) Partially to bond the provisionals in place, teeth are spot etched. The important issue is to try to keep the spots on the same horizontal level. This will ease the cleansing of the bonded area just before actual PLV bonding. The tooth is then covered with adhesive. (b) A flowable composite (Luxatemp) is then loaded into the translucent silicone template and placed over the prepared teeth.

Free Hand Carving

A very quick way to fabricate the provisional intraorally is by the freehand carving technique whether it is for a single veneer or two to four veneers.

When the restorative result is no longer dictated by the remaining tooth structure, manipulation of free hand composite resin enhances creative skills and familiarizes the clinician with different sensitive build-up techniques that are advocated in clinical practice for achieving predictable results.[25,276] The experience also develops spatial visualization, perception of forms and volumes, and the ability to discard rigid esthetic standards and discover creativity.[28] For improved clinical/laboratory communication, the use of free hand composite resins can familiarize the dentist with different dental designs, surface textures and anterior teeth positioning, learned through a unique craftsmanship process, to address the challenge of replicating natural esthetics.[28] The tooth can be spot etched and the bonding agent applied and light cured. Then the necessary amount of hybrid composite, with the desired color that matches the adjacent teeth is rolled between the fingers. The material is then placed and shaped on the tooth, with the help of the index finger. If the surface texture or extension of the provisional to the interproximal is required, then

special instruments can be adjunctively used and light cured. In this technique, the dentists have the maximum control to themselves.

If it is to be placed on a single tooth, the adjacent teeth can be used as references in terms of length, tooth axis and color. However, if two to four teeth are being provisionalized, than the incisal length and position can be adjusted freely, paying the utmost attention to function and anterior guidance. Since these provisionals are being placed one by one, the interdental contacts can be left separated in order to leave space for easy cleaning practices.

Translucent Template or Silicone Impression

The second intraoral technique; is the fabrication of provisionals with the help of the transparent template which closely mimics the wax-up that the lab technician produced at the very early stages of treatment planning. Instead of the template, the dentist may prefer to make a translucent silicon impression (Clinicians' Choice) of the stone models of which wax-ups have been made. To build the provisionals intraorally the dentist can use that impression instead of the template.

Once the teeth are prepared, they can be spot etched and then the adhesive is applied and light

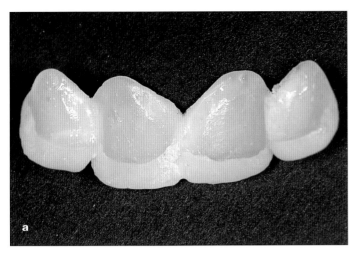 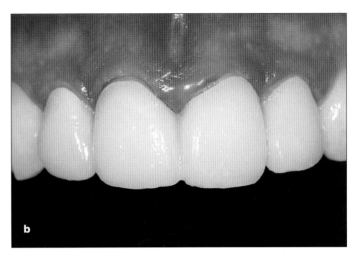

Fig 7-58a, b (a) The provisionals that come out with the template are trimmed down and polished. (b) The provisionals are in the mouth. They should be cemented with either a flowable luting resin or eugenol-free cement.

cured. Next, the template is loaded with a flowable resin, with the color of choice and gently placed over the prepared teeth (Fig 7-57). The nice part of using the transparent template is that it allows the dentist to use light cured composites and they can visualize the voids that sometimes occur during the placement. If the voids are big, the template can be taken out of the mouth, filled with the same flowable composite, and re-inserted. However, if the voids are tolerable it is always possible to restore these areas after the provisional is completely polymerized and cemented.

After the composite is polymerized, two possibilities arise. The provisional either comes out with the template during removal or stays intact on the prepared teeth.

If it comes out, then the margins can be trimmed and polished extraorally and the provisional is then cemented over the teeth with non-eugenol cement or with a flowable composite (Fig 7-58).[277] A flowable luting resin is placed inside the temporary veneers and reseated onto the teeth. Each tooth is cured for 10 seconds with a plasmic arc or laser light, or 30 seconds with a conventional light.

However, if it remains on the teeth, then the provisional is totally polymerized in the mouth and gingival flesh is cleaned with the help of the finishing carbide burs without violating the dento-gingival complex. If voids exist, they can be restored and the final appearance is checked in terms of esthetics and function.

In case any alterations are necessary, they can easily be performed intraorally. Luxa Flow can also be used to repair or add onto the temporary. The areas must be micro etched or roughened with a bur, and a bonding agent should be applied. This represents the treatment phase that enables the dentist to put their artistic skills into practice.

If the provisional from the matrix, does not need to be altered, then the technician can use his/her wax-up for the final PLV build-up as a guide.

However, if any alterations were made, then the dentist should provide the technician with a new impression of the whole arch with the altered design of the provisionals cemented together with the pictures taken.

Laboratory Communication 2

While the availability of novel materials and application techniques in adhesive dentistry have expanded the esthetic armamentarium, it mandates that patient, clinician and technician remain in close communication in order to maintain a high level of performance, incorporating their combined knowledge and artistic ability.[278]

Understanding each other through shared experiences, successes and failures, and being in harmony enables the dentist and ceramist to communicate well. The more subjective side of the triad is the communication between the dentist and patient that relies on trust, dialogue, consensus and complicity.[5]

A solid collaboration between the dentist and laboratory is essential to achieve the desired esthetic result.[279] However, in order to develop the highest level of communication, both the dentist and the technician should be knowledgeable in current trends while ensuring that they keep the communication line between them open at all times. This alone is not enough, as the restorative team must work together (dentist-technician) to develop common goals, interests, values, abilities and desires by improving the dentist's understanding of the laboratory phase, and the technician's cognizance of the clinical aspect of dentistry.[300]

Patient Expectations

Esthetic dentistry-although scientific in nature remains an art form that requires patient approval of the definitive outcome.[278] They are naturally more concerned with the final esthetic result than whether or not the fabrication was difficult. Consequently, there is no point in the dentist explaining the difficulty of the procedure to the patient if the patient is not satisfied with the result. This often leads to the technician feeling forced to make compromises in materials and technology.[283] Laboratory communication is of prime importance in achieving predictable and pleasing results in esthetic PLV cases. "A chain is as strong as its weaker link." No matter the amount of time spent with the patient or the knowledge of the dentist or the efforts of the technician, the result will only be as successful as the strength of the lab-dentist communication link that ensures that all the data is transferred properly. Consequently, the dentist should not expect miracles to happen in order to obtain an esthetically successful result. Therefore, the process in the past that only sent the impression to the laboratory technician without very clear directives about the transfer's color is no longer a feasible communication tool. Beautiful smiles can only be created through sound communication.

Photography

In the case of anterior esthetics, a picture, and all that it is able to convey, is priceless. Using slides, prints or intraoral photographs enable the dentist to easily communicate invaluable information concerning the shape and texture of the teeth. The more sophisticated video imaging is also good at conveying information about the desired form.[96] Pictures make it easy for the laboratory technician to actually see the tooth contours, the translucencies within the incisal edge, hypoplastic spots, enamel staining and the actual intensity of the characterization.

Polaroid photographic prints of the try-in stage or composite mock-ups can be used along with the necessary information written on them to be sent directly to the lab. Instant film development is possible with digital photography, allowing the dentist and technician to review images via email, no matter the distance, and in only a few seconds.

Color Communication

Perhaps the most sensitive and critical area of communication is that of color. It requires very close communication of concise information between the dentist and technician, in order to select the most accurate color (see shade selection). An unsuccessful result is often due to the incorrect choice of color that may be due to the unclear communication and poor correspondence between the parties.

Ideally, the technician should be involved in the selection process along with the dentist and patient. When this personal contact is not possible, photographic images serve as the next best effective way to communicate information on color and esthetics. It is not very easy to convey the exact color by observing a slide, but if a shade tab is placed next to an image of the tooth, quite a lot of information is supplied to the technician about the translucency, texture and luster, along with the chroma, value, hue and the shape of the tooth.

Shade Tabs

The photograph should include the shade tab that has been chosen. A photograph and whatever information it conveys is dependent on the camera, the flash, the film etc. However, it is possible to correctly assess the color if the tab is included and the differences between the tab and the teeth are accurately recorded.[16] In order to correctly assess the color, the tab and the teeth should be on the same plane and placed edge to edge. If the tab is not observed from the same plane then the value may appear different than it actually is.[284] The tab levels must be placed so that they can clearly be seen and if possible, more than one tab should be included. The color is then adjusted according to the differences that have been recorded on the slide. In the comparison of different values, black and white photographs are most useful.

Translucency

With color, communication of the translucency and texture are important parameters that play an important role in the value of the teeth. Transforming the incisal details necessitates highly developed photography techniques. When photographing the mamelons there will be too much reflected light if the camera is held perpendicular to the labial surface. To avoid this, the camera must be held high at a 30-degree angle downwards. To record the translucency the teeth should be photographed clenched and opened. The thickness of the enamel layer and any crack lines can be seen in the photographs taken at a 30-degree side angle.

Full-face Pictures

The photographs should not only be limited to 1:1 intraoral pictures, as full face pictures are very useful and should always be taken and utilized. This is the best way to communicate with the lab in terms of teeth and lip relationships and the relation of them to the whole face. Pictures should be taken before, during and after the preparation and the provisionals. In addition to all the techniques explained for positioning the correct incisal line, photography will have a great input on the issue as well. Pictures of the provisionals should be taken, even if they may not be perfect. At least it helps the dentist, patient and technician by providing something to discuss in terms of reaching the desired esthetic goal that this triad is working towards.

Points of Reference

The technician may need to have one or several reference points in order to place the new incisal length and the new anterior position of the teeth. If intact teeth in the area exist, they will have no problems in using them as guides or references. However, in the case of a new smile design, with many worn or damaged teeth, it is best to use the provisionals as a master guide. The last photographs of the before and after (with provisionals) and stone models should be included.

The impressions should be delicately wrapped and sent to the laboratory in order to avoid any deformation (see impressions).

Facebow Transfer

Some of the other supportive tools of communication are the accurate bite registration and the face bow transfer. However, the face bow transfer does not always necessarily transfer the correct esthetic information. Care should be given to transfer the incisal line position (see Chapter 13).

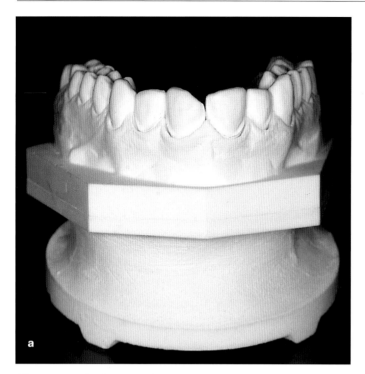 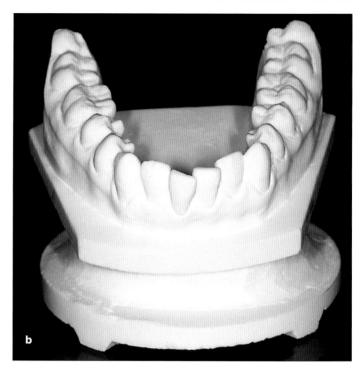

Fig 7-59a, b Model of intact gingival (Geller) with removable refractory dies (front view).

Detailed Prescription

Although there are several ways of communicating information to the laboratory technician, the standard practice is to send a detailed prescription form with sufficient, objective information[285] so that it can easily be translated into a subjective result. A detailed written instruction sheet[286] should incorporate a comprehensive description of the patient and their expectations, as well as the dentist's comments. In this way, all pertinent information is communicated to the technician in a clear, concise manner.[5]

In addition, hand drawn diagrams, such as sketches of the hypocalcification spots, translucency patterns, crazing or even intrinsic shade mapping, will have great value in shade communication.

The details should be discussed, after the technician receives all the information together with the photos, models etc., in order to avoid any conflicts.

Dentist-Technician Collaboration

Once, tooth preparation techniques, new materials, technical procedures, esthetic concepts, and smile design are mastered by the clinician and the ceramist, a higher standard of service can be provided to the patient[287] thereby producing restorations that are mechanically, biologically and esthetically sound.

Improving the dentist and technician's mutual understanding of each other's work and total awareness of the steps they each take as this procedure develops, can only enhance the details of this process of interdisciplinary communication.[288] If the dentist is well trained, or at least has solid knowledge of the technical aspects of the laboratory procedures, he/she should recognize the limits of the dental technician, especially in PLV cases where the maximum thickness of the porcelain will be as thin as 0.5-0.7 mm

On the other hand, the technician should also be dedicated to their profession, having adequate current knowledge of the materials, techniques and their own artistic abilities in order to be able to produce the details that the esthetic dentist has transferred to them (Figs 7-59 to 7-77).

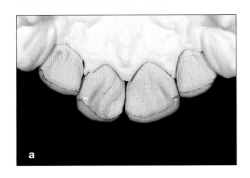
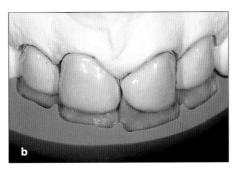

Fig 7-60a, b (a) Model of intact gingival with removable refractory dies (palatal view). (b) Model of intact gingival and silicone matrix on diagnostic volume of teeth.

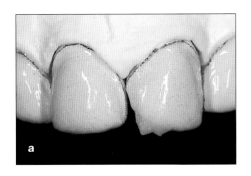
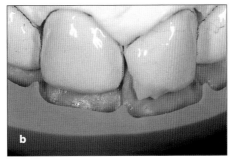

Fig 7-61a, b (a) Material for rebuilding and to tie in with the volume of the preparations in between. (b) Check with silicone matrix. Note the mesioincisal addition on tooth #21(9).

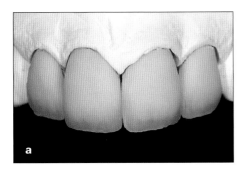
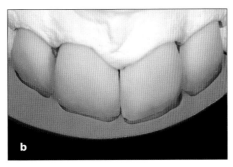

Fig 7-62a, b Principal bake, checked with silicone key.

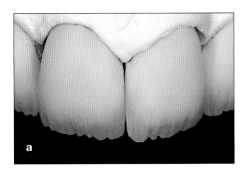
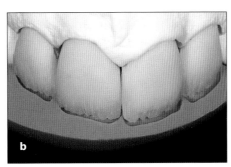

Fig 7-63a, b Cutback with drift. Checked with silicone matrix.

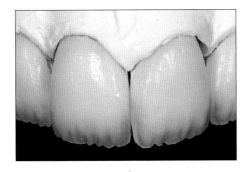

Fig 7-64 Deep characterization with internal stain and ceramic. This is very important in order to achieve a natural-looking PLV.

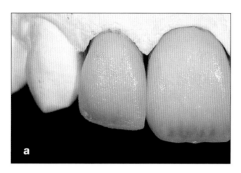 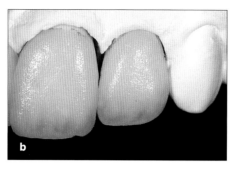 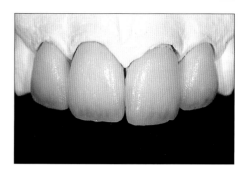

Fig 7-65a, b Opalescent and translucent enamel skin. The amount of translucency should be well controlled. If too much translucency is applied, the PLV will exhibit a grayish color.

Fig 7-66 Second bake correction.

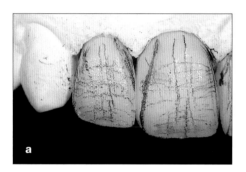 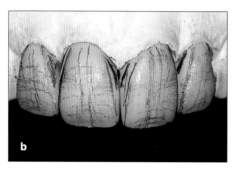 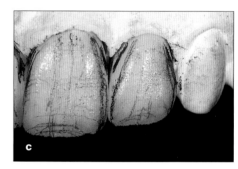

Fig 7-67a-c Adjustment shape with transition lines (front view). These lines, incorporated with the surface texture, are extremely important. The author believes that this may be more important than the color itself.

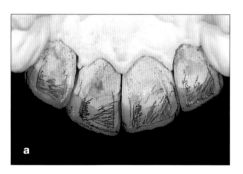 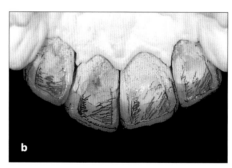 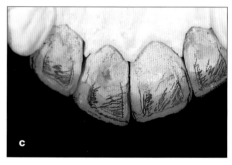

Fig 7-68a-c Visible adjustment on refractory dies (palatal view). The anatomy of the palatal surface plays an important role is establishing the anterior guidance.

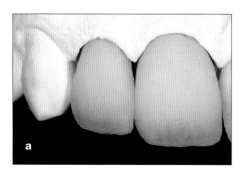 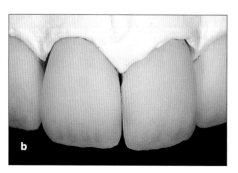 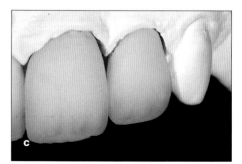

Fig 7-69a-c Surface before glazing. All the necessary texture and form adjustments must be finalized at this stage.

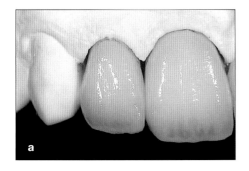
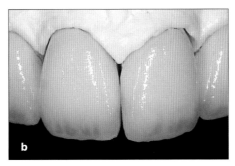
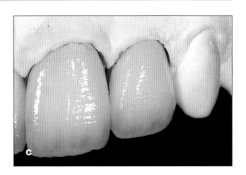

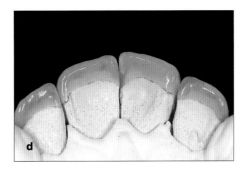

Fig 7-70a-d Surface before being baked with glazing liquid.

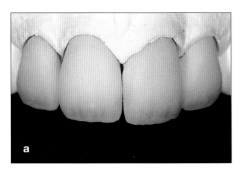
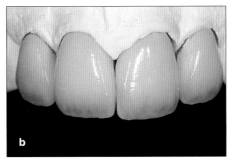
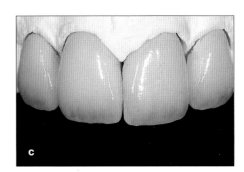

Fig 7-71a-c After bake and mechanical polishing.

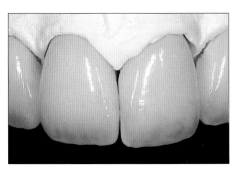
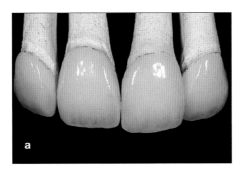
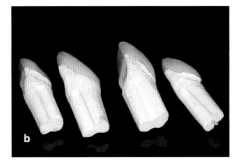

Fig 7-72 Finished crowns on the model before refractory separation.

Fig 7-73a, b Laminates on refractory dies. Note the refractory dies are prepared for the multiple-die technique.

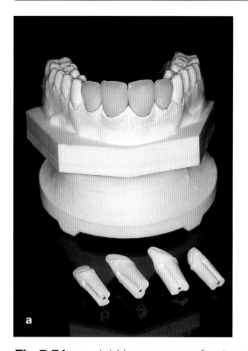
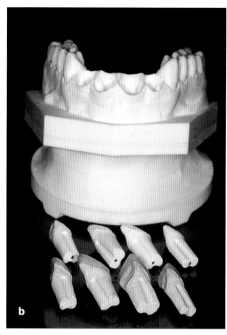
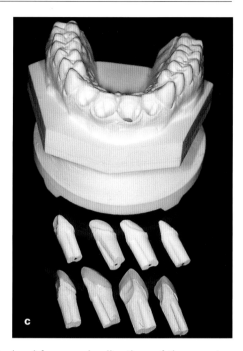

Fig 7-74a-c   (a) Veneers on refractory dies for the model. (b) These dies are derived from a duplication of the master dies and they can be inserted into the model. (c) Detail of model (*Geller*).

Fig 7-75a-c   Final work on the model (Ceramist *Michael Magne*).

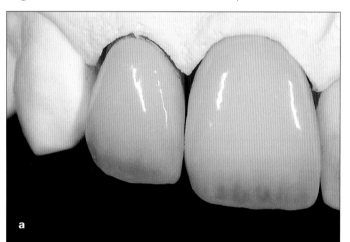
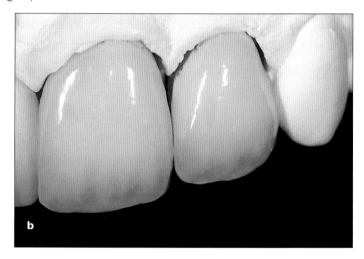
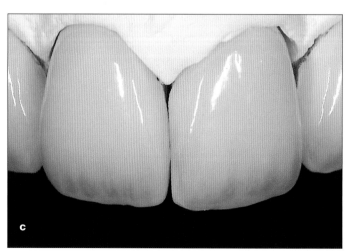

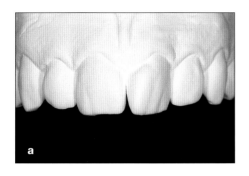
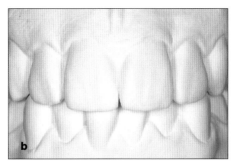
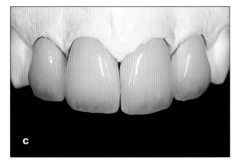
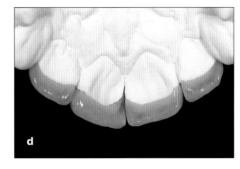

Fig 7-76a-d (a) Before wax-up. (b) After wax-up. Note the lengthening of the incisal edge that changes the individual tooth proportions. (c, d) Final work on the not-fragmented model in frontal and palatal views. Frontal adjustment of the contact.

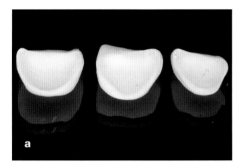
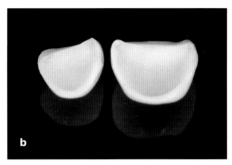
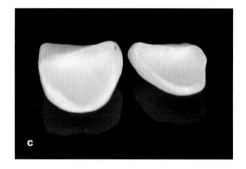

Fig 7-77a-c Finished veneers out from refractory and etched.

Try-in

The veneers should first be tried-in before they are bonded to eliminate unexpected surprises.

When the patient arrives for the final appointment the teeth are first anesthetized for the comfort of the patient. (This is especially true if the dentin is not hybridized at the first appointment) however, one should not forget that the try-in stage will be the final decision making process before the final esthetic outcome. In other words, the dentist and the patient should strive to improve both the esthetic appearance and the new smile design, at the try-in stage (before the PLVs are bonded), while the possibility for improvement still exists.

Therefore, it is not a good idea to numb the area together with the lips because, as it has been explained (see Chapter 2) before, the teeth position and the length and their relation to the lips have a great influence on the smile design and hence the overall appearance. In such cases, it is wise to use a palatal injection, very sparingly, to numb the target area while being careful not to numb the lips.

A vital component in achieving success for the holistic management of the esthetic patient is to conduct the entire treatment in a virtually painless environment. Despite the monumental advances in almost all the procedures related to esthetic case management, the one area that has potentially remained unchanged for as much as

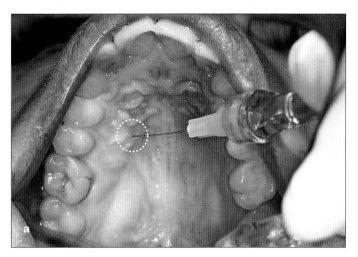
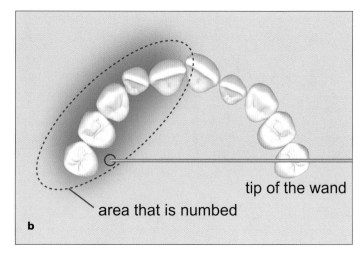

Fig 7-78a, b The tip of the needle is placed into an area (circled) midway between the first and second premolars. The handle should be held between the other premolar to achieve a 90° insertion path way. The whole anterior segment can be numbed without affecting the lips.

150 years (*Charles Pravaz*, Paris 1853) is that of the anesthetic delivery device. The traditional hand-held syringe systems are limited by their linear principles of application and as a result have largely determined the techniques we have chosen to use in the past.

The supra-periosteal buccal infiltration can result in an unwanted hamartoma (rich vascular supply), discomfort for the patient, inability to smile (motor effect), "swollen" lip (anesthetic volume) and resultant inaccuracy in the determination of the smile-line. Added to this, is the need to use more than one site of injection and larger quantities of anesthetic drug when treating the entire anterior arch for veneers in the anterior maxilla.

Aesthetic Anesthetics

Through the introduction of modern drug delivery devices such as the WAND (Milestone Scientific Inc.) 1997 and the CCS (Dentsply) 2001, computer controlled technology is now available to help us and our patients achieve successful "esthetic anesthesia". This term was introduced by *Williams*[289] and refers to the concept of achieving profound pulpal and soft-tissue anesthesia with the least possible unwanted side effects as part of the comprehensive management of the esthetic patient. By virtue of the associated anatomy and techniques defined in this concept, the major benefits contained therein are for procedures conducted from the first incisor to the second premolar on either side of the maxillary arch.

Technique

The AMSA block (anterior middle superior alveolar nerve), described by *Friedman* and *Hochman*,[290] is delivered palatally at a single-site and anesthetizes multiple teeth and related soft tissue. It can be administered to a single-site (unilateral) as well as two-sites (left and right) (bilateral). The exact location of the injection is an area approximately 1 cm in diameter, (i.e. not a point), with the tip of the needle bisecting the first and second premolars; and midway between the mid-palatine suture and free gingival margins. The approach angle for the needle and hand piece should be at a right-angle (90°) to a line drawn across the palatal cusps of the maxillary posterior teeth on the side, being injected (Fig 7-78). Alternatively, approaching the delivery site with the hand piece bisecting the premolars of the opposite quadrant will exact the delivery.

Mechanism of Action

Pain experienced during anesthetic solution delivery into the taught palatal mucosa is largely (if not completely) related to the high pressure that is built up when using the standard hand-held syringe. This pressure, in turn, relates directly to our inability to introduce very small volumes of liquid into these tissues in a consistent and predictable manner. Microchip technology allows for precision controlled flow rates and a resultant reduction in the associated pressure during delivery (current research). It is this marked reduction in pressure that allows for a virtually painless injection into the maxillary palate. The anatomy of the maxillary osseous tissue lends a further, logical explanation to this reduction in pressure and the palatal osseous tissue acts as a sponge when a solution is delivered (drop-by-drop) at controlled (slow) speed (*Hochman* and *Williams*, unpublished).

Structures Anesthetized

Pulps of the mesiobuccal root of the first molar, second and first premolars, canine, lateral and central incisor ipsilateral to injection site, as well as the attached gingiva and mucoperiosteum extending from mid-palatine suture to gingival margin (palatally) and attached gingiva (buccally) can be anesthetized. Although generally co-incidental to the teeth anaesthetized, the extent and direction of soft tissue anesthesia is related to the antero-posterior angulation of the needle/hand piece.

Dosage

Usually 0.6–0.9 ml. depending on the dosage, with a delivery time that varies from 1.5 to 4.0 minutes is enough. The use of a vasoconstrictor in concentrations exceeding 1:100000 may increase the risk of local tissue damage and are discouraged. Once correctly administered the area stays numb for 45 to 90 minutes.

Precautions/Guidelines

Case and drug selection is important in avoiding potential complications. Necroses, although extremely rare, have been reported in cases where patients with a very thin palatal mucosa have been injected. The inability of a thinner mucosa (reduced vascular supply) to rapidly remove a vasoconstrictive drug, the prolonged vasoconstrictive effect of excessive (quantity or concentration) or multiple delivery of vasoconstrictor containing drugs, or the use of inappropriate speed (and resultant high pressure) for delivery of the anesthetic solution to these tissues, may result in necrosis of the soft tissues.

The correct speed of delivery is also important to reduce pain (at commencement and during the injection), reduce the possibility of systemic reaction and to ensure maintenance of physiologically acceptable tissue pressures.

An "anesthetic pathway" should be created and maintained during the insertion procedure by using a controlled rotation-action of the needle. Pain during initial entry into the mucosa can be significantly reduced by correct placement of the needle bevel in relation to the tissue (flat part initially against mucosa—deposit a few-drops of LA then begin to rotate).

P-ASA Block

If only a few anterior PLVs are being tried in, the P-ASA block (palatal approach anterior superior alveolar nerve block) described by *Friedman* and *Hochman*,[290] is a simpler way to achieve anesthesia with a single injection (Fig 7-79). Although similar to the nasopalatine and incisive nerve blocks, the P-ASA differs in that it is described as a primary injection to achieve bilateral anesthesia of the six maxillary anterior teeth as well as the mucoperiosteum and gingiva in the region of the anterior palate innervated by the nasopalatine nerve. As a mucosal landmark the incisive papilla should be the delivery site. The combined advantage of the porosity of the osseous tissue at this site favoring the flow-dynamics of the anesthetic solution (toward the target neural tissue), and the introduction of the drug at slow speed

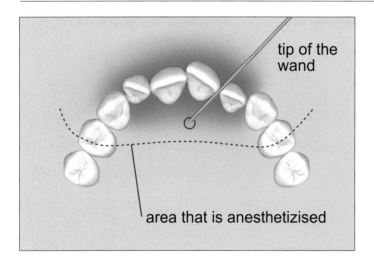

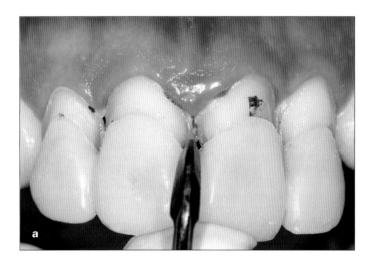
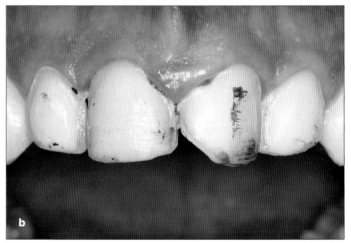

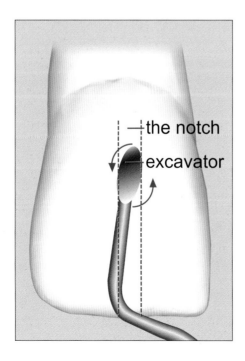

Fig 7-79 With the P-ASA block, only the anterior segment can be anesthetized.

Fig 7-80a, b (a) Usually the veneers can be easily removed with an excavator. (b) Note the microleakage that may occur due to weak bonding.

Fig 7-81 After a notch is created, an excavator is held 90° to the cut and twisted. In most cases the provisional veneer will easily pop up.

(again allowing favorable flow-dynamics with reduced pressure), result in this technique being virtually painless. With the administration to the maxillary central and lateral incisors, maxillary canines (bilateral), the palatal gingiva and mucoperiosteum extending from mid-palatine suture to gingival margin for the anterior 1/3rd of the maxilla and the attached gingiva (buccally) extending from canine to canine is anesthetized.

Debonding The Provisionals

In order to start the try-in, the provisional veneers have to first be debonded. A spoon excavator can help, by levering the provisionals from the proximal wall, which will pop off the veneer at the proximal margin (Fig 7-80).

If the provisional resists dislodgment, then the facial surface can be vertically cut with a tapered fissure diamond bur. This should preferably be done without water spray, as it is easier to visualize the depth of the cut in order to prevent possible damage while entering the facial surface of the tooth. The cut should extend until the depth of the tooth surface is nearly exposed. The spot etched area can be slightly entered into with the diamond bur to enhance debonding. After that, the spoon excavator can be placed into the vertical notch with a torsion movement and the provisional can be broken into two fragments and easily removed (Fig 7-81).

Before the try-in, one of the most frequently ignored stages is the careful examination of the tooth surface itself. The facial and proximal surfaces of the prepared teeth should be carefully examined for any residual resin cement or provisional resin leftovers. If residue is found, it should be carefully removed. It is of vital importance to clarify this, in order to enhance the perfect fit of the PLVs. It is always better to check it with the help of magnifying loops.

If any doubt arises concerning the complete removal of the residual resin luting agent, the suspected area can be etched with 30% phosphoric acid, for 10 seconds as suggested by *Nixon*.[291] The etch enamel surface will display a frosted appearance whereas the residual resin luting

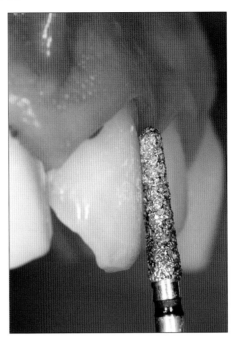

Fig 7-82 The facial surface is cleaned by sandblasting, pumice or with a very light application of a course diamond fissure bur. Care should be taken to use very gentle pressure.

agent will not and so it will be easily detected and cleansed.

Try-in

Now the PLVs can be tried in after the prepared tooth is first cleaned with fine pumice and water (Fig 7-82). A mixture of pumice and mercryl is suggested by some authors and is applied using a rubber Prophymatic cup.[5] This instrument avoids harming the gingiva by its alternating movements that reduce splashing and spilling. Fine metal strips moistened with mercryl are then used to clean the contact area. The tooth must then be thoroughly rinsed to free the tooth of any traces of pumice. Any substances that may cause bleeding should not be used, as bleeding can be detrimental to bonding and, therefore, all use of powder cleaners or brushes should be avoided.

Individual Evaluation

To start with, each veneer has to be tried in individually to evaluate their biologic integration relative to tooth and gingival harmony. Pressure should never be exerted at this stage since the

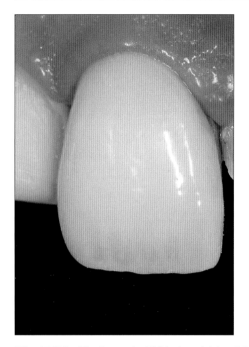

Fig 7-83 First, each PLV should be tried–in individually to check the marginal fit from every aspect, especially at the cervical 1/3rd.

Fig 7-84a, b One of the most important sites to be carefully checked at the try-in stage is the gingivoproximal area, since the marginal openings in that area have been proven to be two to four times larger than midlabially.

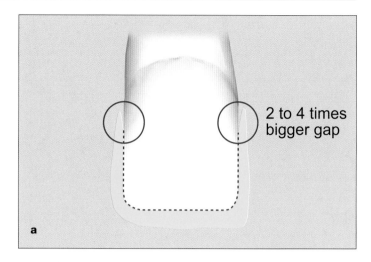

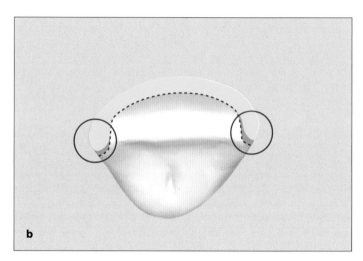

porcelain is brittle before being bonded. Complete seating and marginal adaptation should be carefully checked (Fig 7-83). It must be kept in mind that large marginal discrepancies seen at the try-in stage will result in an unesthetic outcome in cases of supragingival placement or cause periodontal problems in cases of subgingival placement. Shortly after they are bonded the organic matrix of the resin bonder (polymer-matrix composite) is subject to erosion and disintegration in the oral environment.[292] Poor thermal expansion, biocompatibility and plaque adhering properties are characteristic of polymer-matrix composites in comparison to enamel or porcelains. The bonding resin surfaces should be exposed to as little of the oral environment as possible. In order to achieve successful adhesive bonding, a reproducible precision of the marginal fit of complete porcelain is also required.

The delicate quality of porcelain tends to make it rather fragile and therefore it does not lend itself to finishing techniques. Consequently, after a proper margin design is produced by the dentist; the technician is responsible for the quality of the margin that requires their expertise, skill and dedication. Such technicians are able to realign margins and to produce margins very similar to metal or ceramometal restorations.

Checking the Margins

It is better to check the margins without using any kind of try-in gels to enable better, clearer access. Especially for PLVs, when the mesial and distal line angles are placed lingually, checking the gingivoproximal corners individually is of vital importance. Most studies show that the marginal openings at the gingivoproximal corners are two

Fig 7-85 After each PLV is tried-in separately all of the veneers can be tried-in together to see the esthetic integration.

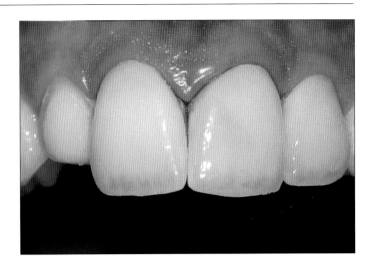

Fig 7-86a, b If the seating problem is due to position shift of the teeth during provisionalization, then a gap will be seen on one side when overlapping of the PLV on the other. Finger pressure can be applied to realign the position of the tooth which has been mesially or distally moved.

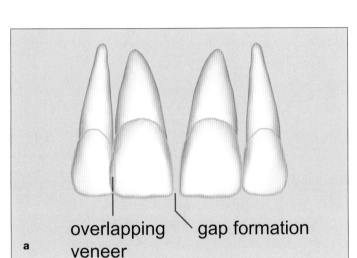

overlapping gap formation
veneer

a

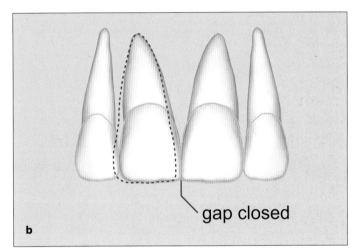

gap closed

b

to four times larger than at the mid-labial portion (Fig 7-84).[50,281,293] This is related to the result of the shrinkage of porcelain towards the region of greatest bulk (the center) and the geometry of the margins. Clinically this poorer fit at the gingivo-proximal corners of the veneers would be further compounded by the difficulty in access for finishing of luted veneers in these regions.[111]

Collective Try-in

Once they are individually checked, all PLVs should be collectively tried-in to evaluate the proximal contacts and contours. This checking of the "esthetic-integration" of the PLVs will be the second stage of the try-in (Fig 7-85).

Under normal circumstances, the veneers should be passively seated on the teeth without any interproximal tightening. If any crowding due to tight contact exists, once it is attempted to place the adjacent veneer, it will move the other one to the side.

When such a problem arises, the lateral or protrusive shift of the prepared teeth during the provisionalization should first be evaluated. If the cause is that two PLVs are pushing each other sideways on their mesial and distal margins, a gap between the others will occur. The gap will close when a little finger-pressure is applied over the two veneers that resisted seating, shifting the teeth back into position and closing the gap between the adjacent veneers (Fig 7-86).

However, if this is not the case, all the other veneers will be in their natural contacts and the veneer(s) with overbuild interproximal contact areas will not be able passively to take its place. The mesial or distal marginal ridge must be adjusted to obtain that passive fit (Fig 7-87).

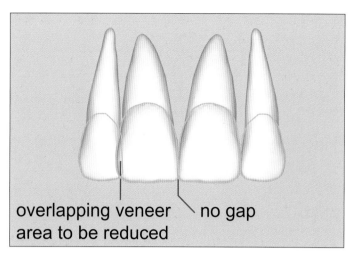

Fig 7-87 If there is no gap between the adjacent tooth exists, then the PLV should be adjusted for passive seating.

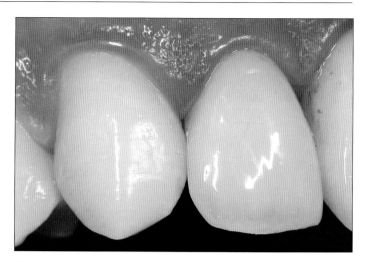

Fig 7-88 After all the veneers are seated, the color is checked. Note the color gradation effect towards the posterior. The canine has a higher chroma.

Most of the prepared teeth are actually unretentive. Therefore, holding six or eight laminates on these unretentive teeth may require a medium to provide stabilization. In order to improve this temporary adhesion and inspect the natural shade of color of the PLV, water-soluble try-in gels or transparent silicone can occasionally be used.[5]

Check the Color

After the veneers are comfortably seated, they should be checked with the shade evaluated under incandescent, fluorescent, and natural light. In order to minimize the effects of metamerism, when choosing a shade, it is best to avoid one that looks good in natural light but appears discolored in artificial light. It is better to opt for a shade that looks reasonably good in all lighting conditions. Before the actual cementation the dentist can allow the patients to moisten the ceramic and adjacent teeth with saliva and to observe themselves in a normal wall mirror for approval.[172]

The final color of the PLV will be affected by different formations and it depends on the laboratory build-up of the color of the ceramic and the color of the underlying tooth. The bonding medium that will be a luting composite may also affect the outcome, due to the thickness or color of its own.

With the advancements both in porcelain material and in the knowledge and artistic skills of the dental technicians, it is now almost possible to alter the dark color of a tooth, with a judicious ceramic build-up, using opaque or translucent dentin and enamel powders in a very natural way (Fig 7-88) (see Chapter 10). Even though the tooth color itself has a role in reflecting its own color and thus affecting the final outcome, the major role is on the delicately layered natural looking masking effect of the PLV itself.

Altering the Color

This shows the importance of reporting the stump shade guide to the lab. It is also very difficult to change the color of the veneer with a thin layer of luting composite. However, some authors[61] alternatively suggest, that a few coats of die spacing should be applied; in order to permit flexible chairside adjustment of value, chroma and to some extent the opacity, thus allowing the color shift. On the other hand, research shows that the thinner the distance between the tooth and the veneer, the better the adhesion and longevity of the PLV.

Additionally, in such instances, the greater the amount of luting resin that is incorporated into the bonding stage, the more polymerization shrinkage will occur that may also lead to marginal leakage.

If the dentist has hesitations about the final color and prefers to use this technique, the choice should be low saturation and opacity. The higher these two factors, the more this layer will act as a barrier to reflect light transmission and hence affect the final color, with unacceptable results. In other words, it may be more advantageous to finish the PLV lighter in color (high value), so that its value can therefore be more easily lowered by the underlying composite. In contrast, it will always be more difficult to lighten a darker colored PLV.

The color of the polymerized luting resin may not always match the color seen when water-soluble, noncuring try-in paste other than transparent is used to visualize the outcome. This phenomenon may take place for several reasons.

The first possibility is that the shade of the try-in paste and the corresponding luting resin are not a precise match. It is also possible that the shade of the luting resin may change after curing or that the cured resin gradually changes over a period of time. One way to minimize this is to bench-cure samples of each luting resin, to place them in water and to note any changes.[96] These notes can help predict the eventual appearance of the final restoration at the time of try-in. It can be assumed that the restoration will be similarly affected if the chosen shade of uncured luting agent or try-in paste is lower in value than the corresponding cured sample and therefore the necessary compensation should be considered. However, to make a reasonable assessment, other factors such as the degree of opacity of the porcelain, the thickness of the luting agent layer and the metameric influence of the porcelain and dentin should be considered.

If the technician realizes that they cannot alter the color of the dark tooth with the veneer that they will be producing, or if there are a few spots on a tooth differently colored than the rest of the teeth (see Chapter 13), then instead of trying to compensate for this at the bonding stage; it is always better to block the dark discoloration of the prepared tooth with the help of an opaque composite at the time of tooth preparation and before impression making. This will not only substantially minimize the shrinkage problem of the luting

cement which will be encountered during the bonding stage, but it will also ease the fabrication of the PLV, in terms of color compensation.

However, the best results are obtained by careful tooth preparation, and good communication with the lab. Consequently, a skillful technician will always be able to obtain the right color match. In such cases, trying the veneers in with water or saliva, or in other words anything transparent, will enable us to predict the outcome in a more reliable way. When it comes to the bonding of these PLVs, in order to augment the light transmission at the interface, the most translucent composite available should be used. A much more natural appearance will be achieved as this transparent layer will transmit light in all directions.[5]

Bonding

Composite resin, acid etched porcelain and etched enamel have been proven in vitro studies to derive from a strong, durable complex (Fig 7-89).[46,294]

The porcelain veneer technique is used to change the color or form of the anterior teeth by bonding a thin porcelain laminate to the tooth surface using an adhesive and luting composite. Therefore, the strength and durability of the bond between the tooth, the veneer and the luting composite is what actually determines the success of the PLV treatment.

In this process of ceramic restoration, the calcified dental tissue, the ceramic and the bonding materials are the three main components, along with the interface between the bonding agent and the ceramics. This well structured ensemble is able to withstand the forces of mechanical stress (knock or mechanical fatigue), thermal stress (mechanical fatigue) or hydric stress (infiltration and sorption) existing in the oral environment.[295]

Chemically, tooth material, ceramic restorations, and composite luting resins are very different materials. A tooth consists of enamel (86% hydroxyapatite, 12% water);[296] dentin (45%

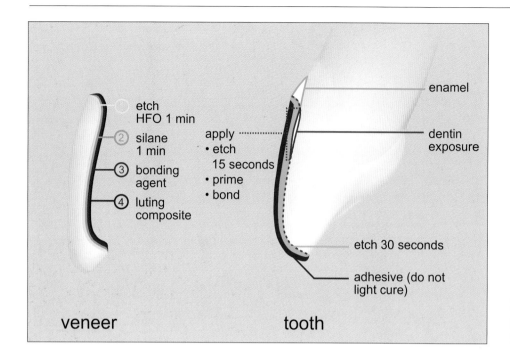

etch
HFO 1 min

② silane
1 min

③ bonding
agent

④ luting
composite

apply
• etch
15 seconds
• prime
• bond

enamel

dentin
exposure

etch 30 seconds

adhesive (do not
light cure)

veneer **tooth**

Fig 7-89 Steps for treating the inside of the PLV and the tooth surface just before bonding.

hydroxyapatite, 30% primarily collagen network, 25% water),[296] the pulp and other structures. Ceramic restorations are purely inorganic.[297] Composites have an organic matrix and inorganic fillers.[298] The composition of these materials explains why it is difficult or impossible to obtain a bond with a direct chemical reaction. *Buonocore's* idea of creating a micro etch pattern by using the acid-etch technique was completely new in 1955.[299] By means of a micro mechanic interlocking, a bond of 20 Mpa was obtained between composite luting resins and purely inorganic enamel.[300,301] The bond strength to etched and silanated ceramics is even as high as 45 Mpa.[302] These bond strength values are high enough to resist tensile and shear forces that are generated by thermal expansion or by shrinkage during the polymerization of composites.[303] To bond the PLV, on the chairside, the inside of the veneer and the tooth surface, have to be treated separately.

Treating the Interior PLV Surface

Acid Etching

Early research indicated that it was possible to chemically bond silica to acrylic or bis-GMA using a silane coupling agent.[304] It was discovered that no bond formed between the glazed porcelain and composite resin, even with silane[305,306] unless the surface was first roughened.[307] These studies done in the early 1980s proved that surface micropores similar to those found on etched tooth enamel are formed under the influence of hydrofluoric acid.[325] Aluminous ceramics apart, this phenomenon occurs because selective silicate compounds are dissolved from the surface.[307,308] An additional property of the hydrofluoric compound is the surface activation of ceramic materials.

Once the PLV fabrication is finished at the lab, the inside of the veneers should be sand blasted and acid etched with a 10% hydrofluoric acid and then sent to the clinic. This preparation can also be made by the practitioner, just before bonding, after taking the necessary precautions for the use of hydrofluoric acid (Fig 7-90). The hydrofluoric acid on its own or together with the sand blasting will enhance the micro retention of the internal surface of the PLV. However, this technique can

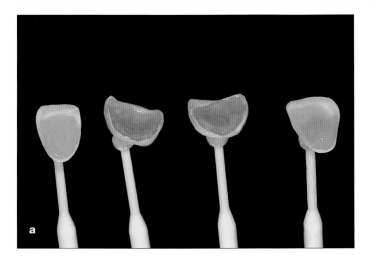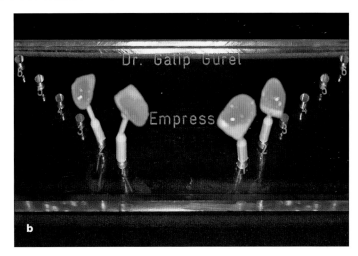

Fig 7-90a, b (a) The veneer should be acid etched with HFA either in the lab or at the chairside after the try-in. Seating veneers on the sticky poles will ease the application of etch, prime and bond. (b) A Plexiglas stand designed by the author. It facilitates the positioning of the PLVs to prevent confusion, especially for the mandibular teeth.

cause abrasion of the ceramics during the sili-coating process that uses airborne particles, and is therefore not recommended, despite its superior bonding strength.[310]

The cohesive strength of the porcelain itself, or that of the bond strength of a luting composite to etched enamel, has been surpassed by the bond strength of a luting composite to the etched porcelain surface which is prepared by etching the inner side of the porcelain veneer with hydrofluoric acid followed by silanizing the etched surface.[46,311-313] Some sort of anchoring is established when etching the inner side of the porcelain veneer with hydrofluoric acid, that creates a relief at the surface of the ceramic with a retentive etch pattern.[312,313] Micro-mechanical interlocking of the resin composite is made possible by the microporosites that have been created on the internal surface area for bonding. The bond strength of the resin composite to the etched porcelain and the micro-morphology of each pattern is determined by the concentration of the etching liquid, the duration of etching, the fabrication method of the porcelain restoration[307,313] and the type of porcelain that is used.[314]

Checking the Etched Surface

After the inside of the PLVs has been etched and 1 to 4 minutes has passed (depending on the concentration of the etch liquid, fabrication of the porcelain restoration), the inside of PLV should be rinsed with a sufficient amount of water. The display of the inside of the PLV should be opaque over the entire surface. If there is, any place that displays a less opaque appearance, than that area should be etched again and the same check should be repeated in that area. A way to check the etched surface is to place a drop of water into the etched surface. If the surface is etched completely, the water will spread all over the internal surface. The cleaning process of the porcelain is aided by the increased wettability of the etched surface (Fig 7-91).[315]

There is no doubt that etching greatly increases the bond shear strength[316] of the porcelain, which is an advantage in that its strength does not diminish over extended periods of time and even surpasses the resin enamel bond strength.[317]

Preparing the Surface

The internal surface of the PLV should be thoroughly rinsed and cleansed after the try-in. To remove any salts from the etching process, the

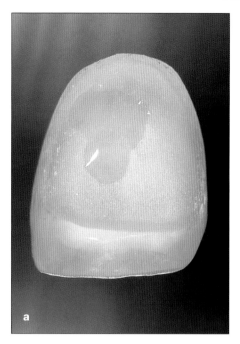 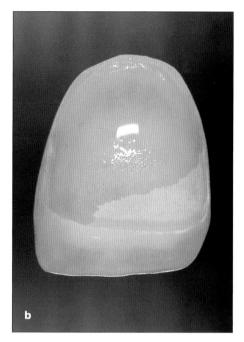

Fig 7-91a, b (a) If a drop of water is placed on the unetched interior surface of the PLV, it will not spread and stays localized. (b) However, when the same amount of water is dropped on the same PLV surface after it has been etched, it will spread over the whole surface.

etched area should be gently rubbed with a wet, cotton pellet and then cleaned with alcohol or acetone to remove any saliva or fingerprint contamination.

Water sorption,[314] fatique[318] and thermocyling,[319] are external factors that have a negative influence on the bond strength of resin composite to a pre-treated ceramic restoration after they are bonded. However, before the bonding process, contamination of the pre-treated surface with die stone,[320] latex gloves,[321] saliva[317,319] silicone-based fit checker paste[322] and try-in paste will also decrease the bond strength. In order to restore the original bond strength several cleaning methods are proposed.[320] Once the inside of the porcelain is contaminated with a try-in gel, cleaning the surfaces with acetone will not suffice. This can only be cleaned with re-acid-etching. However, a study reported that after chemical contamination bonding strength could not be restored.[322]

Re-etching the Surface After Try-In

If the etched surface of the PLV is contaminated with saliva, the surface should be restored with a 15 second application of 37% phosphoric acid.[52] However, it is better to avoid, any other contamination after this stage.

The best result is achieved when the 10% hydrofluoric acid treatment with an etching time of 60 seconds, is done after the try-in. This will minimize the contamination of the acid etched surface, and hence increase the bond strengths. If this technique is used, there will be no need to further acid etch the surface with phosphoric acid. However, if the surface has already been HFA etched at the laboratory prior to try-in, then the interior surface of the PLV should now be covered with 30% phosphoric acid, rinsed and dried. The phosphoric acid will not enhance the micromechanical retentive areas, but rather alter the surface chemistry to make the silane more effective .

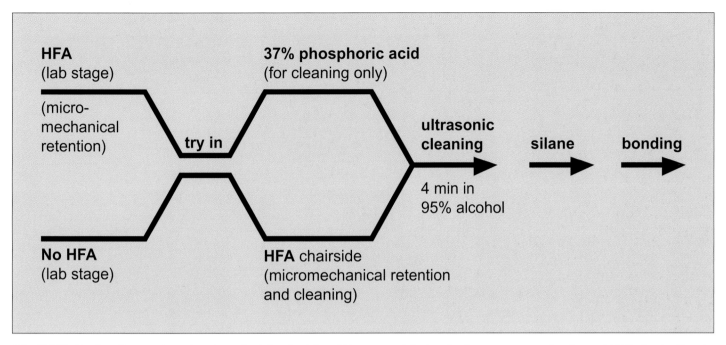

Fig 7-92 During the surface treatment of the inside of the porcelain laminate veneer, application of HFA (hydrofluoric acit) will create the micromechanical retentive surface which will enhance the bond strength. The chairside application of the 37% phosphoric acid, however, will only help to cleanse the contaminated interior surface of the porcelain laminate veneer.

Ultrasonic Cleaning

After acid etching the surface is rinsed and dried, however, SEM studies showed that, even after the etched surface is rinsed with copious amounts of water, a great number of acid crystals still stay deposited on the etched surface that may affect the bonding strength. In order to eliminate this, the veneers should be placed into the ultrasonic cleaner. All residual acid and dissolved debris can be removed from the surface of etched porcelain with an ultrasonic cleaning in 95% alcohol for 4 minutes, or acetone or distilled water. Remineralized salts seen as white residue or deposit[323] must not remain due to inadequate rinsing.[37] Many authors[111,324] agree that the immersion of the etched porcelain in an ultrasonic bath creates the best surface that allows penetrability. However, some have observed[326] no significant differences in surface morphology and bond strength between the hydrofluoric acid etched feldspathic porcelain and that without ultrasonic cleaning.

Silane Application

The bond sheer strength that has been improved from the average 600s to 3000 Mpa by acid etching can further be increased with the silane coupling agent application. The results of the following research best demonstrate the enhanced bond shear strengths when the internal surface of the porcelain is treated with both acid-etching and silane (Fig 7-92). The silane-coupling agent is the second component of the classic conditioning methods for ceramic restoration.[194] Silanizing etched ceramics and their major contribution to restoration techniques has been confirmed by many investigations. This coupling agent makes the retention of the bonded ceramic joints possible with its high wettability and its chemical contribution to adhesion.[295]

Technique

When the inside of the veneer is ready to receive the silane treatment to create a chemical link between the bonding composite and the ceramic, a fine layer of a silane coupling agent is painted over the internal surface of the laminate veneer

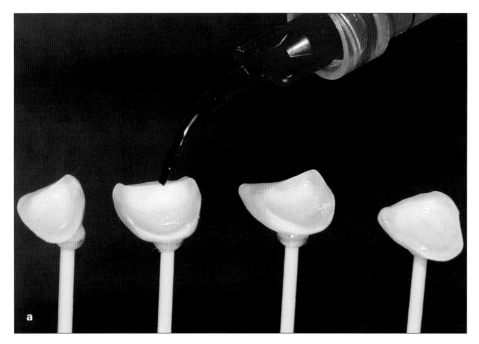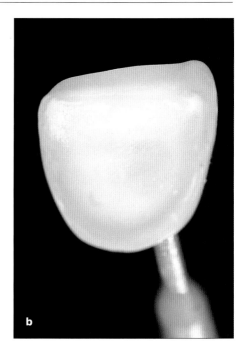

Figs 7-93a and b (a) Silane is applied over the etched surface to increase the bond strength. (b) After a minute the silane is dried with a warm hair dryer to double the bonding effect. A salty-looking appearance should be observed. Once the silane is dried out, the choice of adhesive is applied over the whole interior surface. However, it should not be light cured at this stage but kept in the dark. (Note the yellow color of the tip of the stick, showing through the very thin PLV.)

after it comes out of the ultrasonic cleaner. In the porcelain laminate veneer and the composite resin matrix, it is believed that silanization of the etched porcelain with a bi-functional agent provides chemically bonding to the silica. The silane group bonds to the hydrolyzed silicone dioxide copolymerising with the adhesive resin.[170]

The resin can better wet the surface , as scanning electron micrographs reveal. The silane eliminates the polymerization contraction gap, which forms in etched, nonsilanated and unetched-silanated restorations.[317] The silane is allowed to remain in contact with the etched porcelain for one minute (Fig 7-93). At the end of that time it is dried with an air syringe by blowing the air parallel to and slightly above the veneer and thus allowing the solvent to evaporate completely. At this stage, it has been reported that drying the inside of the veneer, with "warm air" (possibly with a small hair dryer) will enhance the effect of the silane. When the silane-coated porcelain is heated to 100°C it results in bond strength double that of the porcelain where no heat was used.[314]

The numerous silane-coupling agents that exist increase the shear strength of the porcelain to composite resin bond. Single component systems that contain silane in alcohol or acetone are the simplest ways to silanate. However, with 2-component silane systems the two solutions that are mixed with an aqueous acid solution in order to hydrolyze the silane will polymerize to an unreactive polysiloxane and therefore it must be used within a few hours.[150]

Adhesive Application

Once a dry surface is obtained after silanization, the adhesive of choice is applied inside the veneer with the help of a brush or a small cotton pellet. In principle, this could be done in a synchronized manner with the dental assistant while the dentist is applying the adhesive over the tooth surface. The adhesive should be compatible with the composite that is being used as a luting agent. At this stage, the adhesive should not be light cured.

As soon as the bonding is applied, the transparent composite luting agent is preferably placed inside the veneer. If color problems exist,

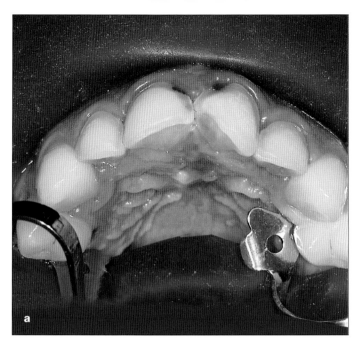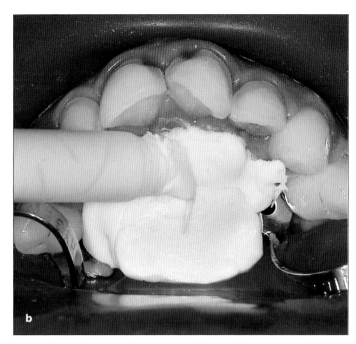

Fig 7-94a, b (a) The sectional rubber dam is applied, clamps are placed on the maxillary molars first, and the rubber dam is seated over them. (b) To provide a complete seal vanilla mousse is applied on the palatinal opening.

predetermined colored composites are used at the try-in stage, and actually, in most cases, light cured composites are used.

If the luting agent has been placed inside the veneer far before the adhesive application to the tooth surface for bonding, than the veneer and the applied luting cement should be kept in an absolutely dark place, to prevent premature light activated polymerization.

Treating the Tooth Surface

The other part of preparation in this process to achieve maximum bonding is the tooth surface. Luting procedures require meticulous attention to every detail. Even though different protocols have been proposed[326-328] if the basic steps are followed properly, the luting procedure becomes quite simple. Since the bonding will primarily depend on adhesion, great care must be taken to work under the cleanest conditions. The area should definitely be kept clean and purified of blood, saliva or oral contaminants (Fig 7-94).

Rubber Dam

A partially sectioned rubber dam application is preferred while bonding the veneers. It acts as a physical barrier to oral fluids, moisture, tongue and cheek movements so that we can manipulate easily in the oral cavity.

It has a good control of the ambient oral humidity thus increasing bonding strengths. Even though the hydrophilic primers like humidity, the hydrophobic adhesives don't. Besides, any kind of contamination of teeth distorts bonding strengths.

This contamination can be avoided with cotton rolls when dealing with a few teeth, but using the rubber dam is so practical and safer. It will prevent inhaling or swallowing dental chemicals.

Cleaning the Surface

The tooth has to be thoroughly cleansed before and after the try-in stage. The water-soluble try-in gels or the temporary cement over the prepared tooth surface should be totally removed. If the

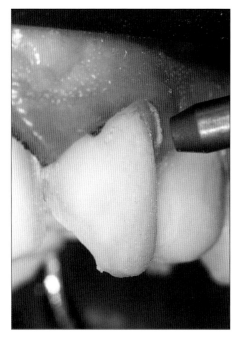
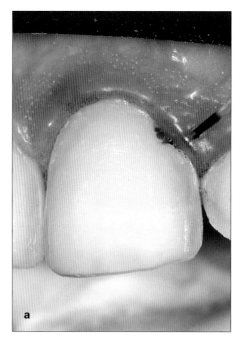
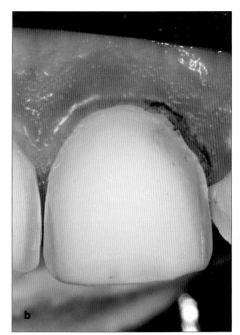

Fig 7-95 The surface is best cleaned with co-jet (Espe). The 30-micron thickness of the material will still let the 80-microns of the adhesive (Optibond) that has been applied at the preparation stage stay in place. Care should be taken not to cause any bleeding of the gingiva.

Fig 7-96a, b (a) The gingiva can easily be recontoured with a diode laser (Biolase), if needed. Note the mesiogingival tissue grown over the tooth due to a small marginal opening on the provisional. (b) The condition of the tissue seconds after laser application

dentin is not sealed at the time of preparation, the whole dentin bonding procedure should be carried out in this appointment. The use of pumice slurry in a prophy cup is to be the procedure for cleaning the teeth prior to etching or prior to conventional cementation of an indirect restoration.[24]

Preparing Hybridized Surface

However, the author prefers, hybridizing the exposed dentin area, just after the tooth preparation when the dentin is freshly cut. If this is the case, upon removal of the provisionals there should be no exposed dentin on the tooth surface, since it has already been sealed with the dentin-bonding agent. Prior to the actual bonding of the PLVs, this surface can either be gently cleansed and roughened with a diamond fissure bur, or even better, sand blasted with air abrasion (Fig 7-95). 30-micron thick particles will only be able to clean the surface of already bonded 80-micron adhesive (Optibond Kerr). If the provisional is bonded to the tooth with the spot etch-

ing method, the point or small area which has been spot etched, should be plotted. The remaining bonding agent on this spot of enamel should be very gently removed with the help of a diamond bur in order to obtain a clean surface for enamel etching.

The tooth surface can then be acid etched with 30%-40% of phosphoric acid, to further cleanse the dentin bonding agent and create micromechanical retention on the enamel surface (see Chapter 3).

Lazing the Tissue

Sometimes the tissue may bleed shortly after the sandblasting or the tissue might have grown over the prepared margin due to a small gap left on the provisional. At this stage, it is best to stop the bleeding with a diode laser (Biolaze). This will immediately stop the bleeding with a highly accurate control of the soft tissue contours (Fig 7-96).

Preparing the Exposed Dentin

However, some dentists may prefer hybridizing the dentin surface at the time of bonding. In other words, dentin etching, priming and application of the adhesive will all be conducted at this appointment, just before the PLV is bonded. In such a case the temporary cement and polluted dentin are best-removed aggressively with brushes and fluoride-free pumice or air-abrasion.[329,330] Current thought suggests that reduced sensitivity by eliminating or minimizing bacterial growth under restorations can be achieved by combining the cleaning step with disinfecting the cavity. Bacteria reaching the pulp can cause sensitivity. Although many may disagree, and although it has not been proven, it is still thought to be best to use a disinfectant to clean the cavity prior to the restoration.

The recommended agent for disinfecting the teeth was benzalkonium chloride (BAC) mixed with EDTA, at the time when the concept of disinfecting teeth was originally proposed by *Brannstrom*. Its purpose was to disinfect and partially remove the smear layer. The current product contains the primary active ingredients of either BAC or 2% chlorhexidine gluconate.

Cleaning

Until the preparation is visibly clean, it should be scrubbed. Antibacterial solution (Tubulicid Red, Global Dental Products, Inc., Consepsis, Ultradent Products, Inc.) is then applied over the etched surface to act as a wetting agent and to decrease bacterial concentration, without having a negative effect to the bond strength.[331] Before placing an adhesive that bonds to the mist/wet tooth structure, these products have also been used to remoisten/rewet the cavity. A residual antibacterial effect can presumably help reduce bacterial ingress because of microleakage.

However, the dentin should not be cleaned with soaps. A study shows that low shear bond strength values of the tested dentin-bonding agents may be the result of cleansing the dentin with soaps after the application of provisional cements. Therefore, it is not recommended to use soaps as a clinical means to remove remnants of provisional cements before adhesive cementation.[136]

Acid Etching Enamel

After this step, the tooth can be acid etched with 30%-40% of phosphoric acid. Gels are favored over liquids due to our ability to exercise more control over the application of a gel than a liquid. An etchant gel should also have a smooth consistency and not be jelly-like.[24]

Acid etching of enamel, which is well known[331] and causes an interprismatic and demineralization, produces adhesive profiles that are more suited to bonding.[295] The creation of a micro etch pattern is the precondition for a successful bond between a composite resin and enamel. The quality of such an etching pattern depends on the morphologic and chemical characteristics of the crystalline structure of enamel. On the other hand, the etching pattern is dependent on the type and on the concentration of the acid used at the time of etching.[136] Different acids have been described for etching the enamel, 37% phosphoric acid as a standard procedure,[299] 10% maleic acid and 1.6 % oxalic acid 2.6% aluminum nitrate,[332] 10% citric acid.[333] The bond strength values obtained with acids are reported to be 40% lower when compared to the 20 MP of bond strength that can be obtained with the standard procedure etching enamel of 60 seconds with 37% phosphoric acid. If the dentin was already sealed at the time of the preparation, this etching will be useful to clean the surface of the adhesive.

Acid Etching the Dentin

Most modern dentin bonding agents use low concentration acids for etching dentin.[334] The interlocking of the bonding agents with the dentin is due to a penetration of the resin into the collagen network of the dentinal surface. This appears to be no deeper than 6 mikrometre.[333] The duration of this application can be up to 30-40 seconds on enamel. However, it should not exceed 15 seconds on the dentin in order to prevent collagen collapse, and thus decreasing the pen-

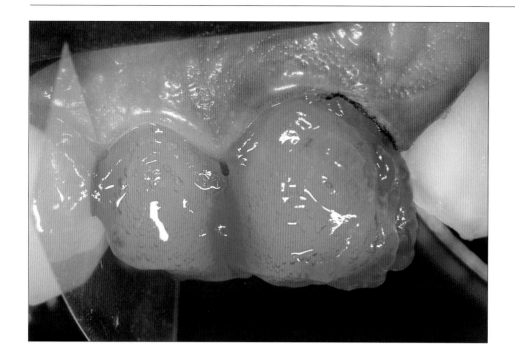

Fig 7-97 37% phosphoric acid is applied on the prepared area. Since the dentin is already sealed, the etch will clean the bonded area. It will also create micromechanical porosities on the enamel. Note the transparent strip, protecting the adjacent canine.

etration of the primer into the dentinal tubule (see Chapter 3).

Etchant should be applied to enamel, keeping it off the dentin, if possible. Etching times on enamel have a wide range; anywhere from 15-60 seconds is acceptable. Whatever the duration for enamel etching that is chosen, the etchant is spread over the dentin with a disposable brush, for the last 15 seconds. Once the etchant is spread over the dentin, an immediate 15 seconds is timed. During this time, the etchant can be further pushed into the restricted areas of the preparation surface, such as the deeply prepared gingivoproximal areas just to make sure the entire preparation is properly coated with etchant. The air-water syringe and suction is kept ready to go. As soon as the 15 seconds is up, the surface is rinsed for as long as is recommended by the manufacturers (Fig 7-97).

Adhesive Application

While the bonding of composite to etched enamel has been clinically proven for many years, the bonding to dentin is the subject of ongoing development. The most current examples of dentin-bonding systems have demonstrated in vitro shear bond strengths that approach the tensile strength of human dentin.[179,335,336] Such a result

would be desirable with use of PLVs when dentin is exposed during preparation, but there is clearly a lack of long-term clinical experience as to its success.

Then the teeth are thoroughly washed and dried. Dentin should only be blot dried with the help of a cotton pellet, in order to achieve "wet bonding".[337] The primer is applied over the exposed dentin area, left in place for 30 seconds and than very gently dried until the carrier of the primer evaporates. This time should be extended if the carrier of the primer is water based, or shortened if it is alcohol or acetone based. Preferably it should be executed with a hair-dryer, keeping in mind that, the air from the air syringe can always be contaminated with humidity or oil coming from the air compressor and thus affecting the bonding strength negatively.

Once the glossy appearance of the primer is achieved (Fig 7-98), than the adhesive can be applied on both the dentin and the enamel (Fig 7-99). The penetration of the resin into the etched enamel seems to be deeper. Enamel bondings can penetrate 15 to 50 micrometer deep into superficial enamel prisms that were etched tangentially to their longitudinal axis. If the prisms are etched perpendicularly to their longitudinal axes, the penetration will only be 5-10 mikrometre.[300] At this stage, it is important that the resin

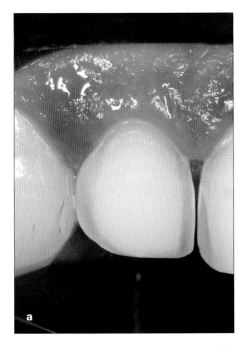
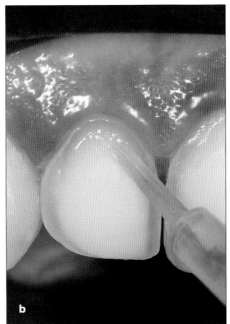
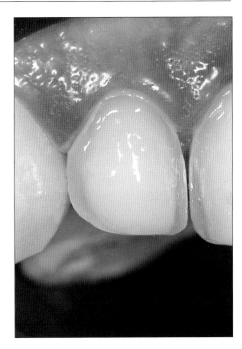

Fig 7-98a, b It has been detected that there is still some dentin exposure on the cervical margin of the lateral. (a) Once the surface is etched, it is blot dried and (b) primer is painted on the exposed dentin area only.

Fig 7-99 After the carrier of the primer has evaporated, adhesive is placed over the whole prepared surface with a brush, giving it a shiny appearance. It is important that the adhesive is not light cured at this time.

should not be light cured until the veneer is seated over the tooth.

Bonding

After the tooth surface and the internal surface of the PLV are prepared, the PLV can be bonded to the tooth surface. A light-curing luting composite is preferred for cementation of porcelain veneers[37] A longer working time compared with dual cure or chemically curing materials is the major advantage of light curing.

In this way the dentist can remove excess composite prior to curing, considerably shortening the finishing time required for these restorations. In comparison to dual-cured or chemical-cured systems, their color stability is superior. The thickness and the opacity of the ceramic[338] affects the transmission of light and consequent micro hardness of the composite.[338-340,342] Although the usual ceramic thickness for the PLV of 0.5–1.0 mm has no significant influence on the hardness of light-cured composite[343] the use of a dual-cure composite might be preferable in certain cases.[342] As mentioned before, if no color adjustments are needed, a transparent luting composite should be

the choice. A light-curing agent should be chosen that is filled in order to increase the resistance and optimize the durability of the bonded joint. In order to obtain wettability of the two substrates, and more particularly of the ceramic, the bonding agent used must not be too viscous. The resin is applied with a brush to the inner part of the restoration. In case a highly filled composite luting agent that is slightly more viscous is being used (i.e. Herculite translucent), it is better to use a spatula to place it inside the restoration.

Technique

When bonding the veneers one by one or as pairs, it is always better to place the luting resin inside the veneer to ease the control. A brush can be used to evenly distribute the composite inside the veneer.

The veneer should be positioned over the tooth very gently and slowly. The author prefers inserting the veneer starting from the incisal edge, and progressively pushing the veneer towards the gingivoapical direction (Fig 7-100). This is one of the best ways of avoiding the formation of voids

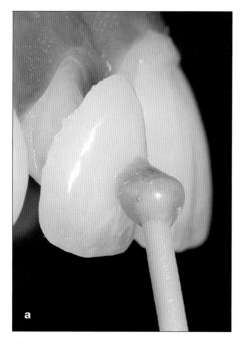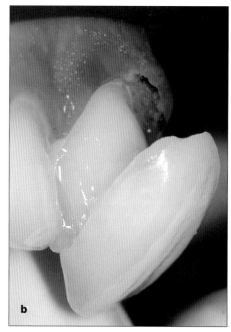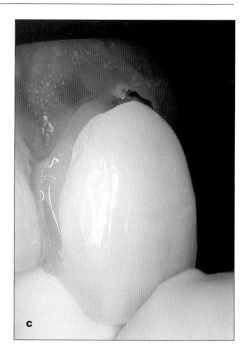

Fig 7-100a-c (a) After the inside of the veneer is loaded with the translucent luting resin (Herculite, Translucent, Kerr), it is brought next to the tooth with the sticky pole. (b) Once slightly seated from the incisal corner (c) it is then pushed apically and palatally with gentle finger pressure. The excess luting resin should be seen on all the margins, confirming that enough material is used.

between the tooth porcelain interfaces. It is also very critical that the dentist must observe the luting resin flash coming out from all the margins, indicating that enough luting material is applied precluding any air residue of air inclusions in the bonding agent.[344,345]

Several significant developments have been achieved in adhesive luting procedures. Of clinical relevance, is the use of ultrasonic energy to assist the placement of the restoration when highly filled luting cement is used.[346] The easy removal of the excess cement with the low viscosity luting resins can also be achieved with these highly filled resins. Even though they have a higher filler load, they have been successfully utilized for many years for the cementation of PLVs.[347] One of the advantages of these resins is their low wear rate. Once the translucent resin with medium viscosity is used, these materials appear to be particularly beneficial, since it provides extended working time and more precision and stability in positioning the restoration.[348] Due to the thixotrophic nature of such resins (Herculite, or Z 100), the veneer will not bounce off the tooth even if gentle finger pressure is released.

However, it is better to keep the veneer seated on the tooth with some sort of gentle pressure, either with the fingertips or with the help of instruments. The pressure should be spread evenly over the entire labial surface. The fingertip is more sensitive and therefore serves better than any instrument in judging the pressure level required.[213] It should be very carefully checked in terms of marginal fit, property seating and its relation with the adjacent PLV or intact tooth. Application of an apically directed pressure on the incisal edge with the help of a second finger will ensure that the PLV will have full contact with the tooth in the cervical area.

Even though the marginal fit was clarified during the try-in stage, sometimes the limited time due to the quick polymerization period of the luting resin may create mental pressure on the dentist. The desire to seat the veneers as quickly as possible may cause some problems in terms of not actually being able successfully to seat the veneers as they should have been and thus ending up with open margins. This is especially a problem for beginners.

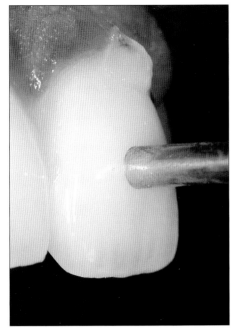

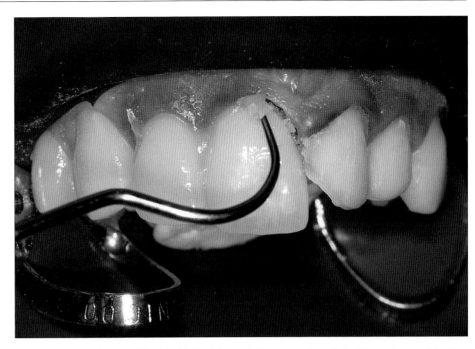

Fig 7-101 When the veneers are completely seated they are spot tacked with a 2 mm turbo tip (Optilux 501, Kerr) centered at the middle 1/3rd. Note the still soft condition of the nonpolymerized luting agent around the margins.

Fig 7-102 After 1-2 seconds of light curing with the 13 mm-diameter curing tip. The excess luting resin that came out of the margins has a jelly consistency and can easily be cleaned with an explorer and brush dipped in a bonding agent.

Seating the Veneers

The author prefers bonding the veneers two by two. This technique does not only ease the control over bonding but ensures that the veneers are seated completely and correctly, without the possibility of inadvertent polymerization due to excess bonding or the chance of luting resin getting on the adjacent preparation prior to veneer placement which would result in an incomplete seating. This will minimize placement challenges and time expenditure while optimizing the results.[349] However, some practitioners prefer bonding them all at once. In doing so, the dentist and their team must be very experienced in using this technique.

Diverting the operatory light from the preparations will eliminate inadvertent polymerization of the adhesive before veneer placement. The veneers are tacked into place after the seating is completed using the 2.0 mm turbo tip light guides (Optilux 501) (Fig 7-101). The tip should be placed centrally at the middle 1/3rd. of the veneer. To provide an inward/upward directed pressure and to ensure complete seating while eliminating

hydraulic pressure from lifting the veneer off the preparation, finger pressure o blunt instruments are applied at the incisal edge and gingival margin. Spot tacking the veneer into place will act like an anchor that will completely stabilize the veneer in its final seated position.

At this stage, the important aspect is that the composite flash that came out from the margins is still soft in nature.

The second stage will be applying the curing light with a 13.0 mm tip over the margins for only a few seconds. This is very important, since this makes the excess composite partially polymerize into a jelly consistency which can then be easily removed without injuring the soft tissues, while at the same time minimizing the post-bonding finishing and polishing procedures (Fig 7-102).

The further removal of the excess of nonpolymerized composite cement should be carried out with a brush moistened with bonding resin. This will reduce the tendency of the resin to drag out of the marginal gap and ensure a smoother margin that is polishable.[350] Meanwhile the interdental contact areas and the gingivoproximal

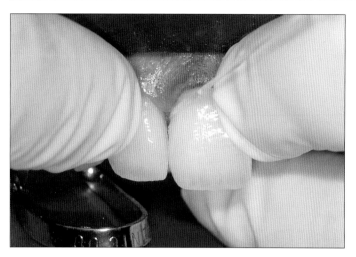

Fig 7-103 Before the luting resin is completely polymerized the interdental contact areas and gingival embrasures are cleaned with the help of dental floss. During this procedure the veneers should be held in place with the help of finger pressure.

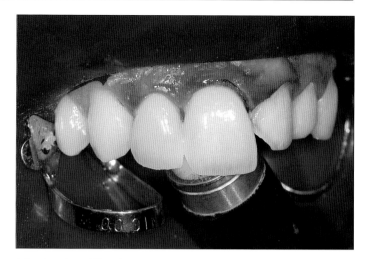

Fig 7-104 The luting agent is completely polymerized with a 13 mm-diameter curing tip (Optilux 501, Kerr) from both palatinal and facial 60 seconds each. The light should be applied to different areas from different angles to avoid overheating of the tooth, thus preventing postoperative pulpal sensitivity.

corners should be gently cleaned with the help of dental floss. The rubbing motion should preferably be towards the palatinal in order to prevent dislodgement of the veneer from its tacked position (Fig 7-103).

Light Curing

The resin is photo polymerized intensely after any excess is removed (Fig 7-104). If the maximum light energy is applied,[172] the quality of polymerization will be superior. The porcelain veneer absorbs between 40-50% of the emitted light. There may be two reasons for prevention of light transmission through the porcelain. One may be the thickness of the material. However, the opacity of the porcelain veneer becomes more important during the photopolimerization. Whatever may be the cause, when PLV retards light transmission, the setting time of the luting resin composite must be increased.[339,343] Some authors even suggest to double the recommended exposure time.

Light cured resin composites do not reach their maximum hardness, in the case of porcelain with a thickness of more than 0.7 mm or when the surface is opaqued excessively.[342] In these situations it is advisable to use a dual-cured luting composite, which contains the initiation systems for both chemically and light-cured composites. A stronger bond can be obtained with the porcelain[351] using the latter luting agents. Due to their higher degree of polymerization, higher values of hardness were reported for the dual-cure resin cements than that for the light-cured luting cements.[342,366]

To avoid the development of an oxygen-inhibited layer at the margins, an oxygen inhibition material, such as deox (Ultradent) or glycerin, should be applied prior to the final polymerization (Fig 7-105). Then each tooth's veneer is light polymerized for 60 to 90 seconds on all surfaces.

Once all the veneers are completely bonded, the rubber dam is removed and now the occlusion and protrusive contacts can be truly checked. Interfering contacts during occlusal closure, as well as the anterior and canine guidance should clearly be adjusted, if necessary. Meanwhile; the silicon index that was used since the beginning of the treatment, is used again over the bonded veneers, to verify their facial/outcomes (thickness and volumes) (Fig 7-106). The patient is allowed to see the result in front of a big mirror, so that they are able to see the veneers as well as their integration with the lips and the face as a whole.

An instruction sheet should be given to the patient, explaining the do's and don'ts for the next 48 hours, as well as for the future.

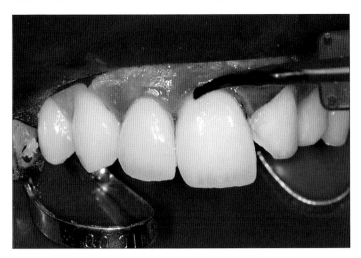

Fig 7-105 Deox (Ultradent) is applied over the margins to prevent an oxygen-inhibition layer and continued light curing.

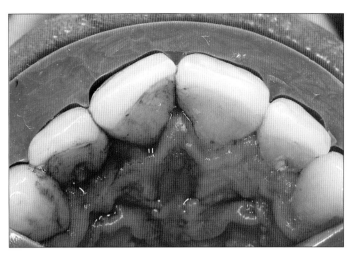

Fig 7-106 The final outcome is double-checked with the silicone index. Notice the precision of the volumetric PLV fit.

Do's
- Use a soft toothbrush with rounded bristles, and floss as you do with natural teeth.
- Use a less abrasive toothpaste and one that is not highly fluoridated.
- Use a soft acrylic mouth guard when involved in any form of contact sport.
- Ensure routine cleaning.

Don'ts
- Avoid food or drinks that may contain coloring.
- Do not use alcohol and some medicated mouthwashes because they have the potential to affect the resin bonding material during the early phase (the first 48 hours).
- Avoid hard foods, chewing on ice, eating ribs and biting hard confectionaries and candy.
- Avoid extremes in temperature.

Finishing and Polishing

Finishing and polishing the bonded veneers is extremely important, especially if special care has not been taken during the bonding stage.

During luting, prime care should be taken in order to avoid marginal discrepancies. They should have been completely filled with the luting composite. This is crucial not only for the sake of preventing the marginal leakage, but also for the ability to polish the cement layer into a smooth margin. However, some authors reported that after finishing procedures, only a small portion of the margins of each porcelain were found to have ideal marginal adaptation microscopically[352] and a considerable amount of excess luting agent at the veneer margins.[293] This can be a problem especially in the cervical regions.[353]

The finishing process of the veneer margins results in removal of the glaze from the porcelain.[315] Glaze is 25- to 100-micron melted porcelain over the porcelain surface.[297] The removal of the glaze of the porcelain restoration during finishing, with microfine finishing diamonds, causes a slight increase in surface roughness at the cervical border. The wear of the antagonistic elements and increased plaque retention along with gingival reaction will occur unless the porcelain can be polished to a smoother surface.

Even though it is claimed that it is impossible to produce a polished surface, which is equal to a glazed porcelain surface with polishing procedures, the author strictly believes in not removing the porcelain glaze at the cervical margin area.[354,355]

Most of these polishing instruments are not well suited for finishing the crucial gingival or interproximal regions of a bonded veneer, however they perform satisfactorily on flat accessible surfaces at high speeds. *Haywood*, et al.[356] evaluated finishing and polishing in these crucial areas in vitro. According to these authors, using finishing grit diamonds followed by a 30-fluted carbide bur and diamond polishing paste, a finish equal or superior in smoothness to glazed porcelain was achieved. Other finishing combinations were not as smooth as glazed porcelain and produced various textures. In contrast to dry polishing, polishing under water spray produced a smoother surface for a given sequence.[357] The effect of these finishing procedures must be evaluated in vitro to assess their effect on the cervical margin of the veneer with their difficult accessibility for polishing instruments.

All of the research above actually indicates the placement of the cervical margin supragingivally, to minimize the possible postoperative problems.

If the preparation's bonding and polishing are properly done, research shows a significant amount of lower bacterial plaque formation immediately after the placement of PLVs.[167]

Postoperative Longevity

When deciding on a type of treatment, the question of longevity is an important issue to consider. The tooth is at a greater risk when the potential treatment requires destructive preparation.[172] Being one of the most minimally invasive techniques, PLV has characteristically been less destructive to the tooth.

If properly prepared, tried-in and bonded, PLVs exhibit a long life span. The durability and survival rate for the PLV seems to range from one month to ten years according to clinical reports that have been published in the last ten years.[142,166,184,358-361] In vitro studies have indicated that when enough intact tooth tissue remains to bond the porcelain veneer, and when occlusion and articulation are not pathological, porcelain veneers are strong and durable restorations.

Clinical studies confirm that the maintenance of esthetics, with porcelain veneers was highly successful in retaining color stability and surface smoothness after years of clinical functioning. Over the years, the author has not witnessed a single patient who was not satisfied with the PLVs bonded and numerous studies confirm this fact. Patient satisfaction ranged from 80-100% while some studies even reported that patient satisfaction actually increased as time passed.[179,380] This increase was explained as a reflection of the patient's continually increasing comfort due to the PLV restorations.

The cervical preparations are usually placed supragingivally. This is beneficial for post-operative longevity. However, even if they are placed subgingivally, providing that the preparation, fitting of the PLV and bonding technique is done properly, the studies reported no changes in the health of the gingival tissues of the restored teeth.[113,142,168,363] However, for those patients with poor oral hygiene habits, some studies reported slight gingival inflammation.[179] Most in vivo studies reported excellent marginal adaptation in a high number of restorations after several years of clinical functioning (65-98%).[168,358,361,364] SEM examinations showed that it was the wearing out of the composite luting agent and the consequent loss of bonding[315] that caused these small marginal defects. In several in vivo studies of porcelain inlays[365] a similar phenomenon was reported as submargination. Replicas of inlays and porcelain laminate veneers in addition to clinical views clearly demonstrated that it was not the bonding agents that were responsible for failure in the restoration, but the fragile nature of the porcelain itself. It is cohesive and not adhesive fractures in the ceramic that show up in the scanning electron.

As mentioned before, the ideal preparation for the PLV should be confined within the enamel margins. However, sometimes due to gingival recession or extended class V caries, the cervical margin may be placed on the dentin or cementum. After the cementation of PLV there have been rare reports of postoperative sensitivity. This may be due to sensitivity in the cervical area where the margins end in dentin and where microleakage may occur. A combination of marginal integrity, the use of a new-generation dental bonding agents and a meticulous execution of the cementation procedure can help to minimize or even prevent this postoperative sensitivity.[5]

The reduction of microleakage of the restoration margins in dentin and enamel is possible with the application of any of the new generation of bonding agents.[5]

If a very thin PLV is placed on a tooth without a masking effect, after some time there may be a color change of the PLV, due to the biologic color alteration of an aging tooth. The darkened color of the natural tooth will reflect, through the veneer, giving the perception that the PLV has changed its color.

After all, properly diagnosed, planned and executed PLV applications have always been satisfactory. When the aesthetic perception of the dentist is enhanced with his/her up-to-date knowledge, together with the artistic skill and devotion of the ceramist, creation of a very natural-looking smile is unavoidable. When details like anterior-posterior color gradation, translucent areas of the incisors, higher chroma of the gingival 1/3rd, surface texture, luster are meticulously applied; the final outcome of the PLVs will be undetectable other than the natural teeth (Figs 7-107 to 7-110).

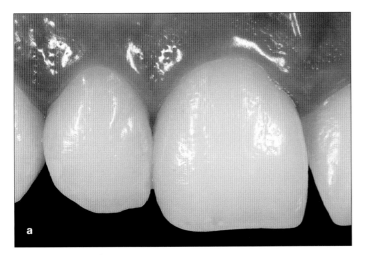 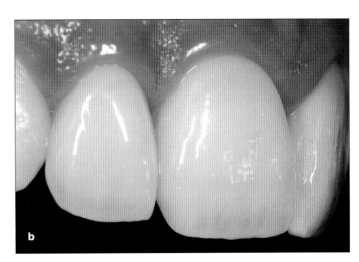

Fig 7-107a, b (a) The protrusive nature of tooth # 21(9) as well as the rotations on teeth 12(7) and 11(8) before the treatment. (b) The final PLVs in the mouth. Note that all the esthetic discrepancies before the treatment have been esthetically and functionally corrected.

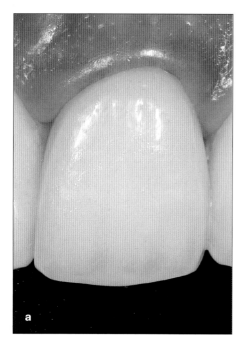 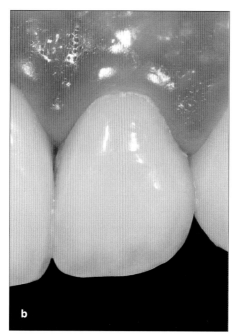 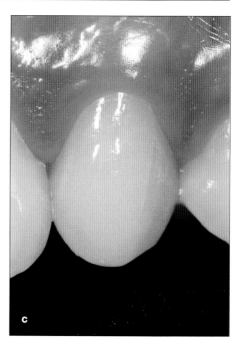

Fig 7-108a-c PLV in the mouth after a year. Note the excellent biologic integration at the cervical 1/3rd, as well as the esthetic integration of the PLVs and natural teeth to each other in terms of form, texture and color. Color gradation of every other tooth within themselves is achieved. The marginal 1/3rd, high in chroma, middle 1/3rd high in value and incisal 1/3rd with all the delicate characterizations. Also note the color gradation from anterior to posterior.

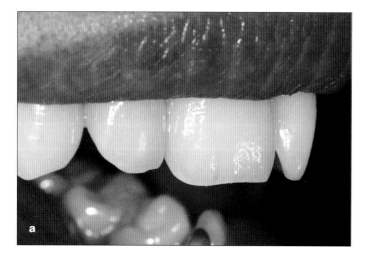 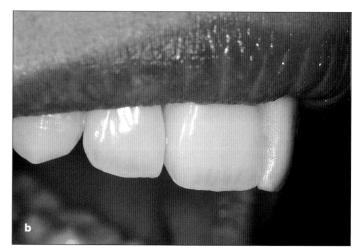

Fig 7-109a, b The harmony of the PLVs with the main frame. The PLVs should be integrated with the lips and the face. Close-up pictures (a) before (b) after. The success of such a natural-looking final restoration is due to careful diagnosis and treatment planning as well as delicate tooth preparation. Communication with the laboratory and the skilful hands of a technician complete the teamwork.

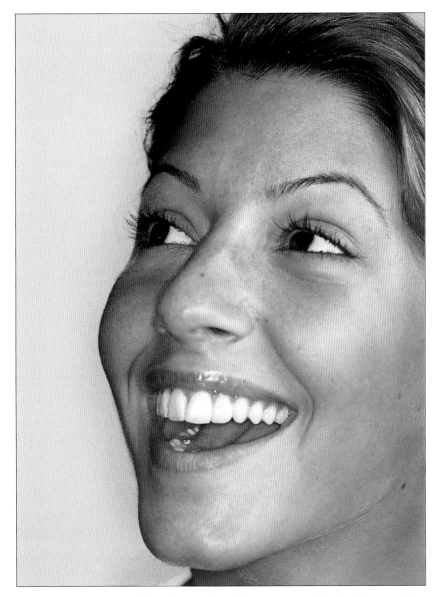

Fig 7-110 A beautiful smile, perfectly integrated with the lips and the face – the color of the veneers as well as the surface textures, form and delicate incisal embrasures adding youthful and beautiful effects to the face.

References

1. Trinkner TF, Roberts M. Aesthetic restoration with full-coverage porcelain veneers and a ceromer/fiber reinforced composite framework: A case report. Pract Periodont Aesthet Dent 1998;10:547-554.

2. Narcisi EM, Culp L. Diagnosis and treatment planning for ceramic restorations. Dent Clin North Am 2001;45:127-142.

3. Chiche GJ, Pinault A. Esthetics of Anterior Fixed Prosthodontics. Chicago: Quintessence, 1994.

4. Magne P, Versluis A, Douglas WH. Rationalization of incisor shape: Experimental-numerical analysis. J Prosthet Dent 1999;81:345-355.

5. Touati B, Miara P, Nathanson D. Esthetic Dentistry and Ceramic Restorations. New York: Martin Dunitz, 1999.

6. Magne P, Kwon KR, Belser UC, Hodges JS, Douglas WH. Crack propensity of porcelain laminate veneers: A simulated operatory evaluation. J Prosthet Dent 1999;81:327-334.

7. Rufenacht CR. Fundamentals of Esthetics. Chicago: Quintessence, 1990.

8. Schönenberger AJ, Di Felice A, Cossu M, The Esthetic Potential of the Ceramic-Fused-to-Metal Technique. In: Fischer J. Esthetics and Prosthetics. Chicago: Quintessence, 1999:31-71.

9. Lombardi RE. The principles of visual perception and their clinical application to denture esthetics. J Prosthet Dent 1973;29:358-382.

10. Cornell DF. Ceramic veneers: Understanding their benefits and limitations. QDT 1998;21:121-132.

11. Frush JP, Fisher RD. Introduction to dentogenic restorations. J Prosthet Dent 1955;5:586-595.

12. Goldstein RE. Esthetics in Dentistry. 2nd ed. Hamilton, ON: BC Decker Inc, 1998:17-49.

13. Morley J. Smile design. Specific considerations. CDAJ 1997;25:633-637.

14. Morley J. The role of cosmetic dentistry in restoring a youthful appearance. J Am Dent Assoc 1999;130:1166-1172.

15. Morley J. Critical elements for the preparation and finishing of direct and indirect anterior restorations. Contemp Esthet Dent 1997;3:1-6.

16. Sulikowski AV, Yoshida A. Clinical and laboratory protocol for porcelain laminate restorations on anterior teeth. QDT 2001;24:8-22.

17. Morley J. Techniques for delivering multiple -unit veneer cases. Rest Quart 1998;7:7-10.

18. Spear F. The maxillary central incisal edge: A key to esthetic and functional treatment planning. Aurum Ceramic Dent Lab News 1998;2:1-5.

19. Kokich V. Esthetics and anterior tooth position: An orthodontic perspective. Part 2: Vertical position. J Esthet Dent 1993; 5:174-178.

20. Miller LL. Porcelain crowns and porcelain laminates. Problems and solutions. Quintessence International Symposium (1991). New Orleans.

21. Rosental L. The art of building a high-profile celebrity practice. Dent Today 1995 May;14:74,76-9.

22. Strub JR, T␣rp JC. Esthetics in dental prosthetics. In: Fischer J, Esthetics and Prosthetics. Chicago: Quintessence, 1999: 11.

23. Magne P, Douglas WH. Additive contour of porcelain veneers: A key element in enamel preservation, adhesion and esthetics for aging dentition J. Adhesive Dent 1999; 1:81-92.

24. Miller M. Reality 2000. Houston: Reality Publishing, 2000.

25. Dietschi D. Free-hand composite resin restorations: A key to anterior aesthetics. Pract Periodont Aesthet Dent 1995; 7:15-25.

26. Vanini L. Light and color in anterior composite restorations. Pract Periodont Aesthet Dent 1996;8:673-682.

27. Roulet J-F, Degrange M. Adhesion. The Silent Revolution in Dentistry. Chicago: Quintessence, 2000.

28. Portalier L. Diagnostic use of composite in anterior aesthetics. Pract Periodont Aesthet Dent 1996;8:643-652.

29. Magne P, Perroud R, Hodges JS, Belser U. Clinical performance of Novel Design porcelain veneers for the recovery of coronal volume and length. Int J Periodontics Restorative Dent. 2000;20:441-459.

30. Bliss CH. A philosophy of patient education. Dent Clin North Am 1960;4:290.

31. Zinner ID, Panno FV, Miller RD, Parker HM, Pines MS. Ceramometal full coverage restorations. In: Dale BG, Aschheim KW. Esthetic Dentistry: A Clinical Approach to Techniques and Materials. Philadelphia, PA: Lea and Febiger, 1993:81-101.

32. Roach RR, Muia PJ. An esthetic checklist. In: Preston JD (ed). Perspectives in Dental Ceramics. Proceedings of the Fourth International Symposium on Ceramics. Chicago: Quintissence, 1988:445.

33. Gehl DH. Investment in the future. J. Prosthet. Dent 1967;18:190-201.

34. Magne P. Perspectives in Esthetic Dentistry. QDT 2000: 23;86-89.

35. Vence BS. Sequential tooth preparation for aesthetic porcelain full-coverage crown restorations. Pract Periodont Aesthet Dent 2000;12:77-85.

36. El Mostehy MR, Stallard RE. Intermediate cementum. J Periodontal Res 1968;3:24-29.

37. Albers HF. Tooth Colored Restoratives. Santa Rosa: Alto Books, 1985 and 1989.

38. Yamamoto M, Miyoshi M, Kataoka S. Special Discussion. Fundamentals of esthetics: Contouring techniques for metal ceramic restorations. QDT 1990/1991;14:10-81.

39. Rosental L. The art of tooth preparation and recontouring. Dent Today April 1997;16:1-4.

40. Rinaldi P. Clinical Topics in Dentistry. Continuing education video (n.d.).

41. Magne P, Douglas WH. Porcelain veneer: Dentin bonding optimization and biomimetic recovery of the crown. Int J Prosthodont 1999;12:111-121.

42. Heymann HO. The artistry of conservative esthetic dentistry. J Am Dent Assoc 1987; (special issue):14E-23E.

43. Magne P, Douglas WH. Design optimization and evolution of bonded ceramics for the anterior dentition: A finite-element analysis. Quintessence Int 1999;30:661-672.

44. Schneider PM, Messer LB, Douglas WH. The effect of enamel surface reduction in vitro on the bonding of composite resin to permanent human enamel. J Dent Res 1981;60:895-900.

45. Black JB. Esthetic restoration of tetracycline-stained teeth. J Am Dent Assoc 1982;104:846-851.

46. Stacey GD. A shear stress analysis of the bonding of porcelain veneers to enamel. J Prosthet Dent 1993;70:395-402.

47. Touati B. Defining form and position. Pract Periodont Aesthet Dent 1998;10:800-803.

48. Baratieri LN. Esthetics: Direct Adhesive Restoration on Fractured Anterior Teeth. São Paulo: Quintessence, 1998.

49. Crispin BJ. Contemporary Esthetic Dentistry: Practice Fundamentals. Tokyo: Quintessence, 1994.

50. Sorensen JA, Strutz JM, Avera SP, Materdomini D. Marginal fidelity and microleakage of porcelain veneers made by two techniques. J Prosthet Dent 1992;67:16-22.

51. Calamia JR. Etched porcelain facial veneers: A new treatment modality based on scientific and clinical evidence. NY J Dent 1983;53:255-259.

52. Horn HR. Porcelain laminate veneers bonded to etched enamel. Dent Clin North Am. 1983;27:671-684.

53. Christensen GJ. Veneering the teeth. State of the art. Dent Clin North Am 1985;29:373-391.

54. Calamia JR. Etched porcelain veneers: The current state of the art. Quintessence Int 1985;16:5-12.

55. Plant CG, Thomas GD. Porcelain facings: A simple clinical and laboratory method. British Dent Jour 1987;163:231-234.

56. McLaughlin G, Morison JE. Porcelain fused to tooth: The state of the art. Rest Dent 1988;4:90-94.

57. Reid JS, Murray MC, Power SM. Porcelain veneers. A four-year follow-up. Rest Dent 1988;5:42-55.

58. Garber DA, Goldstein RE, Feinman RA. Porcelain Laminate Veneers. Chicago: Quintessence, 1988.

59. McComb D. Porcelain veneer technique. Ont Dent 1998; 65: 25-27, 29, 31-32.

60. Weinberg LA. Tooth preparation for porcelain laminates. NY State Dent J 1989;55:25-28.

61. Nixon RL. Porcelain veneers. An esthetic therapeutic alternative. In: Rufenacht CR. Fundamentals of Esthetics. Chicago: Quintessence, 1990:329-68.

62. Garber DA. Porcelain laminate veneers: Ten years later. Part 1. Tooth preparation. J Esthet Dent 1993;5:56-62.

63. Friedman MJ. Augmenting restorative dentistry with porcelain veneers. J Am Dent Assoc 1991;122:29-34.

64. Chalifoux PR. Porcelain veneers. Curr Opin Cosmet Dent 1994:58-66.

65. Troedson M, Derand T. Shear stresses in adhesive layer under porcelain veneers. A finite element method study. Acta Odontologica Scandinavica 1998;56:257-262.

66. Deeks J. Full procedural build-up of a young maxillary left central incisor. QDT 1998;161-169.

67. Brian SV. Sequential tooth preparation for aesthetic porcelain full-coverage crown restorations. Pract Periodont Aesthet Dent 2000;12:77-84.

68. Van Meerbeek B, Peumans M, Gladys S, et al. Three-year clinical effectiveness of four total-etch dentinal adhesive systems in cervical lesions. Quint Int 1996;27:775-784.

69. Van Meerbeek B, Perdigao J, Lambrechts P, et al. The clinical performance of adhesives. J Dent 1998;26:1-20.

70. Lacy AM, Wada C, Weiming D, Watanabe L. In vitro microleakage at the gingival margin of porcelain and resin veneers. J Prosthet Dent 1992;67:7-10.

71. Chalifoux PR, Darvish M. Porcelain veneers: Concept, preparation, temporization, laboratory, and placement. Pract Periodont Aesthet Dent 1993;5:11-17.

72. Kois JC. New paradigms for anterior tooth preparation. Rationale and technique.Oral Health 1998;88:19-22,25-27, 29-30.

73. Magne P, Kwon KR, Belser UC, Hodges JS, Douglas WH. Crack propensity of porcelain laminate veneers: A simulated operatory evaluation. J Prosthet Dent 1999;12:111-21.

74. Magne P, Versluis A, Douglas WH. Effects of luting composite shrinkage and thermal loads on the stress distribution in porcelain laminate veneers. J Prosthet Dent 1999; 81:335-344.

75. Dumfahrt H. Porcelain laminate veneers . A retrospective evaluation after 1 to 10 years of service: Part 1. Clinical procedure. Int J Prosthod 1999;12:505-513.

76. Jones DW. In: McLean JW (Ed.). Dental Ceramics: Proceedings of the First International Symposium on Ceramics. Chicago: Quintessence, 1983:135.

77. Pameijer JHN. Onlays: Is gold still the standard? In: Degrange M, Roulet J-F. Minimally Invasive Restorations with Bonding. Chicago: Quintessence, 1997:139-152.

78. Jordan RE. Esthetic Composite Bonding. Hamilton, ON: BC Decker Inc, 1987, Ch 3.

79. Quinn F, McConnell RJ, Byrne D. Porcelain laminates: A review. Br Dent J 1986;161:62-65.

80. McLean JW, Jeansonne EE, Chiche GJ, Pinault A. All ceramic crowns and foil crowns. In: Chiche GJ, Pinault A. Esthetics of Anterior Fixed Prosthodontics. Chicago: Quintessence, 1994;97-114.

81. Christensen GJ. Have porcelain veneers arrived? J Am Dent Assoc 1991;122:81.

82. Tjan AHL, Dunn JR, Sanderson IR. Microleakage patterns of porcelain and castable ceramic laminate veneers. J Prosthet Dent 1989;61:276-282.

83. Crispin BJ, Jo YH, Hobo S. Esthetic ceramic restorative materials and techniques. In: Crispin BJ. Contemporary Esthetic Dentistry: Practice Fundamentals. Tokyo: Quintessence, 1994:155-299.

84. Symid ES. Dental engineering applied to inlay and fixed bridge fabrication. J Prosthet Dent 1952;2:536-542.

85. Tuntiprawon M. Effect of tooth surface roughness on marginal seating and retention of complete metal crowns. J Prosthet Dent 1999;81:142-147.

86. Smith BG. The effect of the surface roughness of prepared dentine on the retention of castings. J Prosthet Dent 1970;23:187-197.

87. Ayad MF, Rosentstiel SF, Salama M. Influence of tooth surface roughness and surface area on the retention of crowns luted with zinc phophate cement. Austr Dent J 1987;32:446-457.

88. Siegel SC, von Frauhofer JA. Assessing the cutting efficiency of dental burs. J Am Dent Assoc 1996;127:763-772.

89. Siegel SC, von Frauhofer JA. Dental cutting with diamond burs. Heavy-handed or light touch? J Prosthodont 1999;8: 3-9.

90. Ottl P, Lauer HC. Temperature response in the pulpal chamber during ultra-highspeed tooth preparation with diamond burs of different grit. J Prosthet Dent 1998;80: 12-19.

91. Schwartz JC. Vertical shoulder preparation design for porcelain laminated veneer restorations. Pract Periodont Aesthet Dent 2000;12:517-524.

92. Gürel G. PLV A to Z. American Academy of Cosmetic Dentistry. Annual Meeting, San Antonio (1999).

93. Rouse J, McGowan S. Restoration of the anterior maxilla with ultraconservative veneers. Clinical and laboratory consideration. Pract Periodont Aesthet Dent 1999;11: 333-339.

94. Ferrari M, Patroni S, Balleri P. Measurement of enamel thickness in relation to reduction for etched laminate veneers. Int J Periodont Rest Dent 1992; 23:407-413.

95. Liebenberg WH. Porcelain laminate veneers. Preparation and isolation innovations. Gen Dent 1995;43:50-58.

96. Dale BG, Aschheim KW. Esthetic Dentistry: A Clinical Approach to Techniques and Materials. Philadelphia, PA: Lea and Febiger, 1993:123-151.

97. Shillinburg HT, Hobo S, Fisher DW. Preparations for cast gold restorations. Chicago: Quintessence, 1974.

98. Dawson PE. Determining the determinants of occlusion. Int J Periodont Rest Dent 1983;3:17.

99. Jorgenson MW, Goodkind RJ. Spectrophotometric study of five porcelain shades relative to the dimensions of color, porcelain thickness and repeated firings. J Prosthet Dent 1979;42:96.

100. Terada Y, Maeyama S, Hirayasu R. The influence of different thicknesses of dentin color reflected from thin opaque porcelain fused to metal. Int J Prosthodont 1989;2:352.

101. Magne P. Konturanpassung von Keramikveneers. Die Quintessenz 1999;50:1133-1143.

102. Eissmann HF, Radke RA, Noble WH. Physiologic design criteria for fixed dental restorations. Dent Clin North Am 1971;15:543-568.

103. Kourkouta S, Walsh TT, Davis LG. The effect of porcelain laminate veneers on gingival health and bacterial plaque characteristics. J Clin Periodontol 1994;21:638-640.

104. Chan C, Weber H. Plaque retention on teeth restored with full-ceramic crowns: A comparative study. J Prosthet Dent 1986;56:666-671.

105. Koidis PT, Schroeder K, Johnston W, Campagni W. Color consistency, plaque accumulation, and external marginal surface characteristics of the collarless metal-ceramic restoration. J Prosthet Dent 1991;65:391-400.

106. Sheets CG, Taniguchi T. Advantages and limitations in the use of porcelain veneer restorations. J Prosthet Dent 1990;64:406-411.

107. Friedman MJ. Multiple potential of etched porcelain laminate veneers. J Am Dent Assoc 1987;115 (special issue):831-878.

108. Castelnuovo J, Tjan AH, Liu P. Microleakage of multi-step and simplified-step bonding systems. Am J Dent 1996; 9:245-248.

109. Zaimoglu A, Karaagaclyoglu L. Influence of porcelain material and composite luting resin on microleakage of porcelain laminate veneers. J Oral Rehab 1992;19:319-327.

110. Sim C, Neo J, Kiam Chua EK, et al. The effect of dentin bonding agents on the microleakage of porcelain veneers. Dent Mater 1994;10:278-281 (Abstract 215).

111. Peumans M, Van Meerbeek B, Yoshida Y, et al. Porcelain veneers bonded to tooth structure: An ultra-morphological FE-SEM examination of the adhesive interface. Dent Mater 1999.

112. Gaspercic D. Micromorphometric analysis of the cervical enamel structure of human upper third molars. Arch Oral Biol 1995;40:453-457.

113. Pippin DJ, Mixon JM, Soldon-Els AP. Clinical evaluation of restored maxillary incisors: Veneers vs. PFM crowns J Am Dent Assoc 1995;126:1523-1529.

114. Waerhaug J. The location of the restoration margins in relation to the gingiva are governed by histologic conditions. Dent Clin North Am 1960; 4:161-176.

115. Reeves WG. Restorative margin placement and periodontal health. J Prosthet Dent 1991;66:733-736.

116. Silness J. Fixed prosthodontics and periodontal health. Dent Clin North Am 1980;24:317-329; Karlsen K. Gingival reactions to dental restorations. Acta Odontologica Scandinavica 1970;28:895-904.

117. Newcomb GM. The relationship between the location of sub gingival crown margins and gingival inflammation. J Periodont 1974;45:151-154; Jameson LM, Malone WFP. Crown contours and gingival response. J Prosthet Dent 1982;47:620-624.

118. Lang NP, Kaarup-Hansen D, Joss A, Siegrist BE, Weber HP, Gerber C, et al. The significance of overhanging filling margins for the health status of interdental periodontal tissues of young adults. Schweiz Monatsschr Zahnmed 1988;98:725-730.

119. Lang NP. Periodontal considerations in prosthetic dentistry. Periodontal 2000 1995;9:118-131.

120. Richter WA, Ueno H. Relationship of crown margin placement to gingival inflammation. J Prosthet Dent 1973;30: 156-161.

121. Christensen GJ. Marginal fit of gold inlay castings. J Prosthet Dent 1966;16:297-305.

122. Trinkner TF, Roberts M. Anterior restoration utilizing novel all ceramic materials. Pract Periodont Aesthet Dent 2000; 12:35-39.

123. Ahmad I. Predetermining factors governing calculated tooth preparation for anterior crowns QDT 2001;24:57-68.

124. Bichacho N. Cervical contouring concepts: Enhancing the dento-gingival complex. Pract Periodont Aesthet Dent 1996;8:241-254.

125. Nattress BR, Youngson CC, Patterson JW, et al. An in vitro assessment of tooth preparation for porcelain veneer restorations. J Dentistry 1995;23:165-170.

126. Larato DC. Effect of cervical margins on gingiva. J Calif Dent Assoc 1969;45:19-22.

127. Berman MH. The complete coverage restoration and the gingival sulcus. J Prosthet Dent 1973;29:301-304.

128. Stein RS, Kuwata M. A dentist and a dental technologist analyze current ceramo-metal procedures. Dent Clin North Am 1977;21:729-749.

129. Behend DA. Ceramometal restorations with supragingival margins. J Prosthet Dent 1982;47:625-632.

130. Gardner FM. Margins of complete crowns: Literature review. J Prosthet Dent 1982;48:396-400.

131. Goldberg AJ. Deterioration of restorative materials and the risk for secondary caries. Adv Dent Res 1990; 4:14-18.

132. Özer L, Thylstrup A. What is known about caries in relation to restorations as a reason for replacement? A review. Adv Dent Res 1995;9:394-402.

133. Kidd EAM, Beighton D. Prediction of secondary caries around tooth-colored restorations: A clinical and microbiological study. J Dent Res 1996;75:1942-1946.

134. Van Meerbeek B, Peumans M, Verschueren M, et al. Clinical status of ten dentin adhesive systems. J Dent Res 1994; 73:1960-1702.

135. Stambaugh RV, Wittrock JW. The relationship of the pulp chamber to the external surface of the tooth. J Prosthet Dent 1977;37:537-546.

136. Paul SJ. Adhesive Luting Procedures. Berlin: Quintessence, 1997: 67-110.

137. Gwinnett AJ, Kanca J. Interfacial morphology of resin composite and shiny erosion lesions. Am J Dent 1992; 5:315-317.

138. Schüpbach P, Guggenheim B, Lutz F. Human root caries: Histopathology of initial lesions in cementum and dentin. J Oral Pathol 1989;18:146-156.

139. Duke ES, Lindemuth J. Variability of clinical dentin substrates. Am J Dent 1991;4:241-246.

140. Schüpbach P, Lutz F, Guggenheim B. Human root caries: Histopathology of arrested lesions. Caries Res 1992;26:153-164.

141. Van Meerbeek B, Braem M, Lambrechts P, Vanherle G. Morphological characterization of the interface between resin and sclerotic dentine. J Dent 1994;22:141-146.

142. Clyde JS, Gilmore A. Porcelain Veneers: A preliminary review. Br Dent 1988;164:9-14.

143. Levy JH. Ultrastructural deformations and proprioceptive function in human teeth. thesis, 1995. New York University College of Dentistry.

144. Lee WC, Eakle WS. Possible role of tensile stress in the etiology of cervical erosive lesions of teeth. J Prosthet Dent 1984;52:374-380.

145. Paphangkorakit J, Osborn JW. The effect of pressure on a maximum incisal bite force in man. Arch Oral Biol 1997;42:11-17.

146. Heymann HO, Sturdevant JR, Bayne S, et al. Examining tooth flexure effects on cervical restorations: A two-year clinical study. J Am Dent Assoc 1991;122:41-47.

147. Lambrechts P, Van Meerbeek B, Perdiago J, et al. Restorative therapy of erosive lesions. Eur J Oral Sci 1996; 104:229-240.

148. Kippax AJ, Shore RC, Basker RM. Preparation of guide planes using a reciprocating hand piece. Br Dent J 1996; 180:216-220.

149. Xu HHK, Kelly JR, Jahanmir S, et al. Enamel subsurface damage due to tooth preparation with diamonds. J Dent Res 1997;76:1698-1706.

150. Suh BI. All bond - fourth generation dentin bonding system. J Esthet Dent 1991;3:139-146.

151. Prestipino V, Ingber A, Kravitz J. Clinical and laboratory considerations in the use of a new all-ceramic restorative system. Pract Periodont Aesthet Dent 1998; 10:567-575.

152. Rateitschak KH, Rateitschak EM, Wolf HF. Paradontologie. Stuttgart: Thieme, 1984.

153. Takei HH. The interdental space. Dent Clin North Am 1980;24:169.

154. Ramfjord S. Periodontal aspects of restorative dentistry. J Oral Rehabil 1974;1:107.

155. Hazen S, Osborne J. Relationship of operative dentistry to periodontal health. Dent Clin North Am 1967;11:45.

156. Weinberg LA. Esthetic and the gingiva in full coverage. J Prosthet Dent 1960;10:737.

157. Hirshberg SM. The relationship of hygiene to embrasure and pontic design: A preliminary study. J. Prosthet Dent 1972;27:26.

158. Burch J. Ten rules for developing tooth contour in dental restorations. Dent Clin North Am 1971;15:611.

159. Nixon RL. Tooth preparation for porcelain veneers. Forum Esthet Dent 4:5,1986.

160. Williams HA, Caughman WF, Pollard BL. The esthetic hybrid resin-bonded bridge. Quint Int 1989;29:623.

161. Celenza V. Cast Glass Ceramic – Full Coverage Restorations. In: Dale BG, Aschheim KW. Esthetic Dentistry: A Clinical Approach to Techniques and Materials. Philadelphia, PA: Lea and Febiger, 1993:117-122. The finish line must be a well-defined continuous chamfer.

162. Janenko C, Smales RJ. Anterior crowns and gingival health. Austr Dent J 1979;24:225-230.

163. Olsson J, van der Heijde Y, Holmberg K. Plaque formation in vivo and bacterial attachment in vitro on permanently hydrophobic and hydrophilic surface. Caries Res 1992; 26:428-433.

164. Hahn R, Weiger R, Netuschil L, Bruch M. Microbial accumulation and vitality on different restorative materials. Dent Mater 1993;9:312-316.

165. Quirynen M, Bollen CML. The influence of surface roughness and surface-free energy on supra- and subgingival plaque formation in man. A review of literature. J Clin Periodont 1995;22:1-14.

166. Calamia JR. Clinical evaluation of etched porcelain veneers. Am J Dent 1989;2:9-15.

167. Kourkata S, Walsh TF, Davis LG. The effect of porcelain laminate veneers on gingival health and bacterial plaque characteristics. J Clin Periodont 1994;21:638-640.

168. Kihn PW, Barnes DM. The clinical longevity of porcelain veneers at 48 months. J Am Dent Assoc 1998;129:747-752.

169. Walls AW. The use of adhesively retained all porcelain veneers during the management of fractured and worn out anterior teeth. Part 2. Clinical results after 5 years of follow-up. Br Dent J 1995;178:337-339.

170. Peumans M, Van Meerbeek B, Lambrechts P, et al. Five-year clinical performance of porcelain veneers. Quintessence Int 1998;29:211-221.

171. Dumfhart H, Schaffer H. Porcelain Laminate Veneers. A retrospective evaluation after 1 to 10 years of service. Part 2. Clinical results. Int J Prosthodontics 2000;13:9-18.

172. Shillingburg Jr HT, Hobo S, Whitsett LD, et al. Fundamentals of Fixed Prosthodontics. 3rd ed. Chicago: Quintessence, 1997.

173. Hugo B, Stassinakis A, Hotz P. Die Randqualität der Schmelzabschrägung bei adhäsiven Klasse-II-Minikavitäten in vivo. Deutsche Zahnärtzliche Zeitschrift 1995; 50:832-835.

174. Hugo B, Lussi A, Hotz P. Die Präparation der Schmelzrandschrägung bei approximalen Kavitäten. Schweiz Monatsschr Zahnmed 1992;102:1181-1188.

175. Lussi A, Hugo B, Hotz P. Einfluss zweier Finierungsmeden auf die Mikromorphologie des approximalen Kastenrandes. Schweiz Monatsschr Zahnmed 1992;102:1175-1180.

176. Hugo B. Preparation and restoration of small interproximal carious lesions. In: Roulet J-F, Degrange M. Adhesion. The Silent Revolution in Dentistry. Chicago: Quintessence, 2000:153-165.

177. Rouse JS. Full veneer versus traditional veneer preparation with a medium wrap: A discussion of interproximal extension. J Prosthet Dent 1997;78:545-549.

178. Chiche G, Aoshima H. Functional versus aesthetic articulation of maxillary anterior restorations. Pract Periodont Aesthet Dent 1997;9:335-342.

179. Christensen GJ, Christensen RP. Clinical observations of porcelain veneers. A three year report. J Esthet Dent 1991;3:174-179.

180. Dunne SM, Millar J. A longitudinal study of the clinical performance of porcelain veneers. Br Dent J 1993;175: 317-321.

181. Jäger K, Stern M, Wirz J. Laminates – Reif für die Praxis? Die Quintessenz 1995;46:1221-1230.

182. Highton R, Caputo AA, Matyas JA. A protoelastic study of stress on porcelain laminate preparations. J Prosthetic Dent 1987;58:157-161.

183. Magne P, Douglas WH. Interdental design of porcelain veneers in the presence of composite fillings. Finite element analysis of composite shrinkage and thermal stresses. Int J Prosthodontics 2000;13:117-124.

184. Karlsson S, Landahl I, Stegersjö G, Milleding P. A clinical evaluation of ceramic laminate veneers. Int J Prosthodont 1992;5:447-451.

185. Mörmann WH, Link C, Lutz F. Color changes in veneer ceramics caused by bonding composite resins. Acta Med Dent Helv 1996;1:97-102.

186. Hui K, Williams B, Davis E, Holt R. A comparative assessment of the strengths of porcelain veneers for incisor teeth dependent on their design characteristics. Br Dent J 1991;171:51-55.

187. Chpindel P, Cristou M. Tooth preparation and fabrication of porcelain veneers using a double-layer technique. Pract Periodont Aesthet Dent 1994;6:19-30.

188. Meijering AC, Roeters FJM, Mulder J, Creugers NHJ. Recognition of veneer restorations by dentists and beautician students. J Oral Rehabil 1997;24:506-511.

189. Nordbo H, Rygh-Thoresen N, Henang T. Clinical performance porcelain laminate veneers without incisal overlapping 3-year results. J Dent 1994;22:342-345.

190. Crispin BJ. Full veneers. The functional and esthetic application of bonded ceramics. Compend Contin Educ Dent 1994; 15:284,286-294.

191. Gilde H, Lenz P, Furst U. Untersuchungen zur Belastbarkeit von Keramikfacetten. Deutsche Zahnärtzliche Zeitschrift 1989;44:869-71.

192. Friedman MJ. A fifteen-year review of porcelain veneer failure. A clinician's observations. Compend Contin Educ Dent 1998;19:625-636.

193. Tronstad L, Leidal TI. Scanning electron microscopy of cavity margins finished with chisels or rotating instruments at low sped. J Dent Res 1974 53:1167-1174.

194. Fischer J, Kuntze C, Lampert F. Modified partial-coverage ceramics for anterior teeth: A new restorative method. Quintessence Int 1997;28:293-299.

195. Nabakayashi N, Pashley DH. Hybridization of Dental Hard Tissues. 1st ed. Tokyo: Quintessence, 1998:37-39.

196. Olgard L, Brannstrom M, Johnson G. Invasion of bacteria into dentinal tubules. Experiments in vivo and in vitro. Acta Odontologica Scandinavica 1974;32:61-70.

197. Brannstrom M. Etiology of dentin hypersensitivity. Proc Fin Dent Soc 1992;88:7-13, supplement.

198. Ellege DA, Schorr BI. A provisional restoration technique for laminate veneer preparation. J Prosthed Dent 1989; 62:139-142.

199. Rada RE, Jankowski BJ. Provisional laminate veneer provisionalization using visible light-curing acrylic resin. Quintessence Int 1991;22:291-293.

200. Bertschinger C, Paul SJ, Luthy H, Schärer P. Dual application of dentin bonding agents. Its effect on the bond strength. Am J Dent 1996;9:115-119.

201. Paul SJ, Schärer P. The dual bonding technique: A modified method to improve adhesive luting. Int J Periodont Rest Dent 1997;17:536-545.

202. Nikaido T, Burrow MF, Tagami J, et al. Effect of pulpal pressure on adhesion of resin composite to dentin: Bovine serum versus saline. Quintessence Int. 1995; 26:221-226.

203. Cagidiaco MC, Ferrari M, Garberoglio R, et al. Dentin contamination protection after mechanical preparation of veneering. Am J Dent 1996;9:57-60.

204. Cobb DS, Reinhardt JW, Vargas MA. Effect of HEMA-containing dentin desensitizers on shear bond strength of resin cement. Am J Dent 1997;10:62-65.

205. Reeh ES, Douglas WH, Messer PH. Stiffness of endodontically treated teeth related to restoration technique. J Dent Res 1989;68:1540-1544.

206. Degrange M, Roulet J-F. Minimally Invasive Restorations with Bonding. Chicago: Quintessence, 1997:103-153.

207. Nakabayashi N. The hybrid layer: a resin-dentin composite. Proc Fin Dent Soc 1992;88:321.

208. Pashley DH. The effects of acid etching on the pulpodentin complex. Oper Dent 1992;17:229.

209. Kanca J. Effect of dentin drying on bond strength (Abstract 1029). J Dent 1991;70:394.

210. Kanca J 3rd. Improving bond strength through acid etching of dentin and bonding to wet dentin surfaces. J Am Dent Assoc 1992;123:35.

211. Gwinnett AJ. Moist versus dry bonding. Its effect on shear bond strength. Am J Dent 1992;5:127.

212. Manolakis K, Paul SJ, Schärer P. Schmelzhaftung Ausgewählter Adhasiver Zementsysteme. Deutsche Zahnärtzliche Zeitschrift 1995;50:582-584.

213. Mörig G. Aesthetic all-ceramic restorations: A philosophic and clinical review. Pract Periodont Aesthet Dent 1996; 8:741-749.

214. Tjan AH, Castelnuovo J, Liu P. Bond strength of multi-step and simplified-step systems. Am J Dent 1996; 9:269-272.

215. Wakefield CW, Draughn RA, Sneed WD, Davis TN. Shear bond strengths of 6 bonding systems using the push out method of in vitro testing. Oper Dent 1998;23:69-76.

216. Swift EJ Jr, Triolo PT Jr, Barkmeier WW, et al. Effect of low-viscosity resins on the performance of dental adhesives. Am J Dent 1996;9:100-104.

217. Winter RR. Achieving esthetic ceramic restorations. J Calif Dent Assoc 1990;18:21-24.

218. Clark EB. Tooth color selection. J Am Dent Assoc 1933; 20:1065-1073.

219. Miller LL. Organizing color in dentistry. J Am Dent Assoc 1987;115:26E-40E.

220. Sproull RC. Color matching in dentistry. Part 2. Practical applications of the organization of color. J Prosthet Dent 1973;29:556-566.

221. Preston JD. The metal-ceramic restoration. The problems remain. Int J Periodont Rest Dent. 1984;4:9-23.

222. Preston JD. Current status of shade selection and color matching. Quintessence Int 1985;16:47-58.

223. Wasson W, Schuman N. Color vision and dentistry. Quintessence Int 1992;23:349-353.

224. Moser JB, Wozniak WT, Naleway CA, Ayer WA. Color vision in dentistry: A survey. J Am Dent Assoc 1985;110: 509-510.

225. Shillingburg HT, Hobo S, Witsett LD, Jacobi R, Bracket SE. Fundamentals of Fixed Prosthodontics. 3rd ed. Chicago: Quintessence, 1997:419-432.

226. Sproull RC. Color matching in dentistry. Part 3. Color control. J Prosthet Dent 1974;31:146-154.

227. Ubassy G. Shape and Color. Chicago: Quintessence, 1988.

228. Yamamoto M. Technical work and shade taking. Quint Dent Technol 1984;9:428-429 (Japanese).

229. June KS. Shade matching and communication in conjunction with segmental porcelain build-up. Pract Periodont Aesthet Dent 1999;11:457-464.

230. Yamamoto M. Metal-Ceramics: Principles and Methods of Makoto Yamamoto. Chicago: Quintessence, 1985.

231. Marinello CP, Boitel N. Detailwiedergabe Elastomerer Abform Materialien. Eine Rasterelectrobnische Analyse, Schweize Monatsschr Zahnmed 1985;95:1051-1063.

232. Craig RG. Restorative Dental Materials. 7th ed. St Louis, MO: Mosby, 1985:276.

233. Craig RG. A review of properties of rubber impression materials. J Mich Dent Assoc 1977;59:254-261.

234. Herfort TW, Gerberich WW, Macosko CW, Goodking RJ. Viscosity of elastomeric impression materials. J Prosthet Dent 1977;38:396-403.

235. O'Brien JW. Dental Materials and Their Selection. Chicago: Quintessence, 1997;123-145.

236. Keck SC. Automixing. A new concept in elastomeric impression material delivery systems. J Prosthet Dent 1985; 54:794-839.

237. McCabe JF, Wilson HJ. Addition curing silicone rubber impression materials. Br Dent J 1978;145:17-20.

238. Eames WB, Wallace SW, Suway NB, Rogers LB. Accuracy and dimensional stability of elastomeric impression materials. J Prosthet Dent 1979;42:159-162.

239. Johnson GH, Craig RG. Accuracy of four types of rubber impression materials compared with time of pour and a repeat pour of models. J Prosthet Dent 1985;53:484-490.

240. Tjan AHL, Whang SB, Tjan AH, Sarkissian R. Clinically oriented evaluation of the accuracy of commonly used impression materials. J Prosthet Dent 1986;56:4-8.

241. Corso M, Abanomi A, Canzio JD, et al. The effect of temperature changes on the dimensional stability of polyvinylsiloxane and polyether impression materials. J Prosthet Dent 1998;79:626-631.

242. Purk JH, Willes MG, Tira DE, et al. The effects of different storage conditions on polyether and polyvinylsiloxane impressions. J Am Dent Assoc 1998;129:1014-1021.

243. Chai J, Takahashi Y, Lautenschlager EP. Clinically relevant mechanical properties of elastomeric impression materials. Int J Prosthodont 1998;11:219-223.

244. Jennings KJ, Samaranayake LP. The persistence of microorganisms on impression materials following disinfection. Int. J Prosthodont 1991;4:382-387.

245. Minagi A, Fukushima K, Maeda N, et al. Disinfection method for impression materials. Freedom from fear of hepatitis B and acquired immunodeficiency syndrome. J Prosthet Dent 1986;56:451-454.

246. Matyas J, Dao N, Caputo AA, Lucatorto FM. Effects of disinfectants on dimensional accuracy of impression materials. J Prosthet Dent 1990;64:25-31.

247. Herrera SP, Merchant VA. Dimensional stability of dental impressions after immersion disinfection. J Am Dent Assoc 1986;113:419-422.

248. Langenwalter EM, Aquilino SA, Turner KA. The dimensional stability of elastomeric impression materials following disinfection. J Prosthet Dent 1990;63:270-276.

249. Drennon DG, Johnson GH. The effect of immersion disinfection of elastomeric impressions on the surface detail reproduction of improved gypsum casts. J Prosthet Dent 1990;63:233-241.

250. Merchant VA, Herrera SP, Dwan JJ. Marginal fit of cast gold MO inlays from disinfected elastomeric impressions. J Prosthet Dent 1987;58:276-279.

251. Tullner JB, Commete JA, Moon PC. Linear dimensional changes in dental impressions after immersion in disinfectant solutions. J Prosthet Dent 1988;60:725-728.

252. Drennon DG, Johnson GH, Powell GL. The accuracy and efficacy of disinfection by spray atomization on elastomeric impressions. J Prosthet Dent 1989;62:468-475.

253. Merchant VA, McKneight MK, Cibirowski CJ, Molinari JA. Preliminary investigation of a method for disinfection of dental impressions. J Prosthet Dent 1984;54:877-879.

254. Crook WD, Thomasz F. Rubber gloves and addition silicone materials. Current note 64. Austr Dent J 1986; 31:140.

255. Kahn RL, Donovan TE, Chee WWL. Interaction of gloves and rubber dam with poly(vinyl siloxane) impression material. A screening test. Int J Prosthodont 1989;2:342-346.

256. Reitz CD, Clark NP. The setting of vinyl polysiloxane and condensation silicone putties when mixed with gloved hands. J Am Dent Assoc 1988;116:371-375.

257. Council on Dental Materials, Instruments and Equipment: Retarding the setting of vinyl polysiloxane impressions. J Am Dent Assoc 1991;122:114.

258. Chiche GJ, Pinault A. Esthetics of Anterior Fixed Prosthodontics. Chicago: Quintessence, 1994.

259. Stade EH, Hanson JG, Baker CL. Esthetic considerations in the use of face-bows. J. Prosthet Dent 1982;48:253.

260. Shavell HM. Dentist-laboratory relationships in fixed prosthodontics. In: Preston JD (ed). Perspectives in Dental Ceramics. Proceedings of the Fourth International Symposium on Ceramics. Chicago: Quintessence, 1988: 429.

261. Nixon RL. Provisionalization for ceramic laminate veneer restorations. A clinical update. Pract Periodont Aesthet Dent 1997;9:17-41.

262. Roblee RD. Interdisciplinary Dentofacial Therapy: A Comprehensive Approach in Optimal Patient Care. Chicago: Quintessence, 1994.

263. Shavell HM. The Aesthetic of Occlusion: Form, function, finesse. Pract Periodont Aesthet Dent 1993;5:47-55.

264. Dawson PE. A classification system for occlusions that relates maximal intercuspation to the position and condition of the temporomandibular joints. J Prosthet Dent 1996;75:60-66.

265. Dawson PE. Evaluation, Diagnosis and Treatment of Occlusal Problems. St Louis, MO: Mosby, 1974.

266. Seltzer S, Bender IB. The Dental Pulp: Biologic Considerations in Dental Procedures. 3rd ed Philadelphia, PA. Lippincott, 1984:191, 267-272.

267. Mumford JM, Ferguson HW. Temporary restorations and dressings. Dent Pract Dent Rec 1959;9:121-124.

268. Segat L. Protection of prepared abutments between appointments in crown and bridge prosthodontics. J. Mich Dent Assoc 1962;44:32-35.

269. Knight RM. Temporary restorations in restorative dentistry. J. Tenn Dent Assoc 1967;47:346-349.

270. Rose HP. A simplified technique for temporary crowns. Dent Dig 1967; 73:449-450.

271. Meijering AC, Creugers NHJ, Mulder J, Roeters FJM. Treatment times for three different types of veneer restorations. J Dent 1995;23:21-26.

272. Nixon RL. Masking severely tetracycline-stained teeth with ceramic laminate veneers. Pract Periodont Aesthet Dent 1996; 8:227-235.

273. Zalkind M, Hochmann N. Laminate veneer provisional restorations: A clinical report. J Prosthet Dent 1997;77: 109-110.

274. Elledge DA, Kenison Hart J, Schorr BL. A provisional restoration technique for laminate veneer preparations. J Prosthet Dent 1989;62:139-142.

275. Sheets CG, Ono Y, Taniguchi T. Esthetic provisional restorations for porcelain veneer preparation. J Esthet Dent 1993; 5:215-220.

276. Magne P, Holz J. Stratification of composite restorations. Systematic and durable replication of natural aesthetics. Pract Periodont and Aesthet Dent 1996;8:61-68.

277. Christensen G. Temporary cementation. CRA Newsletter, January 1992.

278. Terry DA, Moreno C, Geller W, Roberts M. The importance of laboratory communication in modern dental practice: Stone models without faces. Pract Periodont Aesthet Dent 99;11:1125-1132.

279. Magne P, Magne M, Belser U. Natural and restorative oral esthetics. Part 1. Rationale and basic strategies for successful esthetic rehabilitations. J Esthet Dent 1993; 5: 161-173.

280. Zaimoglu A, Karaagaclyoglu L. Microleakage in porcelain laminate veneers. J Dent 1991;19:369-372.

281. Sim C, Ibbetson RJ. Comparsion of fit of porcelain veneers fabricated using different techniques. Int J Prosthodont 1993;6:36-42.

282. Levin R. Working with your dental laboratory. Dent Econ 1991;81:47-50.

283. Jens F. Esthetics and Prosthetics. Berlin: Quintessence, 1999;31-71.

284. Ban K. Dental Technology Library. St. Louis: Ishiyaku, 1989:157-158.

285. Gillis RE, Jr. Communicating with dental laboratories. Dent Abstr 1997;42:166-167.

286. Leeper SH. Dentist and laboratory. A "love-hate" relationship. Dent Clin North Am 1979;23:87-99.

287. O'Keefe KL, Strickler ER, Kerrin HK. Color and shade matching. The weak link in esthetic dentistry. Compend Contin Educ Dent 1990;11:116-120.

288. Muia P. Bench talk. Paul Muia explains his/her four-dimensional tooth-color system. QDT 1983;7:62.

289. Williams WP. Creating a new perspective on local anesthesia in dentistry. Part 2. Dentistry (UK) 2001;1:29-37.

290. Friedman M, Hochman M. The AMSA injection. Anesthesize the teeth not the face. Contemp Esthet Rest Prac 2000.

291. Nixon RL. Mandibular ceramic veneers: An examination of complex cases. Pract Periodont Anesthet Dent 1995;7: 17-28.

292. Kunzelmann K-H, Deigner M, Hickel R. Dreimedienabrasion von Befestigungskompositen adhäsiver Inlaysysteme. Deutsche Zahnärtzliche Zeitschrift 1993;48:109.

293. Harasani MH, Isidor F, Kaaber S. Marginal fit of porcelain and indirect composite laminate veneers under in vitro conditions. Scand J Dent Res 1991;99:262-268.

294. Dumfart H, Schaffer H. Scherfestigkeitsmessung zur klinischen Bewertung von Keramik verbundssystemen. Deutsche Zahnärtzliche Zeitschrift 1989;44:867-869.

295. Picard B, Jardel V, Tirlet G. Ceramic bonding: Reliability. In: Degrange M, Roulet J-F. Minimally Invasive Restorations with Bonding. Chicago: Quintessence, 1997:103-129.

296. Schroeder HE. Oral Structural Biology. Stuttgart:Thieme, 1991

297. McLean J. The Science and Art of Dental Ceramics. 2 vols. Chicago: Quintessence, 1980.

298. Roulet J-F. Degradation of dental polymers. Basel: Karger, 1976.

299. Buonocore MG. A simple method of increasing the adhesion of acrylic filling materials to enamel surfaces. J Dent Res 1955;34:849-853.

300. Gwinnett AJ. Interactions of dental materials with enamel. Trans Am Acad Dent Mater 1990;3:30-35.

301. Anusavice KJ. Philipsí Science of Dental Materials. 10th ed. Philadelphia: WB Saunders, 1996:139-176.

302. Kern M, Thompson VP. Tensile bond strength of new adhesive systems to In Ceram ceramic. J Dent Res 1993; 72:369 (Abstract 2124).

303. Feilzer AJ, DeGee AJ, Davidson CL. Increased wall-to-wall curing contraction in thin bonded resin layers. J Dent Res 1989;68:48-50.

304. Paffenberger GC, Sweeney WT, Bowen RL. Bonding porcelain teeth to acrylic denture bases. J Am Dent assoc 74:1018-1967.

305. Highton RM, Caputo AA, Matyas J. The effectiveness of porcelain repair system. J Prosthet Dent, 1979;42:292.

306. Jochen DG, Caputo AA. Composite repair of porcelain teeth. J Prosthet Dent 1977;38:673.

307. Simonsen RJ, Calamia JR. Tensile bond strength of etched porcelain. J Dent Res 1983;62:257.

308. Calamia JR, Vaidynathan TK, Hirsch SM. Shear strength of etched porcelains. J Dent Res 1985;64:296.

309. Pape, FW, Pfeiffer, P, Marx, R. Haftfestigkeit von geätztem In-Ceram an Zahnschmelz. Zahnärztl Welt 100 1991;7: 450.

310. Edelhoff D, Marx R. Adhasion zwischen Vollkeramik und Befestigungskomposit nach Unterschiedlicher Oberflächenvorbehandlung. Deutsche Zahnärtzliche Zeitschrift 1995;50:112-117.

311. Calamia JR, Simonse RJ. Effect of coupling agents on bond strength of etched porcelain. J Dent Res 1984;63: 179 (Abstract 79).

312. Lu R, Hartcourt JK, Tyas MJ, et al. An investigation of the composite resin/porcelain interface. Austr Dent J 1992; 37:12-19.

313. Stangel I, Nathanson D, Hsu CS. Shear strength of the composite bond to etched porcelain. J Dent Res 1987; 66:1460-1465.

314. Roulet J-F, Söderholm KJM, Longmate J. Effects of treatment and storage conditions on ceramic/composite bond strength. J Dent Res 1995;74:381-387.

315. Peumans M, Van Meerbeek B, Lambrechts P, Vanherle G. Porcelain veneers: A review of the literature. J Prosthet Dent 2000;28:163-177.

316. Garber DA, Goldstein RE, Feinman RA. Porcelain Laminate Veneers. Chicago: Quintessence, 1988.

317. Nichols JI. Tensile bond of resin cements to porcelain veneers. J Prosthet Dent 1988;60:443.

318. Williamson RT, Mitchell RJ, Breeding LC. The effect of fatigue on the shear bond strength of resin bonded porcelain. J Prost 1993;2:115-119.

319. Müller G. Atzen und silaniseren dentaler Keramiken. Deutsche Zahnartzliche Zeitschrift 1988;43: 438-441.

320. Swift B, Walls AWG, McCabe JF. Porcelain veneers. The effect of contaminants and cleaning regimens on the bond strength of porcelain to composite. Brit Dent J 1995; 179:203-208.

321. Holtan JR, Lua MJ, Belvedere P, et al. Evaluating the effect of glove coating on the shear bond strength of porcelain laminate veneers. J Am Assoc 1995;126:611-616.

322. Sheth J, Jensen M, Tolliver D. Effect of surface treatment on etched porcelain bond strength to enamel. Dent Mater 1988;4:328-337.

323. Della Bona A, Northeast SE. Shear bond strength of resin bonded ceramic after different try-in procedures. J Dent 1994;22:103-107.

324. Jones GE, Boksman L, McConnell RL. Effect of etching technique on the clinical performance of porcelain veneers. QDT 1986;10:635-637.

325. Aida M, Hayakawa T, Mizukawa K. Adhesion of composite to porcelain with various surface conditions. J Prosthet Dent 1995;73:464-470.

326. Dietschi D, Spreafico R. Current clinical concepts for adhesive cementation of tooth-colored posterior restorations. Pract Periodont Aesthet Dent 1998;10:47-54.

327. Garber DA, Goldstein RE. Porcelain and Composite Inlays and Onlays. Esthetic Posterior Restorations. Chicago: Quintessence, 1994.

328. Roulet J-F. Posterior esthetic restoration. In: Dondi dall'Orologio G. Fuzzi M, Prati C (Eds.). Adhesion in Restorative Dentistry. Bologna: Valbonesi, 1995:27-47.

329. Stark H. Does temporary cementing have an effect on bond strength of definitively cemented crowns? Deutsche Zahnärtzliche Zeitschrift 1995;46:774-776.

330. White SN, Yu Z, Zhua XY. High energy abrasion: An innovative esthetic modality to enhance adhesion. J Esthet Dent 1994;6:267.

331. Gwinnett AJ. Effect of Cavity disaffection on bond strength to dentin. J Esthet Dent. 1992;4 (special issue):11-13.

332. Swift EJ, Cloe BC. Shear bond strengths of new enamel etchants. Am J Dent 1993;6:162-164.

333. Van Meerbeek B, Inokoshi S, Braen M, et al. Morphological aspects of the resin-dentin interdiffusion zone with different dentin adhesive systems. J Dent Res 1992;71:1530-1540.

334. Paul SJ, Schärer P. Intrapulpal pressure and thermal cycling: Effect on shear bond strength of eleven modern dentin-bonding agents. J Esthet Dent 1993;5:179-185.

335. Andreasen FM, Flügge E, Daugaard-Jensen J, Munksgaard EC. Treatment of crown fractured incisors with laminate veneer restorations: An experimental study. Endod Dent Traumatol 1992;8:30-35.

336. Shokes AN, Hood JAA. Impact fracture characteristics of intact crowned human central incisors. J Oral Rehabil 1993;20: 89-95.

337. Kanca J. Resin bonding to wet substrate. 1. Bonding to dentin. Quintessence Int 1992;23:39-41.

338. Chan KC, Boyer DB. Curing light-activated composite cement through porcelain. J Dent Res 1989; 68:476-480.

339. Strang R, McCrosson J, Muirhead GM, Richardson SA. The setting of visible-light-cured resin beneath etched porcelain veneers. Br Dent J 1987;163:149-151.

340. O'Keefe KL, Pease PL, Herrin HK. Variables affecting the spectral transmittance of light through porcelain veneers samples. J Prosthet Dent 1991;66:434-438.

341. Castelnuovo J, Tjan AH, Philips K, et al. Fracture load and mode of failure of ceramic veneers with different preparation. J Prosthet Dent 2000;83:171-180.

342. Linden JJ, Swift EJ, Boyer DB, Davis BK. Photo-activation of resin cements through porcelain veneers. J Dent Res 1991;70:154-157.

343. Blackman R, Barghi N, Duke E. Influence of ceramic thickness on the polymerization of light-cured resin cement. J Prosthet Dent 1990;63:295-300.

344. Morig G. Ceramic restorations: medically, aesthetically, and technically. A true alternative? Quintessenz Zahntechnik 1992:18;719.

345. Roulet J-F, Herder S. Seitenzahnversorgung mit adhäsiv befestigten Keramikinlays (Restoration of Lateral Dentition with Adhesively Seated Ceramic Inlays). Berlin: Quintessence, 1989).

346. Noack MJ, Roulet J-F, Bergmann P. A new method to lute tooth colored inlays with highly filled composite resins. J Dent Res 1991;70:457 (Abstract 1528).

347. Besek M, Mörmann WH, Persi C, Lutz F. Die Aushärtung von Komposit unter Cerec-Inlays. Schweiz Monatsschr Zahnmed 1995;105:1123-1128.

348. Dietschi D, Dietschi JM. Current developments in composite materials and techniques. Pract Periodont Aesthet Dent 1996;8:603-613.

349. Hornbook DS. The ìtwo-by-two techniqueî for porcelain veneer cementation: Minimizing time maximizing results. Pract Periodont Aesthet Dent Aug. 1996:8-12.

350. Tay WM, Lynch E, Auger D. Effects of some finishing techniques on cervical margins of porcelain laminates. Quintessence Int 1987;18:599-602.

351. Nathanson D, Hassan F. Effect of porcelain thickness on resin-porcelain bond strength. J Dent Res. 1987;66:245 Special Issue (Abstract 1107).

352. Coyne B, Wilson NHF. The marginal adaptation of porcelain laminate veneers. J Dent Res 1987;66:885 (Abstract 452).

353. Hannig M, Jepsen S, Jasper V, Lorenz-Stucke C. Der Randschluß glaskeramischer Veneers mit zervikaler Schmelz- oder Dentinbegrenzung. Deutsche Zahnärztliche Zeitschrift 1995;50:227-229.

354. Goldstein GR, Barnhard BR, Penugonda B. Profilometer, SEM, and visual assessment of porcelain polishing methods. J Prosthet Dent,1991;65:627-34.

355. Ward MT, Tate W, Povers JM. Surface roughness of opalescent porcelains after polishing. Oper Dent 1995;20: 106-110.

356. Haywood VB, Heymann HO, Kusy RP, et al. Polishing porcelain veneers: An SEM and specular reflectance analysis. Dent Mater 1988;4:116-121.

357. Haywood VB, Heymann HO, Scurria MS. Effect of water, speed and experimental instrumentation on finishing and polishing porcelain intraorally. Dent Mater 1989;5:185-188.

358. Strassler HE, Nathanson D. Clinical evaluation of etched porcelain veneers over a period of 18 to 42 months. J Esthet Dent 1989;1:21-28.

359. Rucker ML, Richter WA, MacEntee M, Richardson A. Porcelain and resin veneers clinically evaluated: 2-year results. J Am Dent Assoc 1990;121:594-596.

360. Barnes DM, Blan LW, Gingell JC, Latta MA. Clinical evaluation of castable ceramic veneers. J Esthet Dent 1992;4: 21-26.

361. Strassler HE, Weiner S. Seven- to ten-year clinical evaluation of etched porcelain veneers (Abstract 1316). J Dent Res 1995;74:176.

362. Meijering AC, Roeters FJ, Mulder J, Creugers NH. Patientsí satisfaction with different types of veneer restorations. J Dent 1997;25:493-497.

363. Jordan RE, Suzuki M, Senda A. Clinical evaluation of porcelain laminate veneers: A four-year recall report. J Esthet Dent 1989;1:126-137.

364. Meijering AC, Creughers NHJ, Roeters FJM, et al. Survival of three types of veneer restorations in a clinical trial: A 2.5-year interim evaluation. J Dent 1998;26:563-568.

365. Gladys S, Van Meerbeek B, Inokoshi S, et al. Clinical and semi-quantitative marginal analysis of four tooth-colored inlay systems at three years. J Dent 1996;23:329-338.

366. Cardash HS, Baharal H, Pilo R, et al. The effect of porcelain color on the hardness of luting composite resin cement. J Prosthet Dent 1993;69:620-623.

367. Garber DA. Porcelain laminate veneers: To prepare or not to prepare? Comp Cont Educ Dent 1991;12:178-182.

368. Burke FJT. Fracture resistance of teeth restored with dentin-bonded crowns: The effect of increased tooth preparation. Quintessence Int. 1996;27:115-121.

8 Failures

Galip Gürel

Introduction

Few successful professionals have not encountered failure in their careers. And, if we are able to learn from them, mistakes or failures can actually be beneficial. Pioneers in any field are bound to sustain failures while seeking to improve techniques. Being human, even dentists are subject to failure, although when this sensitive technique is properly executed, failure rates in the field of PLVs are remarkably low.[1-3]

When PLV was first introduced in the 1980s,[4-6] the physical properties of the materials and the bonding systems that were used, along with some unknowns in the tooth luting resin–porcelain interface, made them prone to failure. However, vast improvements in these materials have minimized such problems. After bonding strength had improved,[7,8] researchers began to investigate why some PLV fractures continued to occur and to address the issues of function and occlusion.[1,9-11] Some more recent concerns include immediate failures resulting from incorrect treatment planning and periodontal problems and long-term esthetic failures, such as blackening of the margins stemming from microleakage at the tooth–porcelain margin interface.

Although only 3% to 4% of PLV applications will end in failure, the author believes that information concerning these failures should be shared with other dentists. This information is especially beneficial for less-experienced dentists, so that they are not discouraged when faced with similar immediate or longer-term failures. Every failure has a reason. This chapter attempts to cover a large selection: esthetic, mechanical, biological and occlusal.

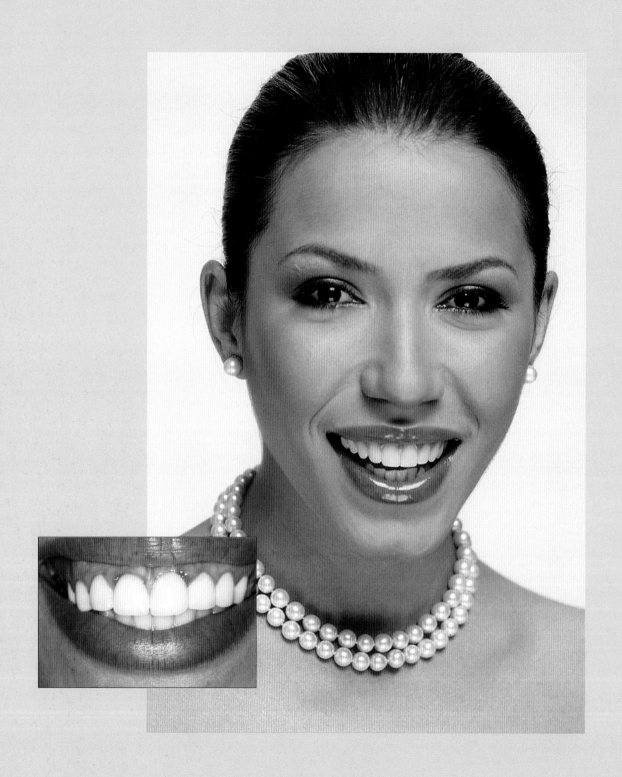

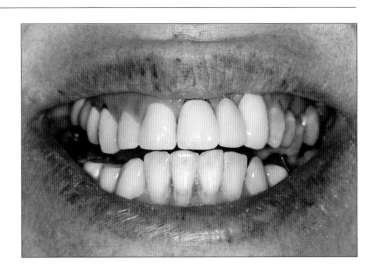

Fig 8-1 An immediate esthetic failure from the start. Attention has been paid to neither gingival harmony nor individual tooth form. The incisal edge silhouette displays a negative smile line and the shapes and positions of the canines are unacceptable. In such cases, achieving the best marginal fit or the strongest tooth–PLV bonding interface will mean little if the smile design is not planned in advance, and treatment will result in an unfavorable outcome.

Esthetic Failures

Esthetic dentistry is based on team effort between the dentist, the specialist, the technician and the patient. If the proper diagnosis or necessary treatment planning have not been carried out, then an immediate esthetic failure will probably occur.

The dentist

The dentist, acting as team leader, ultimately carries full responsibility for the esthetic outcome of any treatment. To ensure success, he or she must have many skills: awareness of the esthetic needs of each case, the necessary esthetic training, the ability to communicate with colleagues and patients, and the judgement to choose the correct team of specialists and technicians while staying up to date on current developments. Not only should the dentist be an expert in the technical and mechanical aspects of PLV, but also be sympathetic to the smile design itself (see Chapter 2).

Failure in smile design

The most important factor in each esthetic case is the smile design. If the dentist does not understand the basic principles of smile design, or is unable to visualize the final result, that treatment is doomed to failure before it even begins (Fig 8-1). The dentist must take into consideration the patient's face as a whole and focus on the relation of the teeth to the lip lines and to the face itself. To avoid failure, the esthetic dentist should be knowledgeable in the esthetic set-up, the incisal edge position, gingival asymmetries and the arch form (all of which are listed in the esthetic checklist).

It is the small details that ensure a successful outcome. Details such as creating deliberate asymmetries, incisal silhouettes, the reconstruction of the related soft tissues, proper usage of the porcelain materials and working with skilful technicians are equally important in achieving success.

Patients may not be aware of all the details involved in their treatment. However, if there is an immediate esthetic failure due to any of these details, then the patient will be unhappy (Fig 8-2).

Incorrect tooth preparation

Incorrect tooth preparation is another reason for esthetic failure, especially since PLVs are only 0.3–0.7 mm thick and are a very delicate form of restoration. The technician can efficiently build up the PLV only if the proper amount of space is supplied during the preparation. This issue is covered in detail in Chapter 7, enabling the dentist to achieve an almost 100% chance of success. However, the softening of the incisal edge needs careful handling, especially if a butt joint preparation is done. If a sharp corner is left at this junction than there will be an unesthetic horizontal line that shows through the bonded PLV

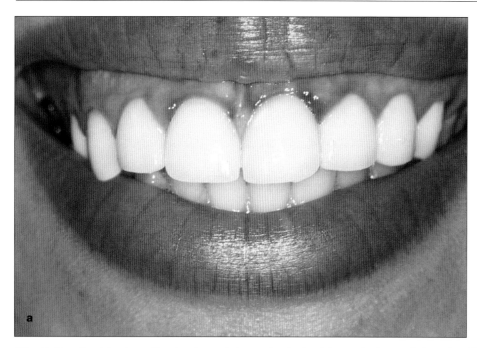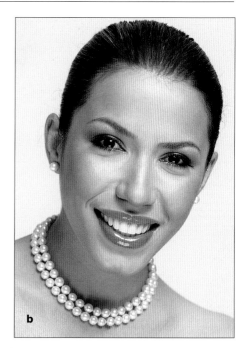

Fig 8-2a, b Most patients do not have technical knowledge of the details that make a smile pleasant, delicate and natural. (a) In such instances they express their feelings about themselves as "not liking the way I smile". The "gummy smile", canted gingival and incisal line and the incisal edge positions of the canines illustrate an immediate esthetic failure. (b) The power of an enhanced smile design on the patient's whole appearance. Not only is the gummy smile treated together with the displeasing canted gingival line but the form, texture and alignment of the teeth are in harmony with the lower lip line.

towards the incisal edge.[5,12] An overbulky veneer, or one that appears too thin, may result from a lack of depth preparation in the facial and gingival areas, thus threatening both the esthetics and the strength of the restoration.

The color of the underlying tooth, the thickness of the gingiva, the position of the lip line and the patient's attitude will all help to set the placement and depth of the preparation line while designing the gingival margin prep.[13] If this is not properly executed, dark discoloration may appear now or in a few months' time, soon after the bonding of the PLV (Fig 8-3). For those patients with a high (or even medium) lip line, an annoying dark zone will be displayed when smiling or speaking.

The placement and finish of the interproximal margins are delicate issues. To avoid visibility of the tooth porcelain interface when viewed from different angles, these procedures must be properly executed. Although no mechanical problems, such as marginal leakage, will arise from misplacement, it remains a reason for immediate esthetic failure (Fig 8-4).

Wrong case selection

Despite the widespread use of porcelain restorations, there are still some contraindications for their use and their esthetic success. For example, PLV alone is not sufficient to close large spaces between teeth as in cases of exaggerated diastema. PLV treatment must in these cases be preceded by orthodontic treatment. A very common mistake in the treatment of a large diastema that exists between the two centrals is to attempt to close the diastema with two veneers placed on the centrals.[14] This will only add another esthetic problem, as the two centrals will then become too wide horizontally, losing their individual proportions (Fig 8-5). As the centrals are the most prominent teeth in the smile, the whole composition will be ruined if they are not in proportion. In order to distribute the visual weights of proportion between those anteriors, it may be wise to include the laterals or even the canines in the treatment planning. If such diastemas also have severe periodontal problems then it may be wise not to treat the case with PLVs at all.

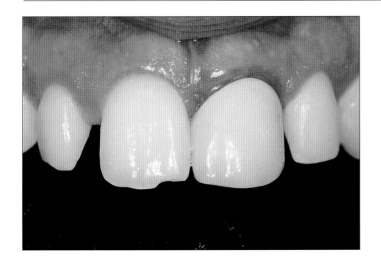

Fig 8-3 A monochromatic single PLV is placed on tooth #21(9). The gingival preparation line is kept level with the soft tissue, without paying much attention to the dark discoloration of the tooth underneath and the possibility of later gum recession. Note the recession after three years and the dark line appearing at the PLV–gingiva interface, illustrating a long-term esthetic failure. This would have been more of an issue if the patient also displayed a high lip line.

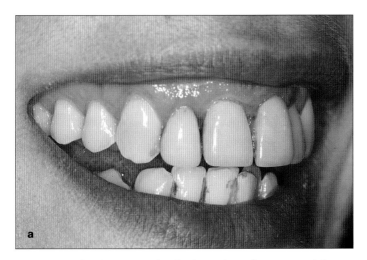
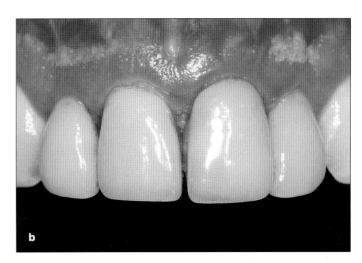

Fig 8-4a, b Improperly designed and prepared interproximal margins. They are kept short of the contact points or areas labially, causing an immediate esthetic failure. Such failures can easily be detected while observing from an angle (a). However, in some extreme failures it can be seen from the facial angle as well (b).

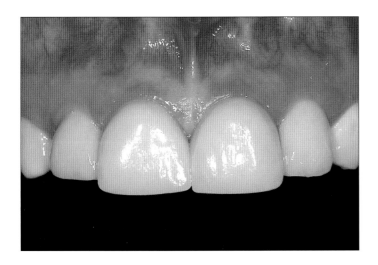

Fig 8-5 A diastema closure case. Even though the four anterior teeth are veneered, the diastema is closed only by enlarging the PLVs on the centrals mesially, creating two disproportionately designed wide centrals.

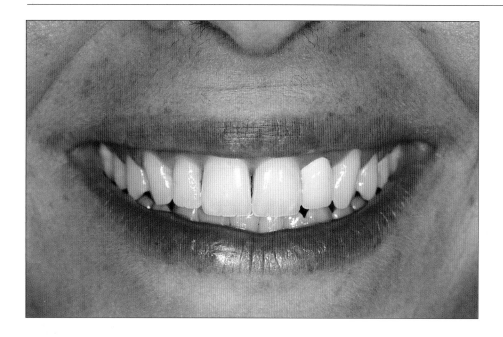

Fig 8-6 Lack of laboratory communication. Tooth #22(10) is treated with a PLV. However, the final result in terms of a color match is a failure owing to the lack of color transfer between the dentist and laboratory.

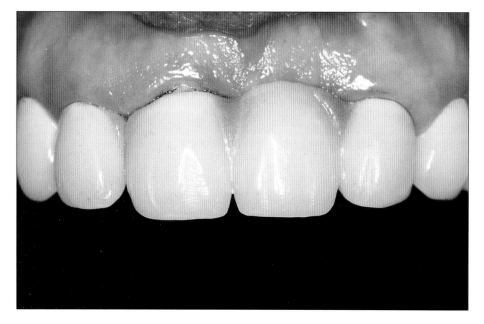

Fig 8-7 Working with an inexperienced lab. Technicians may create esthetic failures. Note the failure of the final esthetic outcome, owing to both the lack of communication and the limited talent of the esthetic technician. The restorations are monochromatic in color, missing all the details in terms of tooth form, texture and gingival architecture.

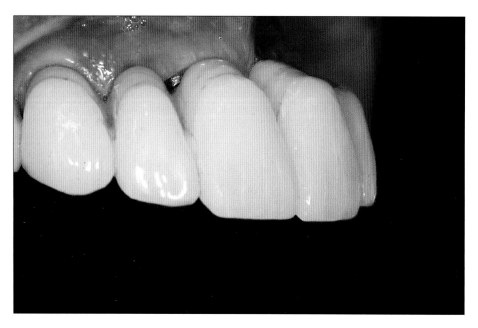

Fig 8-8 A class III type of occlusion esthetically corrected with overbuilt restorations over the implants. It is obvious to see that the dentist ended up with an unacceptable esthetic design because of the patient's unrealistic demands for extra lip support. Such a failure not only appears esthetically unpleasant but affects the occlusal relationship and thus the function as well.

Lack of communication with the patient and the lab

In order to achieve a successful esthetic result, it is vitally important to be aware of your patient's expectations and his or her state of mind. Some of your own treatment proposals may not be suitable for a particular patient and could result in an unhappy outcome for them. So, to avoid unpleasant results that could damage the dentist's reputation, it is best to make good use of all the available tools, such as computer imaging, composite mock-ups, wax-ups, provisionals, etc., to communicate and illustrate your ideas to your patient and to gain your patient's approval before the final veneers are fabricated.

The dentist's skills in communicating with their lab technician are equally important in achieving a successful result. Good rapport with and the full agreement of your patient will mean little if you cannot convey these to the technician (Fig 8-6).

The technician

To ensure success in delicate esthetic cases it is essential to work with a talented, dedicated and knowledgeable ceramist. Your lab technician must be skilful in handling different porcelain materials and techniques, up to date with new developments and aware of all the application indications. The lab technician should be dedicated to excellence, patiently layering the ceramic, while paying attention to form, surface texture, color and especially to function and occlusion. A poor technician will most probably create an open-margined non-characterized PLV that is an esthetic failure – dull and monochromatic (Fig 8-7).

The patient

Patients themselves may be the cause of esthetic or functional failure. Those patients with impossible or unrealistic expectations and no knowledge or understanding of natural beauty may actually lead the dentist to create an unnatural smile design. Some patients may even arrive with pictures cut from magazines displaying the smile of a very young and beautiful model or actress, requesting the same smile even though they have neither the complexion nor the facial outlines or lip size remotely to resemble that person. The dentist who attempts to produce such an unrealistic request is bound to fail.

Every patient has a natural lip position in relation to his or her teeth, even if it is not the most esthetic configuration. Sometimes patients who are not happy with their lip postures, end up in a dental office asking for extremely overbulked anterior teeth forms in order to obtain this missing lip support. Since they are only focused on the issue of lip posture, they may put pressure on the dentist to design an otherwise unrealistic tooth form. If the patient is able to influence the dentist with their unrealistic expectations, the treatment will result in failure and in the long run may even be damaging to the reputation of the dentist (Fig 8-8).

Good communication between patient and dentist enables the dentist to explain to the patient the negative effects of an unrealistic smile design – one that will not blend in with his or her natural facial composition – and will prevent such failures. However, if the patient is adamant with an unrealistic request, the dentist will be wise not to accept the case.

Mechanical Problems

Fracture

The PLV, which is actually a very thin and delicate thin piece of glass, is fragile and may easily break before it is bonded to the tooth surface. So the application procedure necessitates very delicate handling. The dentist or assistant can apply too much pressure on the PLV and may even fracture it (Fig 8-9). The entire esthetic team must therefore exercise great care in handling the PLV until it is bonded. Fracturing after bonding is completed is also a possibility but is due to different reasons.

The enamel and dentin on the tooth surface to which PLV restorations are bonded[15] exhibit different characteristics. The restorations are exposed to external stimuli in the mouth and to mechanical forces, too, as they work under occlusal and functional forces. Mechanical failures may be due to adhesive or cohesive problems, internal or external forces or to faulty design.

Adhesive Problems

Adhesive failure, or debonding, was a serious problem in the past, due to inferior bonding agents. However, with today's improved bonding techniques, it is one of the less likely reasons for failure.[7,8] The thickness and opacity of the veneer will dictate the choice of the luting agent and so the choice of luting cement should be carefully made. Careful analysis of the tooth and PLV is required. If the porcelain is too opaque, or the thickness of the veneer exceeds 1 mm, then a dual-cure composite resin can be a better choice in order to achieve complete polymerization.[16-19] Without complete polymerization, adhesive failure is likely.[7,8]

Tooth–luting resin interface

In cases of debonding, in order to determine the reason for failure, the prepared tooth surface should first be thoroughly checked. If the surface of the tooth is relatively clean and free of bonding agents or luting composite, then it is an indication that the failure is due to a problem at the tooth–luting resin interface. It is probable that a step was missed in the process of treating the tooth surface before the actual bonding of the veneer (Fig 8-10), and so failure may be due to etching,[20] priming,[21] bonding[22] or light curing[19] or to contamination of the tooth surface during any of the bonding stages. The interior humidity of the mouth or exposure to oral contaminants make it likely that a great percentage of the debonding occurs at the tooth–resin interface.

If the PLV is still intact, the PLV can be rebonded. In such cases most of the luting resin will be found on the inside of the PLV (Fig 8-11). In order to use the same debonded PLV, the tooth surface and the inside of the PLV must be recleansed and the veneer tried-in again. If the margin fit is correct, the same veneer can be rebonded to the same tooth (Fig 8-12) (see Chapter 7). However, if any cracks or chipping or marginal gaps are detected, then a new impression must be taken and a new PLV made.

Porcelain–luting resin interface

In the case of debonding, one is less likely to find a very clean porcelain surface owing to the fact that composite bonds react better to etched, silanated porcelain than to the tooth surface.[23,24] However, in some cases it is possible that bonding composite will be found on the tooth surface, indicating that a problem exists between the luting composite and PLV interface (Fig 8-13). The same recleansing techniques can be followed – however, special attention to the internal surface of the PLV will help to ensure more successful and predictable results. Special attention should be given to: careful sand blasting,[25,26] proper etching, avoidance of contamination after etching,[6,23] silanizing,[27,28] adequate wetting of the porcelain surface and keeping the veneer as stable as possible during bonding.

Failures Due to Internal or External Forces

Adhesive or cohesive failure, or any combination of these, may cause fractures so that a part of the PLV may be broken while the other bonded part remains intact.

Adhesive fracture

When a PLV that has been applied with a lack of adhesion gets broken as a result of external stimuli, the fracture itself is displayed as the

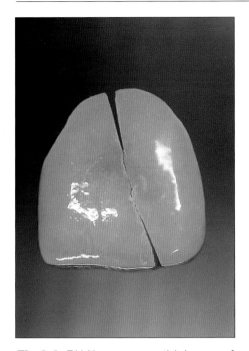

Fig 8-9 PLV has a mean thickness of 0.3–0.9mm and is prone to fracture before being bonded. It will be frustrating for both the dentist and the patient to achieve a result that is a failure at the final appointment, when the patient's expectations are at their highest.

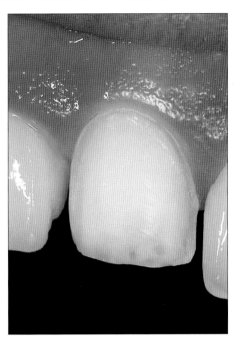

Fig 8-10 Adhesive failure on the tooth–luting resin interface. The clean surface condition of the tooth structure indicates that proper bonding on the tooth surface has not been achieved.

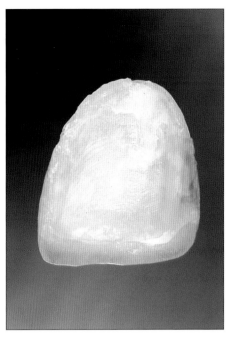

Fig 8-11 Another indication of this condition is the luting resin that stays intact on the inside of the PLV surface. This clearly shows that a mistake was made on the tooth surface preparation during the bonding procedure.

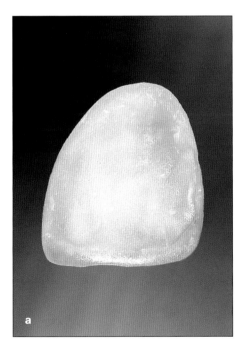

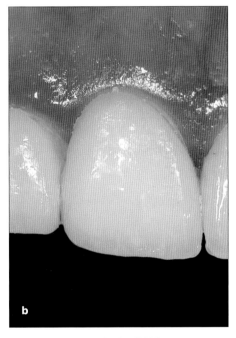

Fig 8-12a, b (a) In most total debonding cases the whole PLV comes out intact. In such cases the PLV should first be tried-in again on the same tooth. If no marginal gaps are detected, then the inside of the PLV can be sand blasted, cleansed and acid etched (b) and bonded on the newly retreated tooth surface. If all the procedures are done in the proper sequence, then this PLV will hold on the tooth, as if a new PLV has been placed. Note the perfect condition of the PLV nine months after being rebonded.

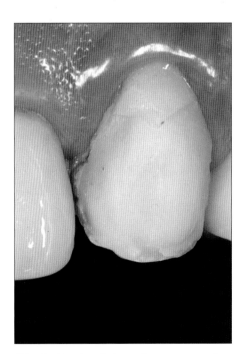

Fig 8-13 In debonding cases, the difficulty is rarely due to a problem at the luting resin–porcelain interface. In such cases, the luting resin will stay on the tooth surface, whereas the inside of the PLV will remain reasonably clean.

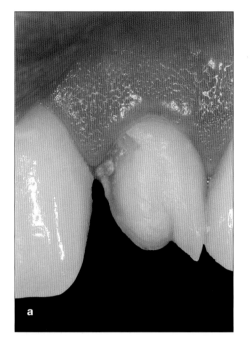
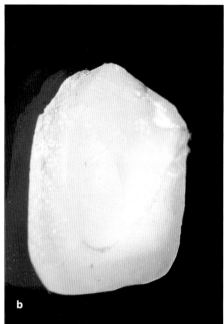
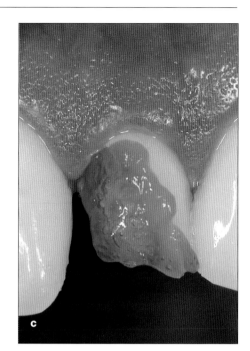

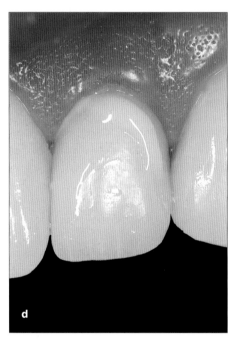
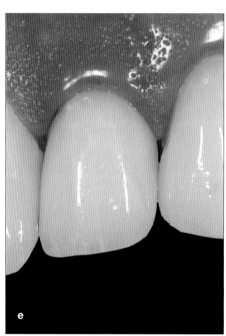

Fig 8-14a-e (a, b) A typical fracture due to both adhesive and cohesive failures. The strongly bonded PLV piece stays intact on the tooth, whereas the other portion is debonded due to lack of proper adhesion and an external stimulus (trauma). (c, d) Both pieces are examined and tried-in again. In emergencies, if the two pieces are kept intact and no marginal discrepancies are observed, then the tooth surface can be cleaned and re-etched together with the PLV surface, and rebonded on the tooth surface. (e) If this repair is delicately executed, it will be difficult to spot the margin where the two pieces are rebonded. Note the almost invisible margin, two years after rebonding.

larger portion of the broken PLV. Although trauma will be the cause, the lack of adhesion results in a larger amount of porcelain debonding while the other smaller portion remains intact on the tooth (Fig 8-14 a and b). The best solution in this case is to remove the small, intact, bonded portion of the PLV, make a new impression and build a new PLV. However, in emergencies, if the dentist believes that the bonded portion is strong enough, then the debonded broken piece of veneer can be sandblasted, acid etched, salinated and rebonded over the tooth again. Even though some marginal discrepancy may be observed between the two pieces at close range, this kind of applications usually presents esthetically pleasant results. Such repair should be closely followed up and if any kind of marginal leakage is observed between the two pieces of porcelain, then the PLV should be removed and a new one fabricated (Fig 8-14 c-e). It is extremely important to determine the cause of the fracture in such cases. If it is due to occlusal forces, it will most probably break again if the necessary adjustments are not made.

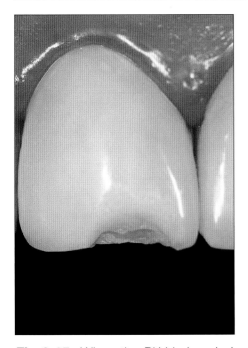

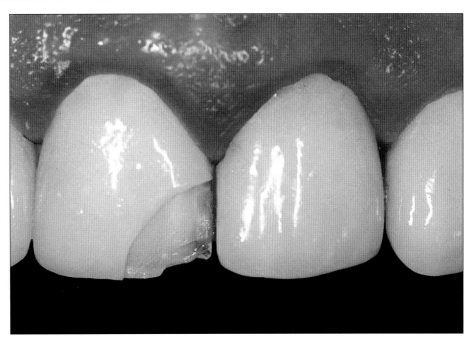

Fig 8-15 When the PLV is bonded strongly on the tooth, a cohesive fracture may occur due to an external stimulus. In such cases, the broken part will be limited to where the trauma is located.

Fig 8-16 When the tooth is not prepared deeply enough, the result will be an overbulked PLV restoration. In order to prevent the esthetic failure, another mistake can be further made by extreme thinning out of the PLV surface, thus creating a chance for adhesive and cohesive fractures. Note the marginal gingivitis due to overbulked emergence profile of the PLVs.

Cohesive fracture

Cohesive fractures may be caused by trauma to the veneer. If adhesion has been successfully completed, only a small part of the PLV will chip off, leaving most of the PLV intact (Fig 8-15). If any mistakes are made during the preparation of the tooth, creating sharp line angles, an internal crack may occur. If the PLV is strongly bonded to the tooth, this internal stress may create only a crack line. However, internal stress can actually cause a part of the PLV to chip off when it has not been properly adhered. Iatrogenic factors may also cause cohesive fractures. If pipe smoking and other similar activities continue, any related areas may exhibit fractures (Fig 8-15). After the cause has been determined, it can either be restored with composite, if the broken piece is limited to only the PLV surface, or a new PLV should be carefully fabricated.

Combination fracture

A fracture that is both adhesive and cohesive is generally related to an iatrogenic origin. Incorrect tooth preparation[9,29] plays a major role in such fractures. Fractures may occur if the surface of the tooth has not been prepared sufficiently to create adequate space for the PLV build up (Fig 8-16).

Support for the porcelain must be taken care of during the preparation of the tooth. In the case of a thin incisal edge, the edges must be included in the preparation limits in order to form a butt joint, avoiding any kind of sharp edges and preventing internal stresses.[29] A thorough check should be made with a silicon index and (a)esthetic pre-evaluative temporaries (APT, see Chapter 7). Excessively deep preparations that expose the dentin will increase the risk of microleakage and postoperative pain.

Too–thick die spacer

A large space between the tooth and the PLV may cause cracking. This may occur when too much

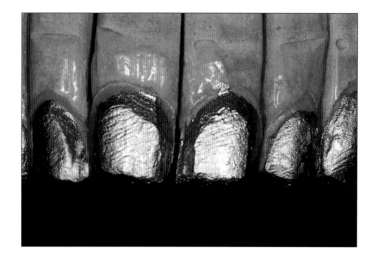

Fig 8-17 Applying too much die spacer on the dies, in order to create more space for the luting resin, may create adhesive–cohesive bonding failures postoperatively. The amount of the thickness of the luting resin should not exceed 1/3rd of the thickness of the porcelain being bonded. Moreover, when too thick a luting resin is required, there may be a risk of marginal leakage due to possible polymerization shrinkage of the high-volume resin.

space has been left for the luting composite at the tooth–porcelain interface. If the thickness of the luting resin is thicker than 1/3rd of the PLV thickness, debonding or fractures are bound to occur (Fig 8-17).[30]

Some dentists prefer a thick luting resin due to their concerns about the final PLV color. In order to have the option of changing the PLV color, if necessary, some dentists or technicians tend to leave too much space for the luting resin. The author believes that attempting to change the color of the PLV at this stage will create other problems which may be related to polymerization shrinkage of the thicker luting resin (see Chapter 7). Therefore, good communication with the lab is essential to avoid problems stemming from an excessively large luting resin space.

Color Change

Luting resin

Mismatching colors or color change may also be reasons for failures. The best way to avoid mismatching the colors of the PLV and natural teeth is to develop good communications with your technician. Stump shade transfer and a brief explanation of the PLV color, texture and form should be supported with pictures, Polaroid photographs and slides.[5,31] If this is done properly, the dentist can then use translucent luting resin for the final bonding stage, thereby creating a perfect color fit that is more natural and stable.

If the final color of the PLV does not match, however, and needs to be altered with a colored luting resin, then the color differences between the nonpolymerized and polymerized state of the resin should be carefully studied to prevent an immediate esthetic failure. It is well accepted that a color difference will most probably occur between the same colored dual- or light-cured resins before and after being polymerized.[17-19] Using a luting resin other than a transparent or translucent one, will also distort the chameleon effect of the margins. A colored demarcation line will be observed at the margins instead of an agreeably blended tooth-veneer interface. If a colored luting resin is to be used, then the cervical margins have to be prepared subgingivally, in order to avoid such an esthetic failure that will be seen at the gingival margin.

Stump shades that have been taken from an overly dry tooth will also cause color-related problems. A dry tooth looks lighter in color than its original stump shade and this is even more obvious on dark, discolored teeth. If the stump shade is taken from an excessively dry tooth surface then the PLV will look darker immediately after bonding.

Since the adjacent teeth dehydrate and appear lighter during the bonding process of one or two veneers, the PLV may appear darker than the

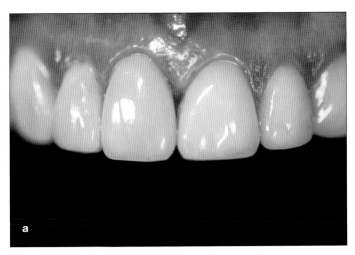
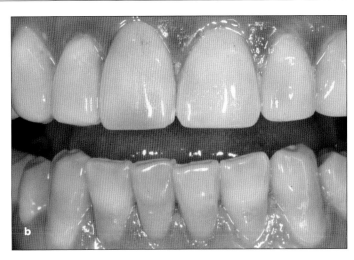

Fig 8-18a, b (a) When ultra-thin PLVs are bonded on teeth, after several years their values can be lowered due to the intrinsic color change of the aging teeth. Even though this cannot be termed a failure, it is a fact that dentist and patient must be aware of in order to prevent further complications. (b) Note the change in value of the PLVs after being in service for fourteen years.

adjacent teeth immediately following bonding. For the inexperienced eye this phenomenon may be perceived as an immediate failure, when in fact it is not. As the adjacent teeth rehydrate, and return to their original color, this mismatch will disappear. However, the dentist should be aware of this fact and it should be specifically explained to the patient that in only a few hours' time, when the teeth rehydrate, the color will match the PLV.

Microleakage at the margins can also be partially responsible for a local color change, limited to where the microleakage is located, and can cause immediate or a long-term failure.

Glazing and Polishing

A detailed sequence of treatment planning and tooth preparation is vitally important in PLV treatment. All problems related to the PLV's length, form and texture, as well as to the smile design, should be corrected at the try-in stage so that the lab can apply the final glaze and polish to the external PLV surface. If these problems are not corrected at the try-in stage, then the corrections will have to be done after they are bonded, result-

ing in a roughened porcelain surface that has lost its glaze[32-34] and is prone to color change from extrinsic colorant. Even though the various intra-oral polishing techniques available to the dentist will be very effective, it will never be the same quality that the laboratory glazed-and-polished surface can produce. Proper application of the whole process of PLV treatment will prevent long-term failures.

Aging

The natural process of aging, which is responsible for the darkening of teeth, will affect the longer-term color of the PLV. Ultra-thin veneers that are bonded with a translucent luting resin will darken in color ten to fifteen years after the operation. However, as it is part of the process that natural teeth will also follow, it will not be perceived as a failure by the patient (Fig 8-18). If the PLVs are made so opaque that the natural change of the color of the teeth cannot be seen though the veneers, then when the natural teeth begin to get darker due to aging, the PLVs will appear high in value (Fig 8-19) and create an esthetic problem.

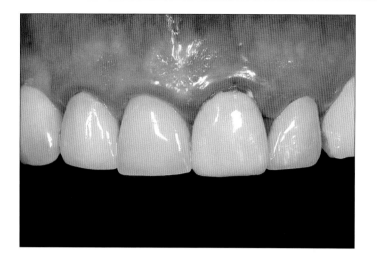

Fig 8-19 Discoloration due to aging. Since the PLVs on teeth #12(7) and #21(9) were built up on an opaque core, they are not affected with this intrinsic color shift, displaying a shade difference with the adjacent PLVs 10 years postoperatively. Also note the marginal gingival inflammation.

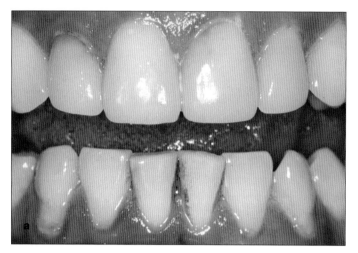
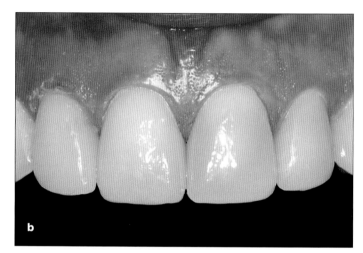

Fig 8-20a, b When microleakage is observed, it is usually seen at the cervical area. This is mostly due to failures created at the time of bonding. Interference of sulcular fluids or blood with the bonding material can cause this kind of internal discoloration at the gingival tooth–porcelain interface, displaying itself as an immediate or a long-term failure. (a) Teeth #12(7) and 21(9) displaying dark internal discoloration due to microleakage. Since the dentin was sealed (etched, primed and adhesive applied) just after the preparation and before the impression is made, no postoperative sensitivity is experienced in this particular case. (b) However, in order to correct this esthetic failure, the existing veneers discolored through microleakage have to be removed, the tooth surface cleansed, a new impression made and the teeth restored with the new PLVs. The case five years after the veneers are replaced.

Microleakage

Microleakage is one of the major causes of an esthetic and mechanical failure and can be related to various factors. Unfortunately, microleakage can only be detected after the PLV bonding is complete and so the only solution to correct this problem is to replace the PLV (Fig 8-20).

Margin Preparation

An incomplete or incorrect margin preparation can be one of the major reasons for failure (see Chapter 7). The cases that require the subgingival margins to finish at the dentin or root surface are more likely to be prone to leakage as these are relatively weaker bonding surfaces in comparison to enamel.[1,35-38] Subgingival margins should be delicately isolated before and during bonding in order to avoid interference of the sulcular fluids with the bonding surfaces which would inhibit or distort the polymerization and thus result in microleakage.

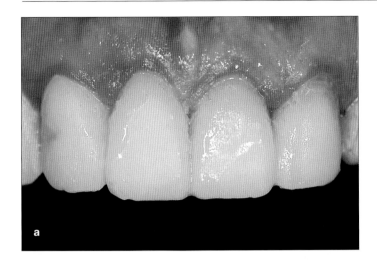

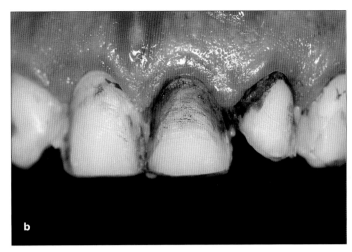

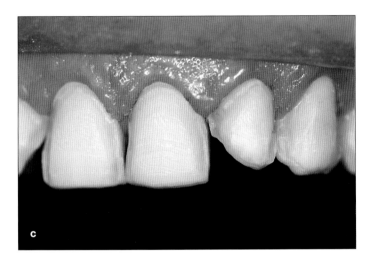

Fig 8-21a-c (a) Microleakage is usually seen at the provisionalization stage, especially if the provisionals are only spot bonded on the teeth. Failure to adapt the margins properly will increase the chances of microleakage. (b, c) This dark staining due to microleakage usually remains superficial and can be easily removed either by cleaning with hydrogen peroxide for a few seconds or by sand blasting.

Provisionals

The critical provisionalzation stage must be carefully handled, with great attention given to ensure that the provisionals are properly cemented, as they may come out easily at this stage. On the other hand, if they are fully cemented, difficulties in debonding or cracks on the prepared teeth may create problems just before the try-in.

Most microleakage occurs at this stage, and no matter what technique is applied, temporary cementation over the unetched enamel is one of the biggest factors. If the margins are not properly fitted, microleakage is inevitable, as the bonding agents used do not produce a true mechanical bond (Fig 8-21a).

If the leakage reaches dentin which has not been properly sealed after the preparation, then the color change may be followed by postoperative sensitivity. Minimal or no postoperative sensitivity is possible if the dentin is hybridized just after the preparation. Leakage can be easily observed when the provisionals are taken out (Fig 8-21b). This can be eliminated if the area is scrubbed with hydrogen peroxide for a few seconds, and, if there is resistance, the next choice is to sand blast (Fig 8-21c).

Lack of Marginal Fit

Precise impressions of the prepared margins should be made and transferred to the laboratory. The same precision should be applied for the porcelain build up, in order to avoid any marginal gaps. The ceramist must check the finished PLV margins on the main plaster model before they are sent to the dentist and the dentist should also do the same check during the try-in session. If a

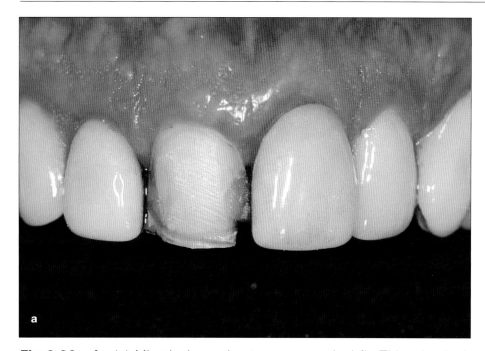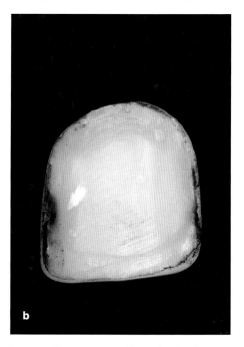

Fig 8-22a, b (a) Microleakage due to poor marginal fit. This microleakage is mostly seen on the gingival area due to the nature of the bonding surface. Thin enamel or preparing subgingivally may result in placing the margins on the dentin or root surface and will increase the chances of microleakage (teeth#12(7) and #21(9)). (b) It is also possible to see microleakage on the interproximal tooth–porcelain interface. The chances of microleakage are higher if the margin is placed on an existing composite.

lack of marginal fit is detected, the wisest option would be to renew the PLV to prevent microleakage and long-term failure.

Even though an attempt to hide or close the gaps with a luting composite may prevent microleakage, color changes in this composite at the tooth–porcelain interface will create esthetic problems in the long term (Fig 8-22).

Tissue Management

Perfect isolation at the bonding stage is vitally important. However, if periodontal health is not perfect or if the removal of provisionals has caused any damage to the tissues, then no matter what precautions are taken to isolate the field, the tissue may bleed, causing a negative effect on bonding. Mechanical force, chemical stimuli and etching agents can also cause bleeding. Not only will it distort the bonding and cause microleakage, but also cause color changes after

the bonding. In order to create a healthy medium for bonding, the bleeding must be stopped with chemical agents, electrosurgery or soft tissue lasers (Fig 8-23).

Isolation

The bonding procedure requires an immaculate working environment. Sectional applied rubber dams[25,26,39] help create an efficient working area for the dentist as well as preventing the teeth from becoming contaminated from the oral environment (Fig 8-24). The dentist should be aware of the effects of humidity on bonding. Humidity may be not only the cause of microleakage but also of the debonding of the PLV, by distorting the interface between the adhesive and the luting resin on the tooth surface.

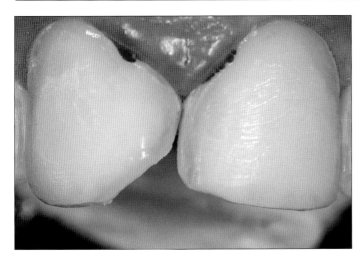

Fig 8-23 Tissue management is extremely important throughout the whole treatment, but especially at the bonding stage. Bleeding tissues or sulcular fluids will distort the quality of bonding. They should be controlled with chemical agents or mechanically (e.g. with diode lasers).

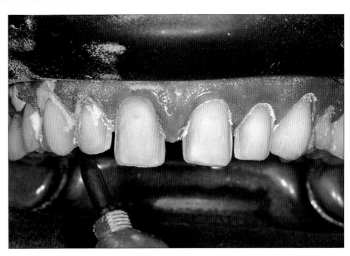

Fig 8-24 Even though it seems or sounds difficult, it is always better to isolate the area with a rubber dam application that will supply an area that is very clean and easy for the dentist to operate in. Contrary to what most dentists believe, this application will not take more than a few minutes.

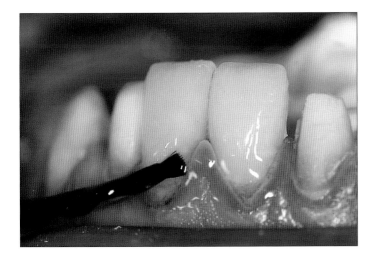

Fig 8-25 Polymerization of the luting resin is one of the crucial steps of PLV bonding. In order to eliminate the oxygen-inhibited layer formation on all the margins, oxygen-inhibiting agents (e.g. Deox, Ultradent) should definitely be applied, and not only limited to the gingival margin but also to the interproximal, palatinal and incisal margins as well.

Incomplete Polymerization

Completely polymerizing the luting resin is vital in preventing adhesive failure. Thick or opaque PLV may prevent light curing penetration. Even if all other precautions have been taken, the light curing mechanism should be checked and should be at a minimum 400–500 mw/cm².

The existence of an oxygen-inhibited area is one of the steps often overlooked by dentists. The oxygen-inhibited area can only be seen at the margins in a PLV case, and, if it is not properly attended to, it may cause postoperative marginal leakage. Therefore, in order to prevent oxygen penetration to the luting resin at the margins, all margins should be covered with oxygen-inhibiting agents and the area completely cured (Fig 8-25).

Biologic Failures

The basic fundamentals must be taken care of to avoid biologic failures, as in any other restoration. If the mistake that has been made is not corrected than it may be irreversible. Three of the most common biologic failures experienced are in the areas of periodontal, marginal and postoperative sensitivity.

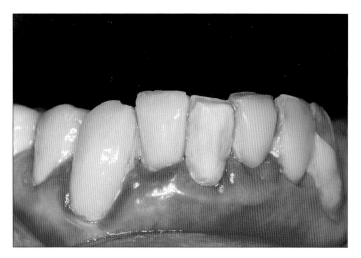

Fig 8-26 A periodontal and esthetic failure. Due to incorrect treatment planning, the gingival asymmetries have not been taken into consideration, creating an esthetic failure. The PLVs are overcontoured and placed subgingivally. Gingival recontouring of the PLV has been attempted after bonding, creating a rough porcelain surface, prone to plaque accumulation, and resulting in a serious periodontal (biologic) failure.

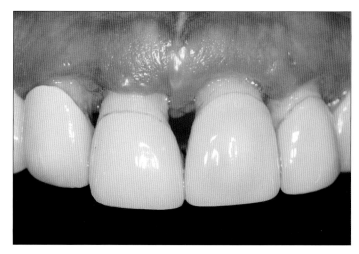

Fig 8-27 Biologic width should be seriously taken care of at treatment planning and respected throughout the preparation stage. Failure to understand the reaction of the biologic width will result in restorations that display black holes at the gingival embrasures and are the reason for an esthetic and biologic failure.

Periodontal problems

In the case of periodontal problems, the least likely restorative treatment would seem to be PLV, especially when compared to porcelain fused to metal restorations.[3] If a serious color change is not desired or if the gingival margin does not need to be extended due to subgingivally located cavities, then PLV is an advantage, as the gingival margins can and should be kept supragingivally.[35] However, problems may arise at the gingival interface if this concept is not given sufficient attention.

Biological width can be negatively affected by excessive luting resin flush left in the sulcus during bonding, or from an excessively overcontoured PLV emergence profile placed in the sulcus. Careful planning of the design of the PLV is, therefore, very important. It can even be worse if an attempt is made to contour[40] the marginal convexity at the gingival 1/3rd after the PLV is bonded. PLV that is properly glazed and polished lessens the plaque accumulation at the margins better than the natural tooth surface.[36,41] When this layer of melted porcelain is removed,[42] the rough surface that is exposed becomes a host

for the accumulation of plaque, and is therefore a prime source for periodontal failure (Fig 8-26).[34,43] Supragingivally placed margins, and avoiding recontouring after the PLV bonding, are the best solutions to prevent such mistakes.

Esthetic failure may occur when there is a biological response by the papilla in diastema closure cases, or in gingival alterations, when attention to the depth of the intercrestal bone is not given and a sound distance of 5 mm from the crest of the intercrestal alveolar bone to the interproximal contact area of the PLVs is not heeded[40] (Fig 8-27). A black hole due to papilla recession, which is not esthetically pleasing, will be created between the teeth if the distance is kept longer than 6–7 mm and the interproximal contact area is not placed apically, as it should be. Close attention to the intercrestal alveolar bone is very important when altering the gingival levels. The existing papilla will disappear if there is unnecessary intercrestal bone removal and the interproximal contact area is too low incisally. An unpleasant esthetic failure will be created due not only to distortion of the PLV form but also the gingival undulation (Fig 8-28).

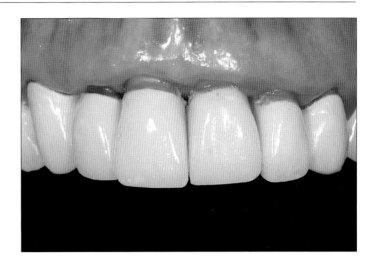

Fig 8-28 Bone is the foundation of the soft tissues. Maintaining proper gingival architecture is only possible when the alveolus bone is correctly recontoured during flap surgery. Extreme attention should be given specifically to the intercrestal bone (see Chapter 12) in order to maintain the papilla. If the intercrestal bone is unnecessarily removed, and the interdental contact areas are kept high towards the apical, the gingival architecture will lose its eye-pleasing undulations, displaying an unacceptable esthetic failure.

Postoperative sensitivity

Bacteria

Postoperative sensitivity is amongst the most annoying failures that can occur in adhesive procedures. Bacteria that remain on the dentin after an adhesive procedure can be one of the major reasons for postoperative sensitivity.[44] When bonding a veneer, great care should be taken in cleaning the tooth surface, especially to achieve a bacteria-free, clean dentin, to avoid such failures. The most accurate preventive method would be to seal the exposed dentin tubules when the dentin is freshly cut, immediately following preparation (see Chapter 7). This technique is not only beneficial in preventing bacterial invasion to the dentin tubules but also in enhancing the bonding, and thus minimizing the risk of postoperative sensitivity, especially in the provisional stage.

Etching-bonding

Postoperative sensitivity can also be caused by improper etching and bonding. The exposed dentin should not be etched for more than 10–15 seconds.[21,45] In order to equilibrate the depth created by the acid in dentin tubules and filled with the primer, the same brand etch-prime and adhesive materials should be used. In this way, debonding failures and postoperative sensitivity will be minimized. Before every application of the bonding materials, the expiration dates of the materials should be checked. Products that have passed their expiration date may be the reason for an unpolymerized interface and cause similar postoperative failures.

Improper Finishing

Polishing

The gingival margin should be cleansed of all excess bonding resin flush. However, if the excess has set, the procedure is not an easy one to accomplish. In a few days' time there is an immediate gingival response around the cervical margin when excess flush remains, especially in subgingival margin placements (Fig 8-26, see Chapter 7). This can be reversed if the excess is limited to the gingival sulcus. The problem can be solved by cleansing the flush by using tungsten carbide burs and polishing with rubber cups. If the gingival tissues are not healthy, gingival inflammation or recession after PLV placement is inevitable, and so the health and esthetic arrangement of the gingiva are very important factors in the treatment process. If unesthetic gingiva levels accompany the problem of unhealthy tissues, an immediate esthetic and biological failure is certain. To prevent scratching the root (or tooth) surface, the use of tungsten burs with no cutting end is vitally important.

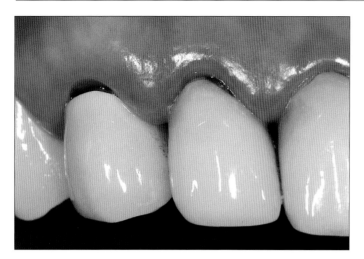

Fig 8-29 A combined carious lesion due to marginal microleakage and bad oral hygiene. The lesion is extended to both the root surface and underneath the PLV on tooth #12(7). The treatment of choice is to replace the PLV by further extending the gingival margin to where the lesion is cleaned.

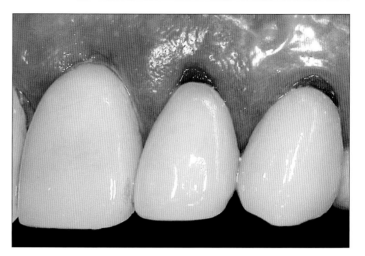

Fig 8-30 Carious lesion limited to the tooth surface only. Bad oral hygiene or a scratch on the root surface during cleaning the excess luting cement flush may cause such a carious lesion. A tight marginal seal of PLV prevents the carious lesion interfering with the PLV–tooth interface. The treatment of choice in such a case will be to remove the carious lesion and replace it with a composite filling without changing the PLV.

Excessive light cure

Correct timing in light curing the luting resin is essential. The pulp may be affected by the energy in terms of heat coming from the tip of a halogen light source. Even though it is suggested that one should apply 30–40 seconds of light curing, caution must be used, since irreversible pulp damage can be caused from application to a single spot. Light curing should therefore be given from various angles so as not to damage the pulp with the heat. Extra care should be given if a turbo tip is being used.

Marginal problems

Marginal leakage, which displays itself as discoloration or postoperative sensitivity, usually stems from poor marginal adaptation. In fact, microleakage can be the cause of carious lesions in the gingival area when the margin of the veneer is located on the dentin or root surface. If the gingival margin is located beyond the cementoenamel junction, the carious lesion may enlarge in the apical direction (Fig 8-29).

If scratches on the dentin or root surface are created iatrogenically while cleaning the excess

luting resin, that may be a serious reason for postoperative carious leasions, especially when combined with poor oral hygiene (Fig 8-30).

Occlusal Failures

If occlusal harmony has not been achieved then it is likely that the PLV will break due to occlusal interference. This is more common when attempting to lengthen the crown heights in patients who exhibit bruxing and grinding habits. PLVs are breakable and cohesive fractures may result from external stimuli or occlusal forces. If there is a broken veneer and no reports of an external trauma (Fig 8-31), occlusal disturbances are a likely cause. Unless the occlusal problem is solved, there is no point in changing the veneer, as it is bound to break in the same spot repeatedly. Therefore, the best solution to the problem is to rebuild a new PLV after adjusting the interferences in occlusion.

The provisionalization period is a useful opportunity to detect occlusal problems. If the provisionals break repeatedly in the same place, it is

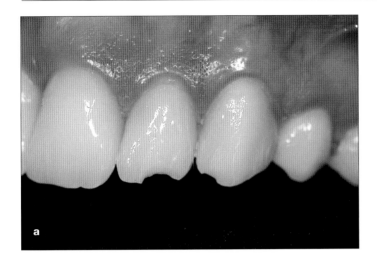

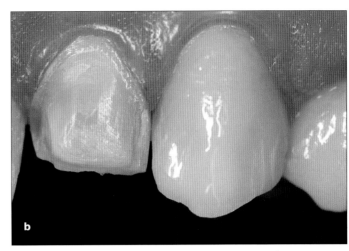

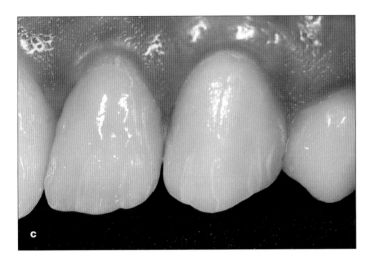

Fig 8-31a-c (a) Broken PLV due to occlusal failure. Care should be given to occlusal adjustments, especially lateral and protrusive excursions. This becomes more of an important issue in patients who exhibit bruxing habits. (b) In such cases, if the fracture is small, it can be adjusted with simple recontouring without affecting the esthetics (tooth #23(11)). However, when the fracture line affects the esthetics, the PLV should be removed and replaced (tooth #22(10)). (c) The final result after replacing tooth #22 (10) and incisally recontouring tooth #23(11). However, this failure will happen again if occlusion is not properly adjusted. It is highly recommended that such patients wear a bite-guard after the veneers are bonded.

only logical to suspect occlusal disturbances at those points. They should be analyzed and this information should be passed on to the ceramist so as to minimize these disturbance points. Careful placement of the occlusal margins of the premolars in onlay veneers and the lingual margins of the maxillary incisors is essential so that they are not located on a central contact point. Otherwise, it may easily result in mechanical failure after bonding as the continuous pressure on the margins may weaken the bond.

Occlusal problems can be minimized if the proper anterior guidance and guided lateral excursions are established.[5,40] The PLV does not necessarily break from the incisal under occlusal force. In fact, breakage at the cervical 1/3rd has been observed. The tooth becomes more flexible and loses its rigidity when it is stripped[9,46,47] of excessive enamel. Tension created in this area

due to tooth flexure provoked by extra occlusal forces and adhesive failures may cause the PLV to break at the gingival 1/3rd (Fig 8-32). The tooth loses its rigidity when aggressive tooth preparation reduces the surface enamel. Excessive occlusal force may add too much pressure and cause the PLV to break at the gingival 1/3rd. The lingual margins of the maxillary centrals should not be placed on the lingual concavities of the maxillary incisors, as there is an accumulation of tensile stress in those areas.

In the attempt to avoid occlusal interferences, the glazed porcelain surfaces are ground down, necessitating examination of the opposing arch, as such a surface may cause wear on the opposing enamel and dentin. If the lingual preparation of the maxillary incisors is overextended and in contact with the opposing arch, this can frequently be seen on the incisofacial surfaces of

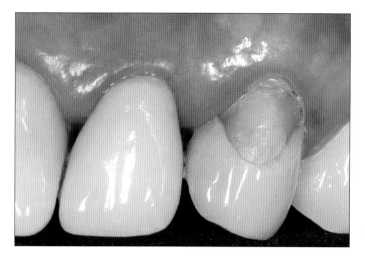

Fig 8-32 Biocompatible preparation for a bonded porcelain restoration is of vital importance. Too much stripping of the enamel at this stage will cause problems and may be the reason for long-term failures. Two major problems are created when unnecessary enamel is removed. One of them is the greater amount of dentin exposure, which may weaken the bonding, and the second is the increased flexibility of the tooth. When these two parameters are gathered then most probably a partial debonding at the facial gingival 1/3rd is seen.

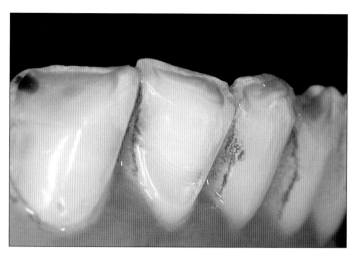

Fig 8-33 When removal of the glaze of the PLV from the palatinal surface is incorporated with an unfavorable occlusal relationship, the teeth on the opposing arch will abrade to various extents, depending on: the nature of the porcelain material used, the amount of intraoral polishing of the porcelain, the severity of the occlusal interference and its duration.

the mandibular incisors (Fig 8-33). Removal of the glaze from the lingual face of the maxillary veneers may result in this. However, these problems can be minimized if the correct selection of porcelain material is made, if close attention is paid to occlusion and anterior guidance and if the process is completed with the proper finishing and polishing techniques.

Conclusion

Failures are a part of any procedure and PLV treatment is no exception. Nevertheless, the longevity of and minimal failures related to PLV treatment have been confirmed in studies.[1-3, 36,48-50] Failures can be minimized provided there is careful treatment planning, proper material and case selection, if effective communication with the lab exists and if close attention to each clinical stage is given.

References

1. Clyde JS, Gilmore A. Porcelain laminate veneers. A preliminary review. Br Dent J 1988;164:9-14.

2. Calamina JR. Clinical evaluation of etched porcelain veneers. Am J Dent 1989;2:9-15.

3. Karlsson S, Landahl I, Stegersjö G, Milleding P. A clinical evaluation of ceramic laminate veneers. Int J Prosthodont 1992;5:447-451.

4. Rosenthal L. Clinical advantages of pressed ceramic restoration technology. Pract Periodont Aesthet Dent 1996; supplement.

5. Touati B, Miara P, Nathanson D. Esthetic Dentistry and Ceramic Restorations. New York. Martin Dunitz Ltd., 1999.

6. Simonsen RJ, Calamia JR Tensile bond strength of etched porcelain J Dent Res 1983;27:671-684.

7. Prati C, Nucci C, Montanari G. Shear bond strength and microleakage of dentin bonding systems. J Prosthet Dent 1991;65:401-407.

8. Triolo PT Jr, Swift EJ Jr. Shear bond strengths of ten dentin adhesive systems. Dent Mater 1992;8:370-374.

9. Magne P. Perspectives in Esthetic Dentistry. QDT 2000: 23;86-89.

10. Gemalmaz D. Use of heat-pressed, leucite-reinforced ceramic on anterior and posterior onlays: A clinical report. J Prosthet Dent 2002;87:133-135.

11. Paphangkorakit J, Osborn JW. The effect of pressure on a maximum incisal bite force in man. Arch Oral Biol 1997; 42:11-17.

12. Tronstad L, Leidal TI. Scanning electron microscopy of cavity margins finished with chisels or rotating instruments at low speed. J Dent Res 1974;53:1167-1174.

13. Lacy AM, Wada C, Weiming D, Watanable L. In vitro microleakage at the gingival margin of porcelain and resin veneers. J Prosthet Dent 1992;67:7.

14. Goldstein RE. Esthetics in Dentistry. 2nd ed. Hamilton, ON: BC Decker Inc, 1998:1:123-133.

15. Schroeder HE. Oral Structural Biology. Stuttgart: Thieme; 1991.

16. Chan KC, Boyer DB. Curing light-activated composite cement through porcelain. J Dent Res 1989;68:476-480.

17. Strang R, McCrosson J, Muirhead GM, Richardson SA. The setting of visible-light-cured resin beneath etched porcelain veneers. Br Dent J 1987;163:149-151.

18. Blackman R, Barghi N, Duke E. Influence of ceramic thickness on the polymerization of light-cured resin cements. J Prosthet Dent 1990;63:295-300.

19. Linden JJ, Swift EJ, Boyer DB, Davis BK. Photo-activation of resin cements through porcelain veneers. J Dent Res 1991;70:154-157.

20. Paul SJ. Adhesive Luting Procedures. Berlin: Quintessence, 1997;67-74.

21. Van Meerbeek B, Inokoshi S, Braen M, Lambrechts P, Vanherlege. Morphological aspects of the resin-dentin inter-diffusion zone with different dentin adhesive systems. J Dent Res 1992;71:1530-1540.

22. Gwinnett AJ. Interactions of dental materials with enamel. Trans Am Acad Dent Mater 1990;3:30-35.

23. Highton RM, Caputo AA, Matyas J. The effectiveness of porcelain repair system. J Prosthet Dent, 1979;42:292.

24. Jochen DG, Caputo AA. Composite repair of porcelain teeth. J Prosthet Dent 1977;38:673.

25. Dietschi D, Spreafico R. Current clinical concepts for adhesive cementation of tooth-colored posterior restorations. Pract Periodont Aesthet Dent 1998;10:47-54.

26. Roulet J-F. Posterior esthetic restoration. In: Dondi dall' Orologio G. Fuzzi M, Prati C (Eds.). Adhesion in Restorative Dentistry. Bologna: Valbonesi, 1995:27-47.

27. Nichols JI. Tensile bond of resin cements to porcelain veneers. J Prosthet Dent 1988;60:443.

28. Roulet J-F, Söderholm KJM, Longmate J. Effects of treatments and storage conditions on ceramic/composite bond strength. J Dent Res 1995;74:381-387.

29. Morley J. Critical Elements for the preparation and finishing of direct and indirect anterior restorations. Cont Esthet Dent. 1997;3:1-6.

30. Magne P, Kwon KR, Belser UC, Hodges JS, Douglas WH. Crack propensity of porcelain laminate veneers: A simulated operatory evaluation. J Prosthet Dent 1999;81:327-333.

31. Lombardi RE. The principles of visual perception and their clinical application to denture esthetics. J Prosthet Dent 1973;29:358-382.

32. Harasani MH, Isidor F, Kaaber S. Marginal fit of porcelain and indirect composite laminate veneers under in vitro conditions. Scand J Dent Res 1991;99:262-268.

33. Hannig M, Jepsen S Jasper V et al. Der Randschluß glaskeramischer Veneers mit zervikaler Schmelz- oder Dentinbegrenzung. Deutsche Zahnärtzliche Zeitschrift 1995;50:227-229.

34. Peumans M, Van Meerbeek B, Lambrechts P, Vuylsteke-Wauters M, Vanherle G. Five-year clinical performance of porcelain veneers. Quintessence Int 1998;29:211-221.

35. Kourkuata S, Walsh TF, Davis LG. The effect of porcelain laminate veneers on gingival health and bacterial plaque characteristics. J Clin Periodont 1994;21:638-640.

36. Strassler HE, Weiner S. Seven to ten year clinical evaluation of etched porcelain veneers (abstr 1316) J Dent Res 1995;74:176.

37. Christensen GJ, Christensen RP. Clinical observations of porcelain veneers: A three-year report. J Esthet Dent 1991; 3:174-179.

38. Gladys S, Van Meerbeek B, Inokoshi S et al. Clinical and semi-quantitative marginal analysis of four tooth-colored inlay systems at three years. J Dent 1996;23:329-338.

39. Garber DA, Goldstein RE. Porcelain and Composite Inlays and Onlays. Esthetic Posterior Restorations. Chicago: Quintessence, 1994.

40. Shillingburg Jr HT, Hobo S, Whitsett LD, Jacobi R, Brackett SE. Fundamentals of Fixed Prosthodontics. 3rd ed. Chicago: Quintessence, 1997;73-81.

41. Meijering AC, Creughers NHJ, Roeters FJM et al. Survival of three types of veneer restorations in a clinical trial: A 2.5-year interim evaluation. J Dent 1998;26:563-568.

42. McLean JW. The science and art of dental ceramics. Bridge design and laboratory procedures in dental ceramics. Chicago: Quintessence, 1980;2:189-209.

43. Goldstein GR, Barnhard BR, Pennugonda B, Profilometer SEM. Profilometer, SEM, and visual assessment of porcelain polishing methods . The Journal of Prosthetic Dentistry 1991;65:627-34.

44. Gwinnett AJ. Effect of Cavity disaffection on bond strength to dentin. J Esthet Dent. 1992;4 (special issue):11-13:995.

45. Paul SJ, Scharer P. Intrapulpal pressure and thermal cycling. Effect on shear bond strength of eleven modern dentin-bonding agents. J Esthet Dent 1993;5:179-185.

46. Schneider PM, Messer LB, Douglas WH. The effect of enamel surface reduction in vitro on the bonding of composite resin to permanent human enamel. J Dent Res 1981;60:895-900.

47. Magne P, Kwon KR, Belser UC, Hodges JS, Douglas WH. Crack propensity of porcelain laminate veneers: A simulated operatory evaluation. J Prosthet Dent 1999;12:111-121.

48. Strassler HE, Nathanson D. Clinical evaluation of etched porcelain veneers over a period of 18 to 42 months. J Esthet Dent 1989;1:21-28.

49. Rucker ML, Richter W, Macentee M, Richardson A. Porcelain and resin veneers clinically evaluated: 2-years result. J Am Dent Assoc 1990;121:594-596.

50. Barnes DM, Blan LW, Gingell JC, Latta MA. Clinical evaluation of castable ceramic veneers. J Esthet Dent 1992;4:21-26.

9   Porcelain Laminate Veneers for Diastema Closure

Galip Gürel

Introduction

A common feature found in the anterior dentition is the presence of diastemas between teeth. They may occur more frequently in certain ethnic groups or be simply due to anatomical differences. They usually distort a pleasing smile by concentrating the observer's attention not on the overall dental composition but instead on the diastema. However, before determining what might be the best treatment, any contributing factors should first be clearly defined. The diastemas can be due to growth and development deficiencies, excessive incisor vertical overlap from different causes, tooth size discrepancies, tooth angulations, pathological conditions, as well as many other factors. In order to close these diastemas, many forms of therapy can be used. A carefully developed diagnosis will lead the dentist to apply the most effective approach to address the patient's problem and to allow them to choose the most effective way of treatment.

Surgical frenectomies can be performed if the cause is the frenulum. They can also be orthodontically corrected if the proportions allow, or they can be prosthodontically corrected with the help of porcelain laminate veneers. If the contributing factors and various treatment plans are not fully considered from the beginning, the results may be discouraging.

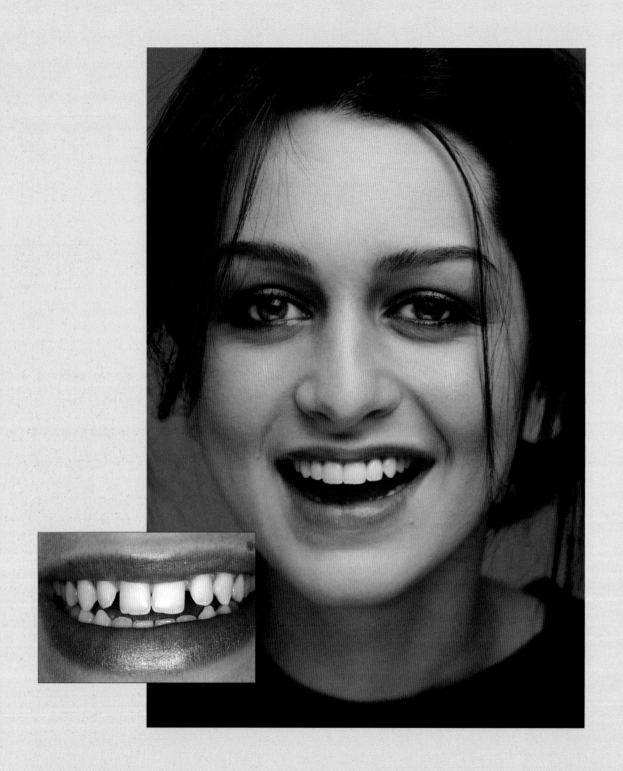

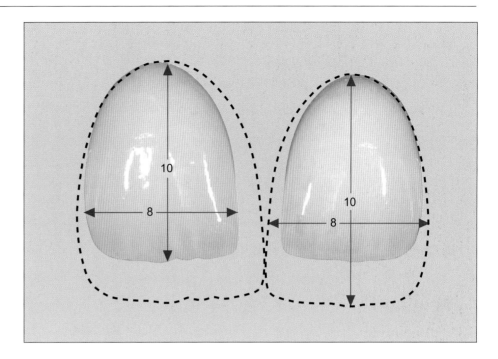

Fig 9-1 While closing diastemas, if the tooth length is also altered, a proportional relationship will be achieved.

Diastema closing is one of the most common indications of porcelain laminate veneers. However, it needs very careful advance planning in order to keep the individual tooth proportions together. The empty space that is determined by the size of the diastema gap should be closed proportionally and distributed amongst the anterior teeth, instead of building up a single or two veneers to close the entire space. Trying to close the gap with one or sometimes two veneers is a common mistake made by some dentists which will result in a return of the original problem.[1] Sometimes it may require correction of more than one or two teeth on either side of the space.

Teeth with identical widths but with different lengths will appear to have different widths.[2] This is an important principle to remember when closing diastemas in the anterior region, as an alteration will be introduced in the length:width relationship and can unfavorably alter the smile.[3] If the maxillary incisors are short and need to be lengthened in a diastema closing case, it is possible to alter the length of the anterior teeth incisally by using porcelain laminate veneers.[4] In this way the teeth will be lengthened as well as widened in order to close the diastema, and the width:height ratio can be maintained. If this is the case, no aesthetic pre-recontouring (APR) will be needed (Fig 9-1) (see Chapter 7).

However, if the dentist decides to maintain the present incisal edge position and there will be no gingival alterations, such as crown lengthening (which means that the teeth have an accepted vertical and horizontal proportion within themselves), then there will be a disproportional height:width relationship after the diastema is closed (Fig 9-2). The way to correct this problem is to arrange the centrals and laterals so that they will maintain their proper width as opposed to their proper height after the diastema is closed. In order to compensate for the horizontal gap between the two centrals and so as to keep the proper proportion of the teeth while closing the diastema, it must be balanced by reducing the distal portions of each central half the size of that gap, providing the midline is in its correct position. The same should be applied to the laterals and extended towards the canines. As the distal portion of the canine is not seen from a facial aspect, due to its position, this gap can be visually distinguished in that region. When this is the case, the dentist must include this illusion and proportion management in his treatment planning (Fig 9-3).

The best way to reduce the distal parts of the centrals and laterals is to make an APR before the actual material preparation within the limits of the wax-up and SI (Fig 9-7a, b). By so doing, the dentist will predict where the distal margins of

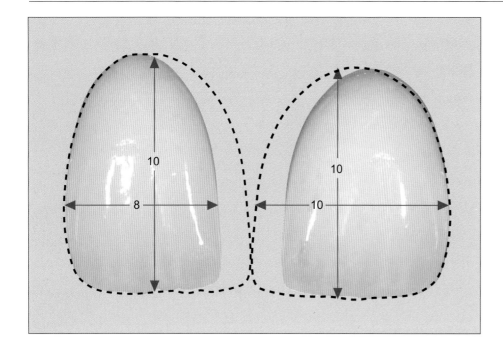

Fig 9-2 If the length is not changed, the veneers look either too short or too wide, losing their natural proportions.

Fig 9-3 When all teeth exhibit favorable proportions within themselves, it is very difficult to close the gap only by altering the centrals. If the size of the gap is x, than the distal margin of the centrals should be trimmed to x/2. This should proportionally be done at the laterals within the limits of x/4 and should be compensated for with the canine width.

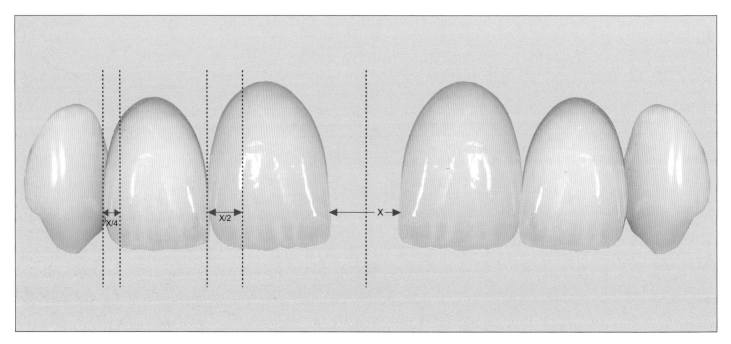

these teeth will be. Later, during the actual material preparation, it will ease the precise location of the interproximal elbows and create an exact space for the laboratory technician to build the porcelain laminate veneers both on the distal aspect of the centrals and laterals and the mesial aspects of the laterals and canines. During this pre-recountouring, the SI, which has been prepared by the lab over the wax-up model, can be used as a reference guide. That will dictate where the distal edges of the centrals and laterals should be placed. If the dentist has not been supplied with an SI, then they can add some composite mock-up on the mesial aspects of the centrals to visualize the proportion of the teeth within themselves and then reduce the distal portion of the centrals continuing in the same way towards the canines.

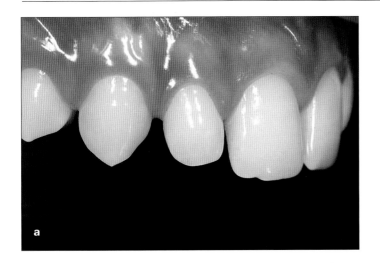
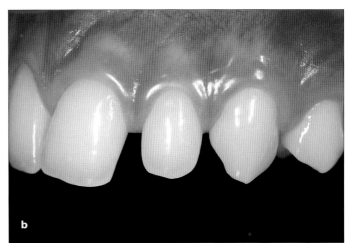
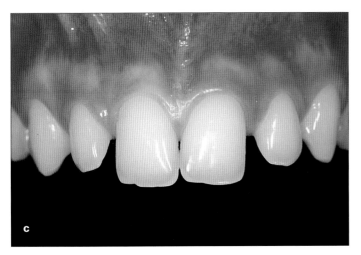
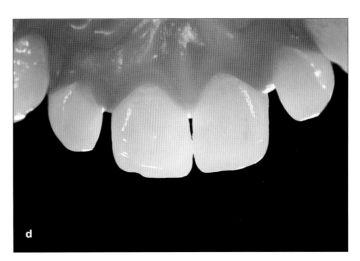

Fig 9-4a-d Diastema closing needs careful treatment planning, especially when more than one diastema exists.

Technique

Each case has to be evaluated as mentioned above. However, when it comes to multi-diastemas, it becomes far more challenging. Now that more than one or two gaps exist, the treatment should be planned in a more advanced way (Fig 9-4). The study models and composite mock-up transfers should be sent to the laboratory, so that the technician will be able to close the diastemas while paying close attention to the issue of function as well as individual tooth proportions.

Examining the smile on a stone model is very different from examining it as a whole with the lips and the face. In cases where some lengthening of the teeth may be necessary in order to compensate for widening the porcelain laminate veneers to close the gaps, the position of the lips in relation to incisal edge position plays an important role. To understand the existing conditions, the basic three positions of the lips – rest, half smile and full smile – should be observed (Fig 9-5). The lab should be instructed whether or not to lengthen the teeth incisally or apically with gingival alterations. Once the treatment option is selected, the lab can wax-up the models (Fig 9-6). SI will be the easiest way to visualize the final outcome when seated over the unprepared teeth, especially in terms of locating the interproximal contact (Fig 9-7). This will also help to identify the protruding portions of the teeth that should be reduced even before doing anything with APR, so that the SI will seat passively on the teeth (Fig 9-8).

The best way of visualizing the final outcome and to prepare the teeth accurately is to make use of the APT over the non-prepared teeth (Fig

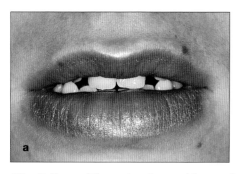
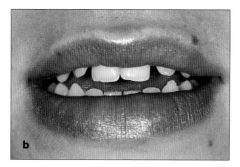
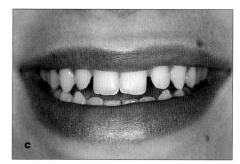

Fig 9-5a-c Three basic positions of the lip and teeth relationship should be studied. (a) Lips at rest (b) Half smile (c) Full smile.

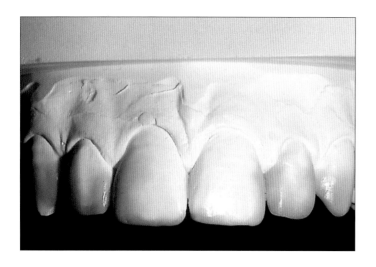

Fig 9-6 The study model must be waxed-up at the laboratory in order to visualize the final outcome, as well as to check the function.

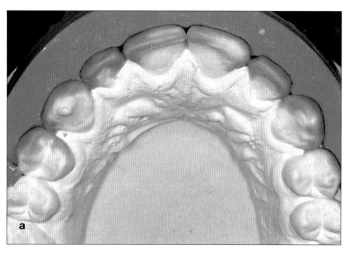
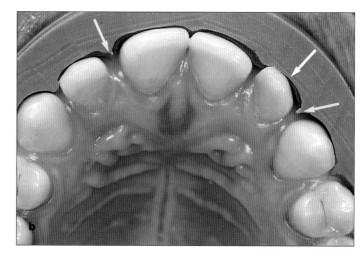

Fig 9-7a, b Silicone index fabricated with the waxed-up positions of the teeth will help the dentist to visualize the final outcome of the teeth. Note that tooth #22(10) is pinching on the SI (white arrow), preventing the index from being fully seated on the arch. Also note the SI is dictating where the interproximal contact areas should be located (yellow arrows).

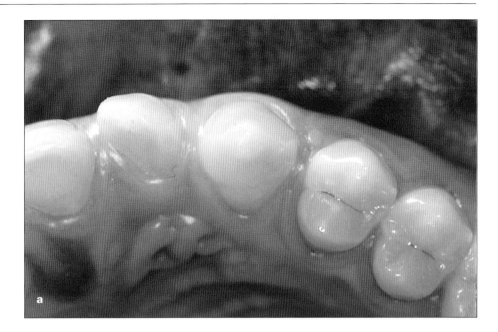

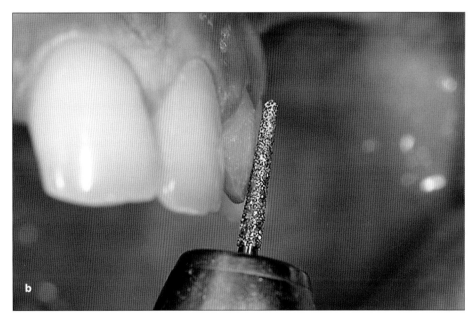

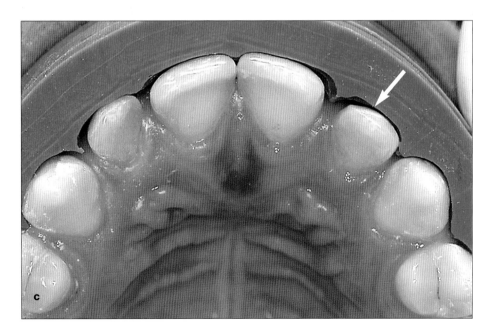

Fig 9-8a-c This will also help the dentist see the protruding corners of the teeth that need to be trimmed down before the actual material preparation. (a) Note the off-the-arch position of the mesial corner of the maxillary lateral. (b) It has to be esthetically positioned correctly. (c) Checking the sufficient amount of tooth reduction. If the SI can passively be seated over the teeth, it is an indication of correct APR.

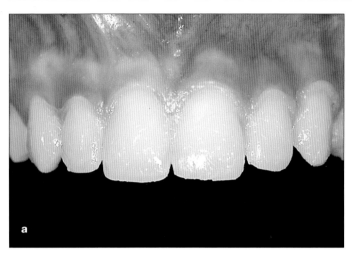
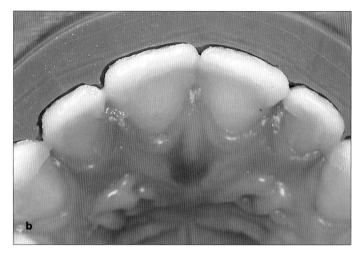

Fig 9-9a, b APT is prepared over the esthetically recontoured teeth. (b) This should be double checked by placing the SI over the APT, because if the template is not seated correctly during the preparation of APTs, facially over-bulked temporaries may result.

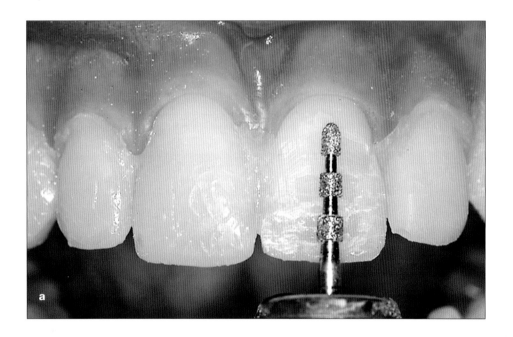

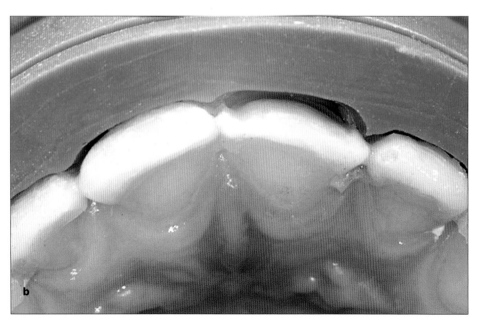

Fig 9-10a, b Once the correct position of the APT is confirmed, the depth cutters are used and the facial preparation can be done through the APT. (b) The required depth is checked with the horizontally placed SI.

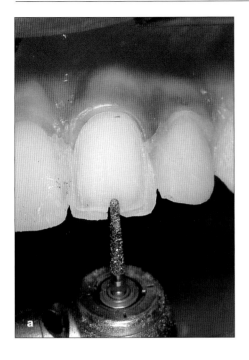

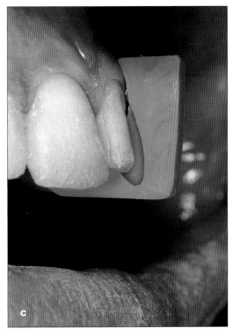

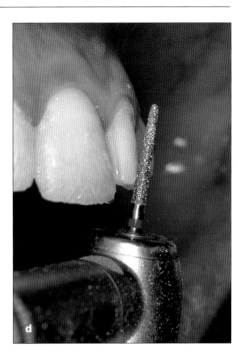

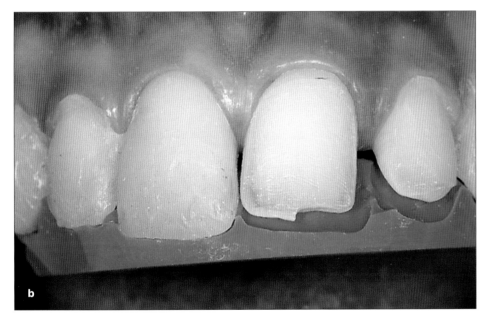

Fig 9-11a-d The APT can also be used while preparing the incisal edge position. Note the minimum incisal edge reduction when the preparation is done through the APT. (b, c) This can be confirmed with the SI from different angles. (d) The incisal corner should be rounded to prevent a distinct demarcation line.

9-9). The depth cutter is used and facial reduction is carried out through the APT. This will ensure the equal and necessary minimum tooth (enamel) reduction from the facial aspect (Fig 9-10). The next step is to prepare the incisal edge while the APT is still on the tooth. This will eliminate unnecessary sound tooth structure reduction, especially when double-checked with the silicone index. It is possible to check the facial depth as well as the incisal with a silicone index placed sagitally (Fig 9-11).

Cervical and Gingivoproximal Preparation

Another important aspect of diastema closing is to create a crisp triangular papilla, which actually stands blunt in a horizontal position when diastema exists. The preparation design of the specific area will dictate the final outcome of the porcelain laminate veneer in terms of creating the shape and position of the papillae. Because of the space between the two adjacent teeth, the papilla changes to a round, flat or even reversed

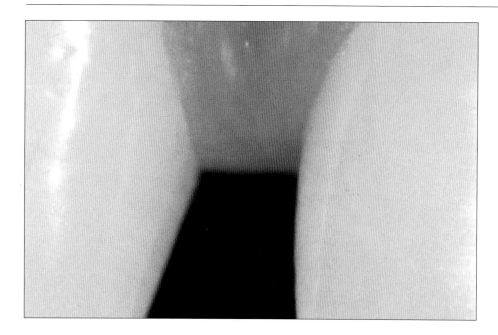

Fig 9-12 When teeth are apart, the tip of the papilla becomes flat or rounded in shape.

form (Fig 9-12). In order to regain the desired papilla form, the soft tissue has to be recontoured either by the tooth itself (orthodontics) or the restoration (prosthodontics). If this is to be done carefully, a new triangular papilla formation can be achieved, providing the tip of the papilla is 5 mm away from the crest of the interproximal alveolar bone.[5] If this has to be done prosthodontically, special care and techniques should be used during the preparation of the cervical and gingivoproximal area.

The technician should have control over the emergence profiles, especially in the gingivoproximal area, to ensure that the soft tissue is recontoured and the interproximal spaces are closed at the end of the treatment (Fig 9-13).[5] The aim must be to create healthy interdental papilla with a pyramid-shape triangle and without the formation of black holes. The cervical margin can be maintained at the supragingival; however, starting from the 1/3rd near the diastema area of the preparation it should be converted to a subgingival preparation, in order to allow the lab technician to establish a progressive emergence profile for the interdental (Fig 9-14) zone of extension.[6] Technically, placing the round-ended fissure diamond bur 0.5 mm into the sulcus is the correct way of handling the preparation and should provide a distance 2.5 mm facially and 4 mm interproximally from the crest of the alveo-

lar bone, and thereby prevent gum recession following the treatment (Fig 9-15).

On the other hand, if the preparation is limited to the facial only, it will be physically impossible to apply this volunteered pressure over the blunt gingiva and achieve the triangular form.[7] Hence, the subgingival preparation should not be limited to the imaginary interproximal contact area, but also be extended towards the palate to create the intentional overcontouring of the porcelain laminate veneer between the buccal and palatinal papillae (Fig 9-16).

The preparation should be extended palatinally, including the "col" area (see Chapter 6). While closing the diastema, the technician should also be aware of this physiological concavity and build the bulk of the veneer accordingly. While influencing the interproximal gingival tissue recontouring to obtain an appropriate papilla, such a build up enhances the shape of the papilla and thus increases the biological integration of the porcelain laminate veneer. It is generally accepted (see Chapter 6) that the "col" area gets larger as it proceeds from the centrals towards the canines and molars.

If this is done carefully, a precise fit will be obtained and the porcelain laminate veneer will create a gentle but dynamic pressure against the free gingival margin. In doing so, a convex tooth form is established within the proximal sulcus,

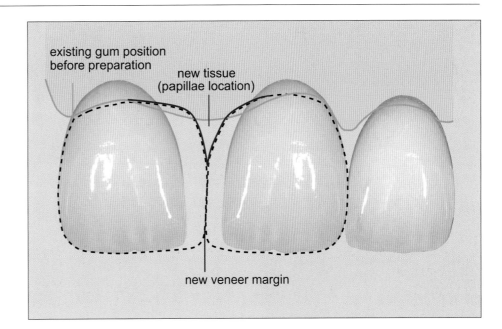

Fig 9-13 The preparation of the gingivoproximal area is very important in diastema closure cases. It should be prepared subgingivally to allow the technician to follow the emergence profile and gently to overbulk the porcelain. This will influence the soft tissue recontouring towards the incisal in order to produce a triangular papilla.

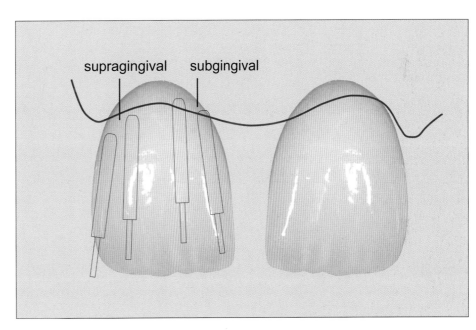

Fig 9-14 The supragingival preparation at the cervical should become subgingival closer to the diastema area.

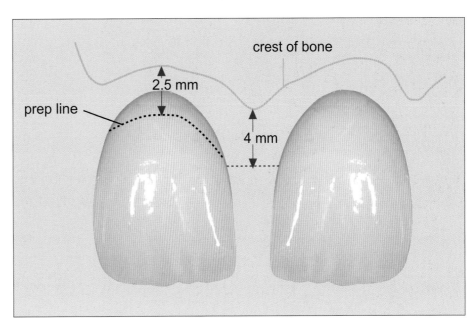

Fig 9-15 A distance of 2.5 mm on the facial and 4.5 mm on the interproximal should be kept with the subgingival preparation margin and the alveolar crest.

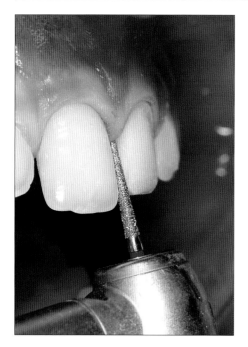

Fig 9-16 The preparation at the gingivoproximal area should be not only extended subgingivally but palatinaly as well.

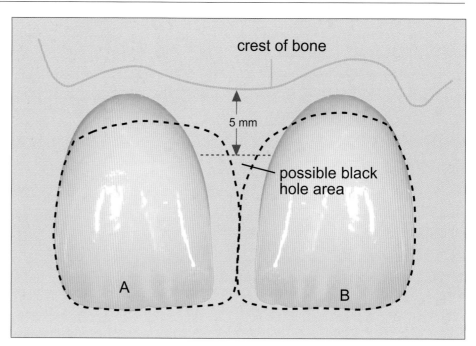

Fig 9-17 When the final porcelain laminate veneer is positioned on the tooth, there is a chance that a black hole will appear between the interdental contact area if the distance between the intercrestal bone and the apical contact point of the veneers is kept more then 5 mms. If this happens, the interproximal contact area should be extended apically to where the red dots indicate.

producing an ideal tooth form for closing the gingival embrasure and maintaining optimal gingival health, while ensuring that the area can easily be dental flossed.[8] These contours will gently push the tissues away from the tooth and in an incisal direction.

Limits

Even though this technique permits the lab technician to alter the emergence profile and establish it without compromising the soft tissue integration,[9] there is a biological limit to how much the papilla can be repositioned. No matter what we do, it should be no longer than 5 mm from the alveolar crest. If it is planned longer it will always have a chance to shrink towards the bone.[10] If such a condition exists, where the interproximal bone stays higher than it should have been, the dentist should define the extension of the interproximal contact area apically, to the technician, in order to prevent the formation of the black hole (Fig 9-17).

Interproximal Contact Area

In order to achieve a natural interproximal contact area the preparation should be extended palatinally in the form of a feather edge, which can easily be prepared with the fissure diamond bur. Care should be paid not to create undercuts while doing so. This will not only ease the lab technician's work, but also provide them with the space to block the dark coloration of the internal mouth space that shows through from the narrow porcelain (Fig 9-18). This will also help the patient to maintain the hygiene of that area more easily.

Lab Procedures with Empress

After all the necessary communication tools are prepared, the case is sent to the lab. The success of any work between the dentist and dental technician is based on their ability to communicate. To use the right technical language is not enough, they must ensure that the chosen medium for

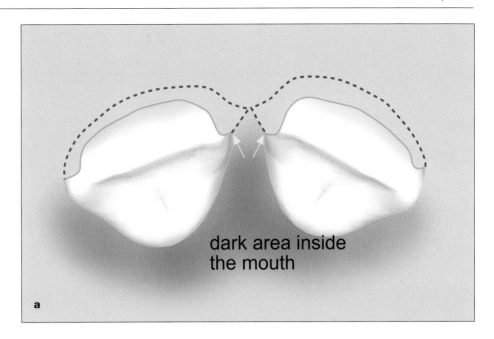

dark area inside
the mouth

a

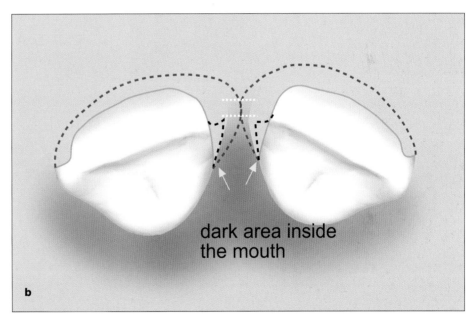

dark area inside
the mouth

b

Fig 9-18a-c If the interproximal area is prepared by conventional methods, the finished PLV will display a thin edge between the two adjacent teeth reflecting the darkness of the mouth from inside out. (b) However, if a feather edge is created towards the palatinal, the technician will have a chance to build up a thick portion of porcelain interproximally (white dots), blocking out the darkness and easing the cleaning of the area for the patient (yellow arrows). (c) Note the feather-edge preparation line of the distal of the central facial diastema (white arrows).

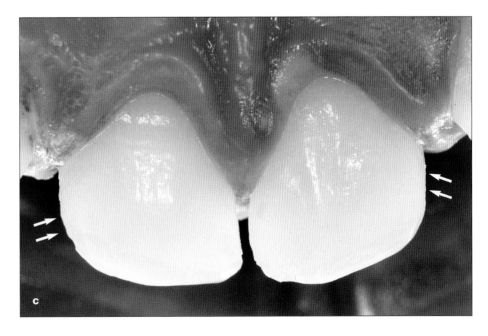

c

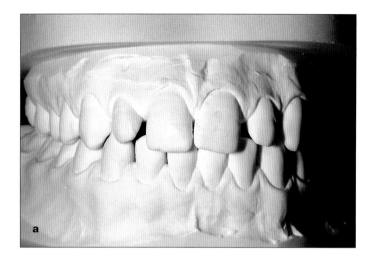
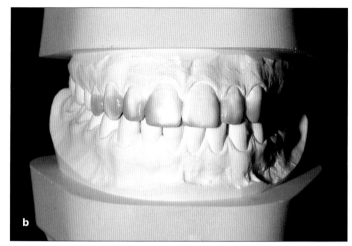
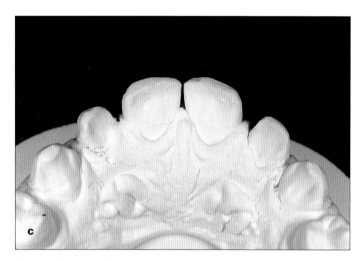
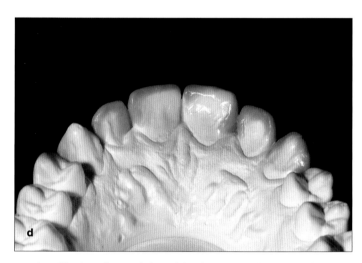

Fig 9-19a-d The technician will have a chance to compare the "before" models with the waxed-up models, to visualize how to close the gaps. (a, c) The "before" models with extensive diastemas. These models are used for the wax-up and to analyze possible adjustments in the esthetic outcome as well as the vertical dimension of the incisal, correction of the empty spaces, rotations and axial corrections. (b, d) Finished wax-up with possible final views. Note that all necessary corrections in form and shape have been made. The modulation in this case has been applied directly to the study model in order to maintain the natural anatomy on the six anteriors.

communication enables clinical requests and received information to be clearly understood. So, all the modern tools for clinic–lab communication must be applied even if the clinic and lab are 3,000 km apart. This is not really verbal articulation. The language is based on understanding the needs of each patient and using the right instruments to transmit this understanding.

Beside the skills and the artistic aspects in such large restorations, the technician must follow the instructions given by the material supplier. High-tech products, such as pressable ceramics, are easy to apply, but in all cases an application error or unforeseen circumstances can increase the

risk of failures. No dental company can foresee that, for example, the instructions for use may only be partially applied. However, the aim of each producer is to advertise the physical and optical properties dependent on the application of specific instructions.

The steps described here are based on long-term experience with pressable ceramic, employing high-tech skills and state-of-the art techniques. *Gerald Ubassy's*[11] demonstrations are always taken from his daily lab work. The steps we see are reproducible at any time (Figs 9-19 to 9-39).

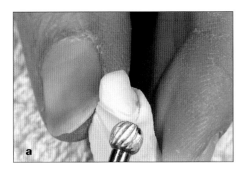

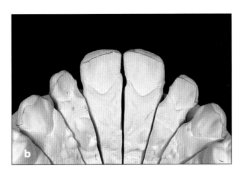

Fig 9-20a, b (a) With a ball–shaped hard metal drill the margins have been exposed and observed. (b) View from occlusal. The palatinal preparation lines are colored with red pencil.

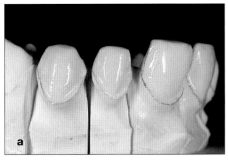

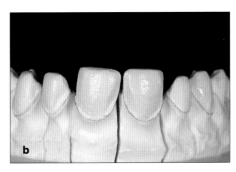

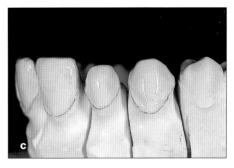

Fig 9-21a-c To apply the spacer is a critical step. The right amount of spacer together with the investment liquid concentration will determine the precision of the fit. According to the instructions, the thickness of the spacer layer should be between 9 and 11 micrometers. However, the shape of the preparation and geometry should be respected by adding or reducing the amount of spacer.

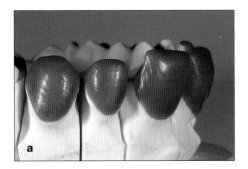

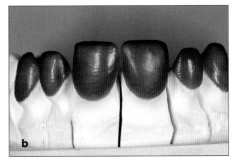

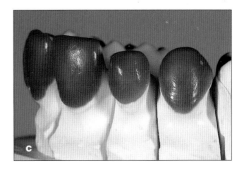

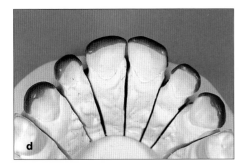

Fig 9-22a-d The modelization of the laminate cores. The core has a minimum thickness of 0.8 mm and the incisal area is harmonized with the expected final outcome, in terms of volume and vertical extension. At this stage the marginal fit should be absolutely exact.

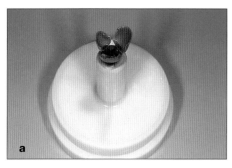 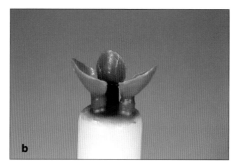 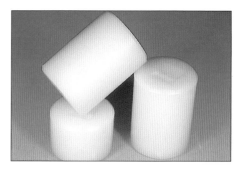

Fig 9-23a, b The core laminates are sprued on the muffle base. To create an easy flow direction of pressable ceramic, the angles of the sprues have to be correctly placed on the sprues.

Fig 9-24 The ingots are chosen according to the shade; only original Empress 2 ingots will guarantee an optimal result.

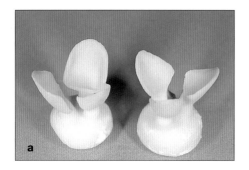 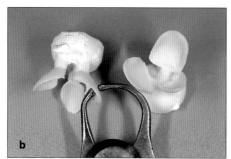 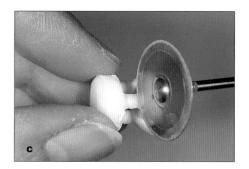

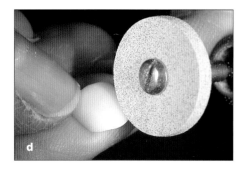

Fig 9-25a-d The objects that are divested by using the sand blaster. With a fine diamond disk the sprues are cut. To ensure that there is no overheating during the processing, a wet sponge can be used. With abrasive silicones the final sprue's connections are eliminated.

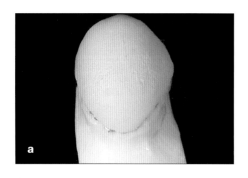 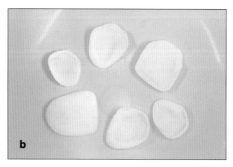

Fig 9-26a, b To remove the reaction surfaces the laminates are placed for 10–20 minutes in invex liquid (>1% HF / >1% sulphuric acid). The surfaces will be sand blasted again.

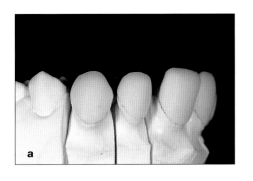
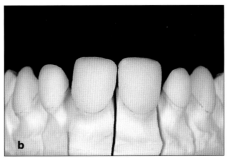
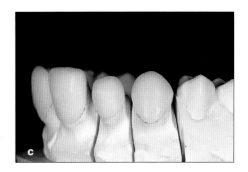
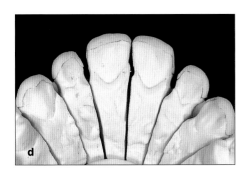
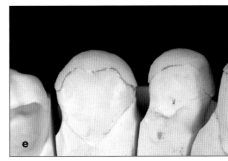
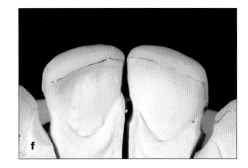
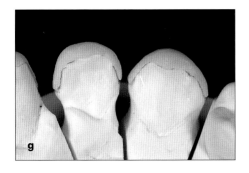

Fig 9-27a-g Through the correct application of the spacer technique, investment, and pressing parameters the result is excellent fit with no margin gaps, no time lost for fitting the cores on the die. All the laminates are now ready to be covered with fluor apatite ceramic.

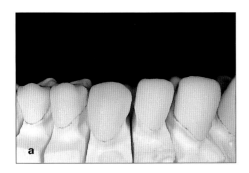
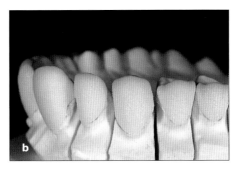

Fig 9-28a, b The restoration is covered with a thin layer of ceramic. This firing process is called foundation firing – it ensure a complete and homogenous interface between frame and ceramic.

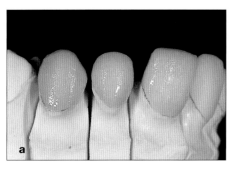 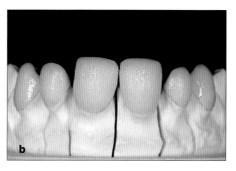 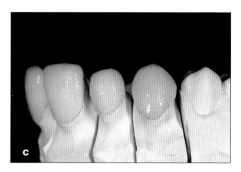

Fig 9-29a-c One additional, very thin coat has been fired using stains mixed with ceramic. This increases the vitality. The canine is observed to be a bit more chromatic.

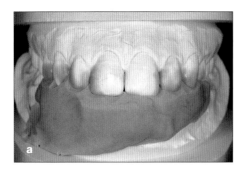 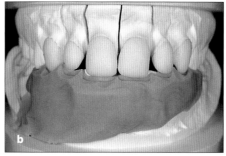

Fig 9-30a, b The wax–up with a silicon key and the pressed cores with the same key as a comparative tool. The key will be used as a guide during the layering.

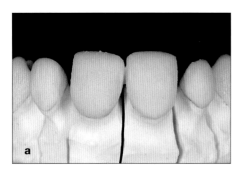 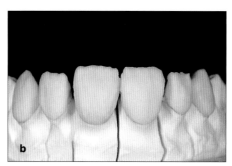 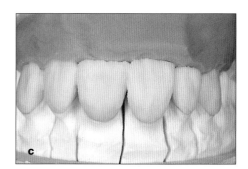

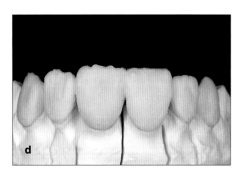

Fig 9-31a-d The picture shows the step–by–step aproach to the final form. In this case the main ceramic has been towards incisal more and more diluted with tranparent neutral. During these steps the silicone key was used as guide line. Different dentins, if necessary diluted with transparent effect, are increasing absorption. Reflection and absorption of light are always in the focus during ceramic modelization.

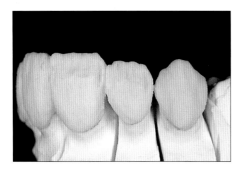

Fig 9-32 The incisal, cut back to provide space for the aplication of effect powders and to bring more life and individuality.

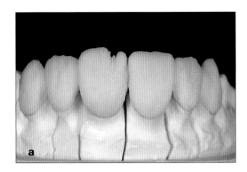
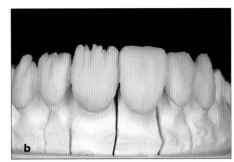
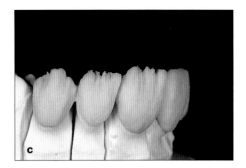

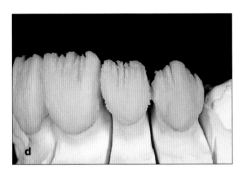

Fig 9-33a-d With very accurate and irregular cut backs in the incisal area, the mamelon and the individual character step-by-step modelized, until the final shape is reached.

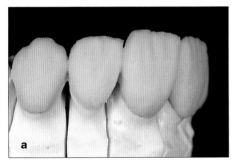
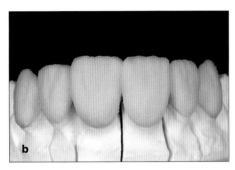
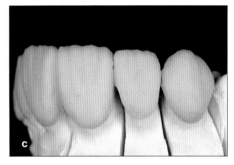

Fig 9-34a-c Final modelized laminates on the master model are now ready to be processed; the dimension is slightly increased to compensate for the shrinkage.

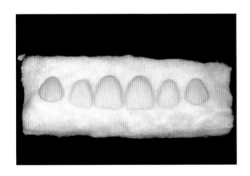

Fig 9-35 The anterior restorations are placed on the firing pillow. A minimum nine minutes of preheating in this stage at a low temperature is recommended. During the modelization, the ceramic should be dried out and always kept in plastic consitency.

Fig 9-36a-c After firing, the surfaces have a slightly shiny appearance. Underfiring or overfiring the laminates would have a negative effect and reduce considerably the esthetic result.

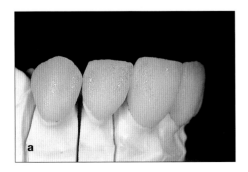
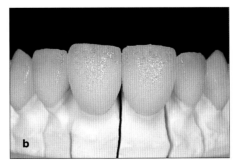
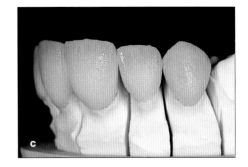

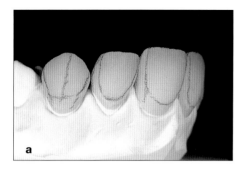
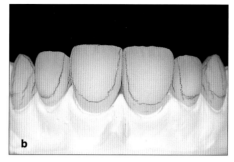
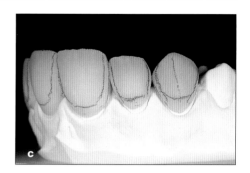

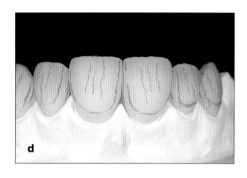

Fig 9-37a-d Shaping is another very important step. Analyzing the surface texture, light determination angle, equator, microtextures, incisal length, abrasions, approximal extensions, all have to be done in a systematic way and without compromise.

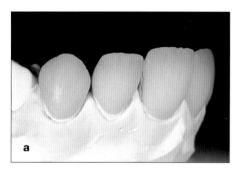
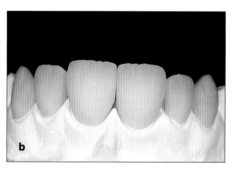
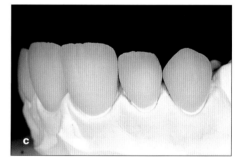

Fig 9-38a-c The surfaces are completly elaborated and ready to be stained and glazed.

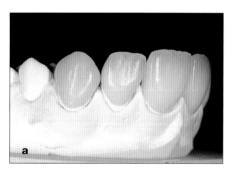
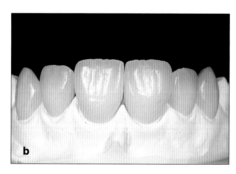
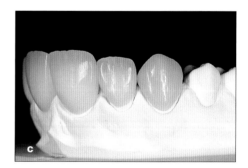

Fig 9-39a-c After the glazing and staining fire, the surfaces have been treated with soft silicone polishing tools in order to increase the shine on the convex and tissue exposed areas, while decreasing the shine on the concave areas.

Bonding

When the veneers are returned from the lab, they are tried-in one by one for the margin fit and then in groups for the esthetic integration. Once the proportions and their relation to each other and final appearance with the face are confirmed, then they are bonded, as explained (see Chapter 7, Fig 9-40).

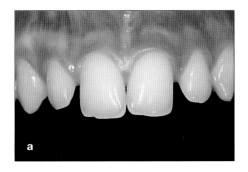
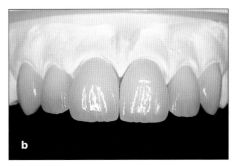
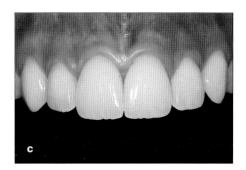

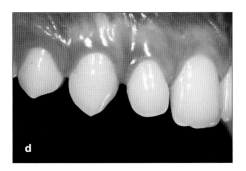
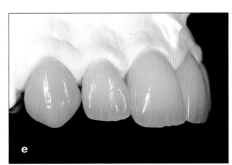
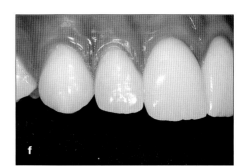

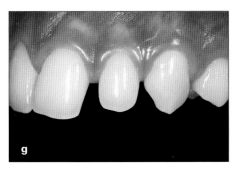
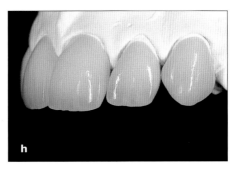
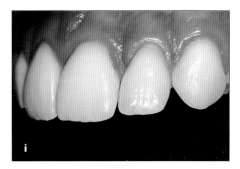

Fig 9-40a-i (b, e, h) The result are anterior laminates with an esthetic and an individual look. The surface shows natural shine. Hue, chroma and value have been adapted to the requested shade. At this stage, they should be perfectly seated on the master stone model. (a, c, d, f, g, i) Once the veneers are returned to the clinic they can be tried-in and bonded, as explained in Chapter 7. When a proper diagnosis is followed by a delicate wax-up and the teeth are prepared exactly to the limits of minimal invasion, the artistic ability and interpretation of the technician come into shape.

Details

It is the details that make porcelain laminate veneers more precious than other veneers. In cases of diastema closing there are many details to be dealt with from the beginning. The case definition, the treatment planning and execution might be different from a normal case. And these details can be observed after the porcelain laminate veneers are bonded (Figs 9-41 to 9-46).

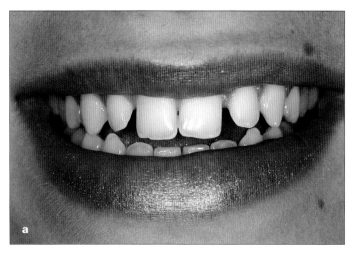
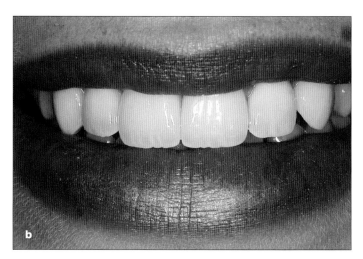

Fig 9-41a, b Note the proportions that are delicately provided by the PLVs, even though there were multiple diastemas at the beginning.

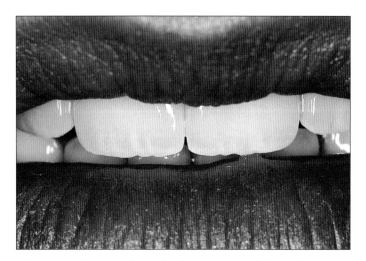
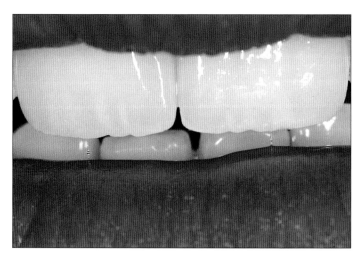

Fig 9-42 The length of the incisors just follow the curvature of the lower lip.

Fig 9-43 The incisal edges of the centrals 3 mm away from the upper lip, and the delicately built-up translucencies inside the PLV, allow a very natural, youthful smile (ceramist: *G. Ubassy*).

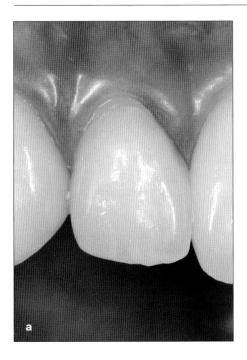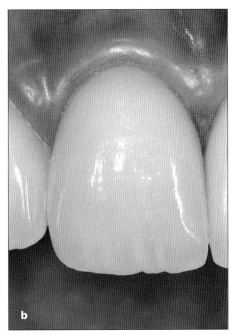

Fig 9-44a, b When every veneer is observed one by one, all the elements that makes a tooth look natural can be seen. The color transition of the tooth within itself is exactly produced. Note the higher chroma at the cervical 1/3rd, the higher value on the middle 1/3rd, the translucencies and mamelons at the incisal 1/3rd.

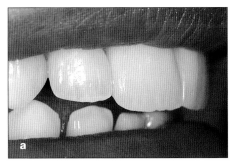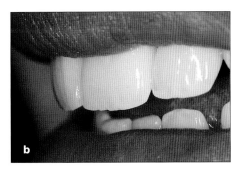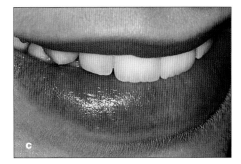

Fig 9-45a-c Viewing the mouth from different angles should not make any difference in the perception of the PLVs which closed the gaps. Note the front-back relation of the centrals, laterals and canines as well as the progression of the incisal embrasures which get bigger and wider towards the canine.

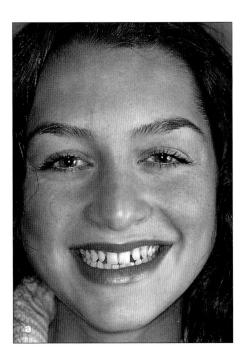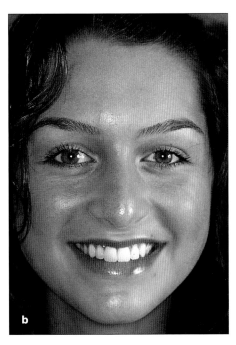

Fig 9-46a, b The impression of a beautiful smile on the whole facial expression.

References

1. Goldstein RE. Esthetics in Dentistry. 2nd ed. Hamilton, ON: BC Decker Inc, 1998:123-133.

2. Yamamoto M, Miyoshi M, Kataoka S. Special Discussion. Fundamentals of esthetics: Contouring techniques for metal ceramic restorations. QDT 1990/1991;14:10-81.

3. Baratieri LN. Esthetics: Direct Adhesive Restoration on Fractured Anterior Teeth. São Paulo: Quintessence, 1998: 35-75.

4. Bichacho N. Controlling the integration—The restoration tooth/implant gingiva. EDAD. Fifth International Congress of Esthetic Dentistry (2001), Istanbul.

5. Tarnow D, Stahl SS, Magner A, Zamzok J. Human gingival attachment responses to subgingival crown placement. Marginal remodelling. J Clin Periodontal 1986;13:563.

6. Belser UC, Magne P, Magne M. Ceramic laminate veneers: Continuous evolution of indications. J Esthet Dent 1997; 9:197-207.

7. Sanavi F, Weisgold AS, Rose LF. Biologic width and its relation to periodontal biotypes. J Esthet Dent 1998;10: 157-163.

8. Cornell DF. Ceramic Veneers: Understanding their benefits and limitations. QDT 1998;21:121-132.

9. Cornell DF. Soft tissue-ceramic interface: True parameter for successful esthetics. J Esthet Dent 1995;7:81-86.

10. Baratieri LN. Esthetics: Direct Adhesive Restoration on Fractured Anterior Teeth. São Paulo: Quintessence, 1998.

11. Ubassy G. Analysis of the New Way in Dental Communication. Brescia: La Nuova Cartografica SpA, 1996; Ubassy G. Shape and Color. Chicago: Quintessence, 1988.

10 Porcelain Laminate Veneers for Tetracycline Discoloration

Galip Gürel

Introduction

The long-term use of certain antibiotics, or diseases such as fluorosis or dentinogenesis imperfecta, may be the cause of a major change in the color of the teeth requiring special consideration when preparing the porcelain laminate veneer (Fig 10-1). With heavily discolored teeth, as in the case of a tetracycline type of dark staining, the dentist and patient may not be satisfied with the result of the porcelain laminate veneer restoration despite positive esthetic results. It is not commonly recommended to use porcelain laminate veneer over seriously stained and darkened teeth because some degree of light will pass through the porcelain, allowing the background of the teeth to be seen through its thinness.[1]

It is said to be impossible to mask a strong discoloration by a thin (0.3 to 0.7 mm) layer of porcelain without making the restoration opaque and lifeless. Consequently, the restored tooth under such conditions is believed never to have the same translucency as the surrounding natural teeth.[2-6] It is even suggested that excessively dark anterior teeth should be treated with ultra-thin metal ceramic full crowns, such as the galvano or captek systems.

However, the author, after many years' experience, believes that if the preparation of the tooth is undertaken properly, using the dentist's common sense together with the artistic abilities and knowledge of an up-to-date technician, it is possible not only to mask strong discoloration but also to achieve a natural-looking result with porcelain laminate veneers. This requires excellent laboratory support and good communication between the dentist and ceramist. In the hands of an experienced dentist and laboratory technician, the tremendous advances in the production of new composite and porcelain materials will overcome this problem. The ceramic technician can create a porcelain veneer using a layered build up of opaque dentin that can mask the discolored tooth. The first approach should be clinically to evaluate the case (Fig 10-2) and to attempt to visualize the final outcome with the composite mock-ups (Fig 10-3).

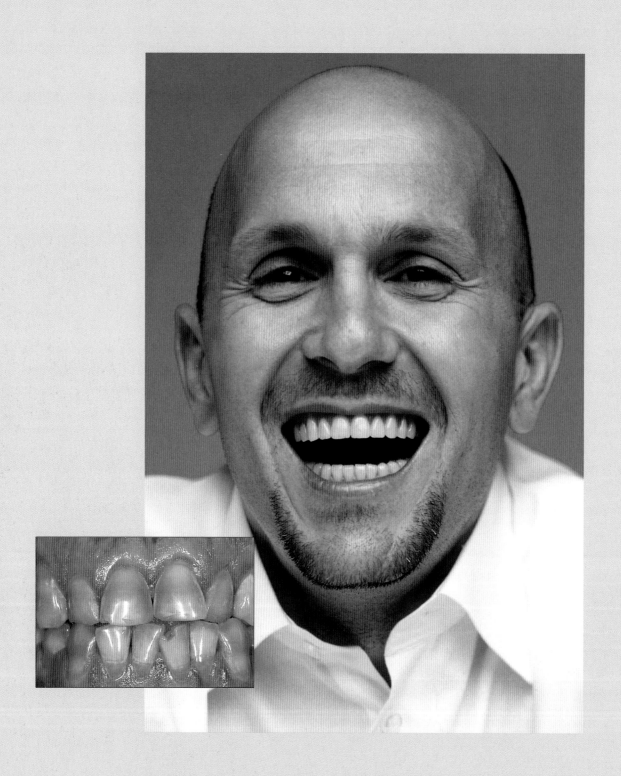

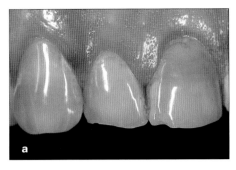 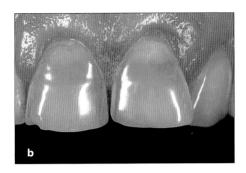 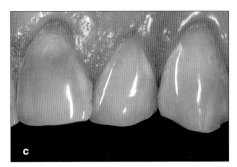

Fig 10-1a-c Heavy tetracycline discoloration owing to the intake of antibiotics.

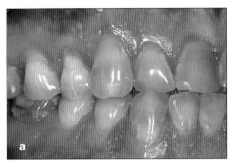 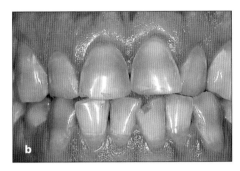 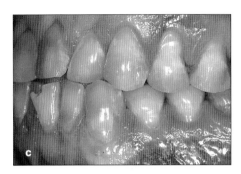

Fig 10-2a-c Natural occlusion and the appearance of the whole mouth. Note the cross-bite on the laterals and edge-to-edge relation of the centrals.

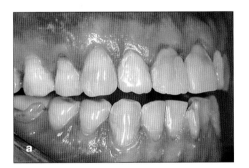 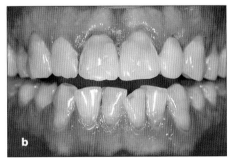 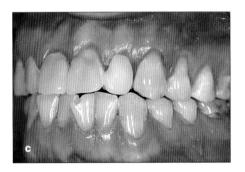

Fig 10-3a-c A quick composite mock-up is applied to visualize roughly the esthetic outcome as well as the functional disturbances.

Laboratory Communication 1

A successful collaboration between the dentist and a skillful technician will be the major factor in designing and executing porcelain laminate veneer preparation on severely stained teeth. With such teamwork, the treatment can be handled without the use of opaque composite luting agents so as to block out discoloration. If, in addition to tetracycline discoloration, the patient exhibits occlusal disturbances and problems related to the teeth's position, then the case can become even more complicated (Fig 10-2).

In such cases, the ability to achieve functional and esthetic restoration offers the dentist and lab ceramist the rare opportunity to transform not just the patient's smile, but his or her entire self-esteem. It is therefore incumbent upon both the dentist and ceramist to work in concert to offer the patient the appropriate procedure and materials, as well as the high level of care and attention that are necessary to create restorations to meet this ambitious goal.

Achieving the incomparable function and esthetics of a premium laminate veneer restoration means beginning with the end result in mind.

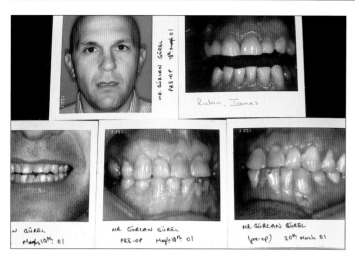

Fig 10-4 The original model with pictures from the patient are sent to the laboratory.

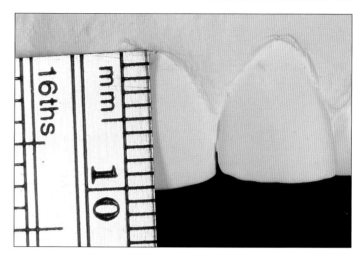

Fig 10-5 The length of the centrals is double-checked at the lab to verify their extended incisal margins on the mock-up.

The dentist and ceramist must think ahead, cognizant that the final result dictates the preparation design. Every detail about the patient and their smile must be recorded properly from the onset to ensure a flawless end result. The following procedure is a full-mouth rehabilitation case that employs this philosophy through every step of the process.

Patient Profile

The patient, a 40-year-old man, requires a full-mouth reconstruction to restore normal function to his bite and esthetics to his smile. This particular case is a prime example of how form must follow function in the pre-planning stages. The ceramist and the clinician work together, mindful of the final function and esthetics of the laminate veneers.

Typically, this lower arch would present itself as a candidate for traditional orthodontics. However, the patient's age and personal preference make braces an unlikely option. Instead, a wireless shaping and laminate technique known as diamond-driven orthodontics will be utilized to correct the alignment, ultimately restoring overall function and esthetics.

The upper arch requires the establishment of an incisal edge positioning and lengthening of the upper centrals. This will enhance esthetics, but, more importantly, it will provide for mutually pro-

tected occlusion. In order to restore group function, canine and anterior guidance must first be established.

To begin with, a chairside composite mock-up technique is utilized in order to facilitate communication with the patient and then with the laboratory (Fig 10-3). Once the dentist has taken a full-mouth impression, a study model is sent to the ceramist along with a facebow transfer and both dentofacial and dental photographs of the patient's smile (Fig 10-4).

Mock-up Design on Pre-op Study Model

Study model, facebow transfer and photographs in hand, the ceramist now analyzes the patient's case by assessing the smile line, articulation, function, wear and color. The ceramist begins to diagnose with a mock-up of the pre-operative study model, indicating where existing teeth should be shaven down to accommodate the laminates. These steps illustrate the careful, systematic thought processes of ceramist *Jason Kim,* with the end result in mind.

First of all, in order to achieve a proper smile line, the patient's upper anteriors must be lengthened (Fig 10-5). Worn canines must be restored to create better guidance, which is now in group function, as well as to protect the lengthened anteriors. The goal of the diamond-driven orthodontic

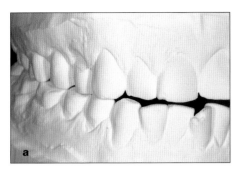 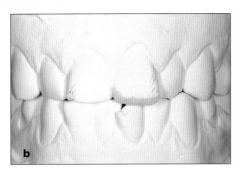 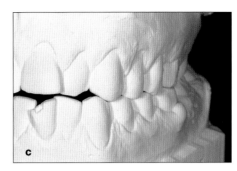

Fig 10-6a-c The lateral and protrusive excursions are evaluated on the articulator.

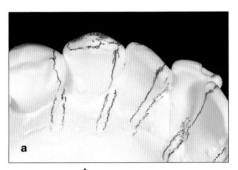 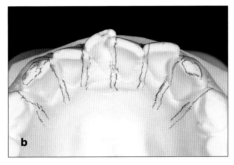 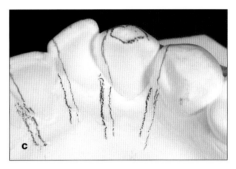

Fig 10-7a-c The mandibular teeth are carefully checked in order to correct their inclinations. The red line is drawn to indicate where the necessary slicing should be done.

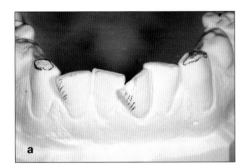 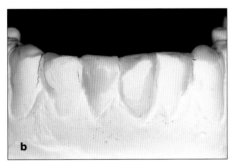 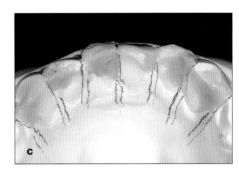

Fig 10-8a-c The arrangements and function of the lowers are arranged to accommodate the upper length. Some conservative grinding is done on the most protrusive elements. The lower canines need to be sliced on the red line in order to gain space in the bicuspid area.

technique is to preserve as much of the original tooth structure as possible with the proper consideration of tooth movement. In such a case, it is practical to save much of the natural tooth with a minimally invasive preparation (Fig 10-6).

In this case, the goal is to straighten out the lower left central incisor without losing the width of the tooth. Due to the overlap, space must be gained distally to compensate for the lingual interference. Therefore, the same must be done to gain space for each successive tooth up to the canine. The blue lines indicate the lines of the existing tooth structure, while the red lines indicate where the slicing should be made in order to gain adequate space for the laminates (Figs 10-7 and 10-8).

Mock-up Model with Function Design

The ceramist uses the Iaformation of the study model from a mock-up made in the clinic by the dentist, indicating where to rebuild the smile once it has been designed. It will ultimately serve as a

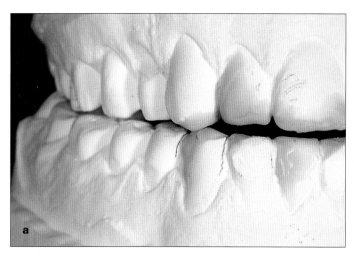 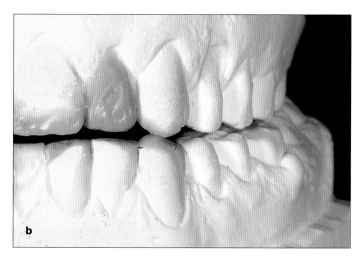

Fig 10-9a, b A rough wax-up is made to determine the tooth size in relation to basic position and function.

blueprint, providing the exact information as to which teeth to slice in preparation to accommodate the laminates. Wax is applied to establish the basic position, function and tooth size. Function is corrected through canine and anterior guidance (Fig 10-9).

Laboratory Study Preparation for Laminate Veneers

The preliminary preparation can be practised on the study cast, using a design mock-up to ensure the feasibility of the final result. The mock-up is also used to communicate the preparation design to the dentist. Furthermore, the preparation design shows how much reduction the tooth requires, as well as the location of the finish line (Figs 10-10 to 10-17).

Actual Teeth Preparation

If the dentist treats a tetracycline case like an ordinary porcelain laminate veneer case, and does not pay attention to both preparation and communication with the lab, the result will most probably be an opaque-looking monochromatic porcelain laminate veneer. There are three major

concerns during the tooth prep for a porcelain laminate veneer that have to be seriously taken into consideration, particularly in a tetracycline case. One of them is the depth of preparation, the other is the cervical margin placement and the third is the extension of the gingivoproximal and interproximal finishing lines.

Depth of the Prep

As opposed to a shallow veneer preparation, where the tooth itself presents almost the same color as the finished porcelain laminate veneer, deepening the preparation is one way of improving the final color match in darkly discolored teeth. If the tooth is not prepared deeply enough, increasing the porcelain thickness will enhance the shade match but will result in overcontouring. At times, although the dentist may be able to select the correct shade of color, they are unable successfully to create the contouring, texture and shape that are essential factors in order to achieve the desired esthetic result.

It is almost impossible to place a veneer that completely hides the background color when there is insufficient tooth preparation. If this has been accomplished, the results will be monochromatic due to the increased amount of opaque porcelain or the amount of opaque composite applied at the time of the cementation. Especially in the gingival area, where the thickness of both

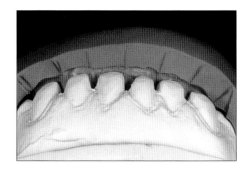

Fig 10-10 The diamond-driven orthodontic technique is used on a duplicate pre-op model. The teeth are now prepared to accommodate the repositioning. The red markings on the cast show where the teeth are to be sliced in order to gain space. A putty index is taken from the mock-up cast and used as a reference to indicate an adequate reduction for the veneers.

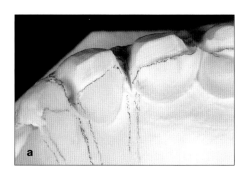

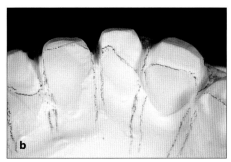

Fig 10-11a, b With the contacts open, it is crucial to have the margin location on the lingual of the proximal wall. This is to ensure masking and proper bonding strength as well as alignment of the lingual overlaps. The slicing and lingual margins of the teeth determine the margin location. The margin will be at the lingual where the contact is open. Note the non-functional lingual area where the tooth finishing line can be lowered to ensure optimal bonding strength.

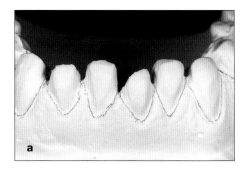

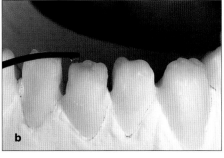

Fig 10-12a-g (a) With the lower preparation design finished, a pre-operative duplicate is made which is then used to form a wax-up duplicate and a preparation guide. (b to e) A fully esthetic lower wax-up is done on a laboratory preparation model. (f, g) The upper mock-up guides the exact incisal position for the lower teeth. This helps to ensure that the integrity of the lower incisal position is preserved at the same position as the mock-up and also ensures the canine guidance and anterior guidance are kept as well. Note the delicacy of the wax-up and note that all the tooth positions have moved distally to achieve optimal alignment.

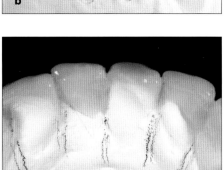

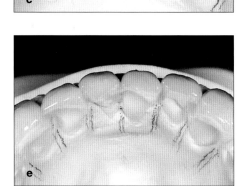

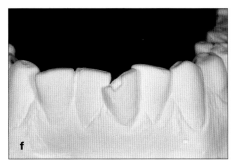

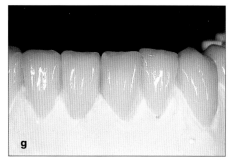

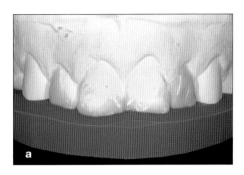
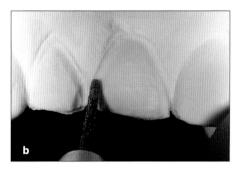
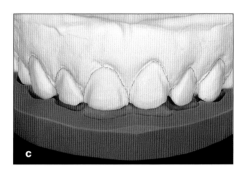

Fig 10-13a-c (a) The upper preparation guide is formed using the putty index from the upper mock-up. (b, c) The putty index provides a proper reference for the uppers to ensure adequate reduction. The upper preparation design is performed using the putty index from the wax mock-up.

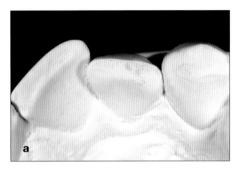
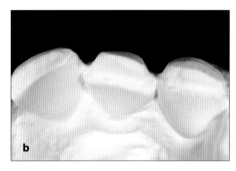
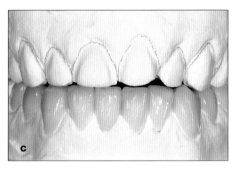

Fig 10-14a-c The pre-op preparation guide indicates the appropriate amount of reduction to be made. Note the finishing line and reduction of overlap on distal centrals. (c) The final upper preparation guide is matched against the lower wax-up.

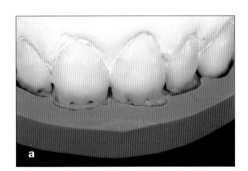
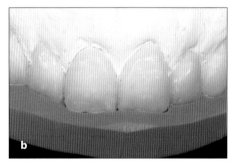
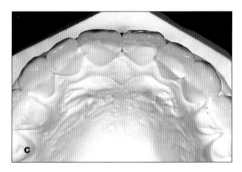

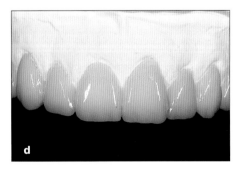

Fig 10-15a-d A fully esthetic diagnostic wax-up is created using the incisal edge position (putty-index) of the mock-up. Note the delicacy of the wax-up. All the incisal translucencies as well as the final contours and texture are created on the wax-up. By using this layering wax-up technique with the same color and layer thicknesses of dentin, enamel and translucent shades, now the technician has a very solid foundation on how and where exactly to place his porcelain built-up layers.(d) Ceramist Jason Kim's fully esthetic complete diagnostic model shows the lengthened centrals and realigned arch compared to the initial position of the teeth.

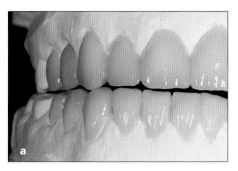 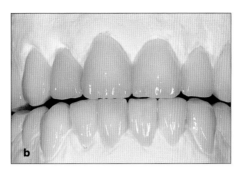 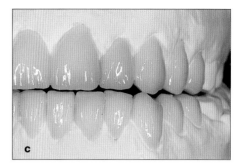

Fig 10-16a-c Note the corrected protrusive and lateral movement. Mutually protective occlusion, the goal from the outset of the procedure, has been achieved.

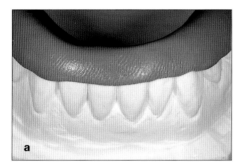 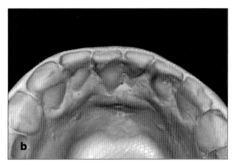 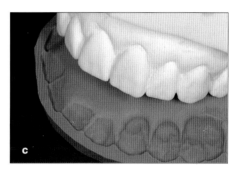

Fig 10-17a-c Duplicate stone models are now made from the final esthetic wax-up model. The clinician can later use a lab putty index and clear plastic stent from this final model to form the temporaries and to guide their preparations.

the enamel and the porcelain is relatively thin, the porcelain laminate veneers placed on such teeth generally appear grayish in color. Deepening the preparation into the dentin labially (see Chapter 7) and placing a subgingival margin to hide the discolored gingival portion of the teeth are usually necessary to overcome this problem (Figs 10-18 to 10-21).

In summary, dark discolorations need deeper preparations. The facial depths can be as much as 0.9 mm, depending on the severity of the discoloration. The chamfer at the cervical margin can be as deep as 0.4-0.5 mm (Fig 10-21). However, one should not forget that tetracycline discoloration is actually deposited on the dentin, which means that the deeper the tooth is prepped, the darker it actually becomes in comparison to the original existing tooth color, owing to the removal of a significant amount of the masking enamel.[7] An experienced eye is able to detect this color change as the preparation goes deeper. Occasionally, some spots appear darker than the rest of the tooth surface. In order to cover the excessively dark stained part of the teeth, the dentist can use a composite of opaque colors just after the preparation stage, before making the impression. This will provide a smooth color distribution on the facial surface.

Margin Prep

The marginal placement of the preparation line needs to be carefully analyzed, as it is a vitally important aspect of the procedure. The cervical margins are kept subgingival in most of the cases concerning the anterior region, due to the need to mask the unpleasant effects of the tetracycline discoloration (Fig 10-21). The preparation margins would end at, or slightly below, the gingival crest and should not be extended deep into the gingival sulcus. Making impressions, checking the temporary restoration, try-in, bonding and finishing are facilitated by this arrangement.[8] A rapid

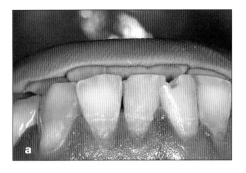
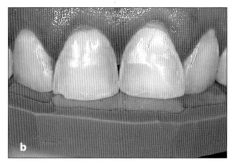

Fig 10-18a, b The silicone index from the lab is used to visualize the final outcome and determine the length and position of the incisal edges.

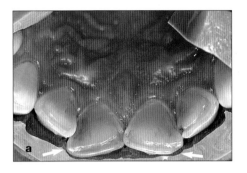
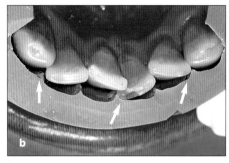

Fig 10-19a, b The protruding edges have to be trimmed down with the help of the silicone index before the actual material preparation.

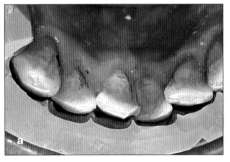
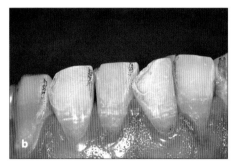
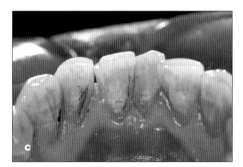

Fig 10-20a-c These edges are trimmed down. The lines that are drawn in the lab are duplicated in the mouth both bucally and lingually with a pencil to determine the slicing areas.

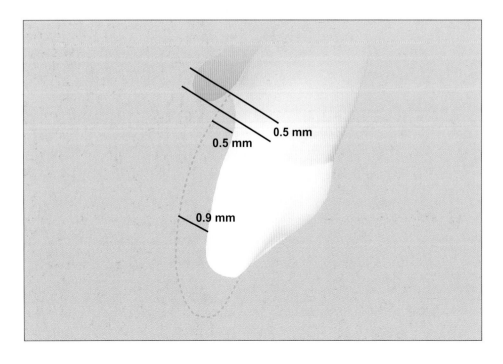

0.5 mm

0.5 mm

0.9 mm

Fig 10-21 The depth of the preparation is usually greater than a regular veneer preparation. It can go as deep as 0.9 to 1 mm at the incisal and middle third and 0.4 to 0.5 mm at the cervical 1/3rd. The cervical margin is placed inside the sulcus at about 0.5 mm.

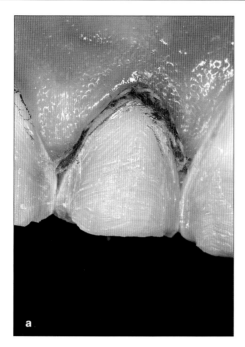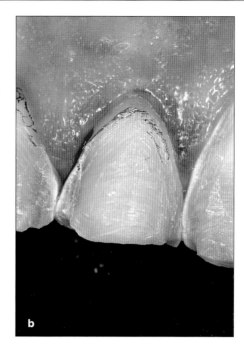

Fig 10-22a, b The preparation depth of the cervical margin is determined and indicated with a pencil before the deflection cord is placed. This line, drawn 0.5 mm under the gingival margin, becomes visible after the deflection cord is placed (a). When the cord is taken out for the ease of preparation, the line already drawn indicates where the cervical margin is to be placed (b). Otherwise, it is possible for an inexperienced eye to overextend the margin apically, as the deflected gingiva will allow a greater space to be prepared.

recovery and ensured longevity of the restoration are made possible by minimizing the biologic violation that results in reduced iatrogenic insult.[9]

If the margins are to be placed subgingivally, a line could be drawn on the cervical margin, before the tissue is deflected (Fig 10-22). Gingival recession, periodontal pockets and the prevention of chronic inflammation are just a few of the factors to be avoided by the careful consideration of the location and the thickness of the porcelain laminate veneer margin. The most important factor in crown margin location is the "biologic width". Ingber, et al. coined the term "biologic width" in 1977, based on original research by *Gargiulo*, et al. in 1961.[10] The sulcus depth has the greatest degree of variation in the dentogingival complex, with a mid-facial depth of 1mm (indicative of a normal osseous crest height) that increases 2.5 mm interproximally (indicative of a low osseous crest height).[9] It is also helpful in enabling long-term monitoring of the tooth restoration seal, satisfying esthetic demands, expediting oral hygiene maintenance procedures, simplifying impressions,

and making and creating a correct porcelain laminate veneer emergence profile. A subgingival margin is necessary for good esthetics, but sometimes at the expense of adequate oral hygiene.

Interproximal Prep

If the contact area is visible during function in the cases that exhibit major tooth color changes, the extension of the interproximal finish line to the approximate depth of one–half the labiolingual dimension of the contact area will be necessary.[7] If the facial surface of the tooth is too convex, then the extension of the interproximal margin halfway between the labial and lingual will be enough. This convexity will block out the remaining unprepared tooth structure when viewed from an angle. However, if the surface is flat, then the interproximal angle should be extended towards the palate in order to prevent the unsightly appearance of the unprepared tooth portion (Fig 10-23).[11]

The gingivoproximal area is also very important in tetracycline discolorations. It should be

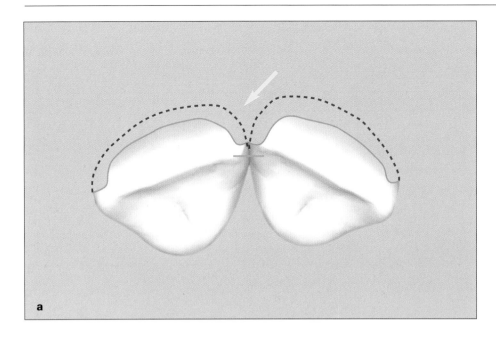

Fig 10-23a, b (a) If the tooth surface is convex when the porcelain laminate veneers are bonded, the interproximal edge may remain short of the contact area when viewed from a different angle (yellow arrow). The mesial bulkiness of the adjacent tooth will hide the interproximal porcelain laminate veneer-tooth interface thus eliminating an unpleasant esthetic outcome. (b) However, if it is flat, the preparation should be palatinally extended to cover this interface.

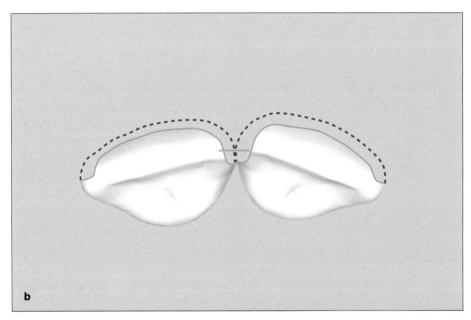

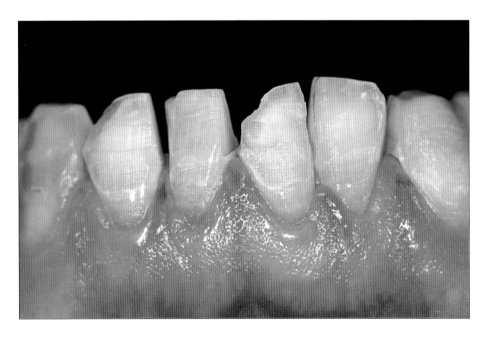

Fig 10-24 The mandibular interproximal areas are prepared similar to the preparations done on the study model.

prepared subgingivally (see Chapter 9) in the form of an elbow or a dogleg, not only to prevent the visible margin connection, but to avoid dark reflection of the tooth color over the papilla. Special care should be paid to the depth of the sulcus and the distance between the crest of the interdental bone and the tip of the sulcus (see Chapter 12). Any violations of the dentogingival complex or miscalculations will result in papilla loss. The shape of the incisor is also vitally important, so that the dentist should preferably not exceed the cementoenamel junction during the preparation. The interproximal contacts are prepared simulating the preparation done in the laboratory (Fig 10-24).

Color Adjustment

If the color needs to be enhanced with the help of opaque composites, the author prefers to do this just after the preparation is finished, and before the impression is made. Even though some dentists prefer to block out dark coloration with the help of relatively thicker placed opaque luting composites over the deeply prepared tooth structure at the time of the actual bonding (into an area which is created with multiple applications of die spacers at the laboratory stage), it should be done right after the teeth are prepared and prior to impression-taking.

Using 6-8 layers of die spacers[12] at the lab stage, and then filling the spaced-out volume with an opaque or any kind of composite during bonding, is another technique. However, since this attempt is often delayed until the porcelain laminate veneer-bonding stage, it may create problems owing to polymerization volumetric shrinkage, especially at the cervical margins.

The restoration tooth interface is the weak link in any bonded restoration whereas the tooth and the composite luting agent interface is the weak link in any porcelain veneer restoration. The bulk of composite resin will have a polymerization volumetric shrinkage in the amount of 2.6-5.7%,[13] when resins are used as a luting agent. This may create loss of the margin seal or create a marginal opening.

The thermal expansion coefficient (TEC) of the luting agent differs quite from the tooth tissue and

the porcelain. To minimize this effect it is always better to keep the luting composite thickness as minimal as possible and to try to get the correct color match through the porcelain laminate veneer build-up.

Finally, composite resins may wear, and the wear will be greatest in the larger as opposed to the smaller gap widths.[14-16] Additionally, dissolution of the resin matrix of composite resin in oral fluids has been demonstrated through in vitro studies.[17,18] Minimizing the composite component and maximizing the porcelain component by adapting the porcelain veneer as closely as possible is desirable.

Technique

Subgingival margin placement should ideally be established 0.5 mm below the free gingival margin and 2.5 mm above the osseous crest to respect the biologic width.[19] Final margin placement can be rendered with a high-torque, low-speed hand piece. The preparation margin is placed at the free gingival margin with or without the tissue retracted (see Fig 10-22). If more than 3 mm of soft tissue exists from the free gingival margin to the osseous crest (the interproximal tissue of the maxillary anterior teeth where the gingival scallop is more pronounced than the osseous scallop), the subgingival margin placement can be greater than 0.5 mm. When subgingival margin placement is not ideal, it is performed according to the biological context for a particular biotype.[20]

Lip Lines

In cases where the root structure is darkly stained (such as endodontically treated teeth), the cervical margin should also be placed subgingivally. In addition to the details concerning the cervical margin preparation, the lip and smile lines must be studied in advance in order to mask the discoloration. One of the conditions in which the gingival margin may not be hidden in a tetracycline case can be when a low lip line position exists. This is also true when the lower lip covers the gingival margins of the lower anteriors. In such cases

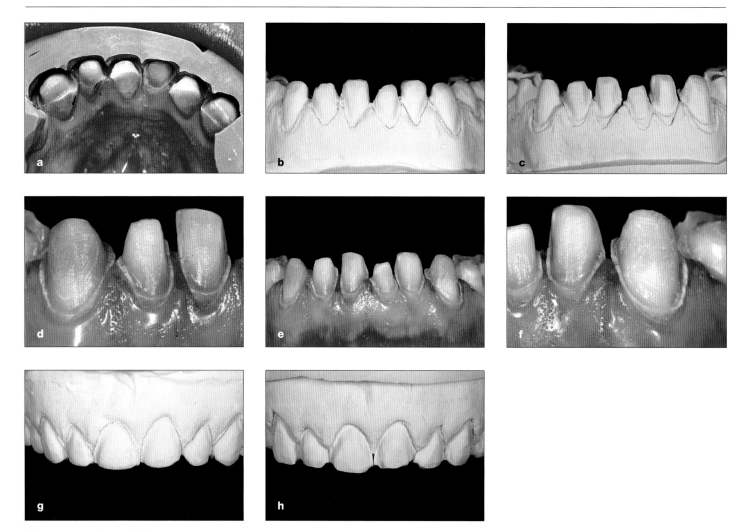

Fig 10-25a-h (a) The mandibular preparations almost duplicate the laboratory preparations. Silicone index is used to verify the necessary tooth reduction. (b, c) The proposed lab model versus the actual preparation model. Note how the preparation guide (white stone model) is utilized to form the actual preparation taken from the patient's impression (beige stone model). (d to f) Actual preparations. Note the supragingivally placed cervical margins. (g, h) Maxillary proposed model versus actual preparation model. Note how closely the preparation guide (white stone model) provided by the technician is duplicated at the actual preparation (beige stone model).

it is virtually impossible to see the porcelain laminate veneer-tooth interface at the gingival margin area. This will not only enhance the bond strengths with the margin being placed on enamel, but the post-op gingival health as well (see Figs 10-25 (d, c, f) and Fig 10-48). However, this is a very critical decision and the dentist must definitely discuss it with the patient in order to avoid the possibility of postoperative dissatisfaction. Some patients with a low lip line and who are not too demanding concerning esthetic details will understand the advantage of limited tooth reduction and accept it. However, patients who are demanding of esthetic results will not be willing to accept visible margins.

In cases where the margins are visible, such as in the medium and high lip line situations, and when gingival recession is expected for various reasons, the cervical finishing line would be extended a fraction deeper, provided that the biologic width is not violated. In order to prevent future conflicts, the patient should also be informed that the margins may become visible in the future owing to biologic gingival recession, which is a result of natural aging.

Iatrogenic factors may be the cause of early tissue recession. Gingival curettage and nicking tissue with the diamond burs while placing the subgingival margin should therefore be avoided. However, the risks and disadvantages of subgin-

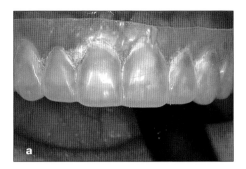
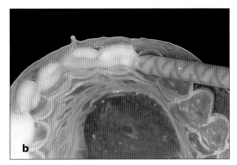
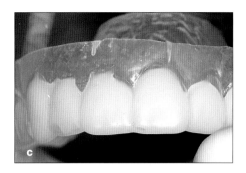

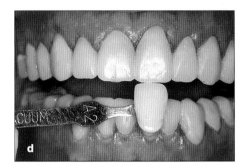

Fig 10-26a-d (a) The transparent template can also be used to double-check the preparations. (b) Then it is loaded with a flowable light curing composite (Luxatemp). (c) It is placed over the prepared teeth. (d) After being light cured, the final color is double-checked with the shade guide. This stage should be the last stage to verify the color, form, surface texture and occlusion. The patient should be given the chance of communicating with the dentist at any time during this stage, if he/she has any concerns about the final esthetic outcome. If any modifications are to be made, these changes should be reported to the lab technician so as to prevent further complications at the try-in and bonding stages.

gival margin placement, as well as the esthetic advantages and possible periodontal risks, should all be discussed with the patient.[16] The teeth in this case are prepared relative to the laboratory diagnostic preparations (Fig 10-25).

Stump Shade Guide

Once the tooth is prepped it is of extreme importance to transfer the stump shade color to the lab. This refers to the existing color of the thin enamel or dentin after the preparation. As mentioned before, as a part of the enamel has been stripped off during porcelain laminate veneer prep, the color of the prepped tooth will appear even darker. That color should be noted accurately and sent to the lab.

A common mistake made at this stage is to take this color when the tooth is dry, or dehydrated. It should never be forgotten that dehydrated teeth appear lighter in color. If the stump shade is taken under dry conditions, the tooth itself will unfortunately appear darker at the bonding appointment when the tooth becomes wet with the try-in paste or bonding agent. To avoid such problems, the prepared tooth must always be kept wet, and the stump shade should always be taken while in a wet state.

Provisionals

To finalize the preparation appointment the provisionals are fabricated. They will be the true test of the functional concerns (Fig 10-26). The fully esthetic wax-up is used to create patient temporaries. An impression (silicone or alginate) made from the wax-up model or using the lab putty index achieves this. The patient evaluates the placed temporary for comfort, esthetics and function. The patient and dentist must communicate fully at this step. Preferably, the patient should also consult with the ceramist better to convey an understanding of esthetic form and color considerations, both of which can be reevaluated and adjustments noted at this time.

Laboratory Communication 2

The laboratory receives the facebow, final impression, photographs and a study cast of the temporaries. The ceramist now prepares the final build-up, utilizing notes on any functional and/or esthetic corrections from the dentist and/or the patient. Again, following these steps carefully with the end result always in mind virtually ensures a superior final result.

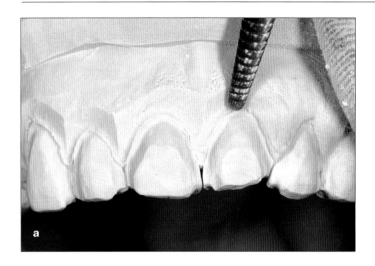

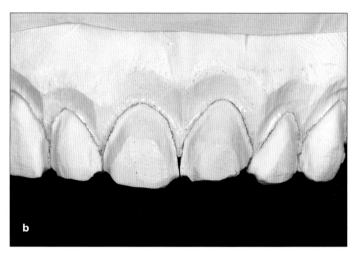

Fig 10-27a, b The margins are prepared for the foiling technique.

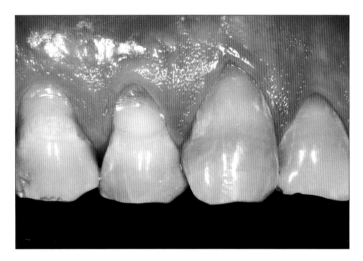

Fig 10-28 The ceramist prefers to use the feldspathic porcelain in order to mask such discoloration, without creating an opaque look.

Feldspathic Porcelain over Foiling Technique

Once the master model is obtained, the margin is then prepared to start the fabrication of porcelain laminate veneer restorations (Fig 10-27). Because of the severe tetracycline discoloration in the patient's teeth, the ceramist employs feldspathic porcelain. This allows for maximum light transmission while enabling the ceramist to customize the final opacity (Fig 10-28). A more opaque material might mask the discoloration, but the end result would not truly mimic the light transmission and luminescence of natural teeth. In order to mask such a discoloration in a very natural way, various colors should be incorporated with a delicately executed layering technique (Figs 10-29 to 10-37).

Completed Restoration

With corrections made for esthetics and function, the ceramist's artistic talent becomes the final factor in the completed restoration. At this point, every minor detail (i.e. from the patient's personality to skin tone) is taken into account by the ceramist to transform the smile.

Bonding the Veneers

When the veneers are received from the laboratory, they are tried in, checked for the marginal adaptation, and, most importantly, for the color fit. It is amazing to see the color difference created in a very natural-looking way through the ceramic without opaque composites that are used at the preparation stage to cover the dark discoloration (Fig 10-38). The veneers are tried with water and bonded with the translucent luting agent (see Chapter 7) (Figs 10-39 to 10-43).

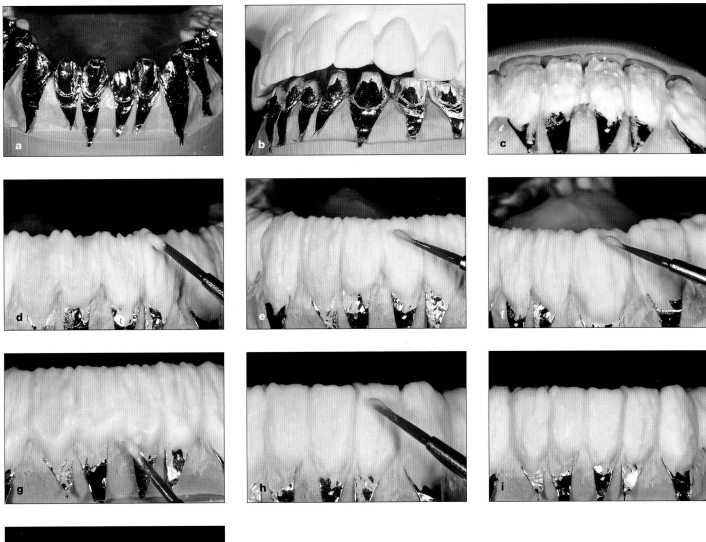

Fig 10-29a-j (a, b) The lower porcelain veneers are built against a cross-mounted duplicate of the upper temporaries. The folio is neatly adjusted over the prepared teeth. (c) The putty index from the incisal edge of the temporaries can also be utilized. (d-i) The layering technique is used incrementally to block out the discoloration as well as to create a natural-looking smile. (Ceramist: *Jason Kim*.)

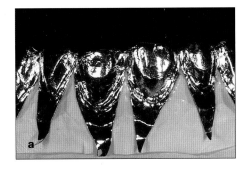

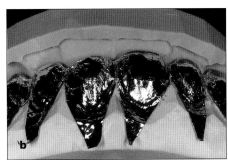

Fig 10-30a, b The uppers are built using the same cross-mounting technique. A putty index is generated from the temporaries to ensure the correct incisal edge position of the upper anteriors.

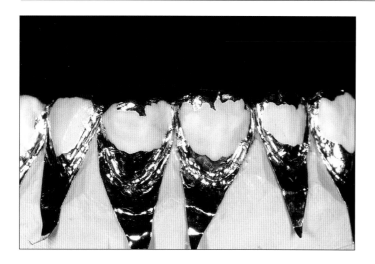

Fig 10-31 To create the closest imitation of nature, ceramist *Jason Kim* has used *Willie Geller's* Creation feldsthethic porcelain with which his artistic hands have the best possibility of controlling fluorescence and opalescence while masking the darkest tetracycline stain on porcelain laminate restorations. To cover tetracycline stain, OD A3 was used. It is a strongly fluorescing material and at the same time has the ability to block tetracycline stain with enough opacity.

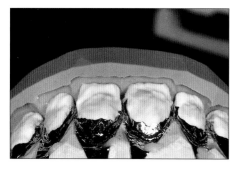

Fig 10-32 Incisal matrixes indicate the lengthening of incisors. As the incisal area does not have the support of natural dentin, OD A1 was used to block the free admittance of light.

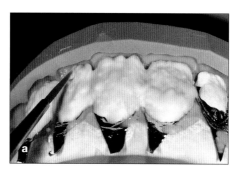

Fig 10-33a, b Dentin A1 as base color, A2 for canines, and California White was used in centrals and #8217 body area to brighten the value.

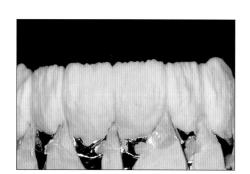

Fig 10-34 Enamel and #8211;57/58. 59 for canines.

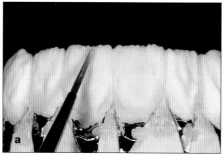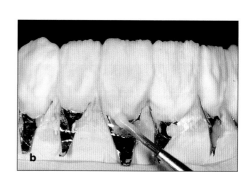

Fig 10-35a, b For mamelon imitation, MI 64, 65, 61 White was mixed with Dentin A1 (to lower the opacity) and fluorescent stain in Nova #3, 4 was used to chromatize. For cervical material, HT 52 and HT 52+ 53 (for canines) that have strong fluorescence were used to increase chroma with translucency.

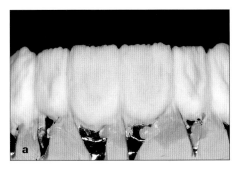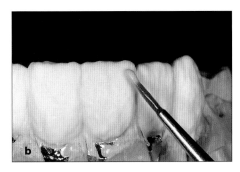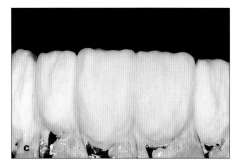

Fig 10-36a-c In layering labial materials, various TI SI was used to create the opalescent effect. SI2, SI4, SI2/CLO, TI3, TI1, OT, TI4, TI2, 58/CLO were applied in a segmental build–up technique.

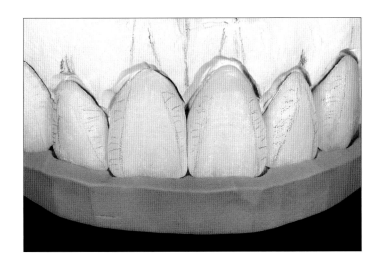

Fig 10-37 The incisal index from the original wax-up model is used for contouring esthetics and to guide incisal edge position. The ceramist contours the veneers, paying careful attention to the highlights of the contours. The contouring of the upper porcelain veneers is finalized. The correct position of the incisal edge is maintained by carefully referring to the incisal edge index.

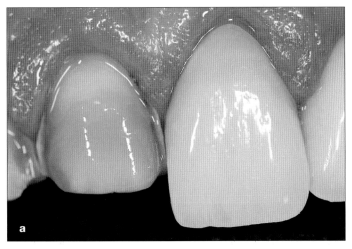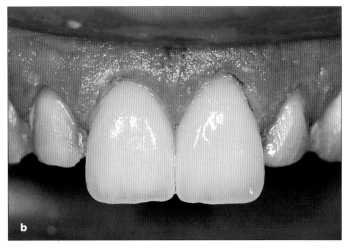

Fig 10-38a, b The veneers are tried in one by one and in pairs. (a) Note the extremely natural color-masking of the porcelain veneer as compared with the prepared tooth color. The holding medium is water, which only means that no color alterations need to be made by colored opaque luting resins. (b) A sectional rubber dam is applied for ease of cementation.

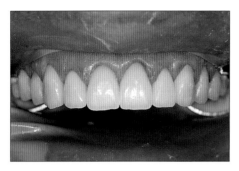 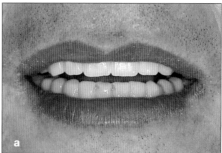 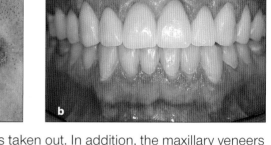

Fig 10-39 Applying the actual bonding procedures, all the maxillary veneers are bonded.

Fig 10-40a, b The rubber dam is taken out. In addition, the maxillary veneers are evaluated, together with the mandibular provisionals. Note the exellent harmony of the maxillary porcelain laminate veneers with the mandibular provisionals, in terms of both esthetics and occlusion. This can only be achieved with properly communicated treatment planning and delicately executed laboratory work.

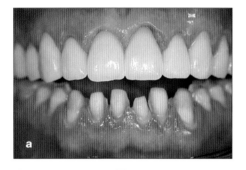 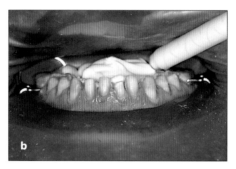 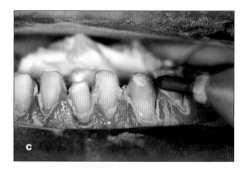

Fig 10-41a-c (a) The mandibular provisionals are removed. (b) Next, a sectional rubber dam is applied. The lingual opening is sealed with Vanilla Mousse (Discus Dental) to stop any saliva contamination as well as intraoral humidity. (c) The prepared surfaces are sand blasted.

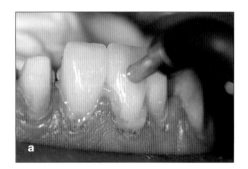 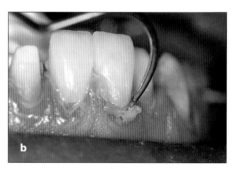 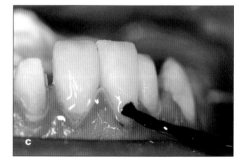

Fig 10-42a-c (a) After etching and adhesive application, the veneers are seated in pairs and spot tacked with a 2 mm turbo tip (Optilux 501, Kerr) at the middle 1/3rd. (b) The still non-polymerized composite flush is removed with an explorer and a brush that is dipped into the adhesive. (c) The margins are coated with DeOx (Ultradent) to prevent oxygen inhibition and the veneers are separately light cured for 60 seconds, from different angles, in order to prevent overheating that may irreversibly damage the pulp.

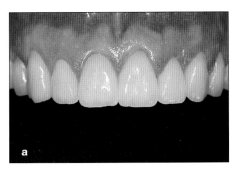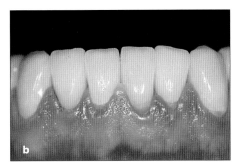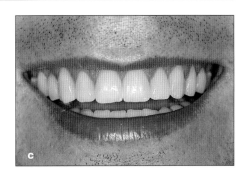

Fig 10-43a-c Finished case with 10 maxillary and 10 mandibular porcelain laminate veneers.

Details

It is important to block out dark discoloration when using porcelain laminate veneers. If special care is not given, in most cases it will be difficult to achieve such results. While doing this, the color gradation within the tooth itself should be mentioned, such as the cervical 1/3rd with the highest chroma, middle 1/3rd high in value and incisal 1/3rd with all the translucencies. The margin placement, both cervical and interproximal, is extremely important specifically in masking dark discolorations, since otherwise any tooth structure showing through these areas will distort the esthetic outcome.

The arrangement of mandibular teeth should be as natural looking as the maxillary teeth. And when all these criteria are met, the results are always pleasant for the patient, dentist and technician (Figs 10-44 to 10-49).

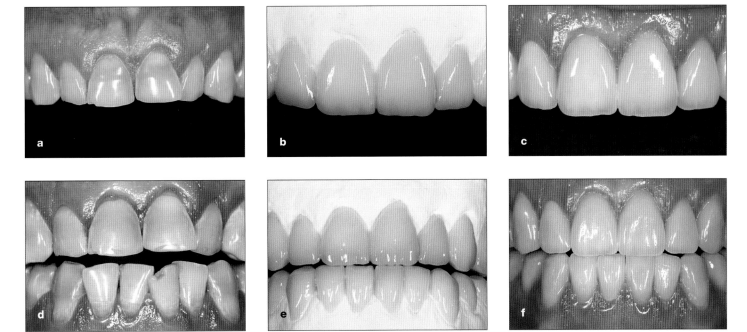

Fig 10-44a-f Transition. (a, d) The teeth exhibiting heavy discoloration. (b, e) The delicate wax-ups produced at the lab that exactly mimic the finished porcelain laminate veneers in terms of form, texture and translucencies. (c, f) The finished veneers. Such a precise collaboration can only be achieved with profound dentist–technician communication.

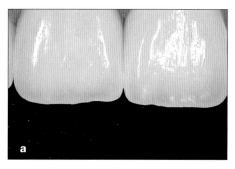 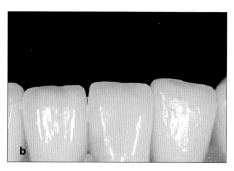

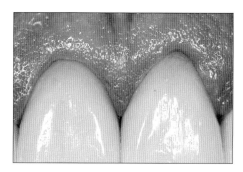

Fig 10-45a, b Note the incisal edge configuration of both the maxillary and mandibular incisors. A very soft transition from the translucencies to the main body shade. The tooth inclinations and incisal edges of the mandibular incisors are deliberately placed in slightly different angles in order to create a natural looking effect (Ceramist: *Jason Kim*).

Fig 10-46 Even though the cervical margins are only placed 0.2 mm sub-gingivally, the dark discoloration is completely blocked out. Note the healthy condition of the gingiva.

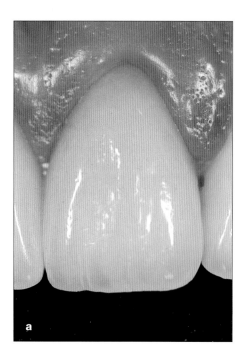 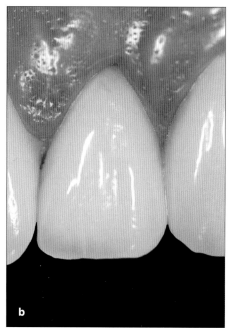

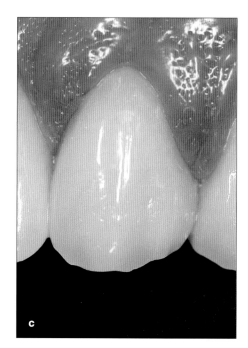

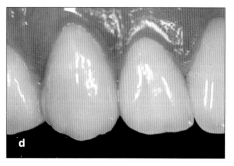

Fig 10-47a-d The central, lateral and canine. Note the interproximal transitions. Owing to correct placement of the interproximal margin during preparation, it is not possible to see the dark color of the teeth from any angle. (d) A color gradation is deliberately achieved. Note the chroma of the canine being higher than the central and lateral.

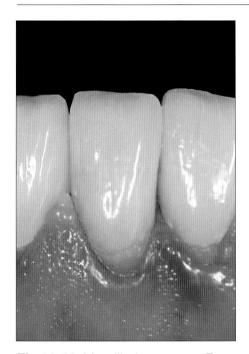

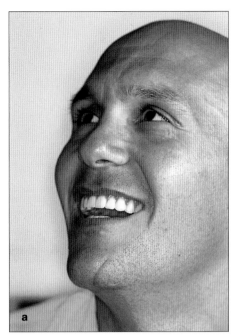

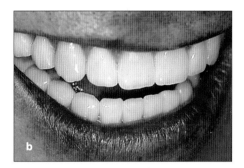

Fig 10-48 Mandibular veneers. Even though this is a tetracycline case, the cervical margins are prepared supragingivally, at least 1 mm away from the gingiva, in order to place the margins in enamel. It is impossible to see this area unless the lower lip is delibrately pulled down.

Fig 10-49a, b The smile from different angles, exhibiting a pleasant arrangement of the porcelain laminate veneers' beautifully blended color, form and texture.

Conclusion

The teamwork and talent exhibited in this case are textbook examples of how the dentist and ceramist can produce a restoration unrivalled in function and esthetics. Careful attention to each step of the process will ensure an accurately placed, comfortable, functional and esthetically appealing smile – not to mention the heightened sense of self-esteem for the patient that will inevitably accompany the restoration.

References

1. Touati B, Miara P, Nathanson D. Esthetic Dentistry and Ceramic Restorations. New York: Martin Dunitz, 1999:161-214.

2. Garber DA, Goldstein RE, Feinman RA. Porcelain Laminate Veneers. Chicago: Quintessence, 1988.

3. McComb D. Porcelain veneer technique. Ont Dent 1998;65: 25-27, 29, 31-32.

4. Clyde JS, Gilmore A. Porcelain laminate veneers. A preliminary review. Br Dent J 1988;164:9-14.

5. Albers HF. Tooth Colored Restoratives: Indirect bonded restorations, Santa Rosa: Alto Books, 1989;1-42, supplement.

6. Peumans M, Van Meerbeek B, Lambrechts P, Vuylsteke-Wauters M, Vanherle G. Five-year clinical performance of porcelain veneers. Quintessence Int 1998;29:211-221.

7. Dale BG, Aschheim KW. Esthetic Dentistry: A Clinical Approach to Techniques and Materials. Philadelphia, PA: Lea and Febiger, 1993:123-150.

8. Touati B, Miara P, Nathanson D. Esthetic Dentistry and Ceramic Restorations. New York: Martin Dunitz, 1999: 215-257.

9. Ahmad I. Predetermining factors governing calculated tooth preparation for anterior crowns QDT 2001;24:57-68.

10. Gargiulo AW, Wentz FM, Orban B. Dimensions and relations of the dentogingival junction in humans. J Periodontol 1961;32:261-267.

11. Nixon RL, IPS Empress: The ceramic system of the future. Signature 1994;1:10-15.

12. Bausch JR, de Lange K, Davidson CL, Peters A, de Gee AJ. Clinical significance of polymerization shrinkage of composite resins. J Prosthet Dent 1982;48:59-67.

13. Shinkai K, Suzuki S, Leinfelder KF, Katoh Y. Effect of gap dimension on wear resistance of luting agents. Am J Dent 1995;8:149-151.

14. McKinney JE, Wu W. Chemical softening and wear of dental composites. J Dent Res. 1985;64:1326-1331.

15. Roulet JF, Walti C. Influence of oral fluid on composite resin and glass-ionomer cement. J Prosthet Dent 1984;52: 182-189.

16. Vrijhoef MM, Hendriks FH, Letzel H. Loss of substance of dental composite restorations. Dent Mater 1985;1:101-105.

17. Becker W, Ochsenbein C, Becker BE. Crown lengthening: The periodontal-restorative connection. Compend Contin Educ Dent. 1998;19:239-240, 242, 244-246.

18. Kois JC. The restorative-periodontal interface: Biological parameters. Periodontol 2000 1996;11:29-38.

19. Sanavi F, Weisgold AS, Rose LF. Biologic width and its relation to periodontal biotypes. J Esthet Dent 1998;10: 157-163.

20. Qaltrough AJE, Burke FJT. A look at dental esthetics. Quintessence Int 1994;25:7-14.

11 Adjunctive Orthodontics, as Related to Periodontics and Aesthetic Dentistry

Frank Celenza, Jr.

Introduction

A complete and thorough consideration of orthodontic diagnosis and treatment is beyond the scope of the central theme of this textbook, and many of the intricacies involved are unrelated to its central theme. However, this book would be incomplete without the inclusion of the essential adjunctive and complementary aspects of orthodontics. Orthodontic treatment, preparatory to restorative and cosmetic therapy, lends substantial benefits to the end result, and the purpose of this chapter is to illustrate these interrelationships. Tooth movement can be employed to harness the body's own reparative and remodeling capabilities prior to restorative procedures and offer a more comprehensive approach to ultimate esthetics. Further, orthodontic tooth movement presents alternative treatment options, particularly as related to difficult restorative circumstances, which must be included in treatment planning when esthetics is the goal. Orthodontic therapy complements and integrates with restorative modalities, but it must also be considered as an adjunct to periodontal therapeutics when treating cosmetic dilemmas. This chapter is intended to identify these interrelationships and explore the orthodontic side of esthetic dental treatment as an adjunct to restorative and periodontal therapeutics. By definition, adjunctive orthodontics is tooth movement used to facilitate other dental procedures essential to control disease as well as restore function and esthetics. The areas in which orthodontic intervention can facilitate cosmetic dental procedures include:

1. Management of disproportionate tooth dimensions and space relationships.
2. Assymmetric or aberrant gingival margin architecture.
3. Incorrect incisal edge and cementoenamel junction (CEJ) positions.
4. Discrepant interdental papilla morphology.
5. Management of restorations with deficient biologic widths.

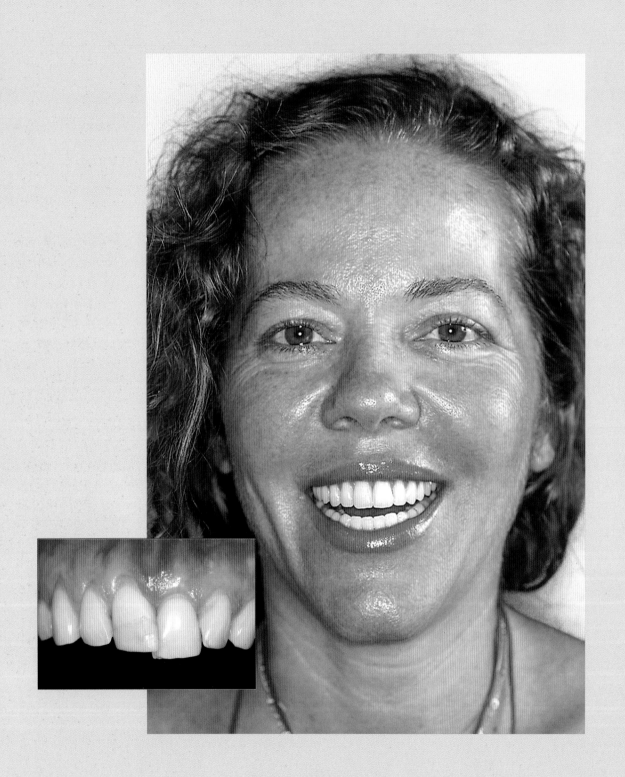

Various forms of tooth movements may be employed to address the above clinical circumstances. These forms include:
1. Bodily mesiodistal movements.
2. Eruptive or incisally directed movements.
3. Rotations.
4. Tipping movements.
5. Torque movements.

It is important for the clinician to understand how these movements relate to and affect the periodontium. From a morphologic standpoint, the periodontal ramifications of tooth position are paramount to this discussion. An overview of the biologic basis of orthodontics is included in this chapter, and the reader will gain an appreciation for the interrelationship between tooth position and periodontal morphology. From a mechanotherapeutic standpoint, there exists a myriad of appliance designs that can accomplish the intended orthodontic outcome. All these appliances can be classified as either fixed or removable. This chapter will review both appliance types, explore the advantages and disadvantages of each, and review new developments in cosmetic and invisible appliances.

Biologic Basis for Tooth Movement

The nature of the attachment apparatus between a tooth and its supporting tissues allows extensive remodeling and alteration of the investing tissues under the right circumstances. This characteristic renders the orthodontic tooth movement possible. There are three zones of attachment between a tooth and the periodontal tissues. They are identified as (from apex to crown) the periodontal ligament, the supracrestal connective fiber apparatus and the junctional epithelium (Fig 11-1). The various ways in which these dentoalveolar and dentogingival junctions impart pressure and tension to their investing tissues can be harnessed via orthodontics to effect beneficial morphologic alterations.

The periodontal ligament is a link between the root surface of the tooth, in which its fibers are inserted into the tooth cementum by virtue of "Sharpey's Fibers" and connect across the ligament space into the alveolar bone. "Wolff's law," which is of paramount importance in orthodontics, states that bone tissue responds to pressure by resorption and to tension by deposition. The periodontal ligament is responsible for providing the pressure and tension stimuli to the alveolar housing of the tooth. It allows a tooth to be moved through the alveolar bone, enveloped in bone that remodels in response.

The supracrestal connective tissue fiber apparatus comprises four groups of fibers.[1] These interconnected and intertwined groups reside in the gingival compartment, just coronal to the alveolar crest (Fig 11-2). The collagen-rich fiber groups originate in the cementum, just apical to the cementoenamel junction, although not all insert into the same tissues. The dentogingival group of fibers inserts into the gingival connective tissues; the dentoalveolar group inserts into the alveolar periosteum (the overlying connective tissue of the alveolar bone); the transseptal group inserts into the cementum of the neighboring tooth; and the circumferential group encircles a tooth, contributing to the connective tissue "cuff" that houses it. These fiber groups may be considered as an intermediary that can impart stimuli to the gingival soft tissues in response to orthodontic forces.

The junctional epithelium provides a unique attachment of the gingival tissues to the enamel of the tooth—it is not a true insertion, but an epithelial attachment or adherence. Using electron microscopy, this epithelial adherence can be visually observed. It occurs by virtue of "hemidesmosomal" structures, which function similarly to the suction cups in morphology. In this manner, the junctional epithelium is subject to certain stresses and strains that are placed onto the tooth. As a result, significant alterations may occur in the gingival tissues.

Two of the attachment zones described above are dentogingival, whereas the periodontal ligament is a dentoalveolar attachment. The two dentogingival zones — the supracrestal connective

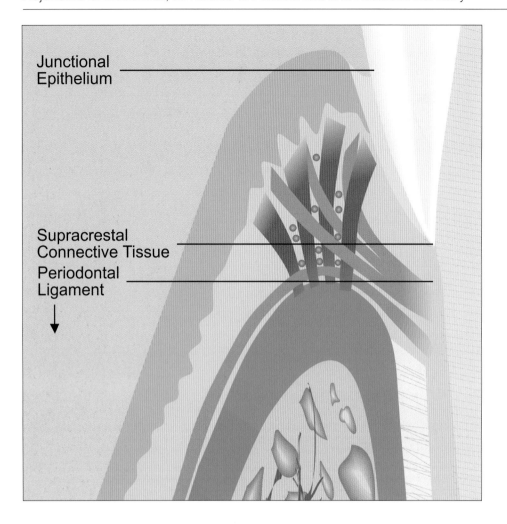

Junctional Epithelium

Supracrestal Connective Tissue

Periodontal Ligament ↓

Fig 11-1 The tooth and its periodontium. The zones of dento-alveolar and dento-gingival attachment are depicted, and include (apicocoronally) the periodontal ligament, the supra-crestal connective tissue fibers and the junctional epithelium.

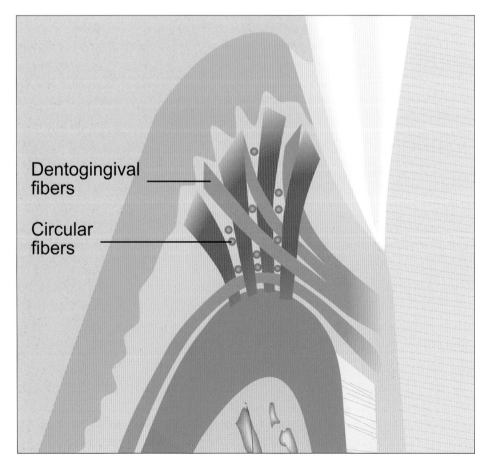

Dentogingival fibers

Circular fibers

Fig 11-2 The two fiber groups of the gingival connective tissue.

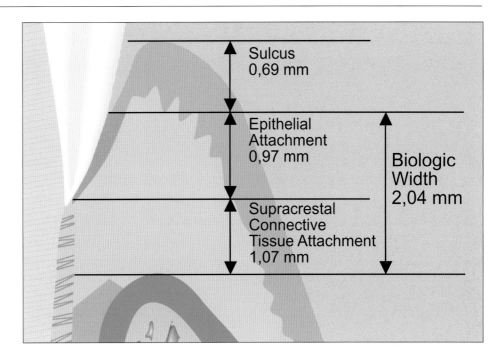

Sulcus
0,69 mm

Epithelial
Attachment
0,97 mm

Biologic
Width
2,04 mm

Supracrestal
Connective
Tissue Attachment
1,07 mm

Fig 11-3 The zone of "biologic width", formed by the supracrestal connective tissue fiber groups and the zone of junctional epithelium. This supra-crestal zone has been quantified and is considered inviolate with respect to proper tooth preparation and restoration.

fibers and the junctional epithelium—have been quantified in their dimension. Together, these zones form what is commonly known as the zone of "biologic width" (Fig 11-3), which has been shown to measure a minimum of 2 mm occlusoapically (each attachment zone contributes approximately 1 mm).[2] The importance of the zone of biologic width cannot be overstated whenever restorative dental procedures are performed. Much has been written about preserving this zone,[3] and measures to prevent violation of this area must be observed in order to respect the periodontal health of the dentogingival junction. Obviously, this is pertinent when performing subgingival restorations.

In a healthy environment that is free of soft tissue inflammation, these various attachment apparatuses can be utilized to effect morphologic alterations of the tissues in which the tooth is housed. These include changes to the soft (gingival) and hard (alveolar) tissues. Conversely, the morphology and nature of the investing tissues are often the result of the position of the tooth, i.e., compromised health or cosmetics. This indicates that cases in which health or cosmetics are compromised are often the result of an incorrect position of the tooth.

If the gingival tissues are to be incorporated as part of the cosmetic picture, as they should be,[4]

and the morphology of the gingival tissue is related to tooth position, it follows that the stability and longevity of the cosmetic result must include a consideration of proper tooth position. Since tooth position influences periodontal morphology, corrective measures to the periodontium may be implemented through orthodontic therapy. As will be shown, orthodontics — as a pre-prosthetic tool — may be utilized to achieve a significantly improved and enduring esthetic result.

For instance, dehiscence of hard or soft tissue can often be demonstrated as position-related. This alteration can be attributed to a tooth that has excessive buccal root torque (Figs 11-4 and 11-5) or even to a tooth with a buccally ectopic position. This type of situation usually involves a tooth or root that lies outside the boundaries of its alveolar housing and exceeds the limits of the alveolar bone that envelops it.[5] Further, the gingival tissues may be similarly exceeded and lack the ability to bridge and cover the root surface. In the case of a dehiscence of hard tissues only, if the gingival tissue is present to cover the root surface, it must be considered as very delicate and friable. There are two reasons for such consideration: If the gingival tissue is present over a root surface that has an underlying bony dehiscence, the periosteum that normally exists on the surface of the alveolar bone is lacking. Consequently, the gingiva will

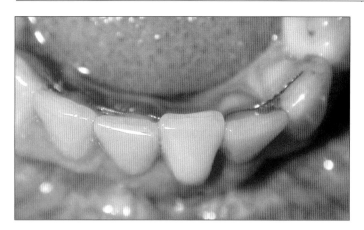

Fig 11-4 Incisal view of post-orthodontic result in which the mandibular left central incisor displays excessive buccal root torque. This results in a very thin, if not nonexistent, labial bone plate, and would predispose the tooth to dehiscence.

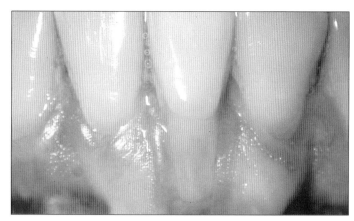

Fig 11-5 Labial view of same tooth as in Figure 11-4. Observe significant soft and hard tissue dehiscence, a consequence of improper tooth position within alveolar housing. Numerous surgical attempts at correction, by gingival augmentation techniques have proven unsuccessful at bridging and covering the root surface.

have no underlying blood supply and must rely upon nourishment from the peripheral areas to be viable. A wider dehiscence is more likely to be accompanied by gingival recession.[6] If a tooth or root is buccally prominent, the gingival tissues will be vulnerable to physical injury, such as toothbrush trauma or scraping during mastication.

When reasonably simple and predictable periodontal grafting and root coverage procedures are utilized, they should be preceded by adjunctive orthodontic procedures to correct the underlying etiology.[7-9] Used in this precautionary manner, orthodontics complements periodontal therapy, and a more stable and predictable end result is achieved. In the case of root dehiscence, application of lingual root torque is often the adjunctive orthodontic procedure of choice. It results in a narrower dehiscence and a less prominent root surface to bridge, which, in turn, aids the periodontal prognosis and surgical outcome considerably.

Teeth that possess discrepant levels of eruption may also pose an esthetic dilemma. The location of the CEJ has a direct impact upon the location of the free gingival margin of a tooth. For the adjacent teeth to display a confluent and harmonious gingival contour, they must have corresponding unified levels of eruption. Adjunctive orthodontic therapy, in the form of selective erup-

tion to harmonize the levels of eruption of the teeth, may have a profound cosmetic effect, particularly in the "cosmetic zone".[10]

It must be remembered that while orthodontics may be employed to impart morphologic alterations to the periodontal structures, tooth movement has never been shown to result in "new attachment" phenomena in the strict sense. This means that while significant remodeling and reorientation of the periodontal tissues (such as bone fill, leveling of defects, coordination of gingival margins and gingival augmentation) may be achieved in response to the tooth movement, repair of a pathologic root surface can never be expected. To a periodontist, new attachment means the formation of new periodontal ligament fibers that insert into a previously diseased root surface by virtue of newly formed cementum and Sharpey's fibers. Controlled orthodontics has never demonstrated this type of regenerative capacity; therefore, it cannot be overstressed that the type of reparative phenomenon described here is limited to a morphologic alteration at the existing level of attachment. Additional considerations of tooth movements related to cosmetics, including case examples, follow in a subsequent section of this chapter.

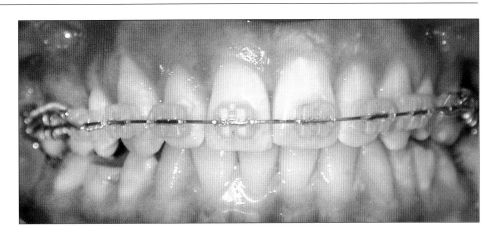

Fig 11-6 Anterior view of a typical fixed orthodontic appliance, bonded to the maxillary arch; in this case, with clear brackets and nickel-titanium archwire. Bracket placement, in terms of apico-coronal location as well as angulation, in conjunction with the labial offset that is built into the bracket base will determine the tooth's ultimate positioning within the dental arch. Modifications can be made by contouring bends made to the archwire.

Basic Appliance Design

In the most basic sense, there are two types of orthodontic appliances—fixed and removable. When selecting appliances, the most important difference to be understood is the specific type of movement required to accomplish the desired result. Due to the nature of removable appliances and the way in which they exert force on a tooth, they are always limited in their ability to affect the highest order of controlled movements. Torquing movements and bodily movements are examples of tooth movements that require higher levels of control, and they are best left to fixed-appliance mechanotherapy. The advantages and disadvantages of the various appliances are reviewed in the following text.

For the purposes of this discussion, we selected a case in which adjunctive movements of a specific nature are being attempted, and the selection of a fixed appliance is appropriate. The modern fixed orthodontic appliance is comfortable and easy to place, manage and remove; the placement is expedient, reversible and predictable (Fig 11-6). Adhesive technology has advanced considerably and allows utilization of fully bonded appliances. While some practitioners still rely on bonded and cemented attachments in posterior areas, this practice remains as a carry-over from the older and more traditional mechanotherapy. Today's fully bonded appliance is sufficiently reliable for consideration as the appliance of choice for adjunctive procedures.

The most common form of orthodontic bracket consists of a double edgewise-winged bracket with a precision-machined slot that engages an archwire (Figs 11-7a to c). The bracket may be fabricated of stainless steel, with a streamlined profile and at a lesser cost, or it can be made of a variety of more esthetic or less-visible ceramic or composite materials. These latter cosmetic brackets are now the industry standard, especially for adult patients, and have replaced the more cumbersome and technique-sensitive lingual bonded brackets.

The edgewise bracket provides a means by which a precise archwire can be fastened to a tooth to effect a controlled guidance. This is accomplished by a sequence of wires that increase in gauge and material stiffness as the treatment progresses and alignment proceeds. The metallurgy behind these archwires is a science in itself, and it is beyond the scope of this discussion. In height and width, the archwires may form the exact dimension of the edgewise bracket slot. When combined with the offset that is built into the bracket base, positional control of a tooth in all three dimensions can be effectively attained. However, the need to utilize full-sized archwires is rare in adjunctive orthodontics, and minor tooth movements can be accomplished easily and effectively by using "light" or even round wires. Various elastic auxiliaries are used to fasten the archwire to the brackets and link or move teeth in the desired fashion. In summary, the primary advantages of fixed mechanotherapy are the ease and efficiency of the use of bonded

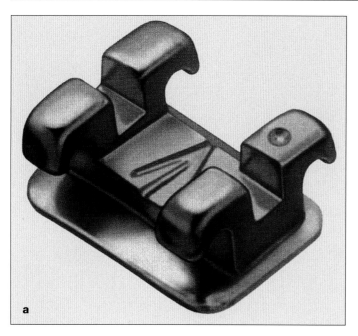

Fig 11-7a Typical edgewise bracket design. Precision horizontal slot will guide movement along the archwire that is inserted into the slot. Wings provide ties to secure the archwire. Correct positioning of bracket is indicated, by convention, by the dot on the tie wing.

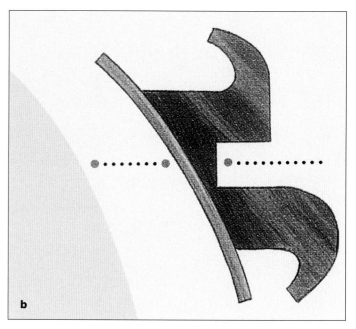

Fig 11-7b Lateral view of edgewise bracket shows how torque and offset are preset into bracket design of straight wire appliance. Each tooth has a bracket that is specifically designed for its contour and anatomy in a pre-torqued and pre-angulated appliance. This serves to minimize the need for operator intervention in the form of wire contouring and shaping.

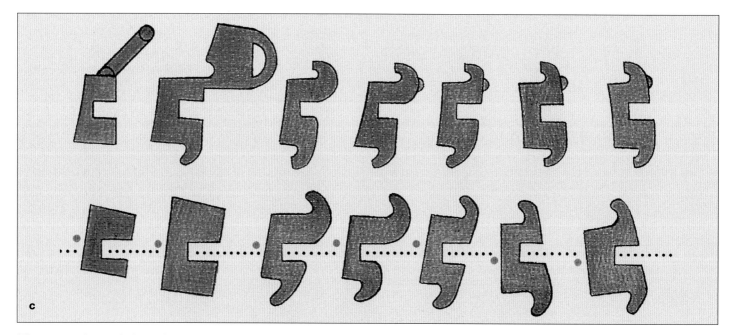

Fig 11-7c Lateral view of maxillary and mandibular quadrant of brackets, illustrating how each tooth in the dentition has a preadjusted bracket, specific to its anatomy and contour.

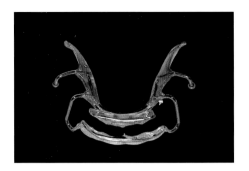

Fig 11-8a Mandibular Spring aligner—a typical removable orthodontic appliance.

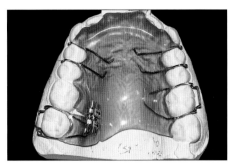

Fig 11-8b Maxillary Sagital appliance—placed here on a maxillary model.

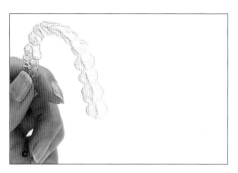

Fig 11-8c The Invisalign appliance. A series of these "aligners" is worn by the patient, in sequence, for two weeks each, to effect tooth movement.

appliances, comfort to the patient, and the fact that they are not as compliance-dependent as removable appliances.

Removable orthodontic appliances, on the contrary, are entirely compliance-dependent. This means that the outcome is dependent upon the patient's willingness and ability to wear the device. Whereas the adult patient is generally considered to be orthodontically motivated, the operator must bear in mind that the removable appliances can often be cumbersome and awkward to wear, especially in a working or social environment. Removable appliances are usually tooth- and tissue-borne, and require contact with large surface areas to achieve stability and anchorage (Fig 11-8a and b). As a result, they often have an effect on the patient's speech. Their ability to move teeth in certain dimensions is compromised, i.e., the application is limited by the ability of the appliances only to tip the teeth. Since most removable appliances exert force on a tooth by virtue of a finger spring or a point of contact, the movement that results is a direct result of the relationship between this point of contact (or force) application and the location of the tooth's center of rotation. Since the center of rotation is almost always located subcrestally, tipping movements are almost always the result. Bodily, torquing and eruptive movements are best accomplished by the use of fixed mechanics.

Generated by the limitations of traditional removable appliances, a new and apparently superior type of removable appliance — the Invisalign System — has been recently introduced (Fig 11-8c).[11] It is worthy of mention, because the early results are promising, and its concept and design are meritorious. The system features a series of clear vaccu-form-type aligners that are precision-manufactured using CAD technology. Computer-generated models emulate tooth movement in small increments upon which clear plastic "aligners" are fabricated. The aligners feature an intimate fit to the entire dentition and are not limited by the point of contact that hampers the more traditional removable appliances. Consequently, more controlled and precise movements are possible. Each aligner differs slightly from the preceding one by the extent of tooth movement that each will accomplish, and which is precisely incorporated into its configuration. Patients wear each set of aligners for two weeks, and then proceed to the next set. The Invisalign system is, therefore, a series of appliances, as adjustments to each are not possible in the traditional sense. The advantages of such a system are the comfort, invisibility and precision of its appliances. The main disadvantage of the Invisalign system is its limitation to adult treatment, since there is no way to "factor-in" or predict an adolescent's growth with this prefabricated appliance. Extensive bodily movements, such as extraction space closure and severe rotations may not be possible. Nevertheless, the system is proving to be a useful treatment alternative for patients who otherwise may not seek orthodontic treatment.

Adjunctive Tooth Movement as related to Aesthetic Dentistry

Forced Eruption

The use of forced eruption as an adjunctive movement is one of the simplest and most effective tooth movements. Well documented in the dental literature,[12] with citing as far back as the 1940s,[13] forced eruption is really a "natural" tooth movement in the sense that, under the right conditions, eruption occurs on its own. If a tooth is taken out of occlusion, for example, it will tend to erupt to the point of reestablishing contact. Use of an orthodontic appliance to accomplish an eruptive movement expedites this movement. Currently, there are four distinct indications for the use of forced eruption.[14] They include:

1. Leveling of isolated infrabony defects.[15]
2. Salvaging a non-restorable tooth.[16]
3. Harmonizing free gingival margins.[9]
4. Implant site development.[17]

This list indicates that forced eruption can be used to alter soft and hard tissue topography.[18] For the purposes of this discussion, the focus is placed upon the second and third indications.

Salvaging a non-restorable tooth

In clinical practice, patients may present with teeth rendered non-restorable by conventional means, either as the result of trauma (i.e, horizontal fracture) or pathology (i.e, external root resorption). These and other clinical circumstances require interdisciplinary dental procedures as a means of restoration. However, on numerous occasions, particularly in cosmetically sensitive areas, the traditional means of rendering such teeth restorable (e.g., through periodontal crown-lengthening surgery) are esthetically unacceptable. The design of such procedures requires that a gingival flap be elevated to expose the underlying osseous tissues and, after the osseous resection, be apically positioned to expose sound tooth structure. In the anterior region, the final result would be unesthetic and unacceptable for three

basic reasons (Fig 11-9). First, root exposure of the adjacent teeth is an unfortunate consequence that arises by virtue of the gingival flap design. The flap must be elongated at least one or two teeth beyond the affected tooth to allow access and proper osseous contouring, which must blend in laterally. Consequently, root exposure (or apparent recession) is the result on the teeth adjacent to the damaged unit, despite the fact that these teeth were unaffected previously. Second, loss of the interdental papilla is a second untoward result of traditional periodontal surgery. Again, this is due to the flap design and the procedure that is followed for crown-lengthening procedures. The resultant "black hole" is esthetically unacceptable, particularly in the anterior region, and currently there exists no predictable means to reconstruct a lost interdental papilla. Third, localized crown lengthening procedures often result in uneven gingival margins with associated discrepancies in tooth length. In these cases, cosmetics may again be significantly compromised.

The use of forced eruption is a compelling alternative in cases where other procedures would yield objectionable results. The orthodontic mechanotherapy is simple, expedient and effective — the attachment apparatus of the affected tooth is relocated to a more coronal position (Fig 11-10a and b). The depth of the tooth's defect determines the required extent of this relocation. By relocating the attachment apparatus or the osseous crest, the "unrestorable" tooth can be manipulated, or its crown lengthened, to be in harmony with the adjacent teeth, thereby obviating the need for resective or invasive involvement of these adjacent teeth. The three undesirable results of the conservative procedures are avoided, and the final esthetic result is often optimal.

The appliance design used to effect forced eruption may be simple. Again, anything that places an occlusally directed force on a tooth will effectively erupt the tooth, provided the occlusal or incisal surface has been reduced. The most commonly employed device for forced eruption consists of a fixed bonded sectional appliance, in which teeth are bracketed to the extent of two teeth on either side of the affected unit. All brackets are placed at the same level gingivo-

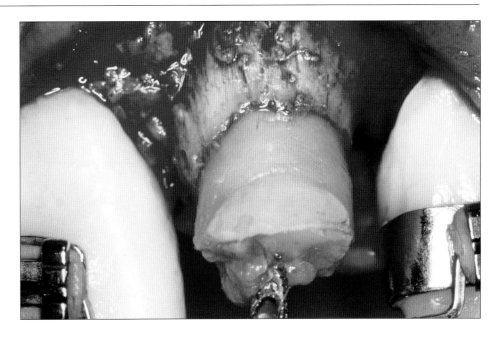

Fig 11-9 Clinical photograph of a gingival flap after forced eruption. Note how alveolar bone has responded to eruptive tooth movement, the spicules of crestal bone denoting the direction of tooth movement and crestal bone deposition associated with the tooth that was erupted. (Orthodontics and Periodontal Surgery, by *Roberto Pontoriero*, DDS, and reprinted with permission.)

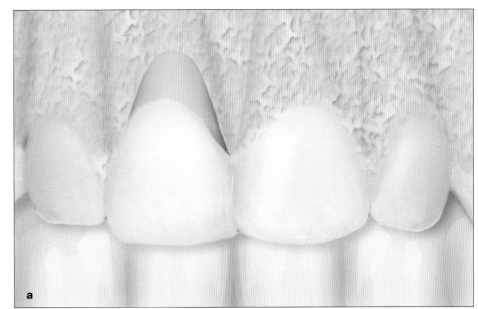

Fig 11-10a Schematic representation of three potential esthetic disadvantages of periodontal surgery in the cosmetic zone: uneven free gingival margins, root exposure and lost interdental papillae.

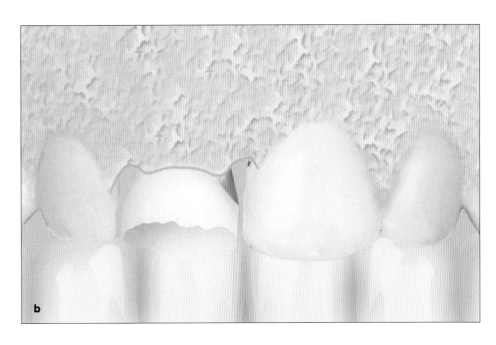

Fig 11-10b Schematic representation of the alteration to the alveolar crest that results from forced eruption. Notice how the alveolar crest of the right central incisor is depicted at a more incisal level than its neighbors, a result of that tooth's response to eruption.

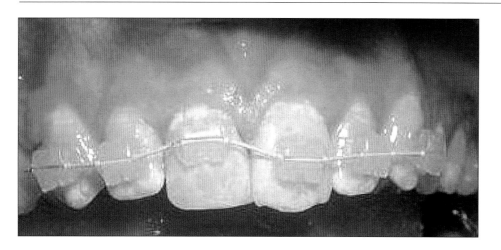

Fig 11-11 Typical set-up for forced eruption, in this case of a maxillary right central incisor. Note bracket placement, with all brackets at same horizontal level, except for the tooth to be erupted, which is more gingival. Activation of the appliance is accomplished by inserting the archwire into the slots of the brackets, and augmented by incisal and lingual tooth reduction as eruption proceeds.

coronally, in passive relationship to one another, except for the tooth to be erupted. The bracket of the defective tooth is bonded gingivally to the others (Fig 11-11), to the extent of the eruption required (usually 3 mm to 4 mm). The affected tooth is reduced, placing it out of occlusion, and a very light wire is inserted into the appliance (usually a braided "memo-flex" or "twisti-flex" type wire).

Patients are seen every 10 to 14 days for the purpose of reactivating the appliance and reducing the occlusal contact. Reactivation is accomplished by inserting more resilient arch wires, in sequence. A commonly employed sequence might be:

Twisti-flex
.016 mm nickel titanium
.018 mm nickel titanium
.018 mm stainless steel

It has been the experience of this author that these archwires, placed at 10- to 14-day intervals, are sufficient to achieve the desired end result. Other means for achieving further eruption include:

(a) relocating the bracket of the tooth to be erupted further gingivally and resequencing the archwires, and

(b) hooking the archwire over the top of the bracket's edgewise wings (Fig 11-12), rather than through the archwire slot, for an additional eruption of 1 mm or more.

Other clinical circumstances may arise that require alteration to the basic appliance design. For instance, the coronal aspect of a tooth may be fractured off completely, leaving no means by which to bond an orthodontic bracket. This condition may be remedied by placing a permanent post and core into the remaining root, onto which a provisional crown is securely cemented. An orthodontic bracket may then be bonded to the acrylic of the temporary crown. It is essential that the provisional crown be cemented securely to prevent the orthodontic force (that will be applied) from unseating the crown, even though this force is comparatively light. Additional deviations may arise and can test the imagination and ingenuity of the operator. There are countless solutions as well, and since forced eruption is not a technically demanding form of movement, a number of modifications to the basic appliance design will meet with success.[19]

When the tooth has undergone sufficient eruption, periodontal crown lengthening may be performed, but the surgical design can be altered by virtue of the alterations that orthodontic movement has caused. Now that the level of attachment of the erupted tooth has been relocated more coronally, resective surgical procedures are required only to reposition the attachment apparatus and gingival margin to their original levels. Significant exposure of sound tooth structure can be achieved, without incurring any of the untoward side effects to the surrounding area, as previously enumerated. The procedure may often

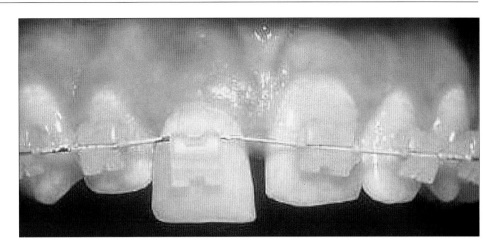

Fig 11-12 Hooking the arch wire over the top of the edgewise bracket affords an extra millimeter or two of eruption. The same effect could be achieved by contouring the archwire with a step-down at the right central incisor, or by rebonding the tooth's bracket further gingivally. (Orthodontics by *Frank Celenza*.)

be performed without surgical invasion of the adjacent areas, thereby reducing the need for surgical access, and the design of the gingival flap can be altered in a minimally invasive manner. In addition to the effective final result, these factors also result in a relatively minor cost in time, financial resources and effort, when compared to any other alternatives.

Alteration of free gingival margin

Confluent and harmonized free gingival margin location is important in achieving an optimal cosmetic outcome. The location of the free gingival margin must be coordinated with the patient's smile or lip line. The dictates of these relationships have been outlined elsewhere in this text. The coordination may be achieved by several means, frequently by periodontal plastic procedures. However, the relocation of the gingival margin can be effected through orthodontic intervention as well: specifically, by employing forced eruption.

The operator must make the diagnosis and determine the appropriate means of correction, confident in the knowledge that alteration of the tooth position will also include a corresponding alteration to gingival configuration. This occurs through a phenomenon known as "sulcular eversion" that was first quantified by *Atherton*.[20, 21] As a result, there is a period during sulcular eversion when a tissue type, known as "Atherton tissue," can be observed.

Sulcular eversion for gingival augmentation can be performed predictably. The process involves the reaction of the junctional epithelium, with its previously described hemidesmosomal adherence to the tooth, responding to the eruption of the tooth (in this case, forced eruption). As the tooth is erupted, the sulcular epithelium — which is not exposed to the oral environment at this stage and is nonkeratinized — everts outwards, and the junctional epithelium is directed coronally. For a short time, this nonkeratinized epithelium becomes exposed to the oral environment and can be visually observed as "whitish" in appearance (Fig 11-13). This tissue then undergoes keratinization, a process which takes approximately 10 days, during which time it appears reddened in color and is known as "Atherton's Patch". The newly formed gingiva augments the zone of keratinized gingiva and relocates the free gingival margin to a more coronal location.

This process of gingival tissue augmentation may be performed predictably to coordinate and harmonize the free gingival margins of dentition for cosmetic purposes (Figs 11-14 to 11-17). The previously described appliance design and management are applicable, although a lesser extent of eruption is usually achieved in this case. Generally, this treatment modality is employed pre-prosthetically, although it can be utilized as a final "fine-tuning" for the eventual post-restoration result. Multiple teeth may be erupted "selectively" to permit gingival augmentation over a wider area.

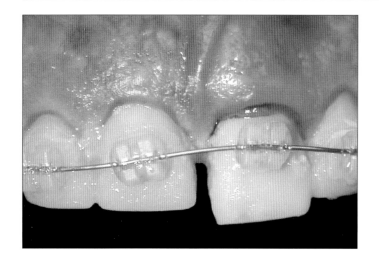

Fig 11-13 Sulcular eversion at the free gingival margin in response to forced eruption. The whitish-appearing marginal tissue represents non-keratinized sulcular epithelium that has everted in response to tooth movement and will undergo keratinization, resulting in gingival augmentation and relocation of the free gingival margin of the left central incisor. (Orthodontics by *Frank Celenza*.)

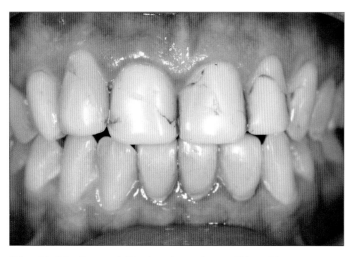

Fig 11-14 Case 1 Pre-treatment condition. Note reverse gingival architecture in which free gingival margins of lateral incisors are located apical to that of central incisors, which lends the appearance of unnatural and unesthetically long lateral incisors.

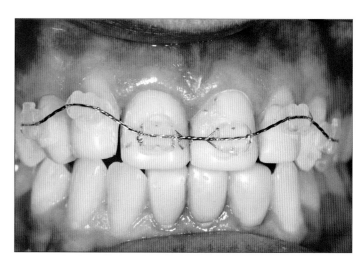

Fig 11-15 Placement of fixed orthodontic appliance. Observe bracket placement of lateral incisors and deflection of activated archwire to effect extrusion of these teeth.

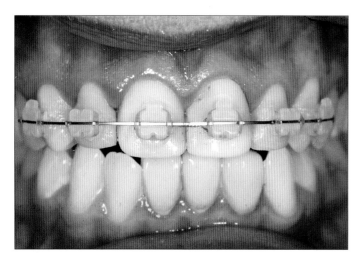

Fig 11-16 Orthodontic result. Archwire is now level, brackets are aligned horizontally, and free gingival margins have reoriented for proper relation, with lateral incisors shorter than central incisors.

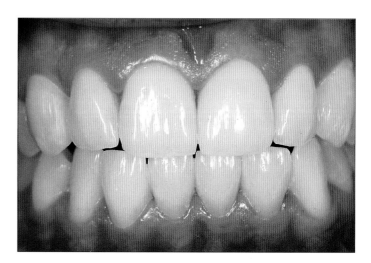

Fig 11-17 Restorative outcome. Note excellent esthetics that result from proper tooth length, proportion, and good coordination of free gingival margins. (Orthodontics and Restorations by *Stephen J Chu*.)

Intrusion Movements

Orthodontic intrusion (as the opposite movement of extrusion) must be regarded as a more difficult movement to accomplish from a mechanotherapy standpoint. Whereas extrusion was previously described as a "natural" form of tooth movement, intrusion is most "unnatural". The fiber orientation of the periodontal ligament is designed to withstand tooth intrusion during normal function, and it follows logically that intrusive forces of orthodontic origin will be similarly impeded. Furthermore, untoward side effects of intrusion have been observed, such as angular alveolar crests and deepened infrabony defects in periodontally involved areas.

Although more difficult to accomplish, intrusion can nevertheless be achieved under favorable circumstances, such as occlusal stability and adequate orthodontic anchorage. The operator is cautioned not to mistake an apparent intrusion for an actual extrusion of the anchor units (the latter often representing the path of less resistance). An example of an instance when intrusion might be preferable is a clinical case where incisal wear has occurred and is accompanied by compensatory eruption (Figs 11-18 to 11-22). In this case, the worn teeth had erupted over time and resulted in a shift of the free gingival margin, giving the teeth an unnaturally shortened appearance. Periodontal crown lengthening surgery is an obvious solution prior to restoration of such area; however, the use of orthodontic alternative of intrusion may have significant advantages. These advantages include:

(a) Better contour of the restored teeth. This results from the greater diameter of the root surface that is preserved by intruding the teeth, rather than resecting the tissue and exposing a tapering root. Papillary implications apply here as well.

(b) Less root sensitivity. Root exposure and sensitivity that may result from surgery is not a factor with orthodontic intrusion.

(c) Greater surface area of enamel to which the restoration is bonded. By intruding the coronal aspect of the tooth, rather than using crown lengthening to expose the root, a more favorable surface for bonding is provided for the restorative dentist.

Mesiodistal Movements

Movements known as "mesiodistal movements" will be described here for (a) their effect upon the position of the tooth, (b) the corresponding effect upon the eventual crown proportions, and (c) the periodontal effect to the soft tissues, specifically, the interdental papilla. Effective mesiodistal movements — if they are to deliver to the clinician the proper environment for optimal esthetic restoration — require controlled and precise crown tip and angulation. Consequently, the comparison of fixed versus removable appliances applies here as well, since the achievement of bodily and alignment movements must be performed carefully, and use of the fixed appliance is, again, the mechanotherapy of choice.

Space management and tooth proportion

Patients may often present for restoration with spaces or diastemata between the teeth. Restoration of a case with these features may result in a smile that is asymmetric, due to the disproportionate mesiodistal width of teeth as a result from closing a space "prosthetically". Due to the same attempt to close spaces restoratively, the teeth will appear to be of disproportionate width in relation to each other.

The "golden proportion" serves as a general guide for the proportion of the anterior teeth, and the dictates of these dimensions have been described in detail elsewhere in this book.[22] It is sufficient to state here that the golden proportion stipulates that the maxillary central/lateral incisor proportion should be 60% of the total width for the central incisor and 40% for the lateral. For example, if a patient presents with central incisors that need to be 9 mm in width, applying the golden proportion the lateral incisors will have to be 6mm in width. When the tooth positions of the patient tat presentation do not allow these proportions in the final restoration, adjunctive tooth movement is indicated as a preparatory step to restoration.

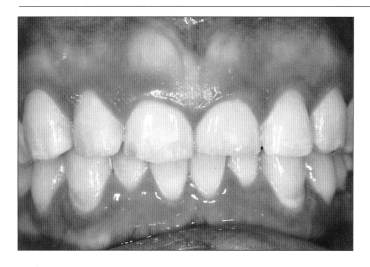

Fig 11-18 Case 2 Pre-treatment situation depicting incisal wear and compensatory eruption of maxillary central incisors. Observe short and wide appearance of central incisor teeth due to inverse relation of free gingival margins to lateral incisors. Central incisor free gingival margins are incisal to that of laterals, which is the reverse of the cosmetic ideal.

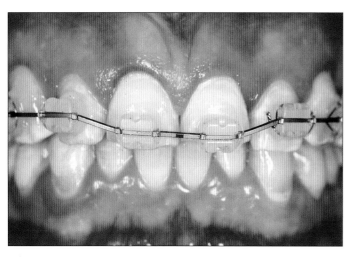

Fig 11-19 Placement and activation of fixed orthodontic appliance. Note bracket placement on maxillary central incisor teeth, located more incisally than the adjacent anchor teeth (the opposite of an extrusion set-up).

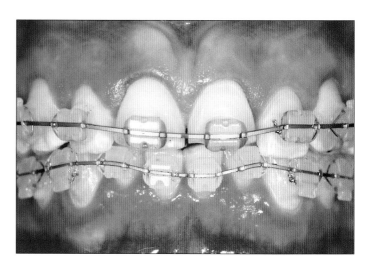

Fig 11-20 Immediate post-intrusion view. Notice change in bracket relations as a result of intrusion of the central incisors and the leveling of the archwire and corresponding reorientation of free gingival margins.

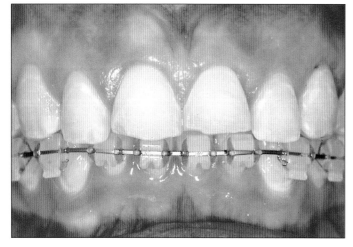

Fig 11-21 Debonding of fixed appliance. Observe the alteration to the free gingival margin relationships and relative changes to incisal edge relationships.

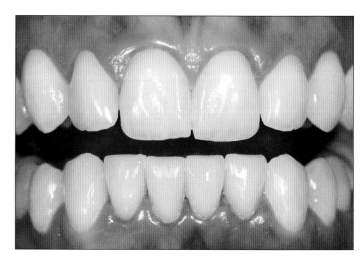

Fig 11-22 Restorative result with porcelain laminates. Note especially the tooth proportion and gingival margin coordination. (Orthodontics and Restorations by *Stephen J Chu*.)

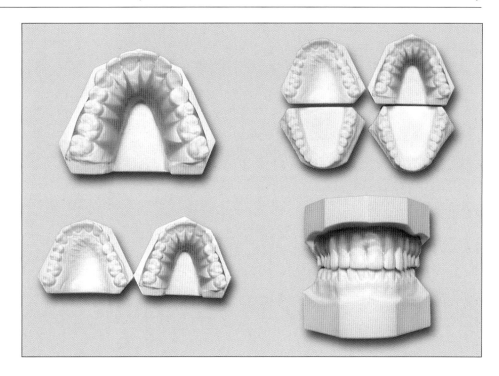

Fig 11-23 Example of a pre-treatment orthodontic set-up. Projected tooth movement is emulated by sectioning teeth off the study model and resetting them in wax to the desired or proposed position. Various treatment options and modifications can be simulated and evaluated before actually commencing treatment. This affords the operator and the patient the opportunity to analyze and evaluate treatment options for optimal outcome.

From a communication standpoint, the various practitioners in the dental team must be in contact with each other and have a clear treatment plan, indicating what each member is supposed to accomplish. A "road map" to the intended outcome can be devised and the time and effort spent in arriving at the desired result minimized. Furthermore, there should be times at critical junctions during the orthodontic set-up at which the restorative dentist should be consulted and asked to direct the orthodontist for final detailing. Such teamwork facilitates the interdisciplinary efforts of the various practitioners and results in a superior outcome. Numerous tools are available to the various dentists for the planning phase of therapy. Examples include diagnostic computer imaging and orthodontic model set-ups (Fig 11-23). These visual aids are designed to direct the practitioners, facilitate their ability to communicate, and lend the patients a means by which they can "foresee" (visualize in their mind) the intended outcome. The patients can provide their own input, participate in the decision-making process and be motivated towards achieving the desired end result.

Reorganization of anterior spacing does not have to include full orthodontic therapy in every case, i.e., a complete rearrangement of the posterior occlusion. When used as an adjunctive means, the goal should be to limit movement to the anterior region, ideally the four incisors exclusively. When the movement can be confined to this region, then the dictates of retention (to be discussed in a later section) are decreased dramatically. The time required to accomplish this type of "limited orthodontics" is fractional. Prior to initiating the restoration, a determination must be made that the patient's occlusion is functional and physiologic; when planning treatment for cosmetic dental procedures, such determination is made routinely.

When mechanotherapy is the treatment of choice, the fixed appliance should be employed to redistribute excessive spaces in the region. For example, if a patient presents with a large midline diastema (Fig 11-24), the restoration required to close that space prosthetically would result in excessive widths of the central incisors and a subsequent unnatural appearance. Periodontal ramifications of grossly overcontoured surfaces would contribute to the undesirable result. The space closure might be accomplished more effectively by distributing this space over multiple dental units, rather than by a midline closure alone. If the orthodontist closes the midline by merely moving the two central incisors together,

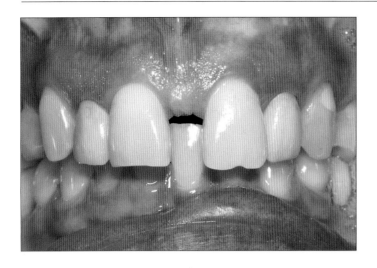

Fig 11-24 Case 3 Pre-treatment view of a patient with large maxillary midline diastema. Restoration of this space by overcontouring central incisors would result in unnaturally wide teeth.

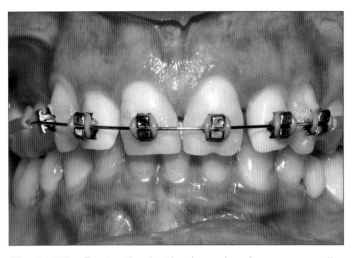

Fig 11-25 Post-orthodontic view, showing space redistribution. Previously large midline diastema has been distributed into smaller spaces among all 6 anterior teeth by virtue of consolidating the teeth toward midline via bodily orthodontic movement.

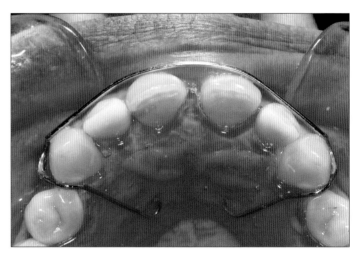

Fig 11-26 Removable orthodontic retainer in place. Notice how palatal acrylic of retainer is scalloped interproximally to maintain the tooth positions achieved in the active orthodontic phase. The retainer is a transitional one, used during the restorative phase of treatment, after which it will be either modified or replaced.

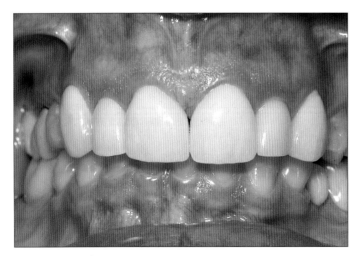

Fig 11-27 Final result; compare to Fig 11-25. Original midline space has been redistributed throughout anterior segment to avoid excessively wide central incisors.

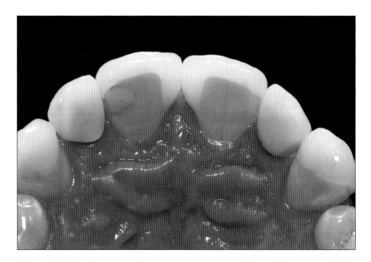

Fig 11-28 Restoration was accomplished by porcelain laminates to central incisors and cuspids, porcelain crowns to lateral incisors (necessary because they were full crowns over peg laterals at outset). (Restorative Dentistry by *Vincent Celenza*; Orthodontics by *Frank Celenza*.)

then all that has been accomplished is the relocation of this space excess to the distal surfaces of the same teeth. The preferable alternative might be a distribution of the original diastema to the distal surfaces of the lateral incisors (Figs 11-25 and 11-26) by moving the central incisors together somewhat, opening space to their immediate distal areas, then moving the lateral incisors mesially into this space. Using this procedure, a single midline space, especially when relatively wide, can be divided and redistributed among four or even six teeth (if the mesial aspects of the cuspids are included as well). As a result, the ability of the restorative dentist to work within the guidelines of tooth proportion is now greatly facilitated, and the final outcome is not punctuated by unattractively wide teeth (Figs 11-27 and 11-28).

Papillary remodeling

Surgical reconstruction of the interdental papilla can be difficult, if not impossible, as explained previously.[23,24] Currently, the profession still lacks reliable and predictable means for surgical reconstruction, while orthodontic means are available by which the correction may be occasionally achieved. Tarnow and colleagues have described the conditions under which papillary tissue has been observed to fill the gingival embrasure area.[25] They observed that when the millimetric measurement from the apical extent of the interdental contact point to the osseous crest (measured radiographically) was 5 mm or less, the interdental papilla was found to fill the embrasure area 98% of the time. When this measurement deviated as little as 1 mm, to the extent of only 6 mm (crest to contact), the papilla was found to be present in only 56% of their cases. An even more dramatic drop off was found at 7 mm, in which instances the papilla was observed to be present only 27% of the time.

The interdental papilla is regarded as a mass of soft tissue, designed to fill the gingival embrasure between teeth. It is a pliable and deformable entity, and its volume is generally considered as constant. Consequently, if the supporting tooth surfaces on either side of the papilla are relocated, the papilla will distend accordingly. It follows then, that orthodontic tooth movement may be employed to "pinch" or "squeeze" the existing papillae, to result in soft tissue closure of the gingival embrasure.

In this manner, the volume of the gingival embrasure area can be manipulated orthodontically. Tipping the apices of teeth towards one another, for example, would decrease the volume of the gingival embrasure between the two teeth by relocating the interdental contact apically (Figs 11-29 to 11-36). A given mass of soft tissue is encouraged to fill the area by reconfiguring the embrasure to more closely reflect the relations outlined by Tarnow and colleagues. The interdental papilla is in effect "pinched" or "squeezed" to fill a smaller space, frequently resulting in an orthodontic solution to a periodontal problem.

More difficult papillary deficiencies occur when a vertical deficiency of soft tissue is present. This deficiency is evident when the interdental peak of soft tissue between two teeth does not coincide with the levels of the adjacent teeth. In such cases, in which a vertical alteration to the gingival embrasure is required, the technique of "forced eruption" can be employed vertically to augment gingival soft tissue. The phenomenon of sulcular eversion, as previously described, can also be of assistance in these instances.

Rotation, tipping and torquing

These tooth movements are reviewed together in this section, since they all occur within the location of a given tooth. These movements are effected not with the intent to relocate a tooth, but rather to reorient it. Such "fine-tuning" will have a direct impact upon the thickness of the eventual restoration and the materials utilized. Teeth with improper orientation in either of these facets will also impart corresponding irregularities on the teeth with which they occlude. Since the opposing arch cannot be addressed properly (Figs 11-37 to 11-41), the restoration of misaligned teeth (the concept of "orthodontic veneers") will inherently limit the outcome.

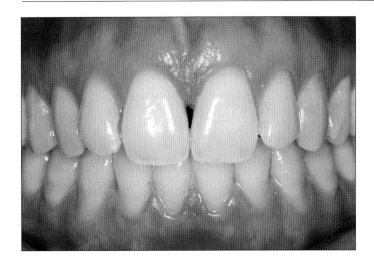

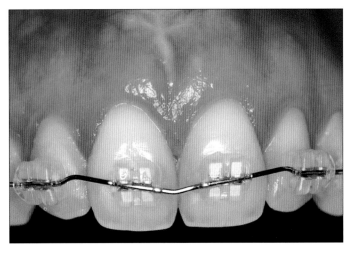

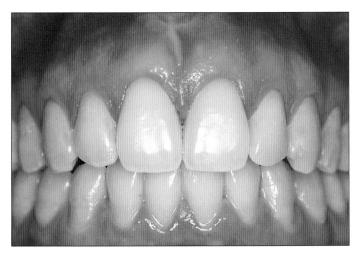

Fig 11-29 Case 4 Pre-treatment view of a patient with midline papillary deficiency. Soft tissue does not fill gingival embrasure, resulting in objectionable "black hole".

Fig 11-30 Fixed sectional orthodontic appliance bonded to maxillary anterior teeth. Note bracket placement and "v-bend" in archwire to effect movement that will tip apices of central incisors toward midline. In effect, the gingival embrasure will be reoriented to allow papillary soft tissue to fill it.

Fig 11-31 Post-treatment result. Volume of gingival embrasure has been decreased by virtue of tipping teeth, interproximal contact point has been repositioned gingivally, and soft tissue now fills interdental embrasure. (Orthodontics by *Frank Celenza*.)

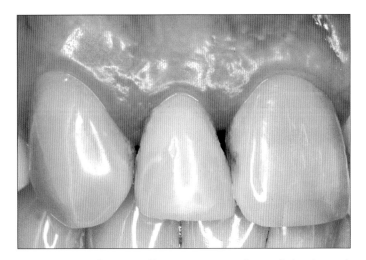

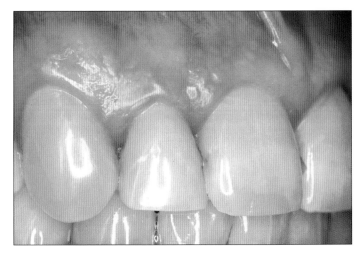

Fig 11-32 Case 5 Pre-treatment view of the lateral maxillary anterior segment.

Fig 11-33 Post-treatment view, showing changes to gingival papilla in response to orthodontic reorientation of teeth to fill gingival embrasure. (Orthodontics by *Frank Celenza*.)

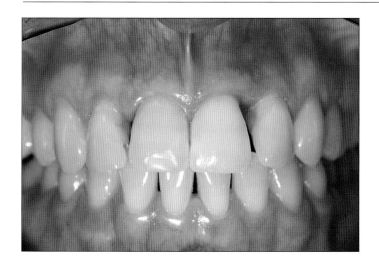

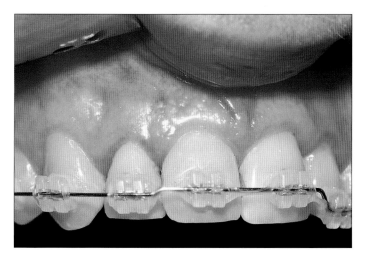

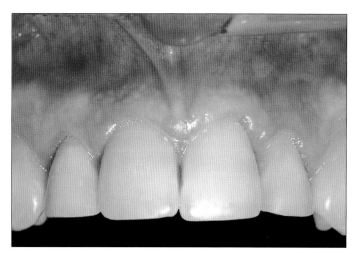

Fig 11-34 Case 6 Pre-treatment view of maxillary anterior segment with multiple papillary deficiencies. Note vertical deficiency between left central and lateral incisors.

Fig 11-35 Mid-treatment view. Observe the vertical step in archwire to cause eruption of left lateral incisor resulting in vertical augmentation of interdental papilla.

Fig 11-36 Post-orthodontic view, demonstrating changes to gingival architecture. Compare to Fig 11-32. The segment is now ready for laminate restorations. (Orthodontics by *Frank Celenza*.)

Therefore, if comprehensive dental therapy is the goal, all these aspects should be considered in treatment planning prior to initiation of the restorative procedure. "Rotation" refers to the location of a tooth, when viewed from its incisal or occlusal surface. If, for example, a central incisor is viewed from its incisal edge, and is found to have a rotation deviating from the ideal, it follows that if a veneer were to be placed on that tooth intending to mimic an orthodontic correction, the restoration will incur certain deficiencies. The material required in the more labially prominent area as a result of the rotation will be thinner than that in the more lingual aspects of the teeth. The restoration will, therefore, incur all the disadvantages of non-uniform thickness, and the cor-

responding misalignment of the opposing arch will have to be incorporated into the restoration as well.

"Tipping" refers to the mesiodistal angulation of a tooth. Teeth have natural angulation that is compatible with health and esthetics. Shifting, due to wear, altered eruption patterns, tooth loss, and parafunctional habits often result in deviations. The ramifications of abnormal or altered tooth location are confined not only to the tooth itself, but also to the surrounding structures, such as the interdental papilla and the contacting and occluding dentition. Restorations that attempt to overcome apparent tipping of teeth will have to be overcontoured and undercontoured on the corresponding dental surfaces. These material

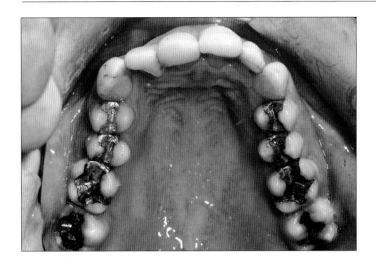

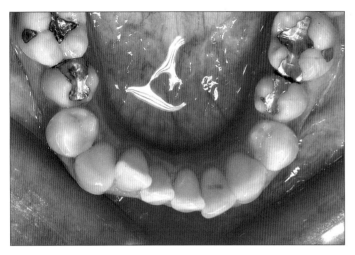

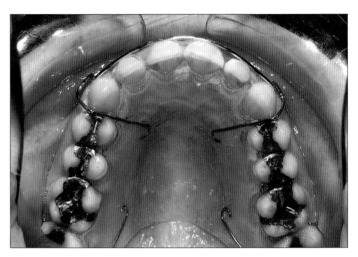

Fig 11-37 Case 7 Pre-treatment incisal view of the maxillary arch of a crowded dentition. The maxillary arch had been previously treated by anterior bonding for cosmetics, without first aligning the teeth.

Fig 11-38 Pre-treatment incisal view of the mandibular arch. Replacement of bonded restorations with labial veneers or full crowns without orthodontic alignment would preclude the ability to align lower anterior teeth, as they must fit within the confines of the maxillary arch form, thereby compromising overall result.

Fig 11-39 Incisal view of the maxillary arch following removal of all labial bonding and orthodontic alignment prior to final restoration.

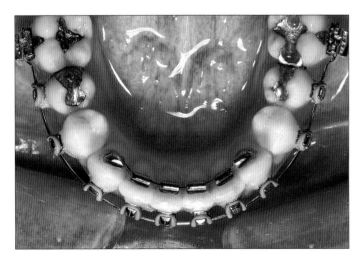

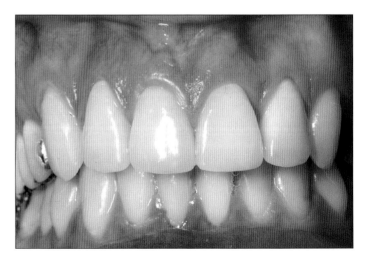

Fig 11-40 Incisal view of the mandibular arch at completion of the orthodontic phase. Lingual bonded retainer is in place, just prior to debonding of labial appliances. This alignment could not be achieved if the maxillary arch were not similarly aligned.

Fig 11-41 The post-treatment final result includes restoration of maxillary anterior dentition and benefits greatly from comprehensive approach, which included pre-restorative orthodontic alignment. (Restorative Dentistry by *Howard Livers*; Orthodontics by *Frank Celenza*.)

manipulations will have cosmetic influences as well as periodontal implications. Simple orthodontic correction prior to restorative intervention can eliminate and correct any of these inadequacies. "Torque", to an orthodontist, is defined as the tip or buccolingual location of a tooth in its alveolar housing when viewed from the interproximal aspect. The effects of torque on the buccal and lingual alveolar bone thickness are very important, and they are addressed in another section of this chapter. Periodontal health, morphology and the contours of the crown of a tooth can be affected by the torque of the tooth. Consequently, if a tooth is to be restored without correcting its orthodontic position, compensation will have to be provided for the same inadequacies as found in altered material thickness in a restoration.

Orthodontic Retention

Although most of the tooth movements described in this section are simple, the importance of effective retention for the end result should not be diminished. It would be foolish to allow the ruin of a beautiful result by the temporary and unstable nature of an orthodontic treatment that does not include retentive mechanisms. In adults, where tissue remodeling may consume more time than in adolescents, the importance of retention cannot be overstated. The importance of retention is greatest at the time when the active appliances are removed. It has been shown that retentive demands decrease, although gradually, as time goes by (months or even years). Therefore, the immediate need for retention must be appreciated and provided for accordingly.

The need for adequate retention is often a disadvantage to the implementation of orthodontic therapy, and the guidelines for it are primarily empirical. The operator is cautioned, therefore, to be aware that if retention cannot be provided, an orthodontic treatment is probably contraindicated, since the time and effort involved will result in a temporary and unpredictable result at best.

As a general guideline, particularly for adult patients, retention should be planned to involve any teeth that are actually moved. When an orthodontic appliance is employed, some teeth that are incorporated in it will serve as anchor teeth, and others will be active (or mobilized) teeth. The inclusion of every tooth in the retentive appliance is not necessary, since the anchor teeth may not have been moved and will not incur a relapse. All active or repositioned teeth should be regarded as requiring stabilization or retention.

An orthodontically treated tooth may tend to return to its preorthodontic position, and an orthodontic relapse may occur. This phenomenon is due to a multitude of factors, not all of which are entirely understood. For one, the fibers that make up the attachment apparatus of the tooth, as previously described, remain under tension until tissue remodeling is completed.[25,26] Consequently, there may remain a very real application of force upon a tooth when appliances are removed, resulting in a relapse of the tooth. A procedure known as the "supracrestal fiberotomy" is frequently employed to sever the supracrestal fiber apparatus, thereby alleviating the tension that results from that area.[27,28] Although proven to be effective, this modality should always be considered only as an adjunctive means of retention, never as an alternative.

In addition, there are environmental factors that must be considered in evaluating the potential for relapse. Habit patterns, occlusal relationships, and other etiologic factors must be evaluated. As a general rule, if the etiology behind the malposition of a tooth is not controlled or eliminated, the potential for a stable and lasting orthodontic repositioning of that tooth or teeth is unlikely.

This author subscribes to two general guidelines for the design of all orthodontic retainers:
1. If a tooth is moved, it requires retention.
2. If a tooth is to relapse, it will do so in the direction from which it originated.

There are two fundamental designs for orthodontic retainers — fixed or removable. All the advantages and disadvantages for fixed and

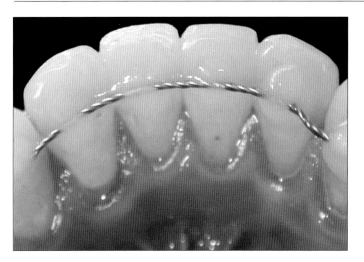

Fig 11-42 Bonded lingual retainer on mandibular arch. Dead-soft twisted wire is formed to the lingual surfaces of the teeth and spot-bonded using light-cured resin. This design results in a retainer that is flexible to allow for physiologic tooth movement, yet not easily deformed, rendering bond failure and tooth migration unlikely.

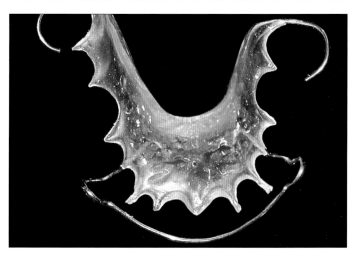

Fig 11-43 Removable maxillary retainer. Note that acrylic can be contoured in anterior region to preserve interproximal spaces as dictated for restoration.

removable active orthodontic appliances described previously apply here as well, particularly with regard to compliance. It can be a particularly sensitive issue to have patients under the impression that treatment is complete when fixed appliances are removed, only to ask them to begin wearing removable retainers, which are often more cumbersome than the active appliance. Therefore, before the treatment has even begun, the operator is advised to discuss the retainers with the patient and describe their function and appearance. This precaution and preparation requires planning and coordination with the restorative colleague ahead of time.

Fixed orthodontic retainer may take the form of a fixed bridge, in which case the permanency is ensured, or it may be a bonded type of retainer. The latter type is used extensively in conjunction with laminate veneer restorations. An extracoronal lingually bonded preformed wire is easy to fabricate and place chairside; it is strong, lasting, and unobtrusive to the patient. It has the added feature of being independent of the veneer restorations. This author uses a braided dead-soft wire that is fabricated and formed directly and is then bonded to the lingual or palatal surfaces using light-cured resin (Fig 11-42). It is sufficiently flexible to allow a limited degree of physiologic

tooth mobility, rather than risk bond failure under function from excessive rigidity. Frequently, these retainers must be placed following veneer restorations to provide interproximal access during the restorative phase of treatment. Removable retainers may be employed on a temporary basis, with the patient informed that this is a transitional phase.

Removable retainers are often used instead of fixed retainers (Fig 11-43). If retention is required for the maxillary anterior teeth, and the patient's bite depth precludes placing a bonded lingual wire, a removable retainer may be the only choice. If retention is required distal to the cuspid tooth (again, any tooth that has been moved requires retention), a removable retainer is often the appliance of choice. Removable retainers can be more effective in retaining transverse or expansive results in the posterior segments, due to the palatal acrylic that is part of their design. Finally, removable retainers are often a better selection than the fixed version because they can incorporate springs and attachments that allow adjustment and can, thereby, double as active or corrective appliances when a minor relapse has occurred or further correction is indicated. In contrast, a fixed retainer is a static appliance that offers no adjustability.

The "static" maxillary or mandibular orthodontic removable retainers include Hawley retainers, vaccu-formed retainers and night guards. The "active" maxillary or mandibular removable orthodontic retainers include Hawley retainers with finger springs or auxiliaries and spring retainers.

The time frame required adequately to retain a tooth is a final consideration relative to retention and its demands. This author subscribes to an empirical scheme. "Double the treatment time" is the often-employed strategy. For example, if the active phase of orthodontic therapy was 9 months, the patient should expect the retention phase to last a minimum of 18 months. The termination of retention is never a sudden one; instead, patients are "weaned off" their retainers, and the transition to function without appliances is a gradual one. During this transition period, patients should be instructed and trained to be observant of any signs of relapse that would be indicative of the need for a longer retention period. In the case of fixed retainers, this transitional period should include the provision for the use of removable retainers when the fixed splint is first removed. In the case of removable retainers, the transition period is a gradual reduction of the hours the appliance is worn.

Conclusion

Orthodontic dental treatment, used as a preparatory procedure in restorative and cosmetic therapy, contributes significantly to the final esthetic result (11-44 to 11-49). In recognition of this capability, the essential adjunctive and complementary aspects of orthodontics have been considered in this chapter. They include biomechanics of tooth movement, basic designs of fixed and removable appliances, adjunctive tooth movements in cosmetic therapy, and post-orthodontic retention. Schematic drawings and photographs from several clinical cases are utilized as visual adjuncts to illustrate and detail the procedures described in the text. It is hoped that the contents of this chapter and the book will in some way contribute to the knowledge of the novice as well as that of the seasoned clinician.

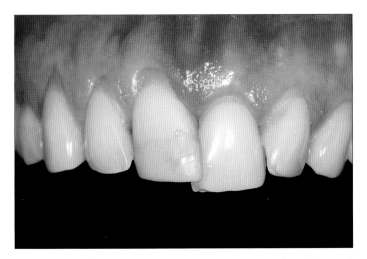

Fig 11-44 Case 8 Anterior pre-treatment view. Central incisors are overlapped at midline and display discrepant gingival margin levels. Recession of three right side anterior teeth is also evident.

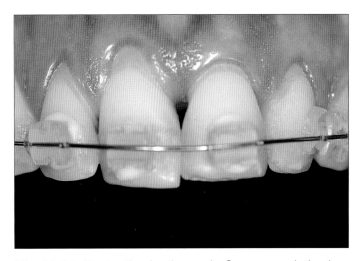

Fig 11-45 Post-orthodontic result. Compare relative levels of incisal edges to Fig 11-44 and observe eruption that was effected upon right central incisor. Gingival margin correction would have benefited from further eruption. Midline papilla deficiency results when overlapped teeth are aligned. Depending upon distance from contact point to interseptal bone, gingival growth, or "fill" can be predicted. If unfavorable, stripping of contact and space closure is advised.

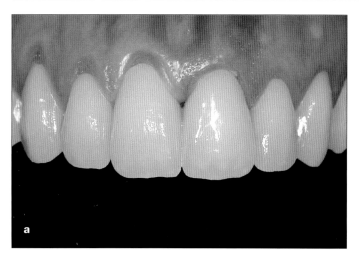

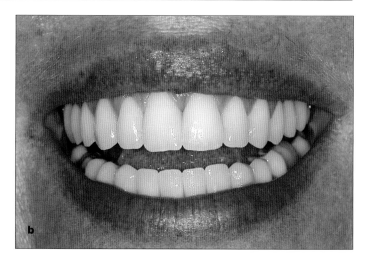

Fig 11-46a, b (a) Final result after porcelain laminates are placed. Prosthetic management of tooth contour and embrasure profile manages papillary area well, but free gingival margin coordination would have benefited from 2 mm more tooth eruption on right central and lateral incisor. (Orthodontics by *Gazanfer Gur.*) (b) However, further tooth eruption to correct that minor discrepancy is deliberately stopped, since the lips are covering that area even in full smile. The mandibular teeth are also restored with PLVs to achieve the same color match. (Restorative Dentistry by *Galip Gürel.*)

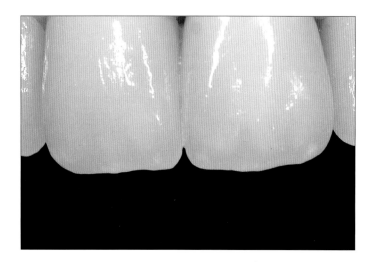

Fig 11-47 Not only gingival balance is obtained but the pleasing incisal edge configuration, as well. One of the main goals of ortho treatment is to obtain leveled incisal edges. However, when ortho is used as an adjunctive treatment to alter the gingival levels, the incisal edge positions may be disregarded. The uneven length of the incisor edges of the centrals (Fig 11-45) are restored and equalized with the PLVs. Butt joint preparation design, that is 1,5 mm short of the final expected incisal edge position, eases the job of the ceramist by leaving him/her the freedom to incorporate all the details to that area. Note the delicate incisal edge effects created by the ceramist *Adrian Jurim*.

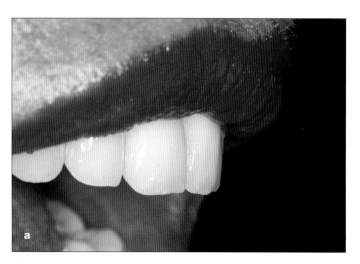

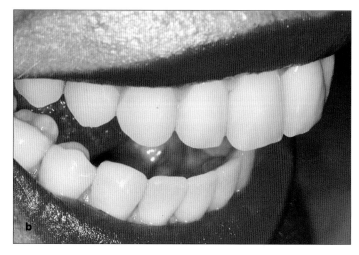

Fig 11-48a, b Final result. The arch, gingival levels are properly aligned with ortho and then delicately restored with PLVs. It looks very pleasing, no matter from which angle you observe the mouth.

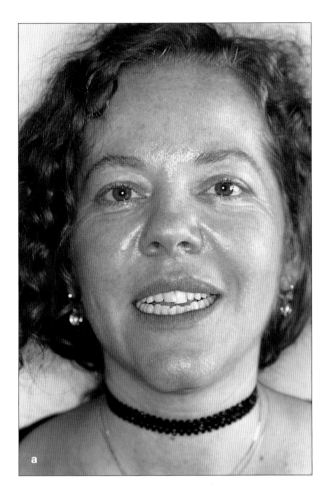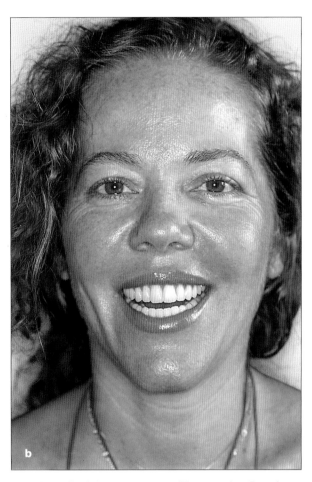

Fig 11-49a, b It certainly has a very positive impact on the whole facial appearance. (Restorative Dentistry by *Galip Gürel*; ceramist, *Adrian Jurim*.)

References

1. Goldman HM, Cohen DW. Periodontal Therapy. St Louis, MO: Mosby, 1973:14-17.

2. Gargiulo AW, Wentz FM, Orban B. Dimensions and relations of the dentogingival junction in humans. J Periodontol 1961;32:261-267.

3. Ingber JS, Rose LF, Coslet JG. The "biologic width". A concept in periodontics and restorative dentistry. Alpha Omegan 1977;70:62-65.

4. Celenza F Jr. Esthetic periodontics. Curr Opin Cosmetic Dent 1995:18-23.

5. Batenhorst KF, Bowers GM, Williams JE Jr. Tissue changes resulting from facial tipping and extrusion of incisors in monkeys. J Periodontol. 1974;45:660-668.

6. Miller PD. A classification of marginal tissue recession. Int J Periodont Rest Dent 1985;5:8-13.

7. Miller PD. Regenerative and reconstructive periodontal plastic surgery. Mucogingival surgery. Dent Clin North Am 1988; 32:287-306.

8. Langer B, Calagna L. The subepithelial connective tissue graft. J Prosthet Dent 1980;44:363-367.

9. Tarnow DP. Semilunar coronally positioned flap. J Clin Periodontol 1986;13:182-185.

10. Ingber JS. Forced eruption: Alteration of soft tissue cosmetic deformities. Int J Periodontics Restorative Dent 1989;9:416-425.

11. http://www.invisalign.com/US/index.html.

12. Potashnick SR, Rosenberg ES. Forced eruption: Principles in periodontics and restorative dentistry. J Prosthet Dent 1982;48(2):141-148.

13. Oppenheim A. Artificial elongation of the teeth. Am J Ortho Oral Surg 1940;26:931.

14. Celenza F. The development of forced eruption as a modality for implant site enhancement. Alpha Omegan 1997;90: 40-43.

15. Ingber JS. Forced eruption. Part I: A method of treating isolated one- and two-wall infrabony osseous defects. Rationale and case report. J Periodontol 1974;45:199-206.

16. Inbger JS. Forced eruption. Part II: A method of treating non-restorable teeth. Periodontal and restorative considerations. J Periodontol 1976;47:203-216.

17. Salama H, Salama M. The role of orthodontic extrusive remodeling in the enhancement of soft and hard tissue profiles prior to implant placement: A systematic approach to the management of extraction site defects. Int J Periodontics Restorative Dent 1993;13:312-333.

18. Celenza F. Orthodontically induced gingival and alveolar augmentation: Clinical and histological findings. Pract Proced Aesthet Dent 2001;13:173-175.

19. Celenza F, Celenza V. Using a fixed provisional as an orthodontic anchor in forced eruption. Pract Periodontics Aesthet Dent. 2000;12:478-482.

20. Atherton JD, Kerr NW. Effect of orthodontic tooth movement upon the gingivae. An investigation. Br Dent J 1968; 124:555-560.

21. Atherton JD. The gingival response to orthodontic tooth movement. Am J Orthod. 1970;58:179-186.

22. Kokich V. Esthetics and anterior tooth position. An orthodontic perspective. Part 3: Mediolateral relationships. J Esthet Dent 1993;5:200-207.

23. Beagle JR. Surgical reconstruction of the interdental papilla. Case report. Int J Periodontics Restorative Dent 1992; 12:145-151.

24. Evian CI, Corn H, Rosenberg ES. Retained interdental papilla procedure for maintaining anterior esthetics. Compend Contin Educ Dent 1985;6:58-64.

25. Tarnow DP, Magner AW, Fletcher P. The effect of the distance from the contact point to the crest of bone on the presence or absence of the interproximal dental papilla. J Periodontol 1992;63:995-996.

26. Reitan K. Tissue rearrangement during the retention of orthodontically rotated teeth. Angle Orthodontist 1959; 29:105-113.

27. Reitan K. Clinical and histologic observations on tooth movement during and after orthodontic treatment. Am J Orthod 1967;53:721-745

28. Edwards JG. A surgical procedure to eliminate rotational relapse. Am J Orthod 1970;57(1):35-46.

29. Pontoriero R, Celenza F Jr, Ricci G, Carnevale G. Rapid extrusion with fiber resection. A combined orthodontic-periodontic treatment modality. Int J Periodontics Restorative Dent 1987;5:30-43.

12 Periodontal Treatment and Porcelain Laminate Veneers

Galip Gürel, Korkud Demirel

Introduction

The health of the soft tissue is of vital importance when a restorative procedure is performed. No matter the kind of prosthetic work to be administered: crowns, bridges, removable dentures or porcelain laminate veneers, the unhealthy condition of the gingiva will jeopardize the final result. However, even if the tissues appear healthy, this does not mean that they are esthetically pleasing (see Chapter 13). The ideal smile should be balanced, with a decent display of teeth and a harmonious gingival architecture.

Gingival asymmetries in the esthetic zone can be corrected with minor periodontal surgery. The goal should be to achieve bilateral symmetry, especially between the centrals, and progressively continued toward the canines. These asymmetries are especially important when the patient displays a "gummy smile". Although it looks like a simple procedure, it needs careful planning and full awareness of the possible effects there may be on the final result (see Chapter 6). Many different factors, such as the incisal edge position, existing crown length, the amount of crown-root ratio, the position of the alveolar bone, the position of the tooth, root angulation and the cementoenamel junction, should all be very carefully analyzed before surgery.

These asymmetries are usually corrected either by crown lengthening or root coverage procedures (see Chapter 13). Another method of treating gingival asymmetries is by orthodontic intrusion or extrusion. If the teeth are intruded or extruded slowly, the overlying gingiva together with the attachment apparatus will follow the direction of the tooth movement (see Chapter 11).

It is well known that the root form gets narrower towards the apex. This is an important factor while trying to elongate the tooth length through periodontal surgery (Fig 12-1). This will not only affect the final form of the tooth but the emergence profile as well (Fig 12-2).

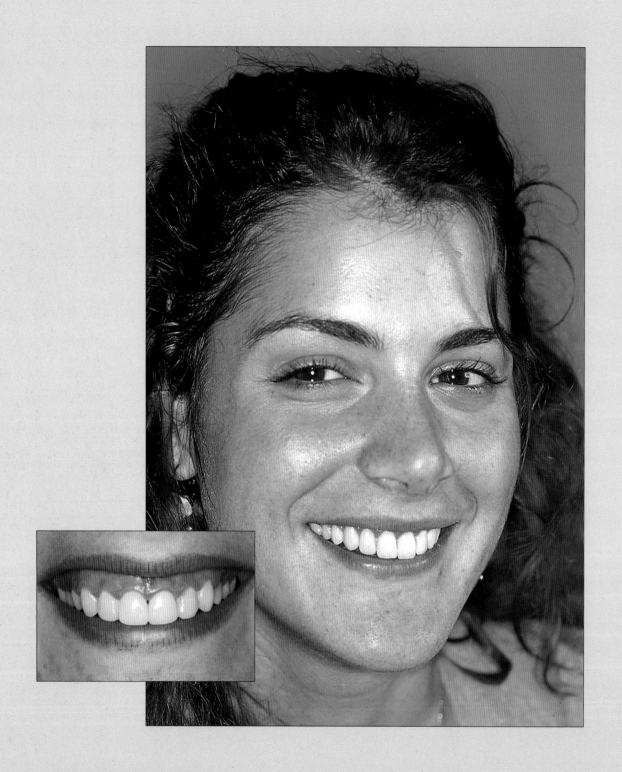

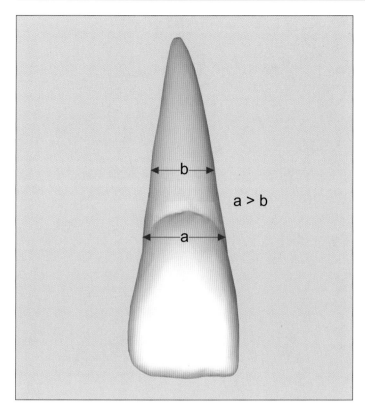

Fig 12-1 The root gets narrower towards the apex. Care should be taken while altering the gingival level apically, since the cervical area will be narrower than the existing diameter.

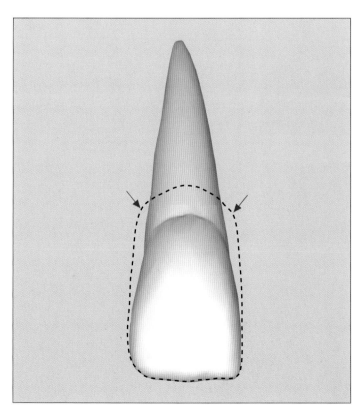

Fig 12-2 An over-contoured emergence profile is needed to compensate for the narrowing of the root structure.

Crown Lengthening

Crown lengthening towards the gingiva is usually utilized in "gummy smile" cases. In such conditions the incisal edge position and the existing tooth length will determine the level of extension as well as the location of the cementoenamel junction.[2]

However, in some cases, even if the patient does not display a truly "gummy smile", crown lengthening can still be executed in order to supply pleasing proportions within the tooth itself and the teeth amongst themselves (Fig 12-3). This is quite common in most of the diastema closure cases. When the dentist decides that the incisal edge position should not be altered, then the choice of direction to elongate the tooth length remains towards the apical, which means a periodontal approach. Many details should be taken into consideration throughout the whole periodontal surgical process. When the basic principles of bone and soft tissue relations (see Chapter 6) are carefully exercised, and excellent communication between the dentist and the specialist concerning the sufficient length to be altered and repositioning of the zenith points (see Chapter 2) relative to the new porcelain laminate veneer position have been established, then the chances for a successful result is very high (Figs 12-4 to 12-10).

Tooth Preparation

After such surgery, a minimum healing period of 6 weeks is necessary before any restorative procedure begins (Fig 12-11). At this stage, the dentist should have been provided with the wax-ups, the silicon index and the template by the laboratory technician (Fig 12-12). The placement of an APT, which can be double-checked with a silicon index, will ease the preparation stage (Figs 12-12 to 12-14). One of the most critical areas in diastema closure is the gingivoproximal area. The preparation should be subgingival. The depth and palatinal extension of the area will be dictated by the size of the diastema and the position and volume of the papilla (Fig 12-15). Such preparation of the area will give the technician the

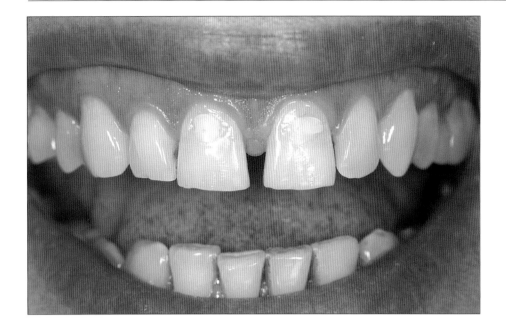

Fig 12-3 A 40-year-old business-woman who runs a top modeling agency is very conscious and concerned with the way she smiles. She has a moderately "gummy smile", mainly owing to an insufficient upper lip (high lip line). The esthetic treatment plan includes periodontal surgery to lengthen the clinical crowns and overcome the slight "gummy smile", but, even more importantly, to achieve a pleasant proportion after the diastema is closed.

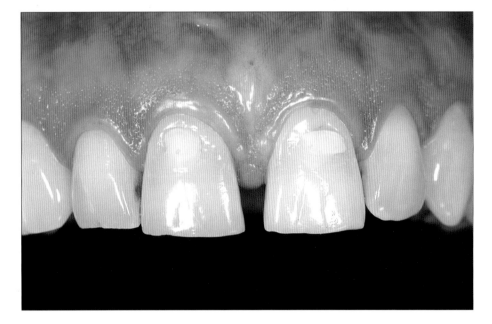

Fig 12-4 Color, surface characteristics and consistency of the tissues reveal a healthy appearance. Note the stippling of the attached gingiva. The gingival margin is moderately scalloped with a significant diastema in the middle. Clinical crowns at the patient's left appear to be longer than the left owing to very little recession originating from brushing trauma. Although interdental papilla between the two centrals does not fill the interdental space, it rises up to the coronal 1/3rd of the crown. Preservation of this volume is crucial for closing the diastema with restorations while expecting the papilla to fill up the interdental space entirely.

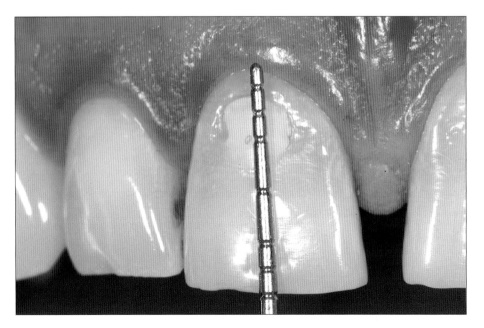

Fig 12-5 The clinical crown is 9 mm long at the mid-buccal. As the diastema will be closed in the restorative phase, the zenith points should be relocated in order to correspond to the distal 1/3rd of the restored teeth. In other words, the existing zenith point of the central should be moved mesially to compensate for the new position and form of the tooth (see Chapter 2, Fig 2-10).

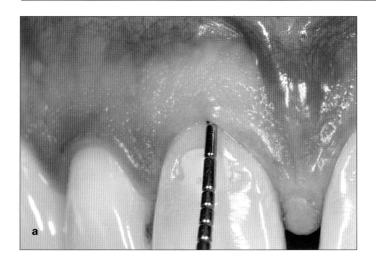

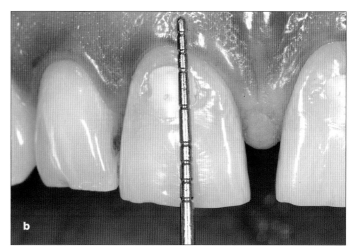

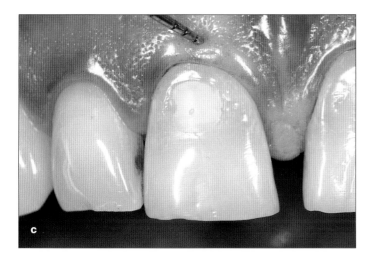

Fig 12-6a-c (a) Sounding of the gingival sulcus reveals a healthy and ideal biologic zone, which is 3 mm from the gingival margin to the crest of the bone. Note how healthy gingival tissue bleaches under probing pressure. (b) The expected zenith points and the optimal clinical crown length are planned before surgery. A 2 mm increase in the clinical crowns and mesial relocation of the zenith will be sufficient for restorative treatment planning. (c) The expected zenith is marked on the gingiva by a bleeding point. This is repeated for each individual tooth to be treated.

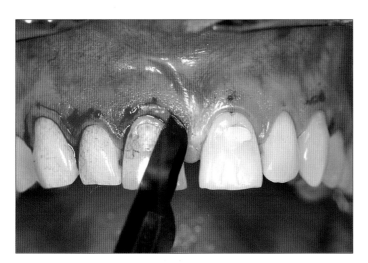

Fig 12-7 A scalloped incision with a #15 blade 2 mm apical to the gingival margin is initiated on the right anterior. Note the incision is closer to the gingival margin at the left lateral to avoid a long lateral that would reverse the marginal harmony of the anterior teeth.

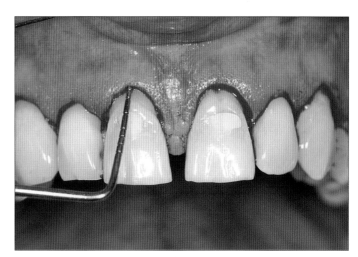

Fig 12-8 Before reflecting the flap, the bone margin should be sounded to find out how much supra crestal space is needed to establish a biologic zone. The distance from the gingival margin to the crest of the bone was found to be 1.5 mm in this case. A minimum of another 1.5 mm is needed for a healthy gingival sulcus as well as epithelial and connective tissue attachments, as a minimum of 3 mm is needed for biologic zone.

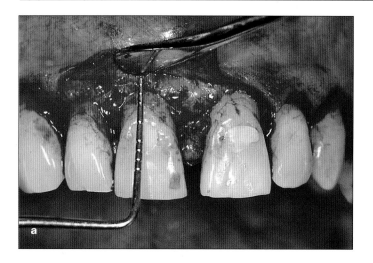
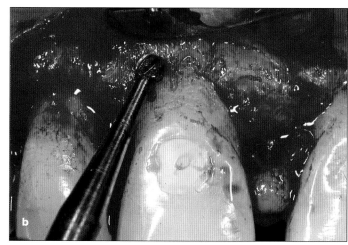
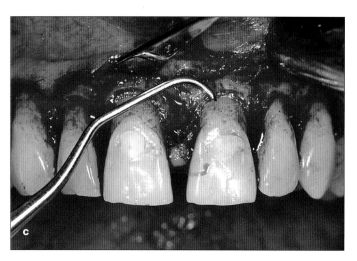
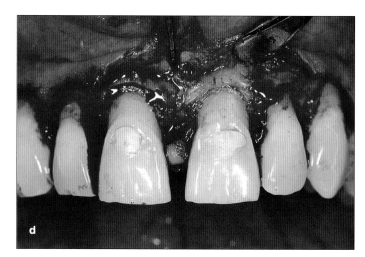

Fig 12-9a-d (a) After flap reflection, the extent of crestal reduction is marked on the alveolar bone. Note that only vestibular flap is reflected and the palatinal side is left untouched. (b) A round bur is used for marginal reduction of the crestal bone at the facial sides. Since the level of the gingival tissue normally follows the architecture of the underlying osseous crest, the location of the gingival zenith should be considered at this stage and a bony zenith is prepared. No osteotomy is performed on the interdental bone supporting the root. Rotary instruments must always be kept away from the root surface to prevent damage. (c) After marginal osteotomy with rotary instruments, the bone margin should be recontoured to establish a knife-edge form. (d) Meticulous planning is advised for the exposed root surfaces to discourage creeping attachment.

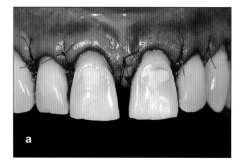
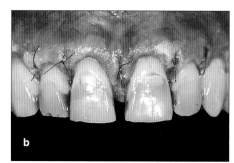
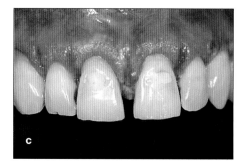

Fig 12-10a-c (a) All measures should be taken for primary closure of the flaps to facilitate predictable healing. 6/0 monofilament nonresorbable sutures are used to secure flaps. Note the height of the interdental papilla is preserved. (b) One week after surgery. Strict adhesion to the principles of atraumatic periodontal surgery resulted in fast tissue healing. (c) 10 days after surgery. Note the mesially displaced zenith points of the central incisors and longer clinical crowns. Healing is not complete before 6 weeks. All restorative procedures can be initiated after 5 weeks but making impressions should be delayed until 6 weeks have passed following surgery.

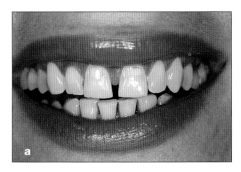
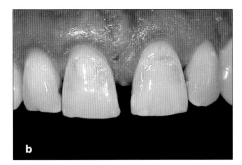
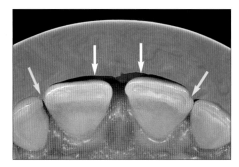

Fig 12-11a, b (a) After 6 weeks, the dentist can start preparing the teeth for porcelain laminate veneers. Note the altered gingival levels. Even in full smile, the "gummy smile" is invisible. (b) The changes after surgery. Note the tapered cervical area owing to the tapered root structure, as opposed to the shape of this area before this procedure was done. The overbulked emergence profile of the veneer will not only help to create the new form, but to push and gently squeeze the papilla, which is presently blunt, thereby creating a triangular shaped papilla.

Fig 12-12 Silicone index over the unprepared teeth. Notice the area that has to be filled with porcelain laminate veneer (white arrows). If this technique were not used, much unnecessary preparation would have been done on the enamel. It also dictates the position of the distal edges of the centrals as well as laterals in order to achieve acceptable proportions (yellow arrows).

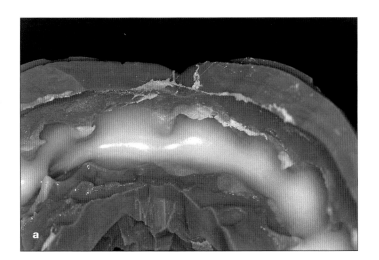
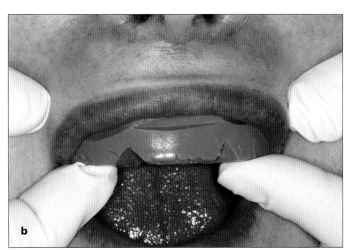
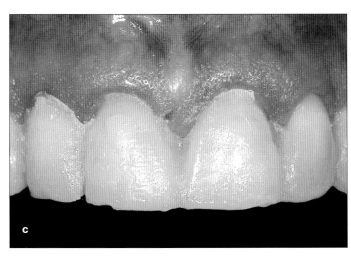
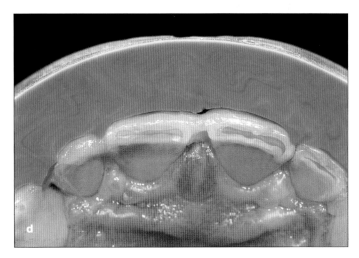

Fig 12-13a-d (a) The easiest way to prepare the (a)esthetic pre-evaluative temporaries (APTs) is to place a flowable composite (Luxatemp) or acrylic into the template. (b) Then place it over the unprepared teeth. (c) With the help of the APT it is possible to visualize the final outcome for both the patient and the dentist. (d) Its final facial volumetric outcome can be double checked with the silicone index.

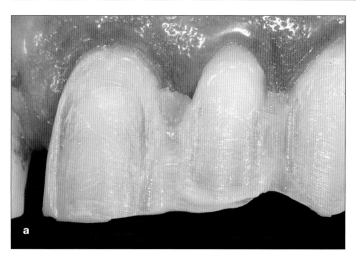

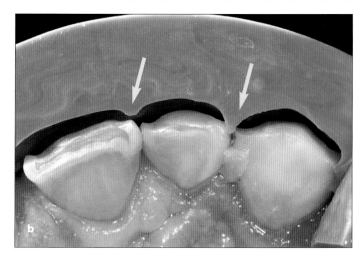

Fig 12-14a, b (a) Preparation through APTs. Maximum enamel structure can be saved when the depth cutter is used through the APT. (b) Double checking the preparation with the silicone index not only confirms the true depth that has been reached but also the amount of distal reduction from the central and lateral to compensate for the area that has to be gained while closing the gap (yellow arrows).

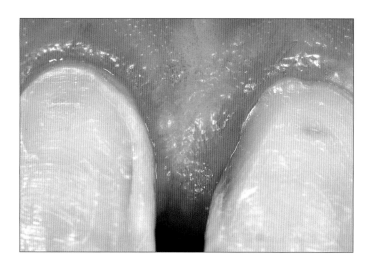

Fig 12-15 One of the most critical areas in diastema closure is the cervical and the gingivoproximal area. Since there will not be a major color change, the cervical margin can be kept supragingival. However, starting from 1/3rd towards the diastema, the cervical margin should be extended to subgingival as well as the whole gingivoproximal area. This will help the technician to adjust the emergence profile in order voluntarily to compress the papilla to prevent the formation of a black hole. The gingivoproximal area of tooth #11(8) is to be prepared whereas tooth #21(9) has already been subgingivaly prepared.

freedom to build up the emergence profile in order voluntarily to squeeze the papilla and push it towards the incisal. In this way, the papilla will be placed between the apical end of the interproximal contact area and the gingivoproximal corner of the porcelain laminate veneer, forming a triangular shape which will fill the area.

After the tooth preparation and impression making, further laboratory procedures and the actual bonding itself is finished (see Chapter 7).

Polishing the Veneers Intraorally

If the bonding procedures are carefully finished, the cervical area will be almost free of leftover composites. However, occasionally, polymerized composite flash may be detected, especially in the subgingival areas. In order completely to clean the area, a non-cutting-ended tungsten carbide bur is used. Finishing tungsten carbide burs come in 8-, 12-, 16-, 20- and 30-fluted designs. If the dentist wants to make a gross reduction, the 8-fluted carbide bur is the best. However, to achieve the smoothest surface, a

Fig 12-16 Once the bonding procedures are completed, the cervical margin should be cleaned with tungsten carbide bur (H50AF Komet) from the porcelain laminate veneer esthetic-finishing bur kit. The rounded tip of the bur is non-cutting and designed to prevent destruction of the root surface. The shape of the bur lets itself enter all areas and especially the gingivoproximal area. The bur should be used dry for better visibility and with very light pressure to prevent overheating. After all the flush is cleansed, a polishing cup (9652 Komet) can now be used to polish the gingival margins. Note that they are used very gently, in order to avoid disturbance of the gingiva.

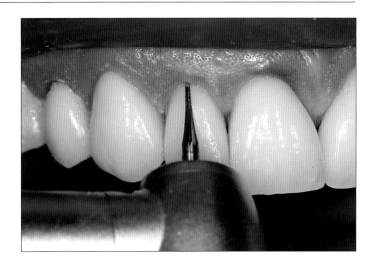

Fig 12-17a, b (a) Finished case with Empress veneers. Owing to the meticulously planned and executed periodontal surgery, not only are the proportions of the centrals perfectly achieved but the proportions of the teeth to one another as well. Note how the blunt papilla is changed to a crisp clear triangular shape. (b) The palatinal view of the feather edge interproximal margins of the centrals lets the technician freely build up the porcelain to close the diastema. The same is done for the laterals.

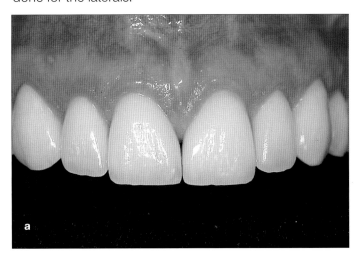
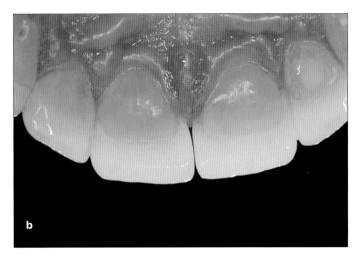

30-fluted carbide bur should be selected. An important point is to avoid the scratches that the bur can create on the porcelain surface; very sharp edged burs should always be used. The dentist with the aid of loops then checks the area with an explorer. If nothing is detected, the site must be polished intraorally with the help of rubber cups (Komet 9555.204.100). The gingiva must not be damaged at this appointment (Fig 12-16).

The most important issue here is not to touch the specifically cervical margin with any kind of diamond burs. There is glaze on the surface which is 25 to 100 microns of melted porcelain. And nothing can replace the glaze in terms of surface smoothness. Once lost, the microporosities at the gingival margin can be the major reason for plaque accumulation and thus gingival irritation in the future.[3] The interproximal contact area can be refined with finishing discs (Flexi Disc Mini Disc, Cosmedent; Sof-lex Extrathin Contouring and Polishing Discs, 3M) or finishing strips (Vision Flex Diamond Strips, Brasser; Flexi Diamond Strips, Cosmedent; Flexi Strip, Cosmedent; Sof-lex Finishing and Polishing Strips, 3M) can also be used. When the contacts are

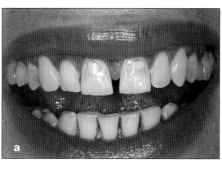
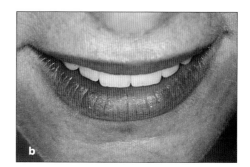
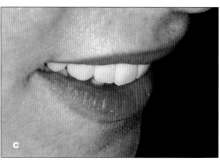
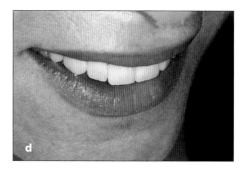

Fig 12-18a-d (a) The smile after the periodontal surgery and before the PLVs are prepared. (b-d)The beautiful smile from different angles in relation to where it started. When the treatment planning is meticulously accomplished, the final results are always rewarding. Full and effective communication between the dentist and the technician that encompasses understanding and expression of the process necessary to achieve a pleasing natural smile, is the foundation of a successful case (Ceramist: *Gerard Ubassy*).

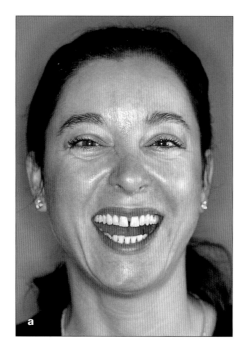
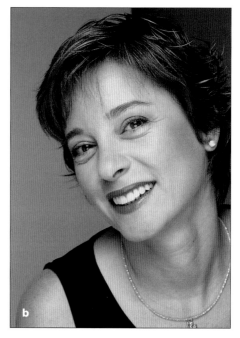

Fig 12-19a, b The patient before and after. The youthful affect of the smile on the face is clearly visible. The most rewarding phrase you can hear from a patient even after such a drastic change is "Everybody thinks I have had a face lift and that I look great. Nobody understands what has changed is my mouth. They don't realize that I changed my teeth and smile, until I say so."

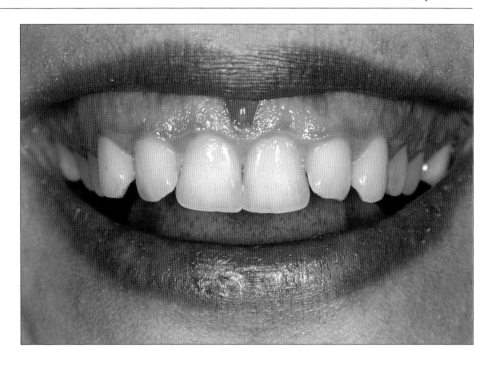

Fig 12-20 A "gummy smile" both anterior and posterior.

very tight, metal strips can be useful (Vision Flex Diamond Strips, Brasser; Flexi Diamond Strips, Cosmodent). Care should be taken not to slide the strip towards the gingiva, in order to prevent unnecessary gingival bleeding.

The occlusion, together with the protrusive and lateral guidances is checked. It is always rewarding when a true, realistic and carefully planned treatment is achieved. However, this can only be conducted with the efforts of the entire team including the dentist, specialists, dental technicians and of course the patient (Figs 12-17 to 12-19).

"Gummy Smile"

In such cases the nature of the "gummy smile" should be evaluated (Fig 12-20). If it is limited to only the anterior, then an orthodontic intrusion may be the choice of treatment. However, if the "gummy smile" is both anterior and posterior, then periodontal or maxillofacial surgery can be carried out according to the severity of the case. In addition, the mouth may exhibit crowded maxillary anterior incisors, where the laterals are protruding out and the centrals are palatinally located.

The treatment plan for such a case is to alter the gingival levels apically to minimize the "gummy smile" with periodontal surgery, and to prepare the teeth for porcelain laminate veneers, while transferring the esthetic plane of occlusion to the lab without making mistakes. With team effort, drastic results can be achieved in creating a natural-looking beautiful smile that changes the whole appearance of the face.

It is now in our hands to create a youthful smile and to enhance the patient's appearance with a delicate touch to their smiles (Figs 12-21 to 12-28).

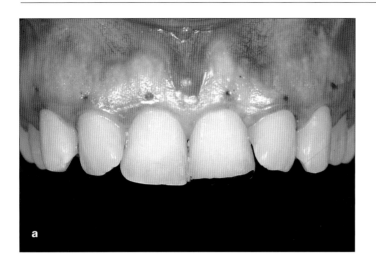
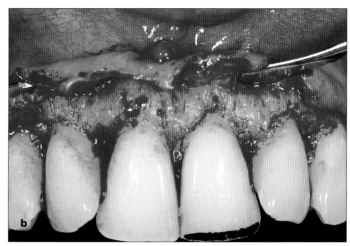
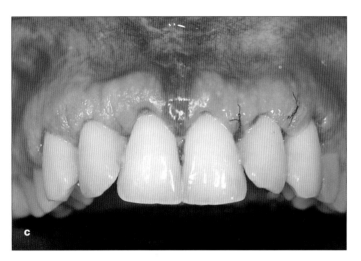
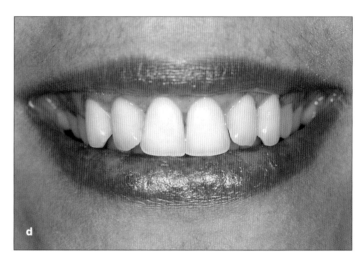

Fig 12-21a-d After a serious consultation between the patient, dentist and the specialist, periodontal surgery is performed to alter the gingival levels apically. (a) The zenith points are subject to vertical and horizontal displacement. (b) The flap is reflected and the alveolar bone is removed to expose 3 mm of root length to the gingival margin on the facial side. This distance between the tip of the interdental bone crest and the imaginary papilla tip is kept 5mm at the interproximal. (c) One week after surgery. Note the "crown lengthening". (d) Even though the teeth still keep their unesthetic configuration; the "gummy smile" has disappeared. Note the lingual position of the premolars that create a large negative space at the buccal corridor.

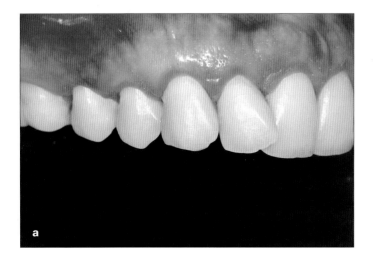
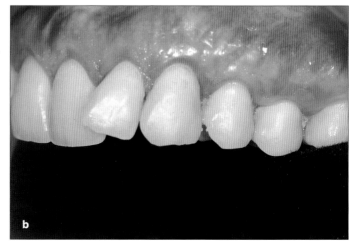

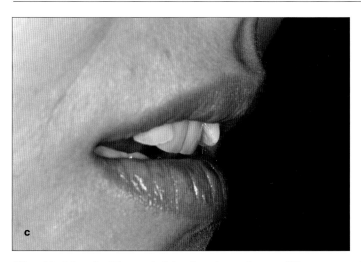

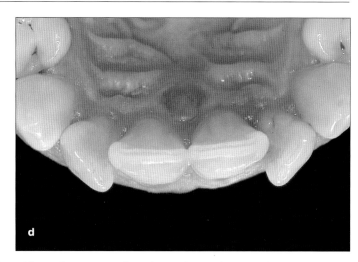

Fig 12-22a-d The axial inclinations from different angles. Note the protruding laterals and extensively lingually positioned centrals.

Fig 12-23a-d The step-by-step progression in cases that seem impossible to correct esthetically. (a) A silicone index is essential when it comes to teeth preparation, in such cases. Note the distance from the facial of the centrals to the inside of the silicon index (white arrows). This is an indication that the facial of the centrals does not need to be prepared except from the cervical 1/3rd. It is also very obvious that the facially protruding mesial line angles of both laterals have to be pre-recontoured (APR) in order to seat the silicon index and the transparent template passively over the dental arch. (b) Diagnostic wax-ups will help the dentist and the patient visualize the final outcome. (c) APT in place. It displays the final outcome instantly. Once the appearance is accepted by the patient and the dentist, the preparation can be made through the APTs. (d) The provisionals after tooth preparation. They already look very pleasant in the mouth.

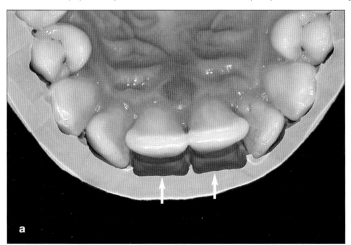

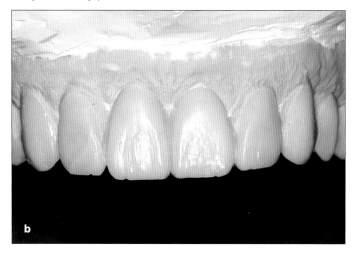

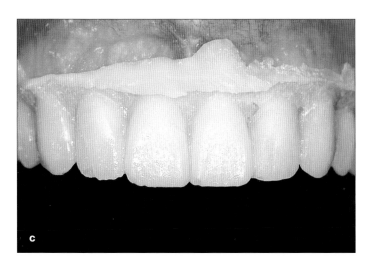

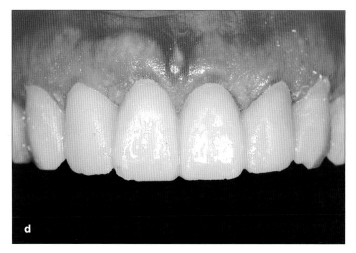

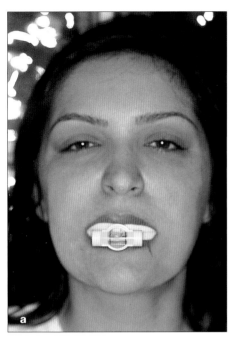
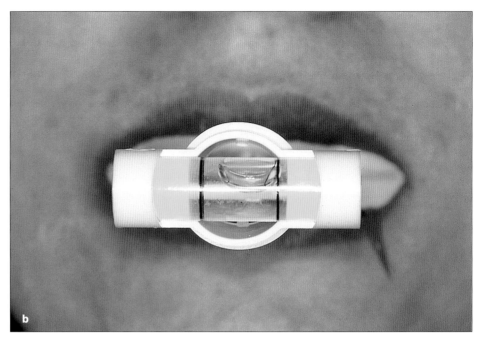

Fig 12-24a, b One of the simplest methods of transferring the esthetic occlusal plane, or in other words the incisal edge position, is by using a hydraulic chamber (Mid-Liner, Vic Pollard Dental Produkts, Westlake Village, CA). After the attached tray is placed and secured in the mouth with the bite-registration material, the patient's head is kept erect while the patient stands upright and the gauge level is adjusted so that the air bubble stays in the middle. This indicates that the incisal edge position is transferred correctly to the laboratory.

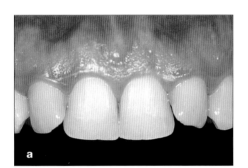
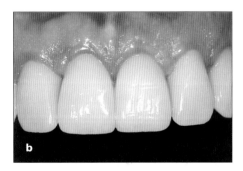
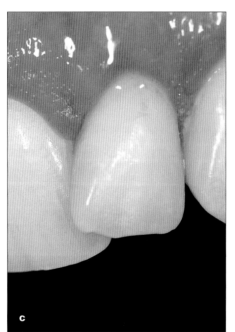
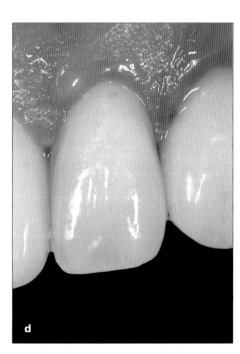

Fig 12-25a-d (a, b) After the veneers are prepared (c, d) they are bonded in the mouth. Note the difference in the tooth axial positions (Ceramist: *Gerard Ubassy*).

Fig 12-26a, b The lip support with the new positions of the anterior teeth adds a very pleasing effect to the smile.

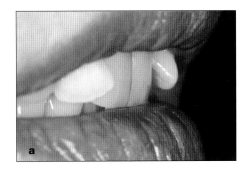 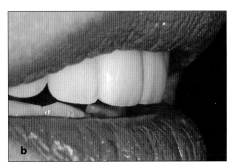

Fig 12-27a, b The drastic change in the smile. Not only has the "gummy smile" disappeared, but the new position of the porcelain laminate veneers has added a totally different feeling to the smile. Note how the smile is completed when the negative space at the buccal corridor is filled with porcelain laminate veneers bonded to the premolar teeth.

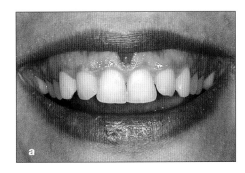 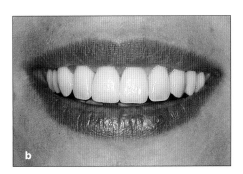

Fig 12-28a, b The new smile and the patient's new facial appearance with added youthfulness and beauty.

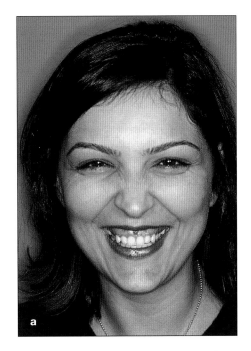 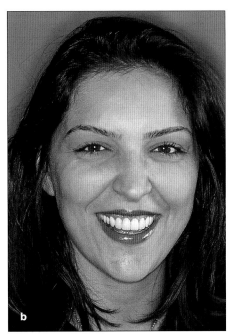

Negative Dental Composition

Undesirable effects of the dental composition may negatively influence the smile. This may be excessive gingival exposure due to supraerupted maxillary teeth. When the anterior dentition is viewed from the front, the teeth should be related to one another and the entire dental composition should relate to the face in a certain proportion. In order to achieve proper esthetic harmony in the anterior dentition, a pleasing repeated proportion between the teeth that progresses from the central incisors to the posterior teeth is critical.[4] The different lengths of the teeth, such as shorter laterals which have already lost their individual proportions, can jeopardize the smile (Fig 12-29).

When this is combined with a "gummy smile", a periodontal approach to begin creating a natural smile is inevitable.

In addition to the negative effects of excessive gingival exposure, a diastema which is closed only by adding composite to the mesials of the central incisors not only destroys the proportions of these teeth but the health of gingiva as well (Fig 12-30). The first step of this procedure is completed with periodontal surgery which alters the gingival levels. Even though the "gummy smile" has disappeared, the esthetic eye can observe that some details are still missing (Fig 12-31).

The dentist must first establish the incisal edge position and the size of the central incisors which will act as a keystone in the smile line. Its measurements should be in proportion to facial width, width of the dental arch, volume of the lips and hence the face as a whole.[5] The first step to this approach should be a delicate wax-up preparation. If this is planned and coordinated well with the dental technician, a successful result will always be achieved (Figs 12-32 to 12-34).

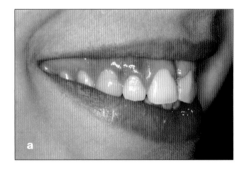 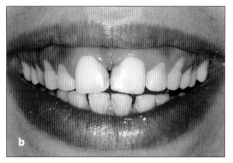 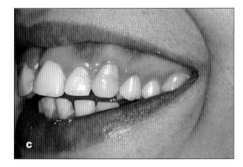

Fig 12-29a-c "Gummy smile", exaggerated with unproportional teeth length. Notice the very short clinical crown lengths of the laterals and premolars.

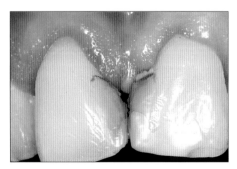 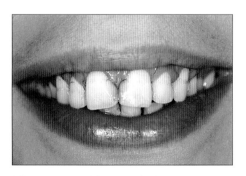

Fig 12-30 Unacceptable pre-existing diastema closure. The whole gap was closed by adding composite only to this area which has totally altered the tooth proportion in a negative way. In addition, the poor design of the filling at the gingivoproximal area is continuously irritating the papilla.

Fig 12-31 After periodontal surgery. Even though the tissue levels are now acceptable, changes should be made in tooth form, position and proportion. The patient displays a negative (reverse) smile line, compared to the lower lip line, with relatively short centrals.

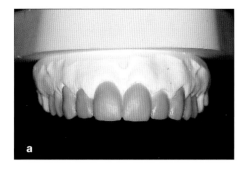

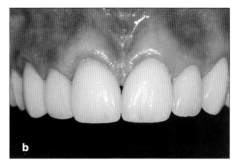

Fig 12-32a, b The proportions and incisal edge position are evaluated and changed with the wax-up. Following the procedures, the veneers are bonded (ceramist: *Gerard Ubassy*).

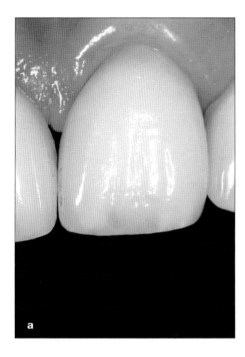

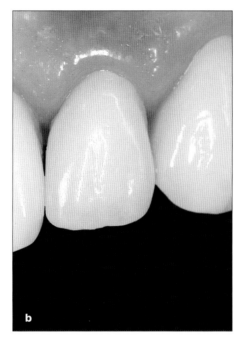

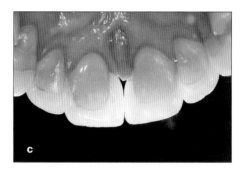

Fig 12-33a-c (a, b) The unesthetic composite is removed and the diastema is closed by removing some material from the distal margins of the central incisors and laterals in order to provide enough space for proportion. Note the change in the shape of the papilla between the centrals. (c) All the teeth are aligned in harmony with each other. Notice the tooth preparation and porcelain laminate veneer distribution from the palatinal view, in order to close the diastema and achieve natural proportion.

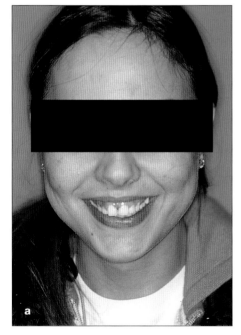

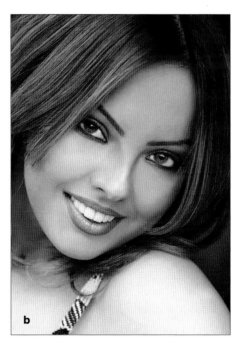

Fig 12-34a, b The concept of beauty often corresponds to harmony in proportion. The dentist's personal interpretation and perception, together with the state of the art approach of a technician, can change the whole appearance of the face in a very positive way.

Excessive Soft Tissue Display

The porcelain laminate veneers are prepared and bonded on the teeth of this top model by respecting all the mechanical criteria in terms of better bonding and retention. However, this may not necessarily mean that an acceptable esthetic result will be obtained. Since the "gummy smile" is not taken into consideration, the smile does not look attractive (Fig 12-35).

Evaluating a case as a whole from an esthetic point of view may indicate that the soft tissue levels should be altered. However, this should be comunicated to the patient in order to share treatment planning of the case. In such instances a "reverse composite mock-up" will help both the dentist and patient visualize the final outcome. The composite is placed over the gingiva, producing the effect of apically positioned crown lengthening. Even through it will produce some bulkiness owing to its placement over the soft tissue, this can easily be explained to the patient.

If the existing teeth seem to be longer than needed, the incisal edges can be indicated with a black marker, giving the illusion of shortened incisal edges (Fig 12-36). If this esthetic set-up also suits the functional needs, than the periodontologist can start apically repositioning the gingival levels.

To avoid a "gummy smile" the gingiva is repositioned towards the apical direction and six weeks later the new veneers are prepared and bonded. There is a drastic change in the patient's smile. Not only is the excessive soft tissue display eliminated, but better proportion in between the teeth and their relation to a beautiful face is also achieved (Fig 12-37).

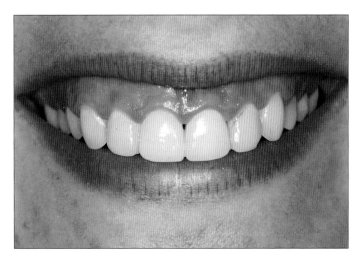

Fig 12-35 Esthetic appearance cannot be enhanced if the gingival levels are not altered in such heavy "gummy smile" cases. Reasonably well-prepared porcelain laminate veneers do not add the necessary beautifying effect to the whole face, since the "gummy smile" still exists.

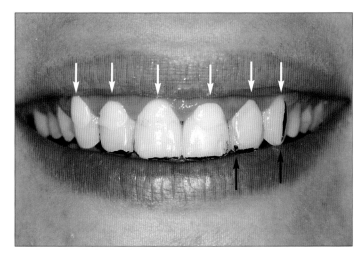

Fig 12-36 A chairside "reverse composite mock-up" is used in order to visualize crown lengthening towards the apical. Small pieces of composite, rolled between the fingers, are placed over the gingiva (white arrows), creating the illusion of apicaly lengthened teeth, thus eliminating the gummy smile. The incisal edges that are planned to be shortened are also painted with a black marker (black arrows). This may be the most important criterion,"the incisal edge position", in determining from where to start the case.

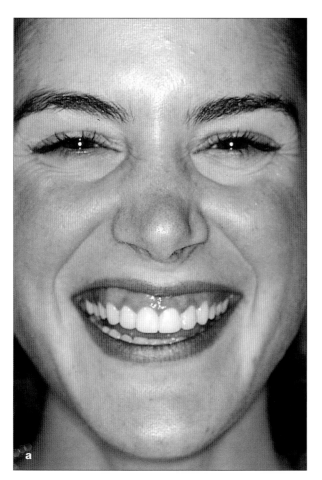 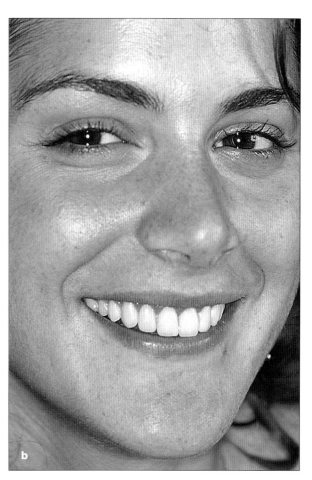

Fig 12-37a, b The veneers are designed after gingival alteration. The facial integration of the new porcelain laminate veneers is so natural and adds so much value to the face. The disappearance of the gummy smile changes the whole perception, thus creating a very pleasant overall look.

References

1. Ingber JS. Forced eruption. Part 1. A method of treating isolated one- and two-wall infrabony osseous defects.
   Rationale and case report. *J Periodontol* 1974;45:199-206.

2. Allen EP. Use of mucogingival surgical procedures to
   enhance esthetics. *Dent Clin North Am* 1988;32:307.

3. McLean JW. The science and art of dental ceramics. The
   nature of dental ceramics and their clinical use. Chicago:
   Quintessence, 1979;1:118-182.

4. Renner RP. An Introduction to Dental Anatomy and
   Esthetics. Chicago: Quintessence, 1985:49-124.

5. Touati B, Miara P, Nathanson D. Esthetic Dentistry and
   Ceramic Restorations. New York: Martin Dunitz, 1999:
   130-160.

13 Special Considerations

Galip Gürel

Introduction

Some cases are more complicated then they at first appear. Esthetics can be jeopardized by different structures and the more structures involved, the more contemporary approaches will be required in terms of teamwork. For the untrained eye, some cases may only seem to exhibit a discoloration problem. However, when carefully analyzed, it can clearly be seen that besides the discoloration there is not only negative visual tension present but gingival asymmetry and incisal edge positions as well (Fig 13-1). When each of the teeth is examined, the complexity of the case begins to reveal itself (Fig 13-2). Such cases must be meticulously planned and the specialist who is involved in the case must approve the treatment plan.

In some cases, a "gummy smile" can be unilateral. In order to improve the esthetics, a canted gingival line should be corrected at the beginning of the treatment. Gingival asymmetry may be attributed to various factors, such as unusual maxillary growth, unilateral overgrowth of a condyle, different arch position or tooth alignment.

If the color of the teeth requires alteration, the case will be more challenging. Although discolorations can be altered with PLVs (see Chapter 10), it is preferable to lighten teeth that are severely discolored because of poor endodontic treatment. This is done by bleaching them to a degree, internally and externally, so that the stump shades display a reasonably even discoloration after the preparation.

When a misaligned incisal edge inclination exists, in addition to a precise facebow transfer, excellent dentist-laboratory communication must be established in order correctly to transfer the esthetic incisal edge positioning and thus the inclination. In esthetics, a perfect earbow transfer does not necessarily guarantee the correct transfer of the incisal edge position.

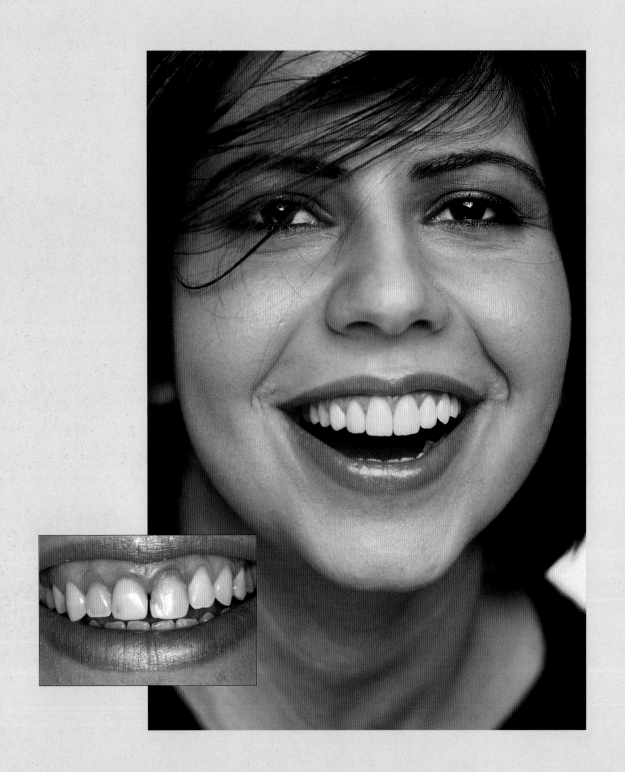

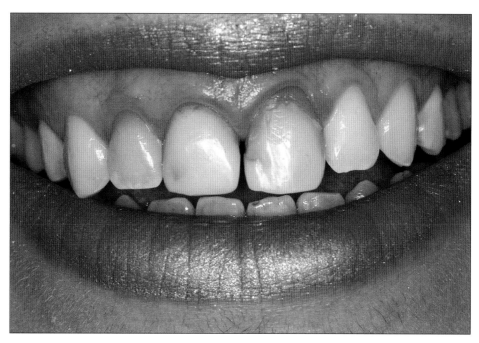

Fig 13-1 When viewed from the facial, a distinct discoloration can easily be seen. In addition to that, neither the gingival line nor the incisal edge position is parallel to the interpupillary line or horizon. A single-sided "gummy smile" can easily be observed on the right side of the patient's mouth.

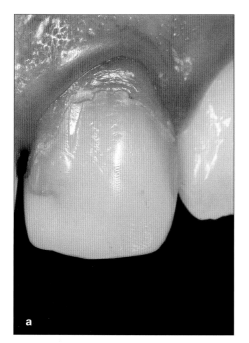 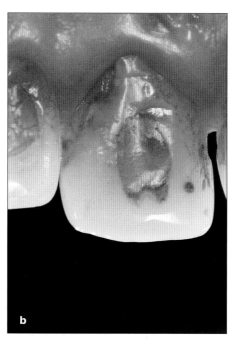 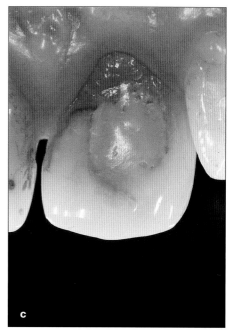

Fig 13-2a-c The discoloration projects a difficult situation. But the amount of existing composite restoration displays an even more difficult condition for the actual material preparation of the bonded porcelain restoration.

Patient Education

In such a complicated case, these problems should be explained to the patient well before the treatment commences.[1,2] It is surprising that the majority of patients have no understanding of the esthetic asymmetries or conditions that they have been living with for years. This is where the importance of patient education comes into play (see Chapter 14). Even though verbal explanations may help the patient to identify any problems, they will always want to visualize everything in order fully to comprehend the outcome that the dentist is designing. Verbal explanations are simply not sufficient.[3,4]

Diagnostic Composite Mock-ups

After years of experience, the author believes that the best way of communicating with the patient is to be able to mimic the final outcome in the patient's mouth before the definitive treatment plan. This way, they will not only be able actually to see what is about to happen in three dimensions, but they will be able to feel the position of the teeth in their own mouth. This will also help the dentist to see and feel the final outcome and its relation to lip position and face (Fig 13-3).

Altering Gingival Levels with the Mock-ups

Before doing anything surgically, the final position of the gingival levels should be approved by the patient. In order to achieve this effect, different colors of composites can be used as mock-ups. A reverse mock-up will help to mimic the tissue as if it is elevated apically or extended incisally. This reverse mock-up will not only let the patient and the dentist visualize the final outcome in advance, but will also help the periodontologist in defining the levels he will be altering during his operation.

Preparing a Surgical Stand

Once the balanced gingival levels are achieved, an alginate impression should be made. The model from this impression will help the dentist and the technician prepare a transparent template that can be used during periodontal surgery in order to alter the gingival levels to their correct positions (Fig 13-4).

Periodontal Surgery

The canted incisal plane and recession (sometimes local) due to toothbrush trauma further complicate a case. The cervical margin of tooth #22(10) is way above the imaginary line between the cervical margins of the central and canine, displaying an unfavorable esthetic situation (Fig 13-5).[5,6] The "gummy smile" and gingival asymmetry due to malpositioning and unilateral maxillary overgrowth must be altered. The surgery should be carefully planned and executed in sections during the operation. After the apical alteration of the gingival tissues on the right maxillary quadrant is carried out, the frenulum that happens to be the cause of the diastema is removed (Figs 13-6 to 13-11). On the other hand, in order to alter the gingival level of the left lateral #22(10) incisally, a semilunar coronally repositioned flap operation is performed (Figs 13-12 to 13-14).

Bleaching the Teeth

The teeth display various discolorations and therefore require bleaching.[7] The reason for the discoloration means that the root canal is retreated (Fig 13-15).[7-9] In some teeth, internal bleaching is administered, while in others, external home and power bleaching is carried out.[7] Extreme care should be paid to seal the root of the endodontically treated teeth while internal bleaching is used, otherwise the teeth will be prone to internal bleaching (courtesy of Dr Cimilli).

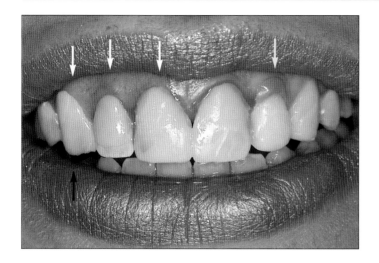

Fig 13-3 Reverse composite mock-up for the visualization of the gingival alteration. Note the composite placed over the gingiva. Tooth-colored composite helps one to visualize apical migration of the gingiva (teeth #13(6), 12(7), 11(8)) (white arrows), whereas pink-colored composite mimics the incisally placed gingiva (tooth #22(10)) (yellow arrow). The incisal tip of the canine (tooth #13(6)) is painted black (black arrow) to mimic the shortening of this edge to equalize its position with the tip of the other canine, thus creating a positive smile line in harmony with the lower lip line.

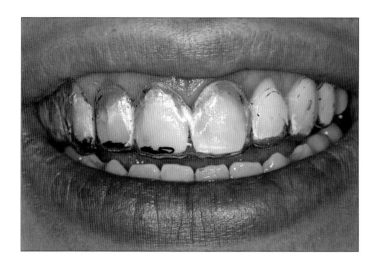

Fig 13-4 A transparent surgical tray can be prepared for use during surgery in exacting the gingival displacement.

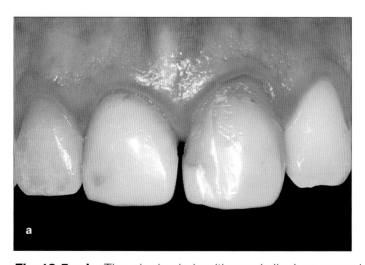
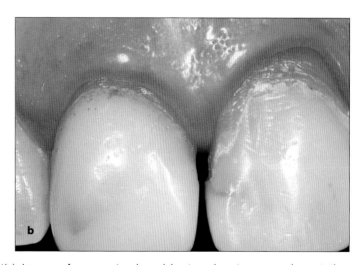

Fig 13-5a, b The gingiva is healthy and displays normal thickness. Asymmetry is evident owing to recession at the left central and lateral incisors. Interdental papilla does not fill the space between two centrals owing to minor diastema.

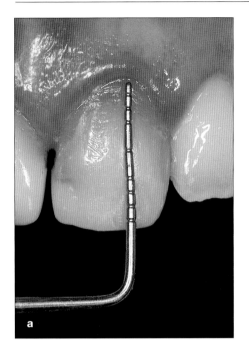

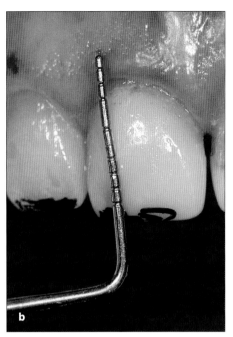

Fig 13-6a, b Treatment planning involves occlusal reduction to correct canting and a crown-lengthening procedure to match crown lengths on the right anterior teeth. Clinical crown length for the central is determined from the left central and projected on the right after marking the planned extent of odontoplasty.

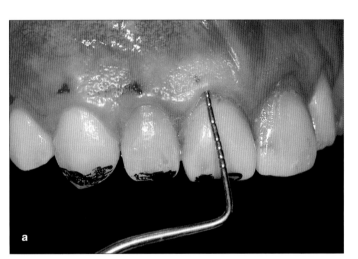

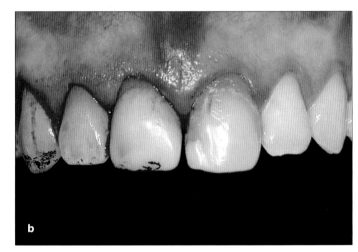

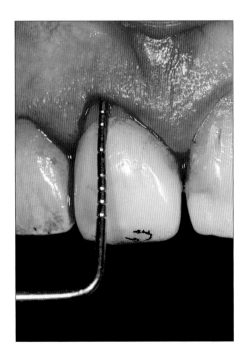

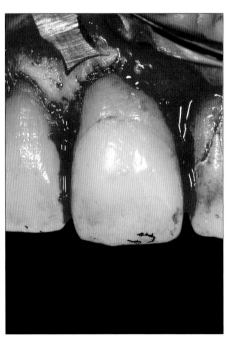

Fig 13-7a, b (above) After the surgical template is placed over the teeth, the zenith points are marked. Removal of the gingival tissue is performed with an incision that connects the bleeding points, indicating the zenith points. Note the incisal edges of teeth #13(6), #12(7), and #11(8) painted black, imitating the shortening of these teeth.

Fig 13-8 (left) Sounding through the newly formed margin indicates insufficient space for biologic zone.

Fig 13-9 (right) Recontouring of the crestal bone is performed by bone chisels until a minimum of a 3 mm space is available from the crest of the bone to the gingival margin.

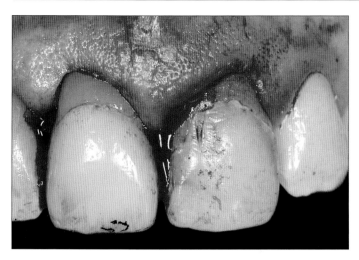

Fig 13-10 With special attention on the zenith points, two identical centrals were created by crown-lengthening procedure.

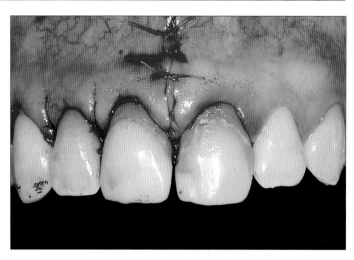

Fig 13-11 The flap is secured from the interdental spaces with 6/0 monofilament non-resorbable sutures, and the median frenum is located apically and sutured with resorbable material. Note the left lateral incisor (#22(10)) with a high gingival margin.

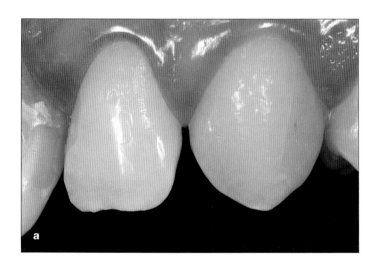

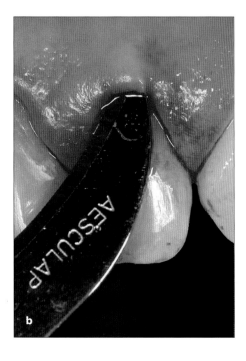

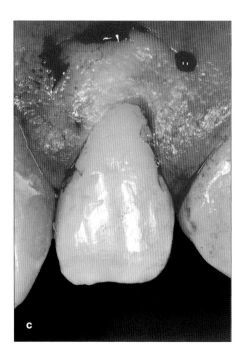

Fig 13-12a-c Recession in the lateral incisor resulted in a long clinical crown comparable with the adjacent canine. *Semilunar coronally repositioned flap.* With one sulcular and a semilunar incision at the mucogingival fold, the band of attached gingiva is released.

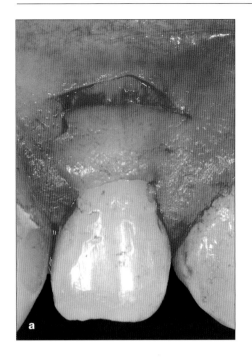
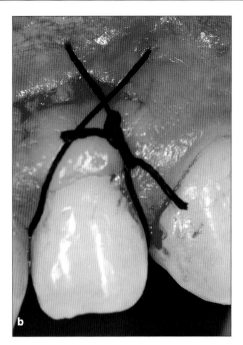

Fig 13-13a, b When the repositioned flap is free of tensional stress; lateral blood supply is sufficient for survival. However, close adaptation of the tissue to the periosteum under–eliminates the formation of fibrin clot under the flap and confirms survival.

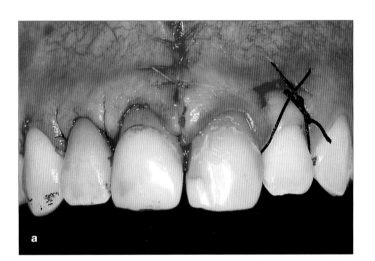
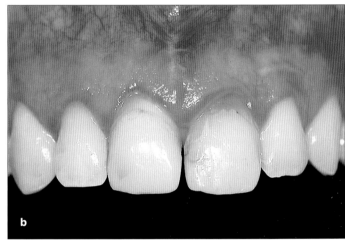
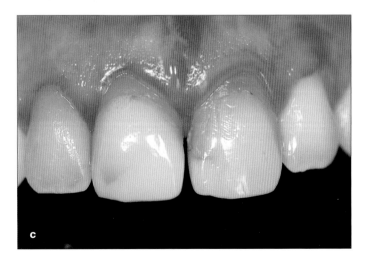

Fig 13-14a-c (a) The final appearance of the case upon completion of surgery. (b) Three weeks and (c) six weeks after surgery. Despite the canted incisal plane, a close match of the esthetically leveled gingival line is attained (Periosurgery by Dr Demirel).

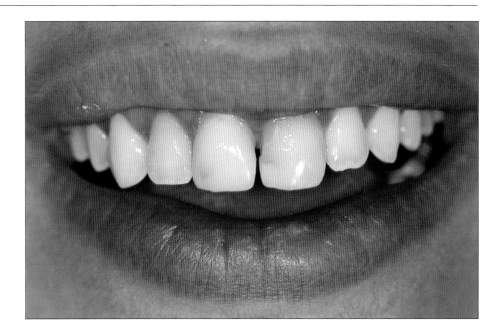

Fig 13-15 Gingival canting is altered to a more esthetic horizontal position. Insisal canting remains. Teeth are bleached and ready for the PLV treatment. Note the slight yellowish discoloration of the centrals owing to $Ca(OH)_2$ that is still inside the teeth (courtesy of Dr Cimilli).

Restoring the Teeth

After the symmetric gingival levels are achieved and the teeth are bleached, a preliminary impression can be made for the wax-up procedure. When the models are completed, they must be mounted and registered correctly together. Currently, most dental work is sent to laboratories without a facebow registration; practitioners take a double-bite or triple-tray impression of the anterior segment to send off.[10] Technicians mount the casts arbitrarily between the frames of an articulator without any information as to an esthetic reference head position, and regularly make the anterior esthetic line of the restorations parallel to the frames of the articulator or tabletop because of lack of information. One of the most serious esthetic errors associated with improperly mounted casts is when the incisal-canine line is made slanted, which causes the maxillary midline (midsagittal) also to slant.

Earbow Transfer

A facebow transfer and a semi-adjustable articulator are essential for proper mounting. The condylar axis that is present in the skull is related to the upper cast with the facebow.[11] One of the simplest methods is to use the earbow, which uses the ear hole on each side as reference, owing to its close relationship to the glenoid fossa.[12] The facebow transfers the occlusal determinants from a functional standpoint and orients the maxillary cast on the articulator, related to the anatomic or obituary candylar axis. In some instances, there may be esthetic misconceptions due to head asymmetries related to the altered position of the condyles.

In other words, facebow transfer may not necessarily record the true esthetic alignment that would be useful to the lab technician, especially when designing the incisal edge position of the PLVs. In the event that one ear is higher than the other (which can occur) the ear bow would also be made slanted in relation to true horizontal, thus giving a false esthetic mounting on the articulator (Fig 13-16). In prosthodontics, the anterior esthetic line has usually been established in the provisional crowns. This is because hand-mounted and facebow mounted casts are not related to the interpupillary line or the true horizontal. Dentists can make any mounted cast work functionally correct at any cant or tilt by changing the morphology of the teeth, but they may not necessarily be esthetically correct.[12] The esthetic plane of occlusion (EPO) must be made equal to the functional plane of occlusion (FPO). This lack of information will be apparent when the restorations are placed in the patient's mouth.

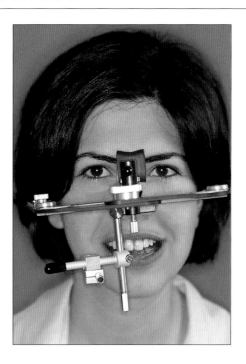

Fig 13-16 All the parameters (horizontal, vertical and sagittal) should be used to relate the restorations to the patient's face. Note the unparallel position of the horizontal segment of the facebow, in relation to the bipupillary line and horizon, due to the asymmetric position of the ears.

The esthetic incisal line of the patient can be transferred from a different perspective if the condyles are not symmetrical. The lab technician will mount the facebow from the recording made from the patient. In these articulators, the arbitrary condylar axis is always parallel to the bench top, which should represent the interpupillary line. However, in cases where head asymmetry exists, the interpupillary line and the intercondylar axis may diverge and thus automatically distort the relationship between the horizontal intraocular line and the esthetic reference plane, which will represent the incisal edge position (Fig 13-17).

Esthetic Orientation

Esthetics is orientated to the horizontal (horizon), vertical (midsagittal), and frontal (coronal) planes as they relate to the patient's cranium. All three planes should be addressed when diagnosing and treating patients during prosthodontics, orthodontics, maxillofacial surgery, restorative dentistry, cosmetic dentistry and periodontics, when gingivoplasty is being performed. Observations of human skeletons with intact teeth show the maxillary incisal-canine line at a right angle to the vertebral column when the skeleton is in the erect position (body standing or sitting). Head posture is of significant concern when trying to establish an esthetic occlusion. Many people's head and facial features are asymmetrical, and so it is preferable to establish an esthetic plane of occlusion parallel to the horizon when the patient is sitting and the head is perfectly erect in a standardized esthetic reference position. The basic problem that a dentist faces is to decide on the proper reference plane or line.

Fig 13-17a-c (a) (chairside) Even though the incisal edge position may be parallel to the interpupillary line; it may not be parallel to the condylar axis owing to one ear being higher than the other. (b) (laboratory) When such an ear bow registration is transferred to the lab and mounted to the articulator, the esthetic plane of occlusion automatically cants. If the technican builds up the incisal edge position parallel to the bench top (which will most probably be the case), (c) (chairside) then the actual restorations will definitely have a different plane of occlusion with canted incisal edge position together with a canted midline (that has been created perpendicular to the faulty incisal edge position).

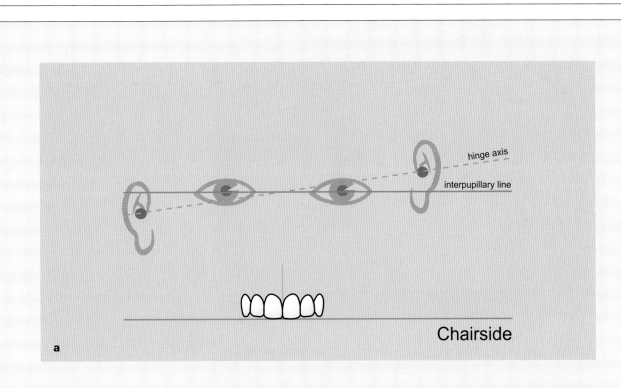

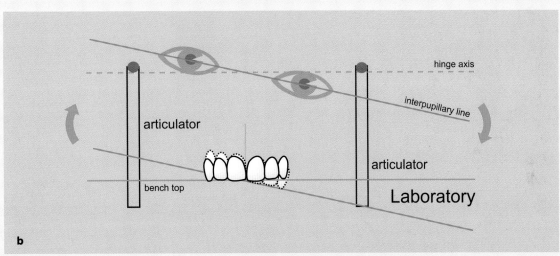

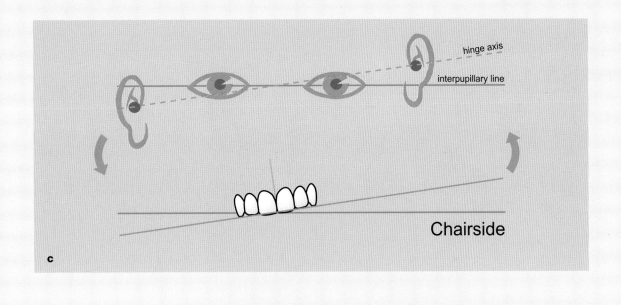

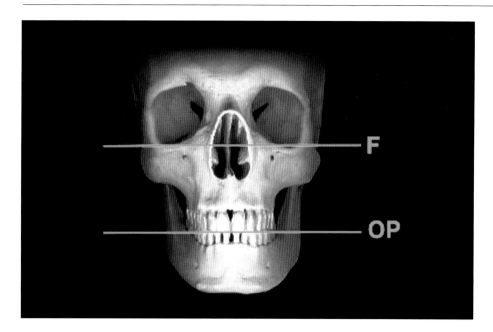

Fig 13-18 The esthetic plane of occlusion should be kept parallel to the horizon.

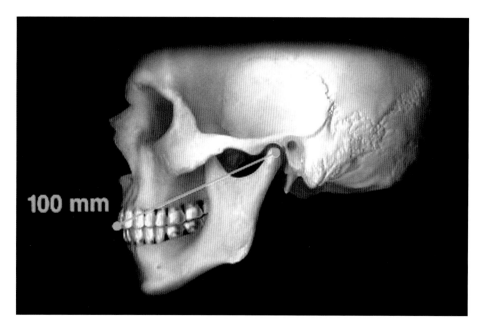

Fig 13-19 The average axis-incisal distance is 100 mm.

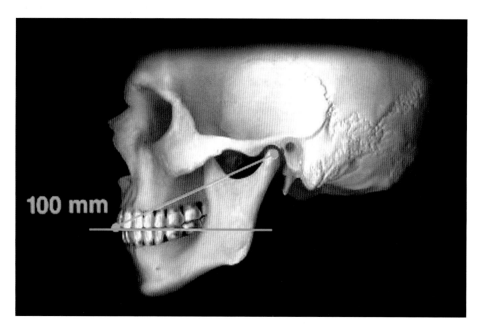

Fig 13-20 The horizontal portion of the analyzer bow registers the incisal/occlusal-horizontal plane of reference (courtesy of Dr J. Kois).

Plane of Reference

Facebows were originally oriented to the Frankfort horizontal plane of reference, from porion (top of the auditory meatus) to orbitale (lower border of the orbit), which is sometimes parallel to the horizon when the head is erect in posture.[13] When a method for locating the hinge axis was discovered, the two posterior points of the reference plane were moved several millimeters down to the transverse hinge axis of the mandible. However, the anterior point of the reference plane (orbitale) was kept at the same level, thus creating the axis-orbital plane of reference.[11] Most facebows are manufactured to a 22–23 mm standardized reference point from nasion (middle of the nasofrontal suture), because it standardizes the system to be used and it is also what orthodontists use in their cephalometrics.[14] Therefore, it may be better to level the facebow on the patient to an arbitrary axis-horizontal or an arbitrary occlusal-horizontal plane of reference in three planes of space, to relate the casts on the articulator for the diagnosis and treatment of function as well as esthetics (Fig 13-18).

The Kois Dento-Facial Analyzer System

What dentistry needs is to have a facebow and articulator system that can be used not only for function or occlusion, but for esthetics as well – a simplified, uncomplicated facebow system with procedures for mounting simple to complex cases into an articulator for the proper diagnosis and treatment of esthetics and function. The *Kois* Dento-Facial Analyzer System (Panadent Corp.), researched by Dr John *Kois*, is based on an average axis-incisal distance of 100 mm (Fig 13-19). This 100 mm distance is supported by *Bonwill's* equilateral triangle, *Monson's* spherical theory (4 inches = 100.12 mm), *Weinberg's* 1963 studies, as well as many others, all showing an average axis-incisal distance of 100 mm. The system registers the steepness and tilts of the occlusal plane in three planes of space. The horizontal portion of the analyzer bow will register an incisal/occlusal-horizontal plane of reference

(Fig 13-20). The vertical rod will register the sagittal plane of reference. The average axis-incisal distance of 100 mm will register the frontal plane of reference. Dr *Kois's* studies were undertaken with male and female patients from different ethnic backgrounds measuring from the hinge axis to the incisal edge of the central incisor. Approximately 80–85% of the patients were found to be within 5 mm of the 100 mm axis-incisal distance, with an average of 100.21 mm.

Registration Procedures

While the posterior portion of the analyzer bow is kept down and out of occlusion, the incisal edge of the maxillary incisors is set to the line or ledge on the index tray to relate to the average 100 mm axis-incisal distance for function. Then the vertical indicator rod is slid posteriorly in the keyway slot of the analyzer bow close to the patient's nose. The vertical indicator rod is aligned to the patient's facial midline to relate the teeth to the sagittal plane for esthetics. While maintaining incisal contact with the index tray, the analyzer bow is rotated up in the posterior until it is level from a profile view. The level gauge can be added to verify that the bow is level (Fig 13-21).

With the steepness and tilts of the occlusal plane in the registration material captured on the horizontally aligned index tray, the analyzer bow can be aligned to the patient's midsagittal for optimum esthetics. In this way, the incisal edge is related to the axis for proper arch of rotation, making eccentric movements valid for optimum function (Fig 13-22).

APT for Preparation

After the true esthetic plane of occlusion is transferred to the lab, a wax-up with the proper incisal edge position is received. APTs can be made over the unprepared teeth for exact tooth preparation. As mentioned in Chapter 7, an APR is also required in this case. The incisal tip of the right canine #13(6) is shortened, so that the template can easily be seated over the teeth to prepare the

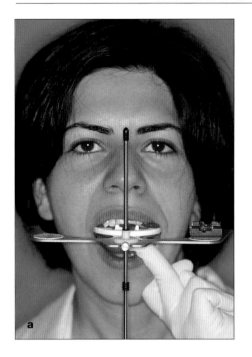
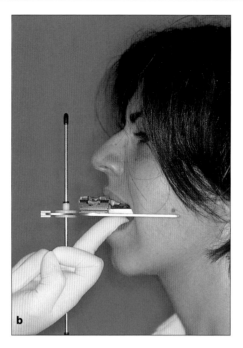

Fig 13-21a, b (a) First the incisal edges are positioned on the analyzer to the average 100 mm distance. (b) Then the analyzer is rotated up in the posterior until it is parallel to the horizon from a sagittal view. Both positions are double checked with a level gauge that is placed on the facial analyzer.

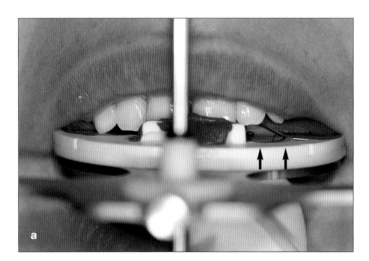
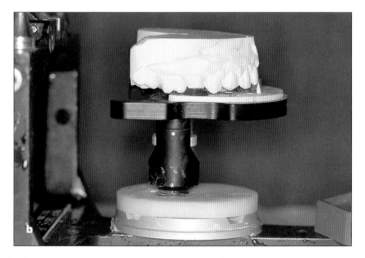

Fig 13-22a, b (a) Note the true transfer of the chanted incisal edge position when the dento-facial analyzer is kept parallel to the horizon. The right canine (#13(6)) is touching the plate, whereas the other canine (#23(11)) is way above this level (black arrows). (b) The model is mounted on the articulator, now that both the EPO and the FPO are transferred

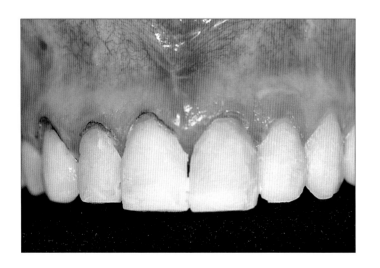

Fig 13-23 APT placed on the teeth before actual material preparation. The canine #13(6) is shortened from the incisal and the gingival tissues are moved 0.5mm more apical to ascertain the gingival symmetry with a diode laser (Biolase Comp.). Since the EPO and FPO are transferred together to the articulator, the wax-up and thus the APT are finished in a predictable way. Note the balance of the incisal edge position.

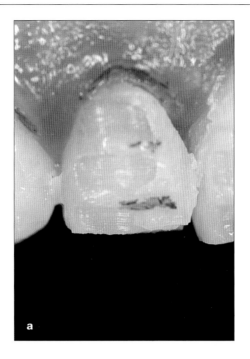
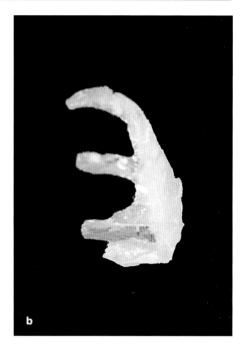

Fig 13-24a, b (a) Using the depth cutter through APT. (b) The leftover composite on the mesial of tooth #12 (7) very clearly defines the amount of saved tooth structure.

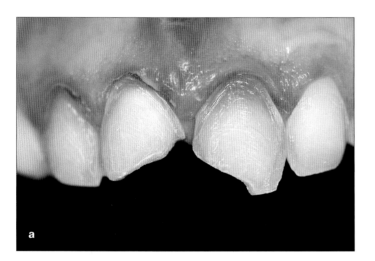
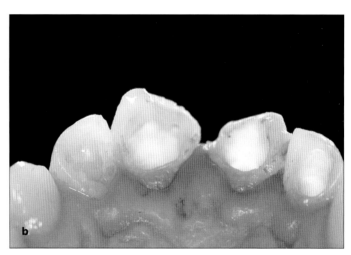

Fig 13-25a, b Tooth preparation and cavity restoration are done at the same time. The lingual preparation line is kept away from the lingual concavity, limiting itself to the incisal 1/3rd only. The cavity that is located in the middle of the lingual concavity is filled with a hybrid composite resin alone.

APT (Fig 13-23). When the teeth are prepared through the APT, the saved sound tooth structure can be easily visualized (Figs 13-24a and b).

Tooth Preparation

The material preparation needs special attention in this case, owing to the opened access cavity for the root canal treatment and bleaching, as well as the existing composite fillings. After the material preparation is finished, the cavity prepared for internal bleaching has to be filled with a hybrid composite (Figs 13-25a and b). Then an impression is made and sent to the lab.

Laboratory Procedures

Once the models are obtained, they are connected to the articulator (Panadent Corp.) with the help of the cast. Now that the technician has both the functional and esthetic orientation, it is much easier to relate the actual esthetic incisal edge position to the model they will be using.

Bonding

Since all these parameters are used during teeth preparation, almost nothing is left to luck. Both the dentist and the technician are aware of the tooth preparation required in order to achieve the most esthetic result with minimum sound tooth tissue loss. After the PLVs are tried-in one by one, they are all seated on the teeth to evaluate the final esthetic outcome. Once this is approved, by both dentist and patient, they can then be bonded.

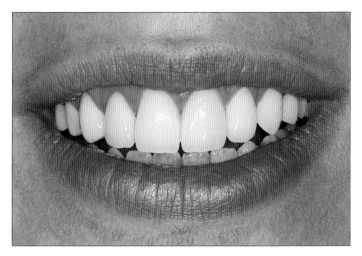

Fig 13-26 The finished veneers. Throughout the whole procedure, excellent communication between the dentist-patient-specialist and the lab technician has been achieved. Note that the unilateral "gummy smile" has disappeared as well as the unfavorable incisal edge position. The new smile line is in harmony with the lower lip line.

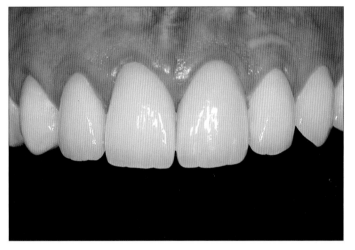

Fig 13-27 The esthetic harmony. All the discolorations are masked. The soft tissue health is excellent six months post-operatively. Note the excellent result of the coronally repositioned flap operation on tooth #22(10). It is now possible to observe the pleasing relation between the gingiva and the teeth in terms of horizontal and vertical harmony, the delicate translucencies, crack lines, surface texture, incisal edge configuration and incisal embrasures created by the dental technician (ceramist *Hakan Akbayar*). These could only be achieved when the EPO is correctly transferred to the laboratory. Shortening or lengthening of the incisal edges of the porcelain (in order to level the incisal edge position) would have distorted the delicacy.

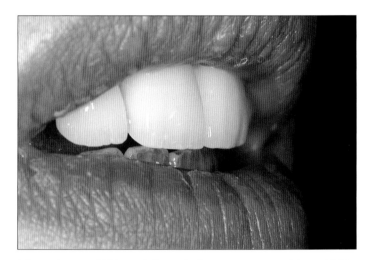

Fig 13-28 PLV and lip relation at rest position. PLVs exhibit a natural blend with the surrounding soft tissues.

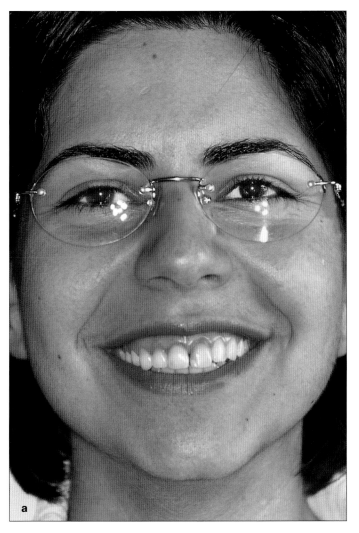
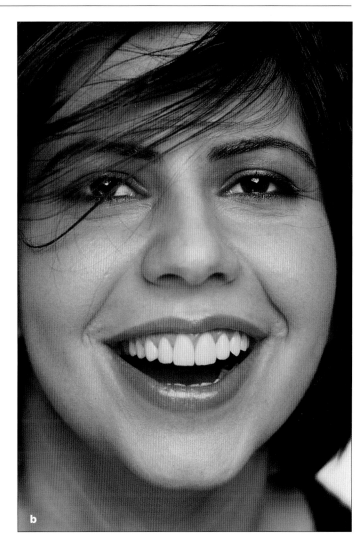

Fig 13-29a, b The integration of the new smile design with the facial composition. The overall positive impact of the new smile on the face has been created with a series of operations. The dull-looking smile has been replaced with an energizing, fresh and healthy one.

Details

When the case is perceived from all angles, treatment enhances not only the function but also the form and esthetics of the teeth, mouth and face. In such a complicated case, almost every aspect one can imagine has been improved. The canting of the gingival margin and the asymmetry have been altered first. Then the necessary teeth are bleached. During the preparation, the canted midline with the incisal edge position has been completely changed (Figs 13-25 to 13-29).

Reverse Color Gradation

Color and color gradation are important criteria in smile design. Teeth usually display individual variations in color. The maxillary centrals are the dominant teeth of the smile and display the brightest color. The laterals are narrower, especially in women, and slightly lower in value than the centrals. Canines have the highest chroma displaying the lowest value. Natural blending creates harmony that is very different from a "whiter than white", Hollywood smile. This natural color gradation is now more favored, especially in Europe. With the introduction of bleaching, more and

481

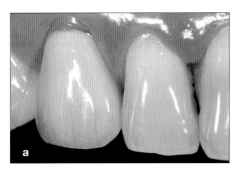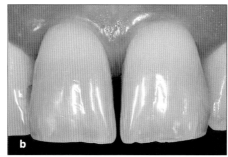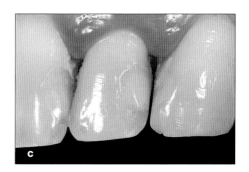

Fig 13-30a-c (a) The teeth should get higher in chroma when observed from the centrals to the canines; however, in this particular case the canines exhibit lower chroma and higher value than the centrals which is an indication that the centrals are darker than the canines. (b) Note the high value on the cervical 1/3rd of the centrals and high chroma on the middle 1/3rd, as opposed to a high chroma at the cervical 1/3rd of a natural tooth. A small diastema also exists between the centrals. (c) PLVs can also be used not only to improve esthetics but also to restore deficient teeth. Note the large class III composite fillings of the left central and lateral, and dark cervical discoloration owing to the gingival recession on the right canine. There is a reverse color gradation both on the centrals as well as on front to back teeth configuration.

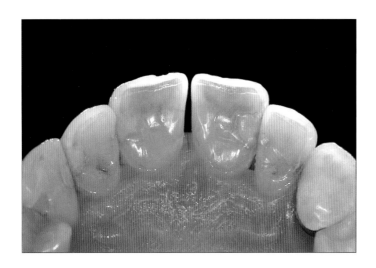

Fig 13-31 The extension of the old fillings towards the lingual surface. It is better to remove the existing fillings first and incorporate with the PLV.

more Europeans demand whiter teeth, but they still respect the anterior-posterior color gradation with higher values.

Every tooth also has a color gradation of its own. Owing to the very thin nature of the enamel on the gingival 1/3rd, the tooth exhibits the highest chroma in this area. The middle 1/3rd displays high value and, in the incisal 1/3rd, translucency. However, it is also possible to see different color configurations from this natural phenomenon. From a dentist's point of view, such cases can be almost too complicated, depending on the nature of the existing teeth and restoration. When the issue of achieving natural tooth form and color comes into consideration, careful communication between the dentist and the lab technician becomes even more important, especially when the natural front-back color gradation needs to be corrected, as well as the color map of every single tooth (Fig 13-30).

When preparing a case like this, all the existing old restorations should be incorporated with the PLV (Fig 13-31). All the existing restorations are removed and replaced with the bonded porcelain restoration (BPR) and, in so doing, the necessary rules and procedures for tooth preparation and bonding are followed. The case is finished in a very natural-looking way. The shape, form and design of the smile are changed without attracting too much attention to the new PLVs. The color-gradation in particular makes the whole smile very natural (Figs 13-32 to 13-49).

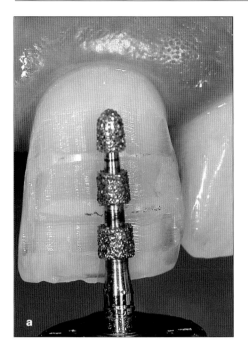
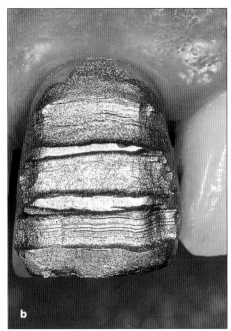
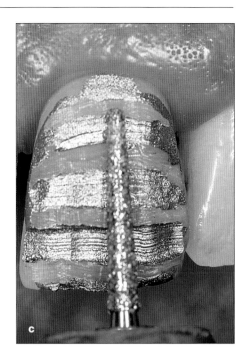
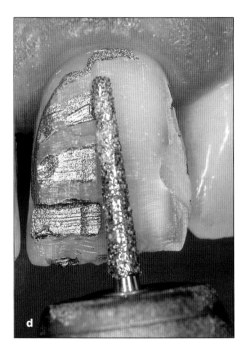
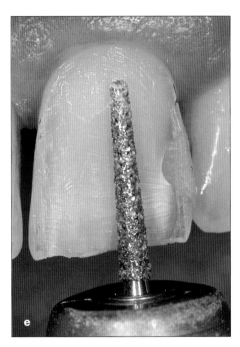

Fig 13-32a-e The author prefers to start the preparation in a regular sequence as explained in Chapter 7. No matter what the condition of the tooth, this sequence will ease the problem of preparing it for such complicated cases. Whether a cavity or a filling exists, the required amount of tooth reduction starts from the facial. (a) Since no facial enamel loss is observed and there will not be too much alteration of the facial outlines, the APT is not used. The depth cutter is applied directly on the facial surface of the tooth. (b to d) The surface prepared with the depth cutter is painted with a water-insoluble paint in order visually to ease the penetration of the round-ended fissure diamond bur. When this preparation is carried out until the coloration disappears, it is a good indication of reaching the correct preparation depth on the facial. (e) The bur should be kept in three different angulations sagitally, in order correctly to follow the facial convexity.

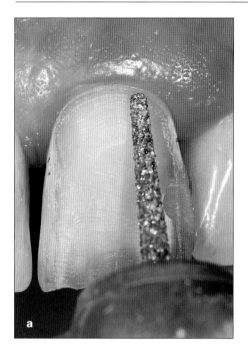
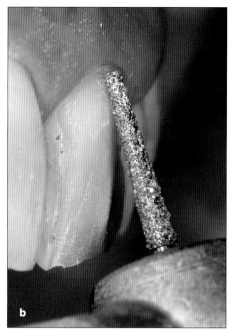
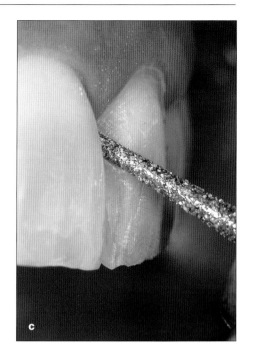

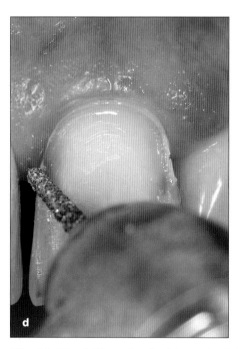
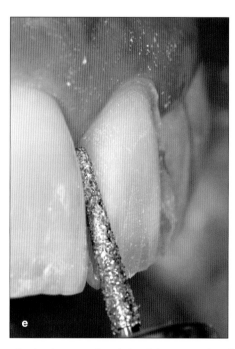
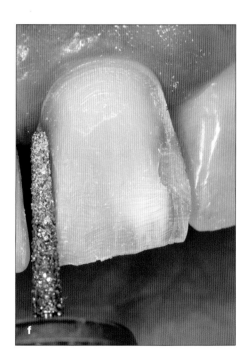

Fig 13-33a-f Then the (a, b) cervical, (c, d) gingivo-proximal, (e, f) interproximal surfaces are prepared. (a) Following the facial preparation the gingival margin is prepared. (b) It is important to hold the bur at an angle that will be parallel to the surface angulation of the gingival 1/3rd of the tooth. It is also important not to go any deeper than the radius of the fissure bur. Depths of more than the size of the radius may cause formation of reverse notches at the gingival margin. (c, d) The angulation of the bur is changed to 60° while preparing the gingivoproximal area. This dogleg preparation will enhance the esthetic outcome of the PLV by hiding the PLV-tooth interface at this junction. This is especially important when a distinct color change is being made. (e, f) Then the bur is uprighted while the incisal-proximal area is prepared. Attention should be paid to the adjacent tooth, especially if it is to be kept intact.

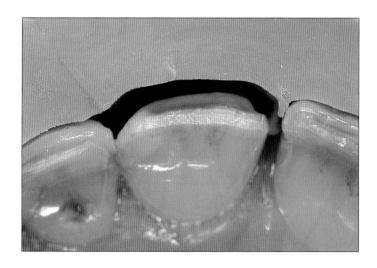

Fig 13-34 These reductions are further checked with the help of the silicone index. Note the equal preparation depth from all angles.

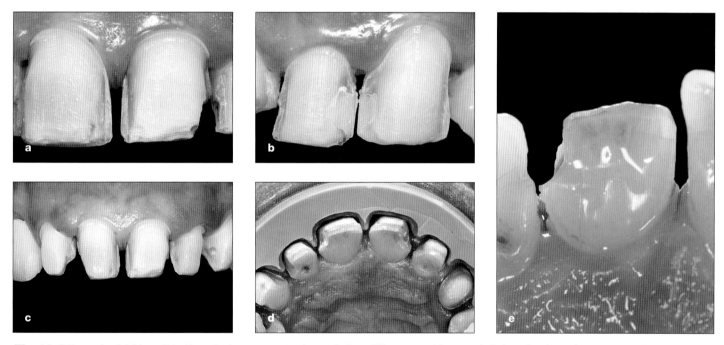

Fig 13-35a-e (a, b) Now it is time to incorporate the existing fillings, cavities or deficiencies into the preparation. (c) First, the fillings must be removed. (d, e) Then the preparation should be extended to the palatinal as much as necessary, paying close attention not to end up in the palatinal concavity, especially on centrals and laterals.

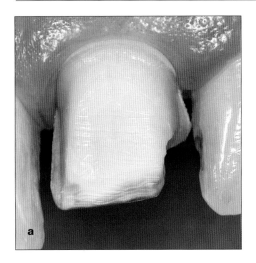
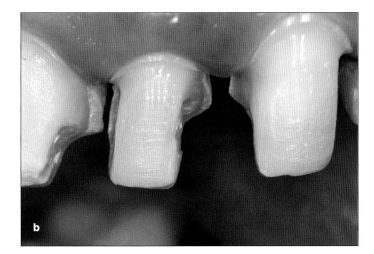
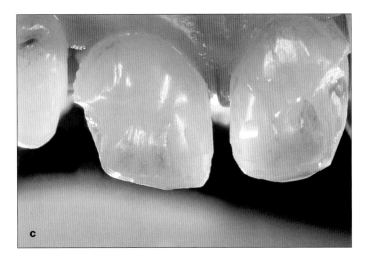
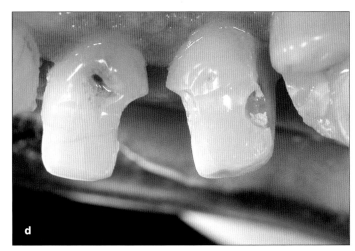
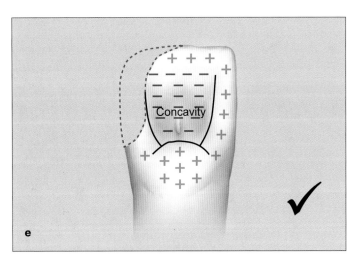
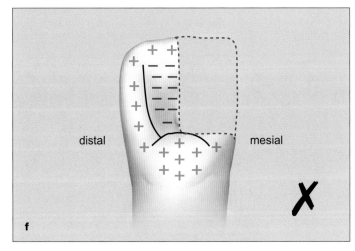

Fig 13-36a-f (a) Even though some adjustments on the mesial and distal surfaces will suffice, like in the centrals, (b) sometimes the size of the deficiency may be so large that the preparation may resemble a three-quarter restoration, like in the left lateral and canine. (c, d) The palatal view. The important factor here is to keep the palatinal margins either on the marginal ridges or on the cingulum. In other words, on the convexities where the tensile stress is minimal (e), illustration to c, d (+) signs show the better placement areas for the PLV margins, whereas (-) signs refer to concavities that are prone to higher tensile stresses. (f) If the lingual margin is located on the lingual concavity, it is better to extend it towards the distal marginal ridge and over the cingulum to minimize the tensile strength that the PLV will face after bonding.

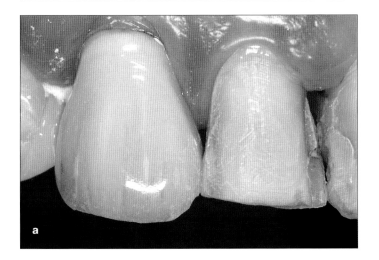

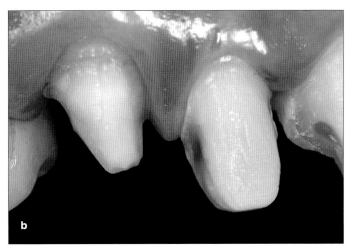

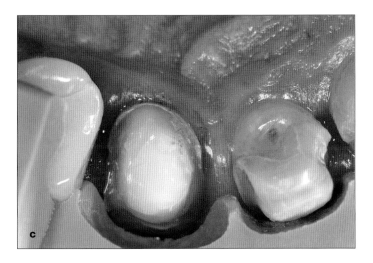

Fig 13-37a-c (a) Once the veneer preparations are finished, the existing crowns can be taken out and the teeth prepared. (b, c) While preparing a tooth for an all-ceramic crown restoration, a 360° chamfer margin is necessary. The canine's preparation depth is obviously different from and deeper than the lateral which is displaying the conservative preparation depth of a veneer.

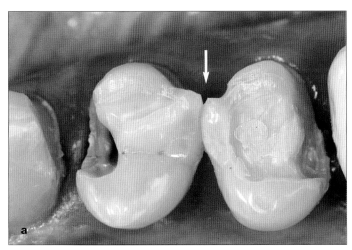

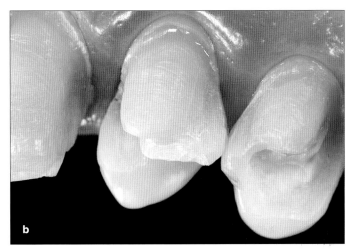

Fig 13-38a, b Similarly, all the restorations and caries defects are removed from the premolars. The choice of restoration in such instances will be the onlay veneers (a) The palatinal interproximal margins are extended to where the ex-restorations were placed. If this margin is located on a centric stop, then it should be carried further away lingually. It is always better to place the centric stops on the onlay veneer or the original tooth surface instead of the porcelain-tooth interface. It is preferable to keep the mesial or distal horizontal cavity floor above the gingival tissue. In addition, if the teeth are in contact, the interproximal contact area should be kept intact, leaving the interproximal preparation margin facial to that area (white arrow). (b) The cervical margins are placed supragingivally in most of the cases, unless a cavity or abfraction extending under the gingiva exists.

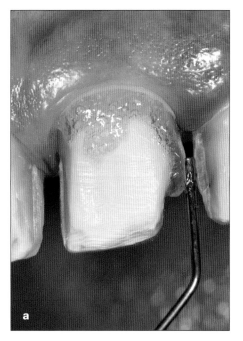 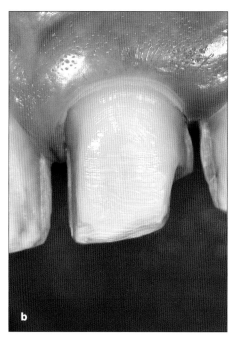 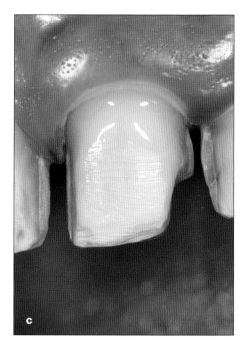

Fig 13-39a-c All the exposed dentin surfaces are (a) etched, (b) primed and (c) adhesive is applied just after the preparation. An 80-micron-thick adhesive (Optiond FL, Kerr) is used with an oxygen barrier (DeoX , Ultradent), to prevent oxygen inhibition layer on top of it, in order to achieve a truly polymerized adhesive on these areas.

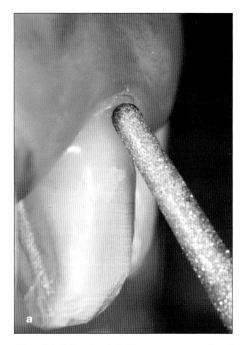 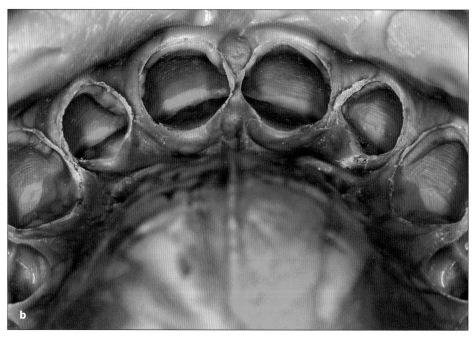

Fig 13-40a, b (a) The excess adhesive that may have spread over the enamel margin should be carefully cleaned with the round end of a fissure extra-fine diamond bur. This will not only clean the enamel surface (b) but also leave a sharp, crisp clear margin on the impression, which can be very easily duplicated by the dental technician.

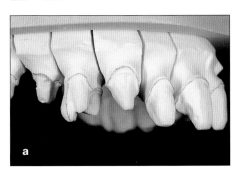 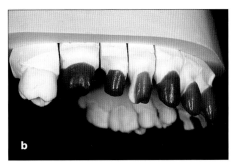 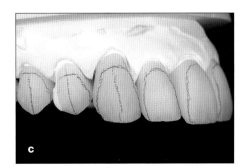

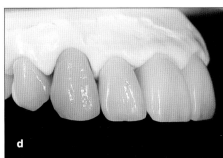 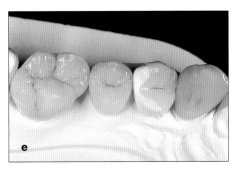

Fig 13-41a-e (a, b) Lab procedures are quite similar to those explained in Chapter 9. (c, d) All the veneers and all ceramic crowns are produced by ceramist Gerard Ubassy, with his layering technique on Empress 2 ingots. Note the internal staining especially on the canine. The chroma is increased at this stage to create the natural anterior-posterior color gradation effect. (e) If possible, it is always preferable to use the same porcelain material on different teeth of the same arch. This will highly minimize the metameric effects. All the restorations (full ceramic crowns on teeth #13(6),# 15(4) and #16(3)); onlay veneer on tooth #14(5), and veneers on tooth #12, 11(7, 8) are built up with Empress II. Note the delicately applied layering techniques to all the restorations creating a very natural outcome.

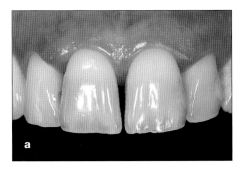 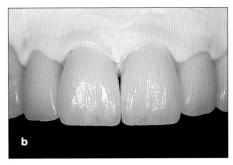 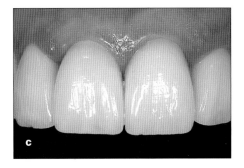

Fig 13-42a-c "Before", "laboratory" and "after" pictures. A very natural change that respects the existing size and position of the teeth can be observed.

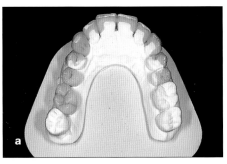 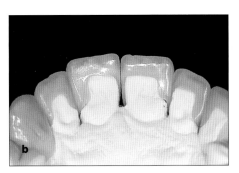 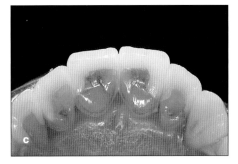

Fig 13-43a-c Special care is taken both in palatinal tooth preparation and laboratory work in this case. The margins are kept away from the concavities and are attempted to be placed on the convex surfaces.

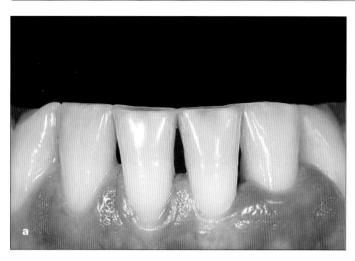 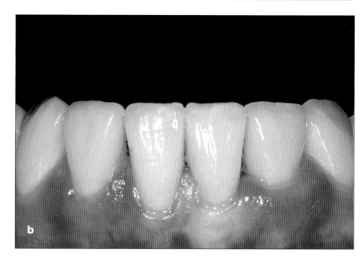

Fig 13-44a, b The same progression is achieved on the mandibular arch. Note how the black gingival interdental holes are closed and incisal embrasures created. Canines are built-up to support the occlusion for the canine guided lateral excursion.

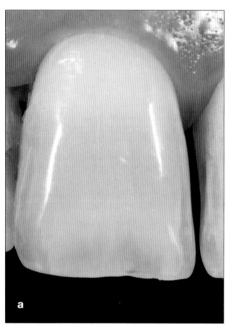 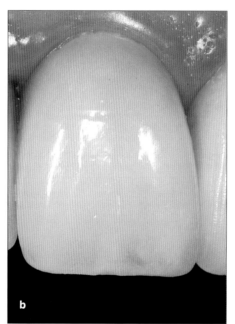

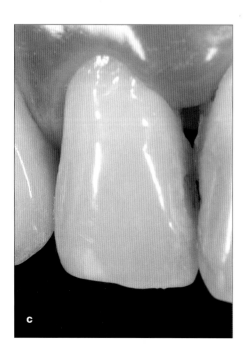 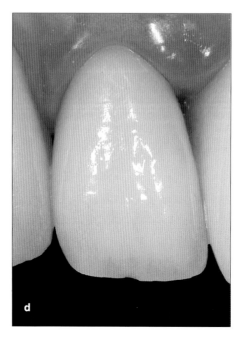

Fig 13-45a-d (a, b) The color and form of the central are drastically changed. However, all the natural effects, such as the translucencies, mamelons and opalescence are respected and reproduced. (c, d) The same delicacy is applied to the laterals.

Fig 13-46a, b Even though the all-ceramic crown needs a thicker application of porcelain, the technician can still adjust the chroma and value with his accuracy in the layering technique. (a) The dark-colored gingival margin is prepared level with the gingival sulcus, and (b) totally covered and blocked out with the Empress II crown.

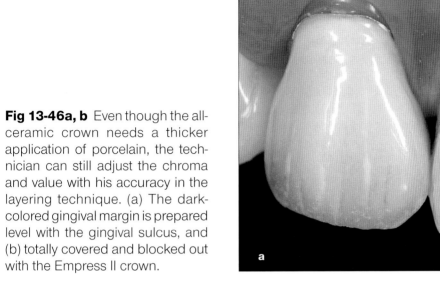
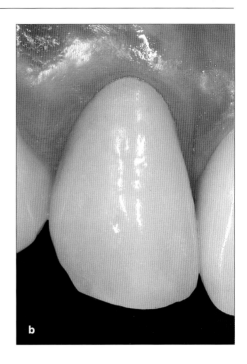

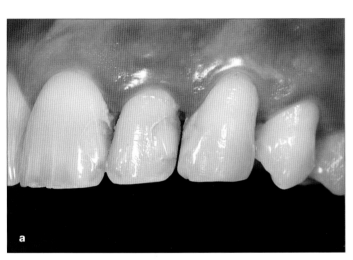
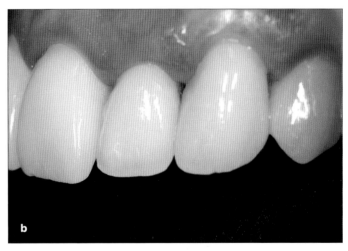

Fig 13-47a, b Old restorations are all incorporated into the preparation and the final restorations. Note the enhanced color production towards the canine. It is hard to identify which teeth are restored with PLV, onlay veneers and all-ceramic crowns.

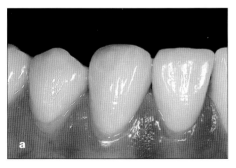
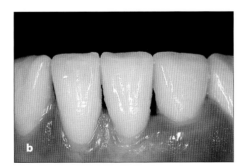
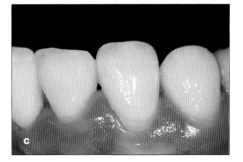

Fig 13-48a-c It is more difficult to build up PLVs on the mandibular teeth owing to the limiting factor of palatinal surfaces of the maxillary teeth. However, when proper preparation is combined with meticulous lab work, very natural-looking mandibular PLVs can be produced. (b) As opposed to maxillary teeth, the mandibular lateral incisors are the most dominant teeth and larger then the centrals. Note how this rule is applied.

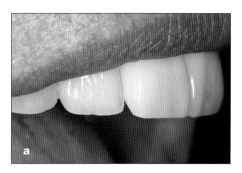 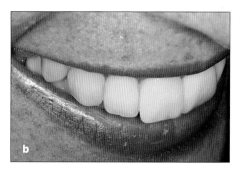 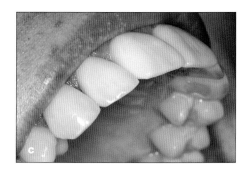

Fig 13-49a-c The teeth should look natural when viewed from different angles. Note how the arch is built up.

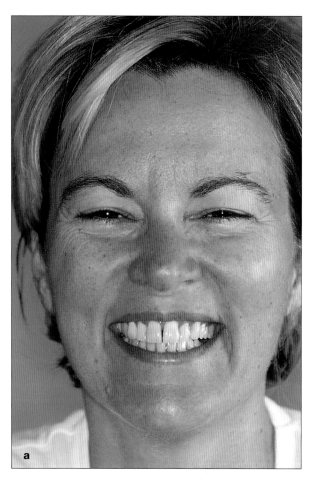 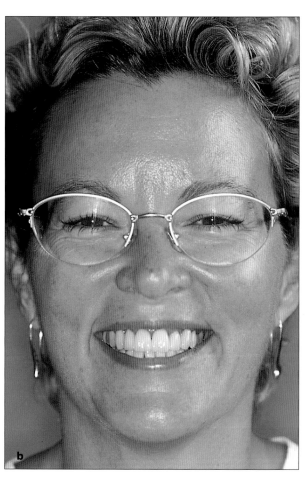

Fig 13-50a, b The change in the facial appearance. It is vitally important that the PLVs are in natural harmony with the lips and facial structures, exhibiting anterio-posterior color gradation. Since the overall value of the restorations is kept high the PLVs exhibit a very natural look that refreshes the whole facial composition.

Multicolored Teeth

One of the most difficult cases is the treatment of multicolored teeth with porcelain laminate veneers. Some patients exhibit different discoloration on every tooth, mostly due to iatrogenic reasons. Sometimes patients can even exhibit five differently colored teeth next to one other (Fig 13-51). The most valuable tool in such a case is the transfer of the stump shade to the dental technician. If they do not have an idea of the prepared tooth color, it will be impossible to match the final PLV colors, which have a maximum thickness of 0.6-0.9 mm.

The case can get even more complicated when secondary caries lesions are detected underneath the existing composite or amalgam restorations. When both the existing restorations and the cavities are cleaned and removed, too little sound tooth structure may remain. However, they can be treated with BPRs, if the margins are located on the enamel (Fig 13-52).

When a patient elects for esthetic work, many of the problems that might have otherwise gone undetected will be diagnosed during treatment. Sometimes the gingival neck may present dark discoloration due to poor endodontic treatment, so, the discoloration shows through the thin gingival tissue. In order to overcome such a problem, the author uses a technique developed by Dr *Nixon*. This technique eases the difficulties that may arise in the laboratory in terms of color, and creates a surface that is identical to the remaining tooth structure (Fig 13-57). The esthetic appearance is also completely changed through operative dentistry, in terms of color, proportion and, more important than all, in its integration to the face (Fig 13-58). This case also proves that "a beautiful smile will add value to a face" (Fig 13-59).[15]

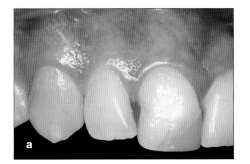
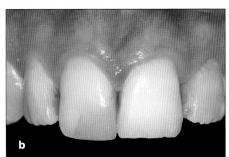
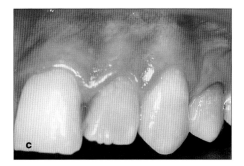

Fig 13-51a-c Teeth presenting different restorations and discolorations.

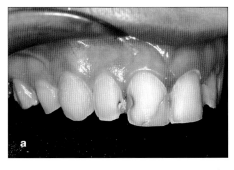
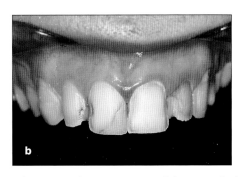
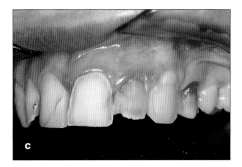

Fig 13-52a-c After the first stage of natural preparation sequence, it is very obvious that teeth # 21(9) to # 25(13) display five major different colors. The most important factor in such cases is to transfer the correct stump shades to the laboratory. Otherwise, it will be impossible for the technician to provide the dentist with satisfactory colors which will match each other.

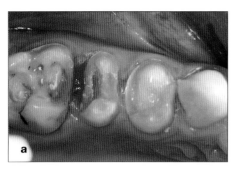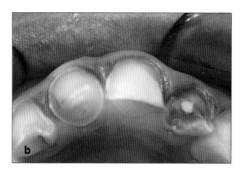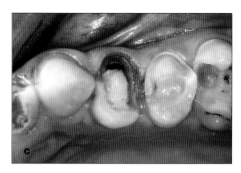

Fig 13-53a-c (a) Note the preparation on the facial surface of tooth #16(3). Only the mesial half of the facial surface is prepared to achieve the desired color, and the distofacial surface is untouched to keep the enamel intact. (b) One central area is prepared for a full coverage all-ceramic crown whereas the other for a PLV. (c) The premolars are ready to receive porcelain onlay-veneers. The cervical discoloration of the lateral #22(10) and the premolar #24(12) is extreme.

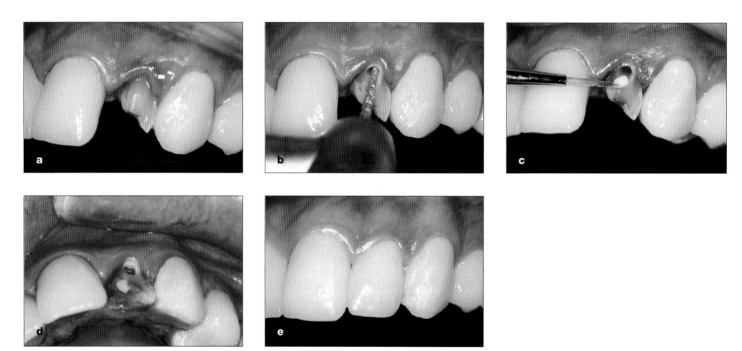

Fig 13-54a-e (a) All the veneers are bonded and the dark discolorations are successfully masked. However, gingiva that covers the lateral displays a slight discoloration owing to the dark color of the root of tooth #22(10) showing through. (b) A practical method, suggested by *R. Nixon* can be used in such cases. A narrow fissure diamond bur is held with an angulation of 10° to the tooth axis and a hole is drilled 1.5 to 2 mm towards the apical direction. It is very important that the margin is not involved and damaged in this operation. (c, d) Then an opaque composite (Cosmodent) is placed deep inside the cavity and light cured. Since this composite intrinsically changes the color of the facial surface of the root, the dark reflection through the gingiva disappears as well. (e) The PLV can easily be bonded over the restored area showing no discoloration on the thin gingiva.

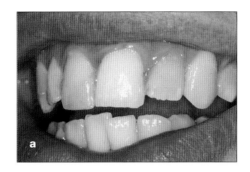
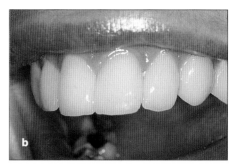
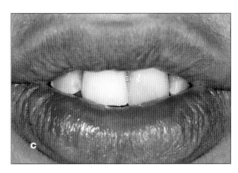
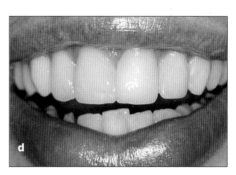

Fig 13-55a-d (a, b) The finished case, with the lips. It is easy to see the color change, especially in the second quadrant. All different discolorations are corrected and matching each other. (c, d) Thick lips, being the main frame of the artwork, are always advantageous in anterior esthetic restorations. In such cases, the dominance of the centrals can be exaggerated.

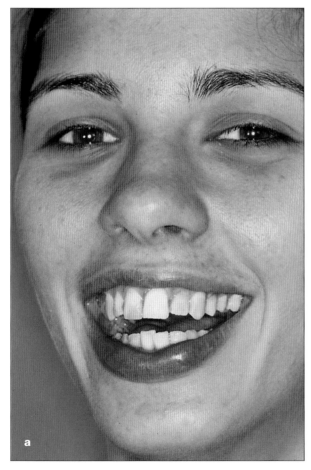
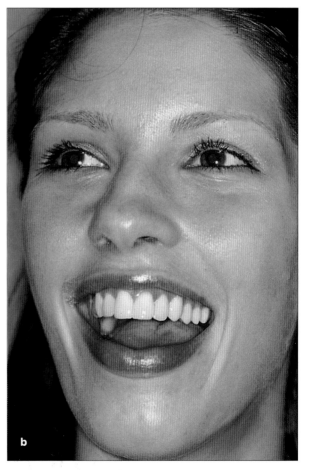

Fig 13-56a, b The truly beautiful effect of an esthetically enhanced smile, that really adds value to a face.

References

1. Narcisi EM, Culp L. Diagnosis and treatment planning for ceramic restorations. Dent Clin North Am 2001;45:127-142.

2. Feeley RT Cosmetics and the esthetic patient and laboratory communication. Oral Health 1995;85:9-12,14.

3. Portalier L. Diagnostic use of composite in anterior aesthetics. Pract Periodont Aesthet Dent 1996;8:643-652.

4. Baratieri LN. Esthetics: Direct Adhesive Restoration on Fractured Anterior Teeth. São Paulo: Quintessence, 1998: 270-312.

5. Wheeler RC. Complete crown form and the periodontium. J Prosthet Dent 1961;11:722-734.

6. Weisgold A. Contours of the full crown restoration. Alpha Omega 1977;70:77-89.

7. Dale BG, Aschheim KW. Esthetic Dentistry: A Clinical Approach to Techniques and Materials. Philadelphia, PA: Lea and Febiger, 1993: 205-225.

8. Van der Burgt TP, Plasschaert AJM. Bleaching of tooth discoloration caused by endodontic sealers. J Endodont 1986;12:231.

9. Sommer FS, Ostrander FD, Crowley ML. Clinical Endodontics. 3rd ed. Philadelphia: WB Saunders, 1966: 489.

10. Chiche GJ, Pinault A. Esthetics of anterior fixed prosthodontics. Chicago: Quintessence, 1994;13-32,53-74.

11. Roach RR, Muia PJ. Communication between the dentist and technician: An esthetic checklist. In: Preston JD. Perspectives in Dental Ceramics: Proceedings of the Fourth International Symposium on Ceramics (1985). Chicago: Quintessence, 1988:445.

12. Lee R. Esthetics and its relationship to function. In: Rufenacht CR. Fundamentals of Esthetics. Chicago: Quintessence, 1990:137-210.

13. Wilke ND The anterior point of reference. J Prosthet Dent 1979;41:488-496.

14. McCullum BB, Stuart CE. A Research Report. Palo Alto, CA: Scientific Press,1955:55.

15. Magne P, Douglas WH. Design optimization and evolution of bonded ceramics for the anterior dentition: A finite-element analysis. Quintessence Int 1999;30:661-672.

14 Patient Education and the Management of Esthetic Dentistry: A Team Approach

Cathy Jameson

"Total Care"

You are care providers. You are commissioned to provide dental services that address the needs of your patients. If you are to be a true care provider, then you must be aware of and deal in "total care". "Total care" means that you address not only the physical needs of a person but also their emotional or psychological needs.

With the phenomenal new advances in esthetic dentistry, you, as health-care providers, can now address the issue of emotional and psychological health through smile enhancement. Different people place different values on their oral health and on smile enhancement. Some people feel great about their smile, but others feel so self-conscious about their smile that their self-image is negatively affected. People can feel so badly about their smile that they fail to take advantage of opportunities because of their low self-image.

Most people do not know what is available to them in dentistry today. In many cases, people are uncomfortable asking questions about smile enhancement because of their embarrassment about their smile. As dental educators and as "total care" providers, you can offer tremendous relief to these people by asking questions that open lines of communication about the person's attitude toward their smile and by informing them of the options available today for smile enhancement.

In this chapter on patient education and the management of esthetic dentistry, the following aspects of integrating esthetic dentistry into your practice will be addressed:
- practice-building and patient education strategies
- effective case presentations
- the use of visual aids
- financial options.

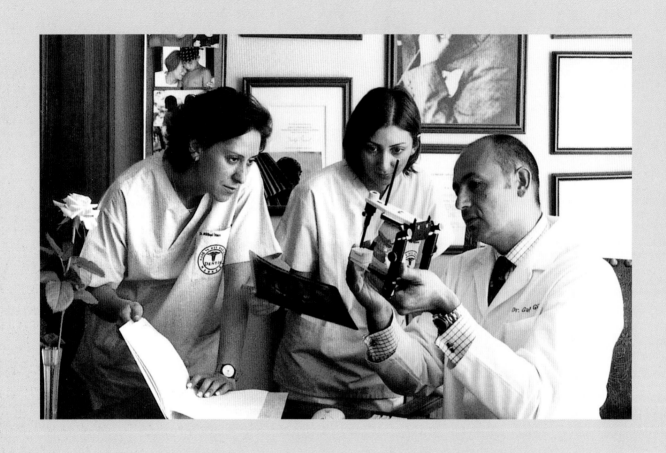

As a healthcare provider, you can expand your services and, indeed, your level of care, through the addition of esthetic options to the treatments you offer. The integration of esthetic dentistry into your practice will require:

- extensive and ongoing continuing education
- careful planning
- energy
- commitment for the entire team

Success does not just happen. You have to make it happen. Consider the benefits – both to you and to your patients – of truly integrating esthetic dentistry into your practice. The end results of such efforts will prove to be worth the commitment.

Practice-Building and Patient-Education Strategies

Practice-building and patient education should be integral parts of the growth of the esthetic portion of your practice: educating people about the opportunities available to them in dentistry today. Most people will have no idea about the range of services offered in your practice. No one is going to educate your patients for you. The responsibility for patient education lies in the hands of the dental team.

Each member of the team should understand his/her role in the building of the esthetic aspect of the practice. Performance responsibilities for each team member must be defined so that everyone is clear about those responsibilities. Then, appropriate training and practice should take place so that they are confident to carry out each task. Each person on the team is vital to the success of a project – the person answering the telephone, the person presenting the esthetic options, the person performing the techniques and the person collecting the fees. Each responsibility is as important as the next. Every person on the team has the opportunity to make or break a relationship with a patient. Getting everyone focused and going in the same direction is imperative for success.

Set goals and design a plan of action

Before any practice-building program is initiated, your team must decide on the following:
- What do you want to accomplish?
- How will you accomplish specific results?
- Who will be responsible for each task?
- What is the time frame for the completion of each task?
- How and when will you evaluate progress and success?

In other words, define a specific set of goals for the implementation of an esthetic program into your practice (Fig 14-1). Here are some proven strategies for educating people about available esthetic options.

Practice-building strategies

"Before" and "after" esthetic photographs

With the written permission of your patients, have beautiful full-face photographs matted and framed. Display these photographs in your reception area, in your corridors, in your treatment rooms and in your consultation room. You will want people to begin thinking about beautiful smiles as soon as they enter your office.

You may choose to display these photographs in albums. These albums can be located in your reception area, in treatment rooms and in the consultation room. People enjoy looking at the various cases where esthetic changes have made a difference in a person's smile and in their total appearance. They can begin to relate to these photographs and may begin thinking of how a change of smile would affect them. Plus, these photographs provide proof that you can accomplish excellent results. If you feel that your photographic skills need improvement, seek a continuing education course on photography or get some coaching from someone whose work you admire.

Before and after photographs provide visual support of your recommendations (Fig 14-2).

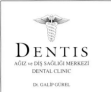

DENTIS
AĞIZ ve DİŞ SAĞLIĞI MERKEZİ
DENTAL CLINIC

Dr. GALİP GÜREL

Projects

Project	Person Responsible	Time Frame	Status

Fig 14-1 Define a specific set of goals for the implementation of an esthetic program into your practice. You can prepare a list of projects.

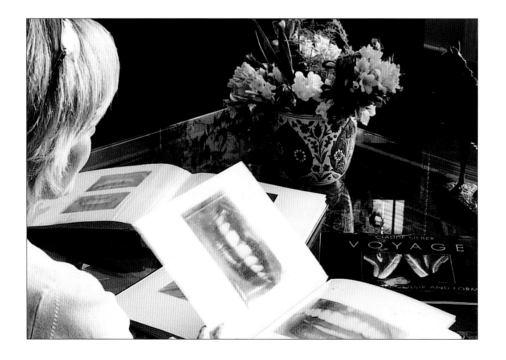

Fig 14-2 Esthetic books, brochures and related literature in the reception area will visually support your recommendations.

500

Smile Evaluation

DENTIS
AĞIZ ve DİŞ SAĞLIĞI MERKEZİ
DENTAL CLINIC
Dr. GALİP GÜREL

1. Do you like the way your teeth look?   Yes ☐   No ☐
   Explain:_____
   _____
   _____

2. Are you happy with the color of your teeth?   Yes ☐   No ☐
   Explain:_____
   _____
   _____

3. Would you like your teeth to be whiter?   Yes ☐   No ☐
   Explain:_____
   _____
   _____

4. Would you like your teeth to be straighter?   Yes ☐   No ☐

5. Do you have spaces between your teeth that you would like closed?   Yes ☐   No ☐
   If so, where?_____
   _____

6. Would you like your teeth to be longer?   Yes ☐   No ☐
   If so, Upper___ Lower_____ Both_____?

7. Do you like the shape of your teeth?   Yes ☐   No ☐
   Explain:_____
   _____

8. Do you have missing teeth that you would like to replace?   Yes ☐   No ☐

9. Do you have old silver fillings that you would like to replace with tooth-colored fillings?
   Yes ☐   No ☐

10. If you could change anything about your smile, what would you change?_____
    _____
    _____
    _____

Fig 14-3 A patient information questionnaire could open doors for you to provide esthetic treatment!

Patient information questionnaire

Develop a questionnaire for new and for existing patients (Fig 14-3). As a part of each new patient's first appointment, ask him or her to complete this questionnaire. For your existing patients, tell them that you are continually trying to improve your services and want to add treatment options to meet their needs. And so, in order to do that, you would like them to take a couple of minutes to complete a brief questionnaire. Present the questionnaire to your patients printed on your practice letterhead and placed on a clipboard with a good pen. Everything you do must say "esthetic".

Make sure that you pay attention to the responses to these questions. This is a wonderful opportunity to let a person feel comfortable sharing their thoughts and feelings about their smile, and could open doors for you to provide esthetic treatment. Patients will be happy to fill out a form if you let them know that you are asking them to do this so as to be better able to serve them.

Patient education videos, CD-ROMs and DVDs

More than 80% of what we learn is a result of visual stimulation. So, the very best way for you to educate your patients is with visual aids. Educational tools help a person visualize the end results of the treatment possibilities. The world is accustomed to TV and movies, so show an educational program in the reception area. This could be running with or without sound.

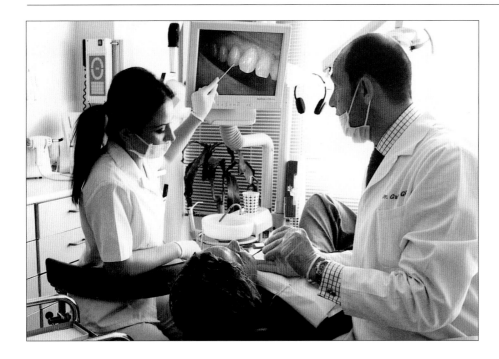

Fig 14-4 An intraoral camera is one of the best diagnostic and educational tools, and supports communication between the patient and the dentist.

A team member can show a video to a patient (or potential patient) before a consultation with the dentist. This can stimulate interest and encourage questions about the treatment possibilities. An educational program can also prove to be useful back-up support for recommendations made by the dentist and a valuable part of the consultation itself. In this case, only that portion relevant to the patient's particular needs would be shown.

Intraoral camera

The intraoral camera is one of the best diagnostic and educational tools that dentistry has yet to incorporate into patient care. Not only can you see things in the patient's mouth that cannot even be seen with scoped eyes, but also your patients will be able to see areas of concern and opportunity much better. Use the intraoral camera on new and existing patients. Photograph areas of concern that need restorative care, and consider taking photographs of various areas of a patient's mouth, showing them to the patient and asking them the following questions:

"What do you like most about the teeth in this area of your mouth?"

"What do you like least?"

"If you could change anything about the teeth in this area, what would you change?"

Make note of any changes that the patient indicates. Then, when you are in the consultation environment, retrieve these images, show the patient the areas in which they indicated a desired change and then illustrate a similar situation and the beautiful results that were obtained (Fig 14-4).

Imaging

The use of digital imaging systems is making the art of visualization a significant reality. When a person can see the possibilities in their own mouth, excitement, motivation and acceptance are accelerated. Either the dentist or a specified team member can provide the imaging. If you have an imaging system, this should be a part of each new patient's experience. Photograph the possibilities designed with the imaging machine. This data will become a part of the patient's record.

If a decision about going ahead with treatment is not made at the initial appointment or at the consultation, send the photographs home with the patient for their family to see and for further discussion to take place. Make sure that a follow-up telephone call is made to inquire about the family response and to schedule another consultation with the dentist to discuss the treatment options. Include the decision-makers in this follow-up consultation.

Notice boards

Notice boards displayed in the reception area, the treatment rooms and the consultation room can be effective in stimulating interest and prompting questions about cosmetic opportunities. Photographs or articles about cosmetic treatment can also be displayed.

On one notice board, display photographs of a particular treatment option, such as bleaching. Place a heading that says, "Ask about whitening your smile!" Put nothing else on the board. This simple but striking display will generate interest and questions. Every few months change the photographs and the heading: stimulate interest in another type of treatment for another particular situation.

Practice brochures

If practice literature is allowed by your licensing authority, a brochure can be used effectively to promote your practice and, specifically, the esthetic aspect of it. It should be educational as well as motivational. Let people know who you are and what you offer, and help them to know that they have made a good decision to choose your dental practice.

Consider including this practice brochure in a welcome pack that you send to a new patient once they have scheduled their first appointment. In this welcome pack, include the following data:

- Your practice brochure.
- An appointment card confirming the appointment.
- The patient information questionnaire and health history (which you could ask them to complete and send back to you or to bring with them).
- A patienteducation newsletter or pamphlet about esthetic dentistry.
- Your esthetic questionnaire.

The patient will know something about you and your ability to provide esthetic treatment before he or she comes for their initial appointment. Plus, if the patient sends you their completed patient-information sheet/health history form and their completed esthetic questionnaire, you will know valuable information about them before their arrival. You will be able to graciously welcome them into your practice.

Esthetic brochures

In addition to the practice brochure, professionally produced brochures about specific esthetic options, such as porcelain veneers, are available. These cost-effective publications are educational tools and should be placed in the treatment room or in the consultation room. They can provide exceptional visual support for the information you are sharing with a patient.

Other ways to use esthetic brochures:
- Include with statements and payment receipts.
- Send to your entire patient list, along with a letter about new esthetic options.
- Include along with your patient education newsletter.
- Send with hygienist appointment reminders. This might give patients an additional reason to come in for their hygiene appointment.

Patient education newsletter

Cost- and time-efficient patient education newsletters can be produced within your own practice with careful planning, or you can commission professionally produced newsletters individualized to your practice. The newsletter can be used to inform patients about the new options available in esthetic dentistry today. Remember that the world is not yet aware of what can be done. You must inform them.

Good marketing dictates that you stay in contact with your customer base every 90 days. Introduce something new to this group every 3 months. If you stay in contact with your patients in a positive way they will think of you in a positive manner.

Cards

Send cards. Very few practices send cards in a systematic manner and with regularity. Tom Hopkins of Tom Hopkins, International says that one of the best ways to establish and maintain a relationship with a client is to "send notes". Establish a protocol for which notes you will send, when you will send them and who will send them.

Examples of cards you might send:

- "Welcome to the practice."
- "Thank you for referral."
- Birthday.
- Special holidays.
- "Thank you for being such a special patient."
- "Thank you for letting us be a part of your new smile" (with "before" and "after" photos included).

Print business cards for all members of the practice team. Have business cards produced that reflect your practice. Have team members give these cards to patients as they are leaving. Tell patients to feel free to call if they have any questions. Always give out two cards: one for the patient's personal file and one to give to a friend or family member. In addition, have the team members carry the cards with them at all times. Let them be ambassadors for your beautiful dentistry. If someone asks who he or she works with and/or if they are asked about their own beautiful smile, let them give the inquirer a card so that they can easily get in touch with your practice.

Provide esthetic dentistry for those team members who need or want treatment. If someone on your team could benefit from a smile makeover, remember that after treatment they will be able to talk knowledgably about the procedures, to reinforce the value of the treatment to their own self-image and to build the patient's trust and confidence in the dentist and in his/her expertise. In addition, dentists, if you need a smile makeover yourself, or if you could benefit from any restorative treatment, go ahead with the treatment. It is imperative that you show your own belief in the dentistry.

Open the doors to esthetic possibilities. People do not know what can be done! You need to let them know what is available. It does not matter how much clinical expertise you obtain. If patients do not know what is available, or if you do not introduce them to these options, you will not be able to provide the treatment you have so carefully studied.

When you tell patients about esthetic options, they get excited. When asked, most people want an esthetic change of some kind in their smile. Most dental professionals just do not ask. So, begin opening your own doors for esthetic possibilities. ASK.

Effective Case Presentations

The fulcrum of your practice is your comprehensive diagnosis, complete and carefully documented treatment planning and excellent case presentations. Introducing new and existing patients to esthetic possibilities is only the first step in building the esthetic aspect of your practice. It is an important step, but it is only the beginning. Getting from the point of the initial appointment to the place where a person agrees to treatment is a sometimes tedious but important journey.

Ask questions and listen

Your initial interview and evaluation are essential for establishing a level of trust with a patient. Confidence and trust must exist if the idea of extensive esthetic treatment is to be accepted. The oral cavity is an intimate zone of the body. The patient receiving the treatment needs, and deserves, a sense of security. After all, you will be recreating that smile.

During the initial interview, open-ended questions relative to a patient's feelings about their teeth and smile need to be gently and caringly asked. An open-ended question cannot be answered with "yes" or "no": it is an invitation for the patient to talk, give you information and begin sharing their feelings with you.

You could ask open-ended questions such as:

"What are your feelings about your teeth?"

"If you could change the appearance of your smile, how would you change it?"

"If you were to tell me what you want most for your mouth, your teeth and your smile, what would that be?"

Asking these or similar questions gives a patient an opportunity to share their true feelings. In order for a patient to share the answers to these questions, they must feel safe, unembarrassed and comfortable. You must ask these questions sincerely, and then you must want sincerely to listen! The most important communication skill you will ever develop is effective listening. Listening is an art form. Of the four things we do with language: reading, writing, speaking and listening, listening is perhaps the most important skill necessary for establishing and maintaining a relationship. However, it is also the least studied and least mastered. Listening to a patient when you ask them how they feel about their smile is the key to discovering their innermost thoughts and feelings. This is the best way to open doors for the sharing of esthetic possibilities between you, as the care provider, and the patient who may yearn for that beautiful smile.

Critical to careful and caring listening is that you do not impose your own values on the patient responding to your questions. As difficult as it may be at times, you must listen and accept a patient's feelings even if they differ from your own. Asking questions, listening attentively and not imposing one's own values is not easy, but so doing may be one of the greatest ways to show respect for a patient. You may think a patient's smile looks fine, but that patient may hate their smile. He or she may be willing to overcome major obstacles to receive a new smile.

I was consulting in the office of a dentist who focused his practice on esthetic dentistry. I was interviewing one of his patients as she was preparing to begin her esthetic treatment. She told me that her husband thought she was "stupid to spend this much money on her teeth". She also told me that she "hated going to the dentist more than anything in the world". She said, "I would love nothing more than to get up out of this chair and go home. But I want this new smile so badly that I would not leave for anything." I asked her about confronting her husband. She said, "I am finally doing something for myself. I have never wanted anything so much. I just know he will be glad once he realizes how great I am going to feel after I have this new smile."

This young lady had two strong deterrents to treatment acceptance: her husband's opinion and her negative feelings about being in a dental chair. However, her positive desire to have the smile she had always wanted outweighed those negatives.

Stop and think about the significance of this example. Do you have patients who would respond in a like manner if they felt that you listened to them? If you educated them about the available options? If they had confidence in your technical abilities? If you epitomized a sincere caring for their unique feelings and attitudes? As the media informs people about the exciting options available through esthetic dentistry, more and more patients will come to you asking for such treatment. But, remember, many people who have negative feelings about their smiles will be uncomfortable expressing these negative feelings. You do them a tremendous service by opening the door, by asking sincere, caring questions, and then getting out of the way and letting the patient express themselves without making judgements or imposing your own values. Ask questions and listen! Listen with honest attention. Then, together with the patient, discuss appropriate options.

- Learn how to ask questions and then listen to your patients' desires.
- Be accepting of the differences expressed by each individual.
- Determine a patient's perceived or felt need.
- Be ready to meet those needs.

Six steps to case acceptance

The presentation of treatment recommendations is your opportunity as a dental educator to inform patients about the benefits of specific dental treatments. This presentation also presents you with the challenge of motivating a patient to accept your recommendations. The purpose of your consultation is to make it possible for a patient to say "yes" to the dental treatment.

Step 1: Build the relationship

Business tells us that in order to attract a new client into your business or to make it possible for a client to become involved with your product or service you must first build a relationship of confidence and of trust. The same need for confidence and trust applies to the dental patient. People will come to your practice and will say "yes" to your treatment recommendations only when they believe in your ability to take care of them, both physically and emotionally. Your ability and willingness to listen will be essential here.

Usually the first person to make contact with a potential patient is the person answering the telephone. The telephone is often considered the most important marketing tool in the dental practice. A potential patient calling your dental practice makes a mental decision about the dental treatment they will receive by the manner in which their enquiry is managed on the telephone. The member of team answering the telephone must be enthusiastic, warm and knowledgeable and must concentrate when answering that telephone (Fig 14-5).

Telephone technique

The initial telephone contact is your first opportunity to encourage a patient to become involved with your practice, and it is your first opportunity to listen to a patient. Listening gives you a chance to determine what a patient's particular wants and needs may be.

Each member of the team who speaks on the telephone must know about the procedures you offer. That team member will have about 30 seconds to help the potential patient make a decision to come to your practice. This initial contact is critical!

An excellent greeting would be:

"Good morning (afternoon), *Dr. Jameson's office. This is Cathy. How may I help you?"*

When delivered with energy, this greeting gives the caller a sense of your own enthusiasm about the level of care you provide and about your pride in your work. Do not underestimate the importance of this very first contact – this first impression. If a patient asks questions about the esthetic dentistry you offer in the practice, be able to answer those questions briefly and in layman's language. I would recommend that you write thirty-second scripts about the main esthetic options you offer. Also write brief scripts for constructive ways you can deal with potential objections or barriers concerning treatment.

An excellent way to answer a question is by asking another question. This will give the caller a chance to give you further information, and it will give the person answering the telephone a chance to clarify, to make sure the caller has been heard accurately.

For example:

Caller: *"I just read an article about esthetic dentistry in a fashion magazine. They talked about porcelain veneers in the article. Do you do that?"*

Business Administrator: *"Are you interested in changing your smile?"*

Caller: *"Yes. I never knew there was anything like this available. I have terrible stains on my teeth, and I wondered if there was anything I could do about them."*

Business Administrator: *"It sounds as if you are uncomfortable with your smile at present and would like to see about improving it."*

Caller: *"Yes. I would be most interested in finding out what I might be able to do."*

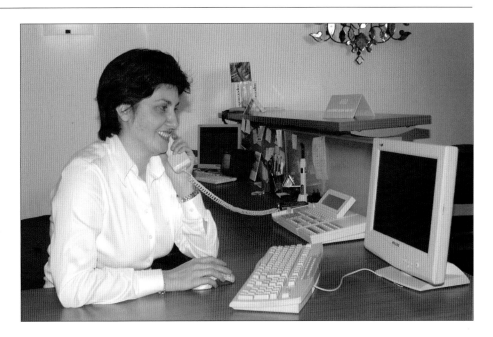

Fig 14-5 When an excellent greeting is delivered with positive energy, this greeting gives the caller a sense of your own enthusiasm about the level of care you provide.

Business Administrator: *"I am so glad you called us. We do provide many esthetic dental options in our practice. We enjoy helping people to acquire the smile they want. Our dentist is wonderful and would be more than happy to talk to you about available options and determine which of these options might work for you. Let me have some contact details and I can schedule a consultation with the dentist."*

Caller: *"That sounds fine. My name is Geraldine Jones."*

Business Administrator: *"Wonderful. Are mornings or afternoons better for you, Ms. Jones?"*

Then schedule a new patient appointment. The key here is to determine her wants before you start answering questions. Filter down to her real issue. If you jump into the answer too quickly, you may answer the wrong thing. You must clarify needs before you try to satisfy those needs. Do this by reflecting back what you have heard or received in the message.

During this initial telephone call, encourage a patient to come to the practice. Once a patient comes to the office, the experience of that initial appointment and the following consultation will encourage him or her to become involved with your practice and your treatment recommendations.

Greeting

The relationship is further developed by the reception received upon entering the practice. The member of staff at the reception desk should stop what they are doing and make a conscious effort to greet the patient by name. An introduction is desirable. (Apply the same etiquette that you use in your home to the dental practice.)

Business Administrator: *"Ms. Jones, welcome to our practice. I'm Cathy. We spoke on the telephone. We are glad you are here. Thank you for sending your health history form and questionnaire to me. I have all the data in the computer, and the dentist and team have reviewed your information. Have a seat, and we will be with you as soon as possible."*

Usually the next person a patient meets is the dental nurse. The dental nurse should also introduce him or herself to the new patient. Address the patient in this way:

Dental Nurse: *"Ms. Jones, I'm Donna. I'm Dr. Jameson's dental nurse. Welcome to our practice. I am so glad to meet you. I will be working with you and Dr. Jameson today. You may come with me now."*

Then the dental nurse escorts the patient to the consultation room or to the clinical area where she reviews the health history, making sure that it is complete, asking some pertinent questions, letting the patient know that she wants to get to know them as an individual and that she notices anything about them that might affect their treatment.

She makes sure that she notes the referral source to establish a point of immediate rapport with the patient. She will also inform the new patient about the procedure of the initial appointment. Always let a patient know what is going to happen before it happens!

If you know that a patient has come to your practice for an esthetic consultation, a patient education video may be played before the dentist is seen. This will answer a lot of questions in advance of the dentist's arrival and will serve to stimulate interest in the benefits of the esthetic treatments available. Upon the entrance of the dentist, the dental nurse makes an introduction. If, for some reason, the dental nurse is not in the room, then the dentist should introduce him or herself. The initial interview begins.

The dentist notes from the patient information sheet some points of common ground upon which to begin establishing a rapport with the patient. On the patient information questionnaire, you have asked questions about their attitude to their smile. Carefully refer to these comments.

Step 2: Establish the need

The second step in an effective presentation is to establish the need. This involves not only determining the clinical needs in the patient's mouth but also the patient's emotional needs. Most people make a buying decision emotionally and will back that decision up with logic. In order for you to help a patient make a decision to go ahead with esthetic treatment (or any other kind of treatment), you must determine their perceived or felt need. People will buy what they want long before they will buy what they need. Your responsibility in your initial interview is to determine that "felt need". You do this by asking questions and listening.

It is now appropriate for the dentist to ask questions about the patient's situation. Ask a question. Then, stop and listen. Do not place your own values or thought processes on the patient, but, rather, listen without judgement. Here is where your open-ended questions will be asked. Once you have asked open-ended questions and have given the patient the space to respond, then reflect back to the patient what you think you hear them saying, to ensure that you are hearing them accurately. The better you listen to the patient, the better they will listen to you when it comes time for you to present your recommendations.

Ask such open-ended questions as:

"Ms. Jones, I notice on your patient questionnaire that you mention that your are unhappy with your smile. Can you say a little more?"

"Ms. Jones, on your questionnaire you have said that you are happy with the shape of your teeth, but that you think they are too yellow. Can you tell me about that?"

"Ms. Jones, how would you like to change your mouth, your teeth and your smile?"

Record the patient's responses so that you can refer to them when you are making your presentation. One of the key issues at this point is to identify the main motivator for this particular patient. What do they want? What is the focus of their visit (Fig 14-6)?

Following the establishment of the patient's felt or perceived needs, the comprehensive oral evaluation takes place. The comprehensive evaluation follows the initial interview. Once you determine the protocol for your comprehensive oral evaluation, do it the same way every time. Your initial appointment should be as precise as any of your appointments. An example of the protocol might be as follows:

- greet
- seat
- review health history and patient information
- initial interview, including cosmetic questionnaire

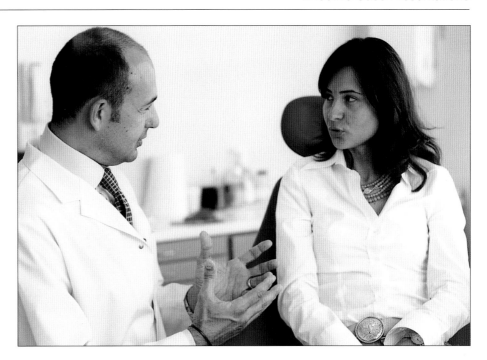

Fig 14-6 In the initial interview you should determine "felt need" by asking questions and listening.

- necessary radiographs
- periodontal evaluation
- oral cancer screening
- head and neck evaluation
- occlusal evaluation
- tooth-by-tooth diagnosis
- tour of the mouth with the intraoral camera
- esthetic imaging
- invitation to come back for a consultation.

At the end of your comprehensive evaluation, set the patient up, roll your chair around, establish eye contact and invite them back for a consultation.

Dentist: *"Ms. Jones, today we have gathered quite a bit of information about your situation. Now, I need to review the data and design a treatment plan that will help us to reach the goals that you outlined for me today. So, I would like to invite you back to the office in about a week so that we can sit down together uninterrupted and discuss the treatment I believe would give you the smile you want. Would that be okay with you?"*

Most people will be happy to come back for a consultation. They will be glad to have your undivided attention! You are going to be changing their smile. They will want to know what you are going to do and will want to be confident in the results you will achieve. Once they have agreed to return for a consultation, ask one last question.

Dentist: *"Ms. Jones, is there anyone besides yourself who will be deciding how you will proceed with treatment?"*

You are trying to find out who the family decision-makers might be. If there is someone who will be helping with that decision, try to make arrangements for him or her to be at the consultation as well. There is no reason to call for a decision when the decision-maker is not there. You will be wasting your time and the patient's time. In addition, it is impossible for a patient to go home and explain the treatment that you have recommended. Dentistry is, for most people, like a foreign language! So, do not send a patient home in the hope that they can make a clear and precise presentation of your recommendations. Much is lost in the translation!

Try to schedule the consultation about one week following the initial appointment. You want to present your recommendations while interest is high. Do not make the mistake of letting too much time pass. Interest may diminish.

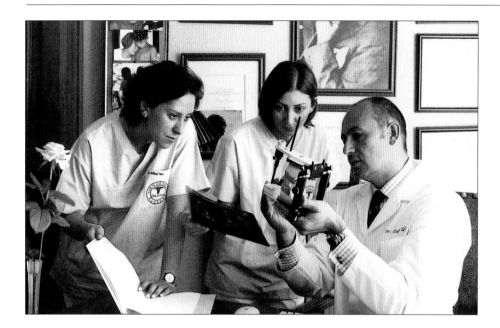

Fig 14-7 Make sure that the case is carefully planned and organized before the patient comes back for his/her next consultation.

Treatment planning

Between steps 2 and 3 of the case presentation comes the treatment-planning phase. Schedule time in your week for case planning. Plan your cases while the information is clear in your mind. Plus, you will want to make sure that the case is carefully planned and organized before the patient comes back for their next consultation. You, your team members and your patient will benefit from careful planning and documentation. Do not expect your team members to be able to make excellent financial arrangements or to schedule succinctly and accurately if they do not have thorough and appropriate information on the treatment plan. If the information is not carefully documented, they will have to guess or to interrupt you to get necessary information. Poor planning will get in the way of case acceptance. And, for the control of stress, the last thing in the world that you want to have happen is to walk in one morning only to have your business administrator or treatment coordinator say, "Doctor, Ms. Jones is coming in at 10:00 for her treatment presentation. Is everything prepared?" and for you to hyperventilate because you have not even thought about the case since the patient came in for their initial appointment. Be prepared. Pre-planning and careful preparation will pave the way for higher case acceptance (Fig 14-7).

Step 3: Educate and motivate

Once you have established the need at the initial interview, the comprehensive diagnosis has been made and the treatment plan has been designed, the next step is to educate and motivate. As dental care providers you are educators of dentistry. People do not come to the dental practice with very much dental knowledge. Education and motivation are critical at the time of the consultation. The consultation appointment is the time when a patient comes to spend quality time with you to review your findings, to hear your recommendations and to find out what you can do for them.

The appointment was scheduled at the end of the initial appointment. You have spent some time carefully designing a treatment plan. Also, spend some time planning your presentation. Your consultation is your opportunity to present. It is at this time that most people will decide whether they are going to proceed or not. This is a critical time in your interaction with your patient, and, perhaps, with the decision-maker. At the consultation appointment, everything in the consultation area is prepared prior to the patient's arrival.

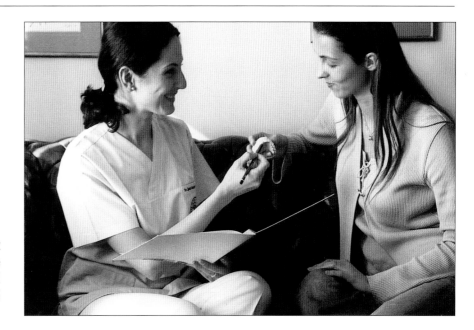

Fig 14-8 Let the patient see what the end results are going to be. The more a patient is involved, the better they will understand the recommendations and they will be placed in a "comfort zone".

The Use of Visual Aids

Since the main mode of learning for most people is visual, it makes sense to make use of excellent visual aids to show a patient the end results and the benefits of the treatment that you are recommending. What people really want to know is: How is this going to affect me? What is in this for me? How is this going to affect my health, my looks, my bank balance, my schedule? You determined the patient's main motivator during the initial interview. Now direct your comments and your presentation toward that main motivator.

Often, dental professionals get so involved with describing the clinical techniques of treatment that they totally lose the patient. The patient becomes confused. A confused patient cannot make a decision. You need to keep the technical aspects simple. Use layman's language. Let the patient see what the end results and the benefits are going to be. That is really what matters to them.

The more a patient is involved, the better they will understand your recommendations. When you are presenting recommendations to a patient, follow this scenario:

Tell/show the patient what they have now.

Tell/show them what you recommend to restore their mouth to health again or to change

their smile. Use your visual aids here. Show them a similar situation. (Have this similar situation ready to show the patient. Remember, prepare for and rehearse this presentation.)

Dentist: *"Ms. Jones, this patient of ours had a situation similar to yours. Can you see the similarity? (Let her respond). I feel confident that once we complete your treatment your smile will look much like this. Is that what you want?"*

Tell/show them the benefits of the treatment you are recommending.

Tell/show them any negative factors or risks that might occur if they choose not to proceed with treatment.

Intraoral camera and esthetic imaging systems

Use of visual aids places a patient in a "comfort zone" that is conducive to learning. This opens the doors to a two-way line of constructive communication. Use of an intraoral camera and/or an esthetic imaging system enhances communication. When a patient can see the possibilities for their own smile, motivation increases significantly (Fig 14-8).

Intraoral camera

Suggested ways to use an intraoral camera effectively are as follows:

Take a tour of the mouth with an intraoral camera with each new patient. Build up a library of photographs from all your patients. For example:

a) Full face, smiling. No lip retractors. Capture the lip line for your laboratory.
b) Smile with lip retractors.
c) Right and left lateral with lip retractors.
d) All four quadrants. (Take photographs of individual teeth within each quadrant where a tooth indicates a need.)
e) Upper and lower arch.

Look at both the upper and lower anteriors. Let the patient focus on the upper anteriors and ask:

"What do you like most about the teeth in the front of your mouth – on the top? What do you like least? If you could change anything about the teeth here, what would you change?"

Then go to the lower anteriors. And so on. Let them begin seeing their teeth in a new way. Let them tell you what they want. Either store these images or run prints. You will want to use these images during your consultation appointment.

Use the intraoral photographs as a way of communicating with your ceramic specialist. When the ceramic specialist from your laboratory can actually see the situation and discuss the case with you, he or she will be much better able to achieve the desired result in their preparations. You will have a visual prescription as well as a written one.

Take "before" and "after" intraoral photographs of every single case you complete. Then, as you are planning your cases and your presentations, you will be able to use these to show similar situations to patients who are considering treatment. Seeing the features of porcelain laminate veneers, realizing the benefits of this type of treatment and obtaining proof that you can access results provide powerful motivation in your presentations.

Consider using the intraoral camera on your regular patients who may be coming to the practice for a dental hygiene appointment. Give the patients the questionnaire. Then, if the door to any esthetic possibility has been opened, take the opportunity to do a tour of the mouth.

Do not hesitate to schedule additional time into your dental hygiene appointments if you choose to include the intraoral camera in the procedures. Your hygienist is an excellent educator. He or she can open all kinds of doors for esthetic opportunities. The time will be well spent and will pay for itself if patients begin to accept esthetic dentistry as a result of the dental education.

Cosmetic imaging systems

Cosmetic imaging systems are becoming more and more popular. They are easily integrated into most practice management software. With the use of cosmetic imaging, you can take an image of a patient's existing smile and digitally change it. You can send the proposed smile makeover home with the patient for contemplation and discussion with family members. Once you and the patient agree on the plan of action to create the desired smile, you can send this image to the laboratory to further enhance your prescription.

As is true with any software and hardware in a practice, comprehensive understanding and use of that system by the entire team is necessary to insure its productivity and profitability. Most prominent esthetic dentists state that an intraoral camera or a cosmetic imaging system is not just an investment in money, it is also an investment in time. But they work. The excitement they can generate for the dentist, for the team and for the patients is unparalleled.

Once you have processed these aspects of your presentation, proceed to the challenging but absolutely essential part of case acceptance: asking for the commitment.

Step 4: Ask for the commitment

The fourth step in an effective presentation is to ask for the commitment. You must ask for a commitment or you will have a lot of people walking out through the door and you will not know if they are going to go ahead with treatment or not. Asking for a commitment means finding comfortable-sounding questions that will either confirm a patient's desire to proceed with treatment or pinpoint any barriers to treatment acceptance that might exist.

Examples of such commitment questions follow:

Dentist: *"Ms. Jones, do you have any questions about the treatment I have recommended to you?"*

Ms. Jones: *"No. I'm pretty clear on what you need to do."*

Dentist: *"Then, if you have no questions about the treatment, tell me, is this the type of smile makeover you would like to receive?"*

Or

"Ms. Jones, have I explained the treatment that I am recommending so that you are comfortable with my explanation?"

Ms. Jones: *"Yes. I'm quite clear about what we need to do."*

Dentist: *"Good. Then, is there any reason why we should not go ahead and schedule an appointment to begin your treatment?"*

Ms. Jones: *"No. Let's book a time."*

Or

Dentist: *"Ms. Jones would having a smile such as the ones we have just reviewed make you happy?"*

Ms. Jones: *"I cannot tell you how happy I would be! I hate my teeth the way they are, and I would love to smile without being embarrassed."*

Dentist: *"Then, let's get started! Are mornings or afternoons better for you?"*

Asking for the commitment gives the patient the opportunity to define for you any barriers to

treatment acceptance. This also gives you an amazing opportunity. If a patient has an objection, you benefit by identifying this objection. Only then do you have the chance to do something about it. If you never know what is keeping a patient from going ahead with treatment, you never have the chance to solve the problem.

Do not be uncomfortable when a patient expresses an objection to you. Think of objections in the following way:
• An objection is a request for further information, indicating that the patient is interested in your proposal.
• If a patient does not present an objection or obstacle, that probably means that they are not interested.
• Objections are the steps necessary to clear the way for a commitment.

Once all clinical and emotional questions have been answered, a discussion of finances takes place. That is the final step of the case presentation: making the financial arrangements. Financial arrangements should always be made before the scheduling of the appointment takes place.

If, at any time during the initial interview, the comprehensive evaluation, or the case presentation, a patient asks, "How much is this going to cost?", answer their question with a question. Make sure that you are hearing what they are asking both clearly and accurately. In addition, make sure to keep the money questions where they need to be. Quoting a fee too early is worse than not quoting a fee at all. If you quote a fee before the patient has made a decision that they want the treatment, they will be preoccupied with thoughts of money and will not hear your presentation.

So, if a patient asks you a money question before you are ready to field those types of questions, answer in the following way.

Dentist: *"Ms. Jones, are you concerned about the financing of your smile makeover?"*

Ms. Jones: *"Yes. I just do not know how much this is going to cost, and I do not know if I can afford it."*

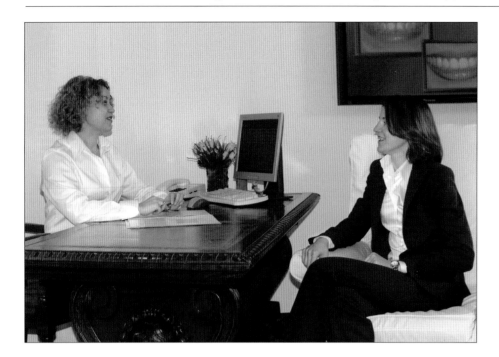

Fig 14-9 All financial arrangements should be conducted by your financial coordinator/business administrator before you go ahead with treatment.

Dentist: *"I can certainly appreciate your concerns. I am going to have Jan, my business administrator, discuss the total fee and the options we have available for payment. She is very experienced. I am sure she will be able to work this out with you. Once we have determined how we will proceed with treatment, Jan will discuss all fee questions with you. However, for now, Ms. Jones, I would like to present to you my recommendations—the treatment that I believe would help you get the smile you want. You are in total control here. You get to say if you want to proceed or not. But, for right now, my responsibility to you is to show you what I believe would be the very best treatment possible. Would that be all right with you?"*

In this example, the dentist acknowledged the patient's concern (his/her objection), but did not start quoting fees. If you begin quoting fees at this point, before the patient has bought into the treatment, you risk getting so involved with the financial aspects of the case that you never get to the treatment. I do not have a problem with the dentist quoting the fee, but I prefer that a financial coordinator/business administrator make all financial arrangements (Fig 14-9). However, make an effort to keep money questions in a constructive place within your presentation.

Once all questions have been answered, and the patient indicates that they would like to go ahead with treatment, you proceed with steps 5 and 6.

Step 5: Financial arrangements

Step 5 of an effective presentation is sorting out financial arrangements. Financing can be a serious barrier to treatment acceptance. No matter how much a patient feels that they want a smile makeover, if they do not think they can afford it, you have an objection to overcome. This objection is not one to avoid, it is real. So, take a potential negative, and turn it around to a positive. Remember: a patient will buy what they want long before they will buy what they need. So, your challenge is to help people want what you believe they need.

Here's the situation:

1. People want and many need esthetic dentistry.
2. Esthetic dentistry can be a source of professional fulfillment for the practitioner and the team.
3. However, many people do not believe they can make a substantial dental purchase.

4. An investment in esthetic dentistry is usually quite sizeable.
5. And so, in order to create a "win-win" situation for both the patient and the practitioner, comfortable financing of the esthetic dentistry must be made available.

There are many people who would benefit from esthetic dentistry. Do not limit yourself or your practice by thinking that only the rich and famous can afford or would want esthetic dentistry. Be more global than that. Do not close your own doors by mentally and financially closing the door to esthetic change to a large segment of your patient family and community.

Financial Options

Consider the following options. You will need to make certain adaptations for your particular country and circumstances. However, be forward thinking. Think outside of your present "comfort zone". Be prepared to find a financial solution for your patients.

- Offer your patients a 5% fee reduction if they pay for the entire treatment plan in full before you begin. You will be ahead if you get the money in the bank before you begin treatment. In addition, people who pay in advance will usually show up for their appointments!
- If a local banking institution will extend a loan to your patients, great! They are in the business of loaning money. You are not!
- Ask for an initial investment of one-half of the fee in order to reserve the appointment and the balance at the time of the preparation appointment.
- If your patient needs longer to pay, ask for an initial investment of one-third of the fee in order to reserve the appointment, one-third at the time of the preparation appointment and the balance at the insertion appointment.
- Suggest that people use their credit cards if they want or need smaller monthly payments with longer to pay.

- In certain countries, lending institutions will offer financing to patients specifically for dentistry. Do your own research to find out if these programs are available for you. If so, gather the information. Learn how to present them to patients, how to overcome objections and how to build the cosmetic aspect of your practice using these programs.

Your goal should be to have all financial responsibilities settled by the time the treatment is completed.

Who benefits from these financial options?
1. The patient who receives the beautiful smile.
2. The friends and family members of the patient. They will feel better about themselves, and their happiness will transfer to others.
3. The dentist and the dental team who provide the esthetic services. Esthetic dentistry is professionally fulfilling. Plus, it is fun to have people say "thanks".
4. The business aspect of the dental practice via increased productivity. You will reap the rewards for work well done. Financial reward will be yours.

Defuse the fear of cost by offering excellent financial options. Learn how to present these options and how to build your practice with them. When you can overcome cost objections, you will overcome a major hurdle. If you have presented your recommendations well enough so that the patient wants the smile makeover, then quote the fee, outline the financial options and get out of the way so that the patient can say "yes".

When you work out the financial aspect of treatment, and the patient agrees to go ahead, you have received the final commitment. You are ready to schedule that first appointment (Fig 14-10).

TREATMENT PLAN

PATIENT'S NAME:_____ DATE:_____

HOME PHONE #_____ BUSINESS PHONE #_____

DATE	TOOTH NUMBER	SERVICE NEEDED	PHASE	TIME BETWEEN APPTS	TIME NECESSARY	FEE	APPOINTMENT TIME	DATE

© Jameson Management, Inc.

Fig 14-10 When you and the patient are ready to go ahead with the treatment, it is time to schedule the first appointment.

Step 6: Schedule the appointments

Step 6 in an effective presentation is to schedule the appointment. The business administrator/financial coordinator makes the financial arrangements and then schedules the first appointment. There is no exception to this rule: financial arrangements are made before the scheduling of the appointment.

In summary, here are the six steps of an effective presentation:

1. Build the relationship.
2. Establish the need.
3. Educate and motivate.
4. Ask for a commitment.
5. Make financial arrangements.
6. Schedule an appointment.

If you follow this six-step process of effective case presentations, you will find that your acceptance rate will increase. The key to this is building the relationship with your patients and helping them feel involved in the treatment decisions.

Conclusion

Communication is the key to successful presentations. Effective communication involves a two-way exchange of information, including the thoughts, concerns and emotions of each participant. Telling a patient what he or she needs and having them immediately accept your recommendation is unlikely, nowadays, to happen. The informed patient of today wants to participate in treatment planning and decision-making. Your presentations must reflect an understanding of and a respect for this.

Finally, study the art and science of esthetic dentistry. Know the techniques. Be comfortable with the materials. Study and practice until your confidence allows you to present the options without hesitation. Integrate excellent patient education and management throughout every part of your practice. Believe in what you do and know that you are adding value to the lives of your patients. Success will happen "when preparedness meets opportunity".

Esthetic dental patients are happy dental patients. Inner joy and pride exude from these people. You will enjoy providing this type of quality dentistry, and your patients will love you!

Index